WP 570 RAO

This book is due for return on or before the last date shown below.

The Infertility Manual

The Infertility Manual

2nd Edition

Editor

Kamini A Rao
DGO DORCP DCh FRCOG (UK) MCh (UK) FICOG PGDMLE (Law)
Medical Director
Bangalore Assisted Conception Centre
6/7 Kumara Kruppa Road
High Grounds
Bangalore–560 001

Co-Editors

Peter R Brinsden
MB FRCOG
Bourn Hall Clinic
Cambridge, UK

A Henry Sathananthan
BSc (Hons) PhD
Monash Institute of Reproduction and Development
Melbourne, Australia

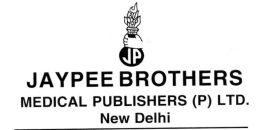

JAYPEE BROTHERS
MEDICAL PUBLISHERS (P) LTD.
New Delhi

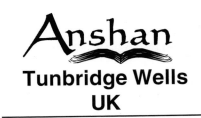

Tunbridge Wells
UK

First published in the UK by

Anshan Ltd
in 2005
6 Newlands Road
Tunbridge Wells
Kent TN4 9AT, UK

Tel/Fax: +44 (0)1892 557767
E-mail: info@anshan.co.uk
www.anshan.co.uk

ISBN 1 904798 160

British Library Cataloguing in Publication Data
A catalogue record for this book is available from the British Library

Printed in India by Gopsons Papers Ltd., A-14, Sector 60, Noida

*This book is dedicated to
the countless infertile couples
from whom we have learnt
so much and who still inspire us
to strive harder*

Contributors

Mala Arora
Noble Hospital
Faridabad, Haryana

Manish Banker
Advanced Fertility and Endoscopic
Centre
Melbourne IVF Gujarat Private
Limited
Ahmedabad

Meenakshi Bharath
Centre for Assisted Reproductive
Techniques
Bangalore

Pushpa M Bhargava
Founder-Director
Centre for Cellular and Molecular
Biology, Hyderabad
Member of Expert Group for
Formulating the National Guidelines
on "Accreditation, Supervision and
Regulation of ART Clinics in India"

RK Bhathena
Consultant
Obstetrician and Gynaecologist
Petit Parsee General and Masina
Hospitals, Mumbai

Reeta H Biliangady
Consultant Obstetric and
Gynaecology
North Star Hospital, Bangalore

Peter R Brinsden
Bourn Hall Clinic
Cambridge, UK

BN Chakravarty
Institute of Reproductive Medicine
Kolkata

Shivani Chaturvedi
Malhotra Nursing and Maternity
Home, Agra

Meena Chimote
Vasundhara Clinic and
Assisted Conception Centre
Nagpur

Natchandra Chimote
Vasundhara Clinic and
Assisted Conception Centre
Nagpur

Michael F Costello
Department of Reproductive
Medicine
Royal Hospital for Women, Barker St.
Randwick, Sydney, NSW
Australia

L Cummins
IVF, Australia
Eastern Suburbs, Australia

Pankaj Desai
Associate Professor and Unit Chief
Department of Obstetrics and
Gynecology (Unit IV)
Medical College
Baroda

Sadhana Desai
Fertility Clinic and IVF Center
Mumbai

Shyam V Desai
Diploma Endoscopic Surgery
(Germany)
Honorary Professor Obstetrics
and Gynaecology
N Wadia Maternity Hospital
Mumbai

A Radharama Devi
Diagnostic Division
Center for DNA Fingerprinting and
Diagnostics
7-18 ECIL Road, Nacharam,
Hyderabad

Herman A Fernandes
Senior Scientist
Christian Medical College Hospital
Vellore

Anna Pia Ferraretti
SISMeR, Reproductive Medicine
Unit, Via Mazzini 12,
40138 Bologna, Italy

Korula George
Professor and Head Reproductive
Medicine Unit
Christian Medical College Hospital
Vellore

Luca Gianaroli
SISMeR, Reproductive Medicine
Unit,
Via Mazzini, 12
40138 Bologna, Italy

Sulochana Gunasheela
Gunasheela IVF Centre
Bangalore

Ashu Gupta
Assistant Professor in Obstetrics
and Gynecology (Unit IV)
Medical College, Baroda

Mehroo D Hansotia
Former Honorary Professor of
Obstetrics and Gynecology
Grant Medical College and
Nowrosjee Wadia Maternity Hospital
Mumbai

Indira Hinduja
INKUS IVF Centre
311, Mehta Bhavan, First Floor
Charni Road, Mumbai

Nikhil S Jani
Consultant
Jeevan Vikas Kendra, Mumbai

R Jayaganesh
Madras Andrology Research Centre
MARC, Chennai

Bharat Joshi
Advanced Fertility and Endoscopic
Centre
Melbourne IVF Gujarat Private
Limited, Ahmedabad

Biraj Kalyan
Infertility Specialist
Consultant
Bangalore Assisted Conception
Centre, Bangalore

Firuza Kharas
INKUS IVF Centre
311, Mehta Bhavan, First Floor,
Charni Road, Mumbai

Nalini Krishnan
Consultant Pathologist
Desai Nursing Home
Bangalore

Pratap Kumar
Professor and Head
Department of Obstetrics and
Gynaecology
Kasturba Medical College, Manipal

Orly Lacham-Kaplan
Centre for Early Human
Development
Monash Institute of Reproduction
and Development
Monash University
Melbourne, Australia

Swee-Lian Liow
Department of Obstetrics and
Gynecology
National University of Singapore
Lower Kent Ridge Road
Singapore

J Lukic
Department of Reproductive
Medicine
Royal Hospital for Women
Sydney, Australia

M Cristina Magli
SISMeR, Reproductive Medicine
Unit, Via Mazzini, 12
40138 Bologna, Italy

Nalini Mahajan
Director
Infertility and IVF Centre
Mother and Child Hospital, Delhi

Jaideep Malhotra
Malhotra Test Tube Baby Centre
A Total Infertility Solution Centre
84, MG Road, Agra

Narendra Malhotra
Malhotra Test Tube Baby Centre
A Total Infertility Solution Centre
84, MG Road, Agra

Riddhi Marfatia
Advanced Fertility and
Endoscopic Centre
Melbourne IVF Gujarat Private
Limited,
Ahmedabad

B Mathiyalagan
IVF Australia Eastern Suburbs
Australia

Jayant Mehta
Scientific Director
Institute of Reproductive Medicine
and Womens Health
Madras Medical Mission
Chennai

Judith Menezes
IVF Australia Eastern Suburbs
Australia

Meheranghiz B Minbattiwalla
Pedieos IVF Center
"Anemomylos" suite 201
8 Karaoli and
Byron Avenue Corner
1095 Nicosia, Cyprus

Sumedha Modi
Clinical Asstt
Mandakini IVF Centre
Chembur, Mumbai

Soon-Chye Ng
Department of Obstetrics and
Gynecology
National University of Singapore
Lower Kent Ridge Road
Singapore

Shreyas Padgaonkar
Director
Shreyas Infertility and IVF Centre
Mumbai

Hrishikesh D Pai
Consultant Gynecologist, Lilavati
Hospital
Scientific Director,
Babies and US Fertility
IVF and ICSI Centre,
Mumbai

Rishma Dhillon Pai
Consultant Gynecologist, Jaslok
Hospital,
Medical Director, Pearl Family
Welfare Hospital
Visiting Gynecologist, Babies and
US, Fertility, IVF and ICSI Centre
Mumbai

Nandita Palshetkar
Consultant Gynecologist, Lilavati
Hospital
Consultant Gynecologist,
Harkisandas Hospital
Medical Director, Babies and US
Fertility, IVF and ICSI Centre
Mumbai

N Pandiyan
Chief Consultant in Andrology and
Reproductive Sciences
(Male and Female Infertility)
Apollo Hospitals, Madras

Mandakini Parihar
Director
Mandakini IVF Centre
Chembur, Mumbai
Hon Asso Prof, KJ Somaiya Medical
College, Mumbai

Firuza R Parikh
Director
Department of Assisted
Reproduction and Genetics
Jaslok Hospital and Research
Center, Mumbai
Founder-Director
Reliance Life Sciences, Mumbai

Pravin Patel
Advanced Fertility and Endoscopic
Centre
Melbourne IVF Gujarat Private
Limited, Ahmedabad

Ameet Patki
Honorary Associate Professor
KJ Somaiya Medical College,
Mumbai
Consultant
Department of Assisted
Reproduction and Genetics
Jaslok Hospital and Research
Centre
Reliance Life Sciences
Mumbai

Contributors

PG Paul
Director, Cochin Gynaecological
Endoscopic Training Centre
36/1919A, Sebastian Road
Kaloor, Cochin

Rohan Potdar
Sr Registrar
KJ Somaiya Medical College
Mumbai

K Prabhakara
Diagnostic Division
Center for DNA Fingerprinting and
Diagnostics, 7-18 ECIL Road,
Nacharam, Hyderabad

Nirmala R
Gunasheela IVF Center
Bangalore

A Rajasekaran
Madras Andrology Research Centre
MARC, Chennai

Arati R Rao
Consultant
Obstetrics and Gynecology
Bangalore Assisted Conception
Centre, Bangalore

Kamini A Rao
Medical Director
Bangalore Assisted Conception
Centre

Radha Reddy
Consultant
Endocrinology and Diabetes
Mallya Hospital, Bangalore

Partha G Roy
Fertility Clinic and IVF Center
Mumbai

Varsha Samson Roy
Gunasheela IVF Center
Bangalore, India

A Henry Sathananthan
Monash Institute of Reproduction
and Development
Melbourne, Australia

Shailaja Gada Saxena
Research Associate
Department of Assisted
Reproduction and Genetics
Reliance Life Sciences, Mumbai

Kamala Selvaraj
Associate Director
Obstetrician and Gynaecologist
CG Hospital, Chennai

Duru Shah
Honorary Obstetrician and
Gynaecologist
Sir HN Hospital and Jaslok Hospital
Mumbai

Jatin P Shah
Director
Mumbai Fertility Clinic and
IVF Centre, Mumbai

PK Shekharan
Former Professor and Head,
Department of Obstetrics and
Gynaecology,
Institute of Maternal and Child
Health Medical College, Calicut

Sanu Maiya Shrestha
Department of Reproductive
Medicine
Royal Hospital for Women,
Barker St, Randwick
Sydney, NSW
Australia

Pankaj Shrivastav
Deputy Director,
Dubai Gynaecology and
Fertility Centre, Dubai, UAE

Rakesh Sinha
Bombay Endoscopy Academy and
Centre for Minimally Invasive
Surgery Research
Gynaecological Endoscopic
Surgeon
Bombay Hospital, Lilavati Hospital
Sir HN Hospital, Bhatia Hospital

Peter Sjoblom
Department of Reproductive
Medicine,
Royal Hospital for Women,
Barker St, Randwick
Sydney, NSW, Australia

Neelam Sood
Senior Consultant and Scientist in
Reproductive Medicine
Indraprastha Apollo Hospital
New Delhi

WD Ratna Sooriya
Department of Zoology,
Colombo University
Sri Lanka

Jaydeep D Tank
Lecturer of Obstetrics and
Gynecology
Seth GS Medical College and
Nowrosjee Wadia Maternity Hospital
Mumbai

Marco Toschi
SISMeR, Reproductive Medicine
Unit, Via Mazzini, 12
40138 Bologna, Italy

Prakash Trivedi
Chief Gynaecologist, Endoscopist
and
Laser Surgeon, Jaslok Hospital
and Research Centre, Mumbai
National Institute of Laser
and Endoscopic
Surgery (NILES), Mumbai
Scientific Director, Aakar IVF-ICSI
Centre, Mumbai

A Trounson
Monash Institute of Reproduction
and Development
Melbourne, Australia

Thankam R Varma
Institute Director
Institute of Reproductive Medicine
and Women's Health
Madras Medical Mission, Chennai

SS Vasan
Uroandrologist
Diacon Institute of Neurourology
and Andrology

Kusum Zaveri
INKUS IVF Centre
311, Mehta Bhavan,
First Floor, Charni Road, Mumbai

Preface to the Second Edition

It is with great pleasure and gratitude that we bring out the second edition of *The Infertility Manual*. The overwhelming response to the earlier edition prompted this endeavor. In addition to some amendments, we decided to complement this book with a CD illustrating the various procedures in assisted reproduction.

Infertility is a problem to a couple, challenge to a physician and a prospect to a scientist, all of whom strive towards one goal—a healthy child. Gone are the days when infertility was studied as a small section of gynecology. Today thanks to various discoveries and innovations infertility is a major specialty in medicine.

There was a time when reproduction inspired awe in religious traditions. It was unbelievable that a human life could be created outside the female body. Since then the march of progress has been relentless. Over the years we have been "wowed" by the milestones of reproduction technology: IVF, LAH, IVM, cryopreservation, ovarian transplants, etc. Two centuries after the discovery that conception results from the contact of sperm and egg, realities as to what makes this possible are still being discovered.

The practice of infertility at the primary/secondary level is not restricted to the domains of an infertility specialist. Hence this book is intended to serve as a reference and a guide to all those involved in the care of the infertile couple. The manual encompasses the entire range of human reproduction, providing important information to both scientists and clinicians at all levels of expertise. The wide range of topics has been contributed by an even wider array of authors, all of whom are experts in the discipline of infertility. Though, emphasis is upon clinical management, the reader will benefit from the detailed aspects of physiology and pathology. It is inevitable that some overlapping of subject matter has occurred, in our attempt to cover every aspect of infertility. We have tried to give the readers a clear perspective of assisted reproduction, its advantages and limitations. We sincerely hope that the book and the CD will accomplish its objective of furthering the readers' insight into infertility.

Kamini A Rao
Peter R Brinsden
A Henry Sathananthan

Preface to the First Edition

Assisted Reproduction is one of the fastest growing areas of medicine, having expanded far beyond the imaginations of those who pioneered the techniques that led to the birth of Louise Brown.

Since we first opened our doors to couples seeking treatment for Infertility, we have enhanced our knowledge of how to provide an opportunity for gametes to join, to begin a new human life. The 90's was an eventful decade for the field of Infertility. Male Infertility was revolutionized with the advent of ICSI while the field of preimplantation genetic diagnosis opened new vistas in gene technology. Important milestones like the use of recombinant FSH and GnRH-a now offer new prospects for controlled ovarian stimulation. Not only has the process of uniting egg and sperm outside the body become a commonly practiced procedure, but we have now entered the era of blastocyst culture and assisted hatching. In such an age when conventional treatment measures are being challenged and replaced by newer innovations, natural wisdom suggests that clinicians keep abreast of the latest developments in the field.

This book *The Infertility Manual* is intended as a reference and learning volume for general practitioners as well as infertility specialists. It encompasses the entire range of human reproduction providing important information for both scientists and clinicians at all levels of training. Though, the emphasis is upon the clinical management of patients undergoing assisted conception treatment, the reader will benefit from the detailed accounts of sperm physiology, stimulation protocols, ovulation, fertilization and implantation as well as the potential gynecological complications of ART. As is inevitable, some overlapping of subject matter has occurred, in our attempt to cover every aspect of Infertility Treatment. We have tried to give readers a clear perspective of assisted reproduction, its advantages and its limitations, and an ability to start an infertility practice with confidence.

The treatment of Infertility in India is fast catching up with the West. The mushrooming of infertility clinics is not confined to the metropolitan cities but has spread to the smaller towns and districts. A contemporary perspective on infertility practice is essential for every physician. This book offers an authoritative and in-depth review available on the treatment of infertility and brings up-to-date the many important advances that have now become an essential part of Assisted Reproductive Technology. We hope that "The Infertility Manual" will be enjoyed by all those of you who read it.

Kamini A Rao
Peter R Brinsden

Acknowledgements

First and foremost we extend our thanks to all the readers of the first edition of *The Infertility Manual*. It is their response, which paved the way to this undertaking.

All the authors, in spite of their busy schedules kept their commitments of contributing to this manual. It is a pleasure to acknowledge a debt of appreciation to them for providing insights and in-depth information on all the concerned topics, without which this book would have missed its mark as a comprehensive infertility manual.

Dr Mamta Dighe was assigned the task of bringing out this edition. Right from revising, formulating and subediting, she has seen the book through to its completion with her consistent and earnest efforts in realizing the same. Our sincere thanks, for her unwavering support to this venture.

Ms Vindhya Subbaiah and Dr Supriya Seshadri have made valuable suggestions and facilitated the proof-reading. We extend our appreciation for the same.

We are grateful to Dr Anu Kottur, Dr Arati A Rao, Mr M Srinivas and Mr Basavaraj, all of whom worked in earnest on the CD, putting in a lot of effort on making it a valuable accompaniment to the manual.

We would also like to thank Ms Gayatri Prashant who was very generous with her time and efforts towards documenting and compiling data and was always willing to help in whichever way she could. A special thanks to Mrs Thelma Swaminathan for her dedicated efforts in helping us throughout this project and also to the entire staff of BACC for their untiring enthusiasm and devotion.

Finally we acknowledge with gratitude our publisher, M/s Jaypee Brothers Medical Publishers Pvt Ltd., for keeping their faith in spite of all the delays that inevitably accompany such a venture.

Contents

SECTION 4 : FEMALE FACTOR INFERTILITY

SECTION 5 : OVULATION INDUCTION

SECTION 6 : ASSISTED REPRODUCTIVE TECHNIQUES

SECTION 7 : LABORATORY MANAGEMENT

SECTION 8 : ETHICAL AND LEGAL ISSUES

CD CONTENTS

- **Assisted Reproductive Technologies**
- **Endoscopic Procedures**
- **Human Sperms and its Contribution to Fertilization and Embryogenesis**

Section **1**

A General Overview

1

Patient Selection Counseling and Management

PATIENT SELECTION

During the last two decades there has been a marked increase in patient population in all infertility clinics the world over; but all infertility clinics may not be sufficiently equipped with the latest technology and expertise essential to offer the best possible help. Hence there is a need for patient selection, in order to categories them in specific groups and then refer them to different levels of infertility care units for step-wise investigations and treatment.

Patient selection for referral and finally for ART should be based on the findings of basic investigations on the causes of infertility. These investigations should consist of the following.

Husband

- Physical examination, both systemic and local, to detect any problem that might be the cause of infertility or that may modify the management of infertility.
- Semen analysis including both morphological and functional tests; if any abnormality is detected, repeat tests should be done after suitable interval. An abnormal finding on a repeat semen examination warrants full-scale investigation by an appropriate specialist to ascertain the cause and then institute the necessary treatment.
- Screening for infections including syphilis, HBV, HCV and HIV, and their appropriate management.

If needed, appropriate endocrinological investigations and therapy.

Wife

- Physical examination, both systemic and local, to detect any problem that might be the cause of infertility or that may modify the management of infertility.
- Detection and timing of ovulation by basal body temperature (BBT), cervical mucus studies, ultrasonography, premenstrual endometrial biopsy and serum progesterone estimation in the mid-luteal phase.
- Assessment of tubal patency by appropriate investigations including hysterosalpingography, sonosalpingography (Sion test), laparoscopy and/or to find out/rule out specific problems and to assess likely response to therapy.
- Screening for local factors including cervical mucus-related problems and lower genital tract infections, and instituting appropriate therapy.
- Screening for reproductive tract infections including syphilis, chlamydia, tuberculosis, HBV, HCV and HIV and appropriate management.

If needed, appropriate endocrinological investigations and therapy.

Any gynecologist not specifically trained in the sub-specialty of infertility care can also complete these investigations.

Based on the results of these investigations, couples should be selected for treatment at different levels of infertility care units. Depending on personnel competence and availability of facilities for investigation and treatment, there should be three levels of infertility care units:

1. Primary Infertility Care Unit
2. Secondary Infertility Care Unit
3. Tertiary Infertility Care Unit.

　　These care units should work in a 'tier' system.

Patient Selection and Categorization of Infertile Couples for Treatment in Different Infertility Care Units

In general, infertile couples can be categorized broadly into three groups: (1) those with single defect in one of the partners; (2) those with multiple defects in one or both the partners; (3) no apparent defect in either partner (unexplained infertility).

Single Defect in One of the Partners

The fault may exist either in the male or in the female partner. The defect may be either treatable or untreatable. For example, in the female partner, a treatable defect could be tough or imperforate hymen, or oligo- or anovulation due to polycystic ovary syndrome or may be a submucous fibroid. The untreatable female partner defects would include premature ovarian failure, absence of uterus, dense pelvic adhesions due to endometriosis, tuberculosis, and pelvic inflammatory disease or as a sequelae of pelvic surgery.

　　Unlike female factor infertility, male factor infertility is seldom easily correctable. Except oligozoospermia without asthenospermia, and sexual dysfunction due to phimosis, no other male factor infertility is easily amenable to simple medical or surgical therapy.

　　If a single defect in one of the partners is correctable, approximately half of the patients will respond with pregnancy to conventional medical or surgical therapy and the other half will not. Further treatment for the unresponsive couples will then consist of counseling and an in-depth investigation, leading to the use of ART; failing which adoption is the only alternative.

　　For an incorrectable single defect, either in the male or in the female partner, the choice would be between ART and adoption. The alternative to

be chosen should be suggested by the counselor after evaluation of the age, financial capabilities and psychological attitude of the couple.

Multiple Defects in One or Both Partners

When multiple defects involve either one or both partners, attempt to correct these defects and hoping to achieve a pregnancy in the natural way is almost always unrewarding. This should be explained by the consulting gynecologist or physician to the couple to prevent unnecessary expenditure by the couple. Judicious and effective counseling plays a very vital role under such circumstances; at least some couples will accept that at this point their treatment ends. A few will opt for adoption, while others might wish to try the challenges of ART procedures.

No Detectable Defect in Either Partner (Unexplained or Idiopathic Infertility)

This is a group most difficult to deal with as, they would have a right to ask that, in spite of every thing being normal, what is standing in their way to achieve conception.

Referral System and Responsibilities of Different Infertility Care Units

The severity in the cause of infertility differs widely in different couples. Sometimes, simple counseling or minor intervention will be all that is necessary. Others may require more aggressive treatment; such cases should be referred to speciality clinics. It is therefore, recommended that infertility treatment should be offered at three levels. The infertility care units should be categorized (and accredited) into three levels and authorized to offer treatments as described below. Patients should be referred by their gynecologist or physician to whom they go first, to specific level of infertility care unit where appropriate facilities for investigation and treatment for that patient would be available.

Primary (Level 1) Infertility Care Units

These would be clinics where preliminary investigations are carried out and the severity of infertility diagnosed. Primary infertility care unit or clinic could be a doctor's consulting room, such as a gynecologist's or a physician's consulting room, or even a general hospital. Depending on the severity of infertility, the couple could be treated at the Level 1 clinic or referred to speciality (Level 2 or Level 3) clinics.

Investigations into the cause of infertility by diligent history taking, physical examination and a simple semen analysis that can detect cases of azoospermia, can determine if the cause of infertility is related to the female or the male or to both the partners. Multifactorial or unexplainable cases should be referred to speciality secondary (Level 2) or tertiary (Level 3) infertility care units.

The responsibilities of a primary infertility care unit would be:

1. Completion of the basic investigations mentioned above.
2. Treatment of minor anatomical defects like tough or imperforate hymen, phimosis or submucous fibroid (Surgical perforation of hymen can be carried out after ensuring that the husband does not have erectile dysfunction. Extreme care must be taken in performing hymenectomy).
3. Treatment of mild endometriosis after confirming its presence by diagnostic laparoscopy carried out by a competent surgeon with adequate endoscopic experience.
4. Induction of ovulation in non-ovulatory women (especially PCOS) with clomiphene citrate, with or without adjuncts like bromocriptine, eltroxin, dexamethasone or spironolactone. (Gonadotropin should not be used at a primary infertility care unit level). Currently metformin (Insulin sensitizing agent) and Letrozol (Aromatase Inhibitors) are being used extensively in clomiphene resistant anovulation women. Gynecologist at level 1 unit should be familiar with the use of these drugs.
5. Correcting minor endocrine disorders such as thyroid disorders or hyperprolactinemia by prescribing appropriate corrective medications.
6. Treatment of oligozoospermia without asthenozoospermia.

7. Detecting infection of the reproductive tract using appropriate diagnostic tests, followed by normal health care steps after carrying out appropriate antibiotic sensitivity tests. (Particular care must be taken to treat the couple and not the female or the male patient alone).
8. Referral of the couple to secondary or tertiary infertility care unit, specially when the woman's age is more than 35, or when the couple has a multifactorial defect, or when patients with single treatable defect have not responded to conventional therapy.

The gynecologist or the physician in charge of a Level 1 infertility care unit should have an appropriate postgraduate degree and be capable of taking care of the above responsibilities.

Secondary (Level 2) Infertility Care Units

These units must have infrastructure for further in-depth investigation and extended treatment of infertility except where oocytes are handled outside the body. Some of the investigations and treatment facilities required for Level 2 care units are detailed below:

Facilities for investigations:

1. Immunological tests for infertility, sperm cervical mucous penetration test (SCMPT), sperm cervical mucous contact test (SCMCT), or antibodies (IgG, IgA) against sperm antigen in cervical mucous.
2. Sperm function tests like hypo-osmotic swelling test (HOST), and assessment for improvement of sperm motility potential with pentoxifyllene co-culture.
3. Assessment of follicular growth and ovulation by serial transvaginal sonography (TVS).
4. Hysteroscopy, laparoscopy and transvaginal sonography.

Treatment Facilities

1. Facilities for semen preparation and intrauterine insemination (IUI).
2. Provision for semen collection in men with a vibrator or an electroejaculator in functional erectile and ejaculatory problems. Currently

sildenafil (Viagra) is available, but should be prescribed cautiously.

3. Conservative infertility surgery either through a laparoscope, hysteroscope or via laparotomy. It should be possible to perform hysteroscopic cannulation of proximal blocked tubes, resection of submucous myoma or uterine septum.

4. Combined medical-surgical therapy by a coordinated team as in endometriosis or some cases of polycystic ovaries (ovarian drilling).

Tertiary (Level 3) Infertility Care Units

Such units will have three functions to perform, viz. diagnostic and therapeutic at the highest level of specialization and with the best of facilities, and research. Some examples of the first two functions are given below.

Advanced diagnostic procedures for male infertility

a. Endocrine assay.
b. Further tests for sperm function and integrity such as acrosome reaction and binding to zona-free hamster oocytes, and sperm-oocyte interaction *in vitro*.
c. Assessment of cell contaminants, debris and infection.
d. Karyotyping when sperm density, morphology and motility are abnormal.
e. Assessment of seminal plasma for viscosity, thinness, blood contamination and bio-chemical constituents.

Advanced diagnostic procedures for female infertility:

a. Endocrine assay.
b. Karyotyping in premature ovarian failure and other varieties of primary amenorrhea like Kallmann's syndrome.
c. Color Doppler for checking growing follicles, functional integrity of corpus luteum and developing endometrium in stimulated or unstimulated cycle.
d. GnRH challenge test in non-ovulation due to hypothalamic pituitary failure.
e. Clomiphene challenge test to ascertain ovarian reserve before ovulation induction or controlled ovarian hyperstimulation.

Advanced Therapeutic Procedures

1. Induction of ovulation in refractory non-ovulation due to PCO-down regulation with a *GnRH-agonist* followed by induction with gonadotropin. Ovulation induction with gonadotropin in PCO women with or without GnRH-a down regulation should only be attempted in tertiary care unit where there are facilities for follicular aspiration in care of unwarranted event of ovarian hyper-stimulation.

2. All varieties of assisted reproductive techno-logies, including ICSI.

3. Special procedures for IUI using split ejacu-late, pooled ejaculate or sperm recovered from post-coital specimen of urine in retrograde ejaculation.

4. Sperm banking and embryo freezing.

The choice of the procedure used, e.g. IVF-ET, GIFT, ZIFT, or ICSI is made depending upon the needs, resources and circumstances of the couple, availability of the facilities, and experience expertise of the gynecologist/embryologist. The commonest procedures of ART used currently are IVF-ET and ICSI.

Selection Criteria for *In Vitro* Fertilization and Embryo Transfer (IVF-ET)

Tubal Disease

IVF-ET can be offered where microsurgical techniques for tubal and peritoneal disease have failed or are unlikely to benefit the patient. The presence of peritubal adhesion, condition of the tubal wall, condition of the ciliary epithelium and degree of fimbrial damage would detect the choice between IVF and microsurgery. Patients who have already undergone tuboplasty and those with inaccessible ovaries would be more suitable for IVF. In case of history of ectopic pregnancy, IVF would be a better option.

Endometriosis

IVF is a suitable option for (a) women with moderate to severe endometriosis; (b) those in whom medical or surgical therapy has failed; and (c) sometimes in cases of mild to moderate endometriosis in the presence of other factors contributing to infertility.

Unexplained Infertility

Couples who have prolonged unexplained infertility would benefit from IVF. Many small, often overlooked infertility problems like subtle ovulation defects, defects in ovum pick up, gamate transport, tubal environment, sperm or oocyte abnormality may come to light when IVF is used.

Immunological Factor

IVF can be used when there are antibodies either in the male or the female and when other techniques such as immunosuppression, use of condom, intrauterine insemination and other therapeutic measures have failed.

Cervical Factor

IVF can be offered for cervical factor defect only if repeated attempts (6 to 8 cycles) of intrauterine insemination have failed and other therapies have not resulted in pregnancy.

Male Factor

IVF-ET is the logical therapy in case of low concentrations of sperm (less than 10 million/ml), low motility (less than 30%), and/or abnormal sperm morphology (presence of > 60 percent abnormal forms). No universally accepted minimal sperm concentration for success in IVF exists. In case of severe male factor infertility, assisted fertilization by means of micromanipulation and sperm injection (ICSI) can be offered even in obstructive and non-obstructive cases. In severe oligozoospermia, teratozoospermia, and azoospermia (obstructive/non-obstructive), ICSI can be employed using either ejaculated, epididymal or testicular sperm.

Ovarian Disorders

IVF-ET can benefit patients with hypogonadotropic anovulation, oligo-ovulation, and recurrent luteinized unruptured follicle syndrome, although IVF is rarely indicated when these disorders exist as isolated conditions. IVF-ET can be used for women with polycystic ovarian disease, but the high-risk of ovarian hyperstimulation syndrome in these women should always be guarded.

Uterine Disorder

Patients with Mullerian agenesis or congenital uterine anomalies, women with severe intrauterine adhesion refractory to surgical lysis of the adhesions, and hysterectomized patients can through IVF, transfer their embryos to a surrogate mother. Multiple fibroids and adenomyosis are not really the contraindications, but the chances of pregnancy in these cases are very limited. Surrogacy, if acceptable, may be an alternate option for these women.

In Association with Donor Eggs and Donor Embryos

Women who have undergone premature or timely menopause and women in the perimenopausal age group who do not show proper recruitment of follicles and who have other existing causes of infertility can avail the option of donor eggs and donor embryos. Women with genetic disorders, those who have undergone radiation therapy, and those with ovaries, which are not accessible by ultrasound due to severe adhesions, can also be advised to avail of donor eggs for IVF-ET.

Selection Criteria for Gamete Intrafallopian Transfer (GIFT)

The experimental background for GIFT is to determine the ability of the fallopian tube to serve as the site for capacitation and fertilization in human beings. Earlier experiments using GIFT were carried on monkeys that had undergone tubal resection and ligation. In 1979, Shettles reported pregnancy after intratubal transfer of freshly aspirated oocytes at the time of tubal re-anastomosis combined with cervical insemination. Asch and Colleagues[1] reported the first pregnancy and birth using laparoscopic GIFT. GIFT is possible when at least one fallopian tube is patent.

Subsequently Robert Jansen from Sydney reported successful pregnancy following the procedure of ultrasound guided transcervical GIFT. With rapid development of good laboratory embryology technique in conventional IVF, the procedure of GIFT is currently not popular as it was a decade ago. Laparoscopic GIFT involves additional interventional procedure of laparoscope and moreover the results of transcervical GIFT are not as rewarding as those achieved by Laparoscopic GIFT or conventional IVF.

Choosing between IVF-ET and GIFT

Decision in regard to which of these techniques should be utilized must be individualized with each patient. The advantages of IVF over GIFT are documentation of fertilization, less trauma and relatively lower anesthetic risk. There is no exposure to excess quantities of carbon dioxide in IVF as happens during laparoscopic insufflation with GIFT. On the other hand, GIFT is more natural as fertilization occurs in the tubal ampulla, the gametes are minimally exposed *in vitro,* and early embryo development occurs in a natural environment. Yet, as mentioned before GIFT, is now not a widely practice procedure. Further, GIFT cannot be compared with IVF, since in GIFT the fallopian tubes (at least one) must be patent, while in majority indications of IVF, the tubes are either damaged or blocked.

Micro-assisted Fertilization (SUZI and ICSI)

Sub-zonal insemination (SUZI), intracytoplasmic sperm injection (ICSI) and assisted hatching need micromanupulation of gametes. SUZI involves sperm injection directly into the oocyte outside the body. This technique has now been virtually totally replaced by ICSI which involves injection of sperm into the cytoplasm of the oocyte and is useful in a variety of cases such as in repeated fertilization failure and in may cases of male factor infertility, and in some clinics this is used as a routine procedure, replacing IVF (to improve fertilization rate). Assisted hatching of embryo by drilling a hole in the zona pellucida is often resorted prior to embryo transfer for improving implantation rates.

COMPLICATIONS

ART procedures carry a small risk both to the mother and to the offspring. These risks must be explained to the couple for appropriate counseling. ART procedures are to be initiated only after patients understand these risks and still want to undergo ART. Some of the most commonly encountered risks are mentioned below (this list is not exhaustive).

Multiple Gestation

The reported incidence of multiple gestation ranges from 20 to 30 percent. Incidence of twin pregnancies in the range of 10-20 percent may have to be accepted, as inevitable, but specific efforts must be made to reduce the incidence of triplets and multiple births of higher order. Therefore, not more than three embryos should be transferred for IVF-ET at one sitting excepting under exceptional circumstances (such as elderly women, previous record of poor implantation, adenomyosis, or poor embryo quality) which should be recorded. The remaining embryos, if any, may be cryopreserved and, if required, transferred in a later cycle.

Ectopic Pregnancy

Ectopic pregnancy rates could be as high as up to 8 percent for ART procedures. The choice of an appropriate procedure, as per guidelines mentioned earlier especially in women with tubal disease, may reduce the chances of an ectopic pregnancy.

Spontaneous Abortion

Spontaneous abortion rates range from 20 to 35 percent. Abortion rates rise with increasing age of the mother and in multiple pregnancies. In cases where more than two fetuses are present, selective embryo reduction should be advised. It is essential that the advantages of embryo reduction (better chances of the survival of other fetuses and the fact that they are likely to be born nearer term and with better birth weight) and disadvantages (the possibility that there might be an increased risk of abortion following the procedure) must be explained to the couple, and their informed consent taken before embryo reduction is attempted.

Preterm Birth

There is a higher risk of premature/low birth weight delivery following ART, especially in the presence of multiple fetuses.

Ovarian Hyperstimulation Syndrome

The use of superovulation for ART entails a risk of hyperstimulation in some women in the range of 0.2 to 8.0 percent. The extent of this risk is determined by the hormonal profile of the woman, the estradiol values (greater than 2500 pg/ml), the dose required for triggering ovulation, the ability to aspirate all the follicles at the time of oocyte retrieval, and several other factors like increased level of VEGF (vascular endothelial growth factor) predominantly found in women with PCO. The program director should be fully aware of the means to avoid hyperstimulation and also its treatment. Careful monitoring and management will reduce this risk as well as the morbidity associated with it.

In addition to these specific complications of ART, couples undergoing various ART procedures are also exposed to the risks associated with the operative and anesthetic procedures involved in ART.

COUNSELING

Counseling of the infertile couple is an integral step in the management of infertility. A busy infertility clinic predominantly devoted to investigation and treatment may not have enough time to look into the emotional factors, associated with infertility while such omission is generally unintentional. Yet it cannot be denied that ignoring the emotional issues may create a vicious cycle, delay the response to specific therapy and aggravate the distress of these couples who have already been victims of sustained emotional stress. Emotional factors may play a significant role in the etiology of infertility. Stress may also be a sequelae of long drawn procedures of investigation and treatment of infertility.

Stress as a Cause or Consequence of Infertility

Several authors indicate that sexual dysfunction may result in the inability to conceive.[2,3] Amenorrhea and other types of endocrine and reproductive dysfunctions have been shown to be associated with psychological stress.[4] It has also been suggested that social factors may be a significant component of the overall psychological distress, which appears to be a causal factor of infertility.[5] Moller and Fallstroms[6] suggest that stress is not only a contributing factor for infertility but may be increased as a result of infertile condition, creating a vicious cycle, which may further impair the couple's inability to conceive. Patients in ART program have a number of significant psychological issues and concerns. These problems create anxiety and stress, often leading to a lack of sense of control over life decisions.

Stress Following Gamete Donation

Use of donor's gamete may have profound impact on the couple as well as on child, which is generated through such procedure. Use of donor's gametes may lead to many adverse psychological problems. The problems relate to future couple relationship, secrecy of the procedure, anonymity of the donor and social attitudes.

Regarding couple relationship, some couples may feel that this alternative is not the solution for their childlessness while others may come to realize that it is the last option for them. Secrecy of gamete donation is the 'Modus Operandi' for couples and medical professionals. But secrecy places a lie at the foundation of a basic relationship, the one between the parent and the child. Whether secrecy is harmful for the child or not is a debatable issue.

Donor anonymity is a concern with regard to gamete donation. In most of the countries this is crucial for maintaining secrecy around this parenting option. This is more true regarding sperm rather than oocyte donation, because there is a lack of legal protection for social fathers and donors in almost all the countries around the world.

Social and religious attitudes of the couples play a significant role in sperm and oocyte donation for conception. Religious prohibitions play an active part in their lives. In this case conception does not involve the conjugal act. Apprehension on the part of the couples, that they may be rejected by their religious community make them more concerned about their decision to maintain secrecy.

Couples in ART programs are in greater emotional crisis. This is because the financial burden is too great and the stress of the procedure creates too much anxiety, depression, disruption and strain.[7] Yet it appears that majority of couples believe that trying an ART procedure is worth the effort.

Stress Originating as a Result of Interaction between Infertile Couple and the Medical Staff

The members of the staff of an infertility clinic which include physicians, nurses, other professionals and administrative personnel may have a profound impact on the sense of wellbeing and significantly increase or reduce the psychological stress that the couple is already experiencing because of infertility. Infertility has profound physiological, psychological and social implications.[8] The health care professionals and medical team must be careful not to add additional stress to already stressed infertile couples. It may be very frustrating, painful and humiliating for infertility patients to wait several hours beyond scheduled appointment time to meet the physician and even then not be given an explanation or an apology. Even a minor negligence on the part of the medical professionals or paramedical staff may have an adverse impact on the couple's psychology who are already emotionally wounded and rendered powerless by their infertility problem.

Guidelines for Counseling Infertile Couples

The following guidelines are few among many which may help in psychologic boosting of infertile patients.

1. Sympathy, understanding and accessibility are of great importance. Emotional components and psychological status of the infertile couples should be realized specially when the investigative procedures are becoming prolonged and protracted.

2. Physicians should counsel and treat infertility as a couple's problem regardless of the fact that who has diagnosed the medical defect.

3. A clear investigative and treatment protocol should be initially discussed with the couple; then the order in which investigations, medications, options for treatment, to be carried out are to be discussed. The cost, prognosis and time schedule are to be informed. For majority of couples, time is pressing both physically and psychologically.

4. Couples should be encouraged to ask questions. Information is very helpful for psychological wellbeing of the couples. Information increases the feeling of effectiveness and also promotes positive self-approach.

5. At the outset, couple should be informed that all possible efforts will be taken to help them to achieve a viable pregnancy but despite every one's best efforts results cannot be hundred percent. At the same time, investigations cannot continue forever. They should be advised to end treatment or seek a second opinion without the fear of embarrassment or a sense of inferiority complex.

6. Before proceeding with physical examination, the physician must be conversant with the medical records of the patient. The patient becomes distressed meeting the physician when undressed, lying or sitting on an examination table.

7. The various treatment procedures with their potential side effects are to be explained to the couple in advance. If they know what and how much to expect, they respond respectfully with less risk of confusion.

8. Infertile man and woman are in great need of sympathy and support. There should be an infertility support organization comprising of mental health professionals. They can offer positive help to these couples who find it

difficult to adjust with the life crisis of infertility and sometimes its long drawn and complicated treatment.

MANAGEMENT

It has already been mentioned earlier that from management point of view, infertile couples can be broadly categorized into three groups:
  i. Those with single defect in one of the partners.
  ii. Those with multiple defects in one or both partners.
  iii. No apparent defect in either partner (unexplained).

Approach to management protocol with regard to nature of defects may be summarized as follows:

Outline of management protocol of infertile couple

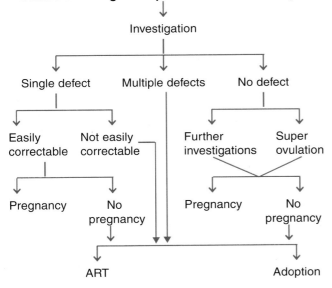

Hence overall management protocol should be outlined on the basis of the nature of infertility problem or problems with which the couple presents for treatment. Five types of management options are available: (1) Medical, (2) Surgical, (3) Medical/Surgical combination, (4) Assisted Reproduction and lastly, if everything fails or not applicable (5) Adoption.

Medical Management

Medical management is expected to work satisfactorily, if there is a single treatable defect in one of the partners or no defect in either partner (Unexplained infertility). The commonest situations in which medical management is likely to be effective are anovulation specially associated with PCO, early endometriosis (minimal and mild) hypogonadotropic azoospermia/oligospermia and some cases of male sexual dysfunction.

Medical Management for Non-ovulation

About 75 percent of women presenting with the problem of no-ovulation will at any one point of time develop full blown clinical and biochemical features of polycystic ovarian syndrome.[9] Medical management consists of administration of clomiphene citrate with or without an adjunct like dexamethasone, bromocriptine, eltroxin or sprionolactone. Metformin (Insulin Sensiting agent) has been used for obese hyperinsulinemic, hyperandrogenic PCOS. Letrozol (Aromatase inhibitors) is a new introduction and showing promise in clomiphene resistant hyperestrogenic PCOS. In non-responders, gonadotropin with or without GnRH-a down regulation may be tried. But use of gonadotropin should be restricted to only those centers, where there is a facility for follicular aspiration (Tertiary care unit). Because ovarian hyperstimulation syndrome may be an adverse and sometimes critical consequence of gonadotropin stimulation in PCOS.

Non-ovulation, other than PCO may be due to hypogonadotropic hypogonadism or premature ovarian failure. For dysfunctional hypogonadotropic anovulation, programable portable minipump was initially introduced for GnRH administration in a pulsatile fashion. The reported pregnancy rates were excellent (80% after 6 cycles and 90% after 12 cycles).[10] Despite the advantages, GnRH pump has not received wide acceptance by patients because of its complexity of use and alternative better management with gonadotropin stimulation. There is no definite medical management of premature ovarian failure responsible for non-ovulation. A small subgroup may respond occasionally to medical management. This group consists of impending and autoimmune ovarian failure. Sequential estrogen progestogen, GnRH analogs for down regulation of elevated FSH followed by gonadotropin stimulation combined with corticosteroids for immunosuppression have been sporadically reported in the literature for this small subgroup and the results have been claimed to be encouraging.[11-13] These groups of anovulatory women should be treated at a tertiary care unit.

Medical Management for Endometriosis

Endometriosis irrespective of its stage certainly reduces fertility potential of a woman. But medical management alone seldom improves the chance of conception. Even in the early stages (Minimal or Mild) hormonal preparations may not offer any advantage in promoting conception.[14-16] Perhaps this lack of enhancement of fertility may be due to less number of estrogen-progesterone and/or androgen receptors in the endometriotic lesions compared with normal endometrium. Alternatively the exact mechanism by which early endometriosis prevents conception in a woman is still not very clear and therefore the hormonal treatments employed for treating infertility in endometriosis are not specific. The drugs used to treat early endometriosis and have a doubtful role to improve fertility potential are Danazol, Progestins and GnRH-agonists. These drugs have been proved to be cytoreductive rather than cytoablative.

Danazol

Danazol is a synthetic derivative of 17- α ethinyl testosterone and was introduced for treatment of endometriosis in 1971.[17]

Danazol acts in three ways: (a) Inhibits GnRH secretion; midcycle LH surge is ablated, but the basal gonadotropin concentrations are maintained, (b) Direct androgenic and anti-progestational effect on the endometriotic implant, (c) Creates a hypoestrogenic and hypoprogestational environment antagonistic to endometriosis.

Side effects of Danazol are too many and are usually dose related. These include weight gain, muscle cramps, decreased breast size and vasomotor symptoms. Danazol is an excellent drug for relief of pain in endometriosis but its role

in improving fertility has been questioned. Recent studies concerning use of Danazol for minimal, mild or moderate endometriosis could not substantially establish any therapeutic benefit in enhancing conception.[15, 16] Moreover attempts at conception are delayed while the patients are receiving the medication.

Progestogens

Combination of high dose of estrogen-progestogen regimen was introduced in late 1950s for symptomatic relief of pain in endometriosis. Because of multiple side effects and potential risk of high dose of estrogens in some patients, progestogen only (medroxy- progesterone acetate; MPA) regimens have gained popularity. High dose of progestogens inhibits pituitary release of LH and thereby suppresses ovarian steroidogenesis and also promotes decidualization of ectopic endometrium and finally atrophy. Side effects include break through bleeding, weight gain, edema and irritability. Like danazol, conception rate is not significantly increased, when compared with control group.[18]

GnRH-Agonist

GnRH-a is a recent introduction in the medical management regimen of endometriosis. Some of the frequently studied analogues include buserelin, triptorelin, goserelin, leuprolide and nafarelin. Continued administration of the analogues leads to desensitization of the pituitary gonadotropin receptors and a reversible down regulation of the pituitary ovarian axis.[19]

The effect of GnRH analogues on endometriosis-associated infertility is difficult to assess due to lack of expectant management control group in most of the studies.[20,21] The pregnancy rates reported in majority study groups which range from 0-60 percent have been achieved in trials based on the stage of the disease.[22]

Medical Management for Unexplained Infertility

Ovulation inducing drugs are used emperically. Further indepth investigations are suggested only to allow time for spontaneous conception. Because while these couples are under the regime of emperic treatment and experimental investigations, approximately 30 to 35 percent will conceive following ovulation induction, bromocriptine, steroid, antibiotic therapy and combination.[23] The remaining patients are to be advised for superovulation followed by IUI or ART. ESHRE multicentic trial has shown that application of ART increased the chance of pregnancy by nearly two times more than that obtained by superovulation alone.

Medical Management for Male Infertility

There is no convincing evidence that medical management improves the deficiencies responsible for male factor infertility. Oligo or azoospermia due to gonadotropin insufficiency or leydig cell inefficiency may respond to either clomiphene citrate, low dose androgens (Synthetic androgens, mesterolone or testosterone undecanoate) or gonadotropin. Use of growth hormone may accelerate receptor responsiveness to endogeneously produced or exogeneously administered androgens. Bromocriptine may help to improve functional sexual disorders in male partner especially when hyperprolactinemia is associated. Local injection of papaverine have been used for erectile problems of male infertility. In extreme degrees of these functional disorders, vibrators and electroejaculators may help in erection and ejaculation. The sperms thus recovered may be frozen for subsequent use for artificial insemination. Recently, Sildenafil (Viagra) has been used extensively in psychogenic erectile dysfunction with encouraging results. For pyospermic semen samples, antibiotics and vitamins (Vitamin E) are to be used for a prolonged period of time. Leucocytes in semen liberate free oxygen radicals which are harmful for the normal sperms. Vitamin E in particular, has an antioxidant role.

Asthenospermia may be due to chronic prostatitis and when infection is adequately treated, sperm motility may improve. In unexplained asthenospermia, motility may be improved *in vitro* by pentoxifyllene co-culture followed by the procedure of artificial insemination. In practice,

however, results of this procedure have not been very encouraging.

Oligo-terato-asthenozoospermia (OTA Syndrome) most frequently has a genetic background. Rarely, this may be due to infection. When infection is the etiology, antibiotics may help.

Except for GnRH-a treatment for endometriosis and some specialized treatment for male infertility, all other patients can be treated at the primary care unit. In case, the response to treatment is delayed the couples should be referred to secondary or tertiary care unit.

SURGICAL TREATMENT

There are two groups of infertile couples who require surgical treatment for improvement of their fertility potential. In one group, surgical treatment is obligatory and in the other this is complimentary.

Obligatory Surgical Treatment

The indications for which surgical treatment becomes obligatory involve mostly the female partner. These indications include: tough or imperforate hymen, cervical stenosis or atresia, submucous fibroids, other varieties of fibroids (Cervical intramural, subserous, broad ligament) grossly distorting pelvic anatomy or uterine cavity, big benign ovarian tumors and endometriomas more than 3 cm in diameter. Surgical correction of these defects in the female partner is obligatory because: (a) the treatment may improve the chances of natural conception (b) there is no specific medical management of these disorders (c) unless the defects are corrected, alternative treatment of assisted reproductive technology cannot be attempted.

Complimentary Surgical Treatments

Surgical treatment in this group is considered complimentary because apart from its own therapeutic value, it helps the effectiveness of medical management or alternative procedures of assisted reproductive technology. Indications include both male and female partner defects.

Female partner defects include: Laparoscopic drilling and cautery or open laparotomy for wedge resection of polycystic ovaries, endoscopic ablation, vapourization, cauterization of endometriotic implants and adhesiolysis in moderate or severe endometriosis, and synechiotomy for mild and moderate grades of uterine synechiae. Hysteroscopic resection of uterine septum may help achieving pregnancy either spontaneously or by subsequent medical management.

Complimentary surgical treatments for male partner defects include, correction of phimosis, hypospadius, varicocele, hydrocele and vasoepididymeal anastomosis. Patients in these groups should be referred to secondary infertility care unit.

Combination of Medical and Surgical Therapy

The objective of the combination therapy is to improve the response to one therapy by instituting another modality of treatment. The common situations in which such combination therapy is expected to work effectively are endometriosis and polycystic ovaries.

In endometriosis, preoperative medical therapy may reduce pelvic vascularity, size of endometriotic implants thus minimizing intraoperative blood loss and minimize the amount of surgical resection needed. Postoperative medical therapy is advocated to eradicate residual endometriotic lesions. This is applicable for patients who had extensive endometriosis and resection of all implants was not possible or advisable at the time of primary operation.

In minimal or mild endometriosis, if endoscopic surgery has already been performed at the time of initial diagnostic laparoscope, there is no justification of adding postoperative medical treatment. This attitude perhaps applies to moderate endometriosis as well because postoperative addition of medical therapy might delay the chances of conception. In advanced stages of endometriosis however, there may be justification for combined therapy.

There is only one study which has convincingly demonstrated that use of postoperative danazol improved fertility.[24] Majority of other reports, however, failed to demonstrate beneficial fertility improving effect of preoperative or postoperative medical therapy.[25, 26]

Medical treatment prior to ART in advanced endometriosis has been reported to yield better pregnancy rates compared to when ART is performed without prior medical treatment of the disease. Hormonal suppression with GnRH-a for six months followed by ART resulted in increased number of oocyte retrieval, transferable embryos and ongoing pregnancies.[27]

Combination of medical surgical treatment may also be necessary in some cases of polycystic ovaries resistant to medical treatment only. The basis of treatment of polycystic ovaries is to reduce androgens and to increase estrogens. If following wedge resection or laparoscopic cauterization, spontaneous ovulation does not occur, clomiphene may be added. Pregnancy rate following combination therapy of polycystic ovaries resistant to single therapy has been estimated around 60 percent.[28] Obviously combination therapy is possible in secondary or tertiary infertility care units.

Assisted Reproductive Technology

The procedures are exclusively carried out in tertiary care unit. The most frequently and currently practised Assisted Reproductive Technologies are: (a) *In Vitro* Fertilization and Embryo Transfer (IVF-ET) (b) Intracytoplasmic Sperm injection (ICSI) and (c) Intrauterine Insemination (IUI). By strict criteria of definition, IUI should not be included under the heading of ART, as the procedure does not involve direct retrieval of oocytes from the ovaries. But since extracorporeal male gamete manipulation is involved with superovulation of the female partner, majority clinics consider IUI as one of the technologies of assisted reproduction.

In Vitro Fertilization and Embryo Transfer (IVF-ET)

The procedure involves six essential steps: (a) Indication and selection of cases; (b) Stimulation and monitoring; (c) Ultrasound guided oocyte retrieval; (d) Fertilization and cleavage in laboratory under optimum environment; (e) Embryo

Transfer and (f) Post transfer hormonal support. Since the introduction of this revolutionary technology in human reproduction in 1978, the procedure of IVF has passed through several changes and modifications. The objectives were to (a) expand the indications (b) simplify the procedure (c) reduce the cost (d) improve the result and in the process (e) to acquire further knowledge in many unknown fields of human reproduction.

Brief account of significant changes are summarized as follows:

a. Expansion of indications and criteria for patient selection:

  • Originally IVF evolved as the treatment for irreversible tubal damage. Since 1980s the treatment has been extended to individuals with male factor infertility, unexplained infertility, endometriosis and immunologic causes of infertility. Subsequently success has been achieved using donor oocyte in women with premature ovarian failure. Selection depends on age, pelvic pathology, and presence/absence of systemic infection and base line FSH, LH and E_2 levels.

Stimulation Protocol

The first baby by IVF treatment was the result of fertilization of an oocyte retrieved in natural cycle. Although non-stimulated cycles are still used sporadically with decreasing expenses, the delivery rate per retrieval is approximately 5 percent.[29]

In early 1980s, clomiphene citrate and gonadotropins were introduced in the stimulation protocol, which improved the result but at the same time increased the number of cancellations due to early luteinization and premature LH surge. This problem to a large extent was solved by the introduction of GnRH-agonist in late 1980s. Use of GnRH agonist increased treatment cost as it increased the amount of gonadotropin necessary to stimulate the follicular growth. But the positive advantages included (a) Improvement of results (b) Reducing cancellation rates (c) more flexibility in scheduling necessary interventions.

In 2001, GnRH antagonist has been introduced. This has helped to reduce the cost and shorten duration of treatment. The protocol is still in the learning curve and the reported pregnancy rate is relatively lower compared to what is achieved in GnRH-agonist protocol.

In order to achieve competent cohort of follicular growth following gonadotropin stimulation, the nature, quality and source of gonadotropins have also changed over the years. Initially, urinary human menopausal gonadotropins were used. It was realized that LH component in HMG was detrimental in early follicular phase. Highly purified FSH (Metrodin-HP-Serono) was introduced. But this product also contained some amount of LH and other urinary protein contaminants. Recently, recombinant gonadotropin has been made available commercially. This product is being widely used in stimulation protocol of IVF in many centers. Though cost is high, results are encouraging.

Monitoring the Cycle for Adequate or Poor Response or Hyperstimulation

Commonly accepted monitoring parameters include, measurement of serum estradiol and ultrasound imaging of ovarian follicular response. Adequate response indicates growth of at least 3-4 co-dominant follicles with diameters 14 mm or greater combined with estradiol levels of approximately 150 pg/ml per large (14 mm) follicle. The objective is to retrieve 6-12 oocytes of which at least 3-4 should be mature.

Abnormal response includes hyperstimulation and poor response. In general, more than 11 intermediate follicles (less than 9 mm in diameter) with serum estradiol levels of more than 4000 pg/ml are the predictors of impending ovarian hyperstimulation syndrome—(Schenker 1993). Poor response to ovarian stimulation will be evident when (a) not more than one dominant follicle develops (b) growth pattern of follicle/follicles is arrested or retarded (normal: 1 mm increment/day) (c) estradiol level is less than 500 pg/on HCG day and (d) endometrial growth velocity lags behind follicular growth.

Embryology

Though the basic principle remains the same, there have been many changes in the constituents of fertilizing and growth media to produce better quality embryos, and allow them to grow in culture for longer period (blastocyst culture) to facilitate effective embryo-endometrial interaction and embryonic implantation. Blastocyst culture and transfer on day 5 is a relatively recent concept. This allows the embryo produced *in vitro* to enter the uterine cavity on the day and at a stage similar to those, which occur with embryos generated in *in vivo* conception. Embryo transfer in the blastocyst stage may improve success rate in poor responders, women beyond 38 years of age and where endometrial development is poor on day 2 post pick-up.

Embryo Replacement

Transfer technique should be absolutely atraumatic. Currently 2-3 good quality embryos are transferred to reduce the risk of multiple pregnancies. The surplus embryos are cryopreserved for future transfer, in case, the index cycle fails to produce a pregnancy.

RESULTS

Success after IVF is now reported in terms of delivery rate perretrieval and delivery rate percycle initiated. Data of uniform reporting is not usually available. Many clinics are achieving delivery rates in the 35 percent range, specially in women under the age of 35 years.[30]

Multiple pregnancy rate is approximately 35 percent (30% twins, 5% triplets and 0.6 percent higher multiple). Three percent pregnancies achieved through IVF are ectopic and the incidence of heterotropic pregnancies is 1 in 100 pregnancies.[31]

Micro Manipulation

The previous technique of zona drilling to facilitate sperm entry and injection of sperm into the perivitelline space has been replaced by intracytoplasmic sperm injection (ICSI).

ICSI is indicated in severe oligospermia, azoospermia, in situations like presence of antisperm antibodies, poor fertilization despite normal semen quality and also for refractory unexplained infertility. In azoospermic subjects, sperm for injection can be obtained by microsurgery from epididymes (MESA) or from the testis (TESE).[32] Sperms may be obtained through percutaneous aspiration or open biopsies. Even the sperm precursors have produced successful pregnancies through ICSI.[33] In women under the age of 34, pregnancy rate per transfer has been reported to be as high as 49 percent.[34]

However, there are concerns regarding transmission of genetic abnormalities in the newborns delivered through the procedure of ICSI. Male with azoospermia and severe oligospermia should have genetic screening because the risk of genetic abnormalities in these individuals is higher than men with mild sperm impairment.

INTRAUTERINE INSEMINATION (IUI)

The procedure of IUI has the advantage of placing the sperm in close proximity of the oocyte, thereby enhancing the chance of fertilization. At least one fallopian tube must be patent. There has been a sharp decline in the demand of donor insemination (therapeutic donor insemination–TDI) because the alternative procedure of intracytoplasmic sperm injection (ICSI) into the oocyte, currently used is more acceptable for many couples who can afford to bear the cost.

Indications of artificial insemination using husband's semen include unexplained infertility, mild oligospermia without asthenospermia, ovulatory dysfunction, early endometriosis, cervical factor defect, immunologic infertility and unilateral tubal defect.

To be practiced correctly, IUI involves detailed scans, endocrine assessment, aspiration of excess follicles and proper sperm washing to avoid placing seminal plasma in the uterus. Results of IUI are far superior in stimulated than in unstimulated cycles.[35]

Adoption

Couples who are refractory to the usual treatments of infertility should be advised alternative treatments like ART or adoption. Most infertile couples in India are reluctant to accept adoption as an alternative procedure but at the same time cannot afford the expensive treatment of ART. Couples desiring adoption have a range of choice namely, social agency adoption, private adoption or international adoption. Lawyers should be approached regarding the adoption laws in individuals'countries. For this, 'support and counseling units'are essential specially at the tertiary care unit.

REFERENCES

1. Asch R, Balmaceda J, Ord T, Borrero C, Cefalu E, Gastaldi C, Rojas F. Oocyte donation and gamete intrafallopian transfer as treatment for premature ovarian failure. Lancet 1987;1:687.
2. Berger DM. The role of the psychiatrist in a reprod. Biology Clinic Fertil Steril 1977;28:141.
3. Palti Z. Psychogenic male infertility. Paychosom Med 1969;31:326.
4. Barnea ER, Tal J. Stress–related reprod. Failure. J In Wit Emb Trans 1991;8:15.
5. Wasser SK, Sewall G, Soules MR. Psychological Stress as a cause of infertility. Fertile Steril 1993;39:685.
6. Moller A, Fallstrom K. Psychological consequences of infertility, a longitudinal study. J Psychosom Obstet Gynaecol 1991;12:27.
7. Lasker JN, Borg S. In search of Parenthood: Coping with infertility and High–tech reprod. Boston. Beacon Press 1987.
8. Appleton T. Counselling, Care in infertility; the ethic of care. Br Med Bull 1990;46:842.
9. Franks S. Polycystic Ovary Syndrome, New Engl J Med 1995;333:853.
10. Brast DD, Schomaker R, Schomaker J. Life table analysis of fecundity of intravenously gonadotropins–realizing hormone–treated patients with normo-gonadotropic and hypogonadotropic amenorrhoea, Fertil Steril 1991;55:266.
11. Blumenfeld Z, Amit T, Barkey RI, Lundnfeld B, Brades JM. Ann: NY Acade Sci 1991;626:250-65.
12. Baber, Abdallahi, Studd JWW. The Premature menopause, Progress in Obst and Gynec Churchill Livingstone, 1991;9:209-26.
13. Chakravarty BN. J of Obst Gynec, of India, 1991;41:129-35.
14. Seibel MM, Berger MJ, Weinstein FG, Taymor ML. The effectiveness of danazol on subsequent fertility in minimal endometriosis. Fertile Steril 1982;38:534-37.
15. Hull MGR. Epidemiology of infertility and Polycystic Ovarian disease; endocrinological and demographic studies Gynaecol Endocrinol 1997;1:235.
16. Telimaa S. Danazol and medroxy progesterone acetate inefficasious in the treatment of infertility in endo-metriosis. Fertil Steril 1988;50:827.
17. Green RB, Dmowski WP, Mahesh VB, et al. Clinical studies with an antigonadotropin danazol. Fertile Steril 1971;22:102.
18. Hull ME, Moghissi KS, Magyar DF, et al. Comparison of different treatment modalities of endometriosis in infertile women. Fertile Steril 1987;22:102.
19. Maldrum DR, Clang RJ, Lu J, et al. 'Medical Oopho-rectomy' using a long acting GnRH agonist–a possible new approach to the treatment of endometriosis. J Clin Endocrinol Metab 1982;54:1081.
20. Henzl MR, Lason SL, Moghissi K, Buttram VC, Berquist C, Jacobson J. Administration of nasal nafarelin as compared with oral danazol for endometriosis. A multicenter double blind comparative clinical trial. N Evol J Med 1988;318:485-89.
21. Dmowski WP, Radwanska E, Binar Z, Tummon I, Pepping P. Ovarian suppression induced with buserelin or danazol in the management of endometriosis: A randomized comparative study. Fertile Steril 1989;51:395-400.
22. Hesla SJ, Rock AJ. In JA Rock, AA Murphy, HHW Jones (Eds): Fem Reprod Surg 1992;11:205-44.
23. Navot D, Rosenwaks Z, Margalioth EJ. Prognostic assessment of female fecundity Lancet II 1987;645.
24. Wheeler JM, Johnston BM, Malinak LR. Postoperative danazol therapy in infertility patients with severe endometriosis. Fertil Steril 1981;36:460.
25. Ronnberg L, Jarvinen PA. Pregnancy rates following various therapy modes for endometriosis in infertile patients Acta Obstet Gynecl Scand 1984;123(Suppl):69-72.
26. Donnez J, Nisolle M, Clercks F, Casanas F. Evaluation of preoperative use of danazol, gestrinane, lunestrenol, buserelin spray and buserelin implant, in the treatment of endometriosis-associated infertility. Prog Clin Biol Res 1990;323:427-42.
27. Dicker D, Goldman JA, Levy T, Feldberg D, Ashkenaz J. The impact of long-term gonadotropin–realizing hormone analogue treatment on preclinical abortions in patients with severe endometriosis undergoing in vitro fertilization–embryo transfer. Fertile Steril 1992;57:597-600.
28. Campo S. Ovulatory cycles, pregnancy outcome and complications after surgical treatment of polycystic ovary syndrome. Obstet Gynec Surgery 1998;53:297.
29. Clamans P, Domingo M, Garner P, Leader A, Spene JEH. Natural cycle in vitro fertilization–embryo transfer at the University of Ottawa; an inefficient therapy for tubal infertility. Fertile Steril 1993;60:298.
30. Speroff L, Glass RH, Kase NG. Assist Reprod, An overview of the Asst Reprod Tech 6th edn. 1999;1139.
31. Mollay D, Deambrosis W, Keeping D, Hyues J, Harrison J, Mashiach S. Multiple–sited (Heteropic) pregnancy after in vitro fertilization and gamete intrafallopian transfer Fertil Steril 1990;3:1068.
32. Silber SJ, Nagy Z, Liu J, Tournaye H, Lissens W, Ferce C, Liebaers I, Devroey P, Van Steirteghem AC. The use of epididymal and testicular spermatozoa for

intracytoplasmic sperm injection; the genetic implantations for male infertility. Hum Reprod 1995;10:2031.

33. Tesarik J, Mendoza C, Testart J. Viable embryos from injection of round spermatids into oocytes. New Engl J Med 1995;333:525.

34. Oehninger S, Veek L, Lanzendorfs, Maloney M, Toner J, Muashher S. Intracytoplasmic sperm injection, achievement of high pregnancy rates in couples with severe male factor infertility is dependent upon female and not male factors. Fertil Steril 1995;64:977.

35. Zeyneloglu HB, Arici A, Olovi Dl, Duleba AJ. Comparison of intrauterine insemination with timed intercourse in Supervulated cycles with gonadotropin; a meta–analysis. Fertil Steril 1998;69:486.

• Narendra Malhotra • Jaideep Malhotra

2

Transvaginal Sonography in Infertility

The application of transvaginal ultrasound in the evaluation and assessment of the infertile couple is expanding each day. The transvaginal ultrasound picture depicts accurately the pelvic anatomy of the scanned area safely, quickly and reproducibly.

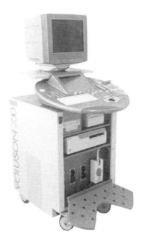

FIGURE 2.1: USG machine and probes

The quality of depiction of the pelvic anatomy is dependent on the ultrasound equipment being used and the experience and proficiency of the person performing the scan.

It should be mandatory for the person performing the scan to know about the female endocrinology and be well versed with the causes and management of infertility, specially with the ovulation induction protocols.

Till date there are no known adverse biological effects of transvaginal ultrasound on the patient, on the oocytes or on the ultrasound operator (AIUM).[1]

Transvaginal ultrasound today is the modality of choice in evaluating male and female infertility as a first step investigation and should be used by the clinician in the consulting chamber along with pelvic examination. It is like marrying palpation with imaging.

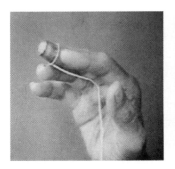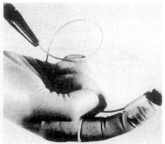

FIGURE 2.2: Fingertip probe

ULTRASOUND ASSESSMENT OF THE MALE PARTNER

Male factor infertility today comprises of almost 40 percent of the causes. In an infertile male the modern life style and additives in food have became a major environmental cause of oligo astheno spermia. The function of male genital system encompasses the central nervous system (hypothalamus and pituitary), the adrenal glands, the testes, the epididymis, the seminal vesicles and the prostate gland. Any malfunctions of any of these may affect the male reproductive capacity.

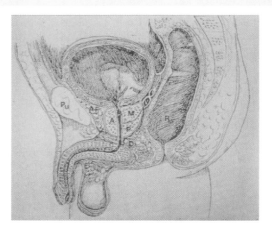

FIGURE 2.3: Male reproductive system

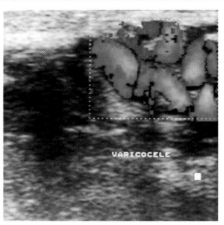

Varicocele

In suspected male factor infertility ultrasound imaging of the ejaculatory system and of the testis is necessary to rule out structural anomalies. Scrotal and transrectal (TRUS) are used in evaluation of the reproductive tract disorders. Color flow imaging is used for assessment of varicocele. 3-D is used for testicular volume and seminal vesicle and prostate evaluation. Computed tomography and endorectal Magnetic Resonance Imaging can also be used.

Scrotal sonography is performed with patient in supine position using a 7.5–10 MHz linear probe. This can evaluate the testis for size, shape, hydrocele, benign tumors, atrophy, malignancy, orchitis, torsion, hemorrhage, focal lesions, etc. Ultrasound imaging is very sensitive in testicular evaluation.[2-5]

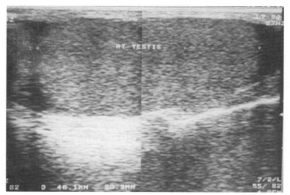

Testis

Transrectal ultrasonography (TRUS) is an excellent approach for visualising the seminal vesicles, prostate and ejaculatory ducts. With TRUS we can assess obstructions, absence or hypoplasia of seminal vesicle and ejaculatory ducts. TRUS is an excellent screening test for ejaculatory duct pathologies and is indicated in all men with severe oligospermia and a low volume ejaculate.[5]

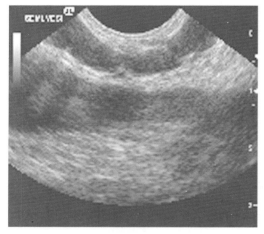

FIGURE 2.4: TRUS seminal vesicle bow tie picture

Assessment of the Female Reproductive Tract

The female is responsible for 40 percent of causes of infertility and contributes in another 20 percent of mixed causes in the couple. Out of this the ovulatory dysfunction (30%) and tubal factor infertility (25%) are major factors.[6] The female reproductive tract is usually evaluated by the busy gynecologist by a per speculum and a per vaginum examination and then an HSG is usually ordered and then a transvaginal scan is ordered and later followed with other tests. These usually take time and frustrate the patient and the doctor.

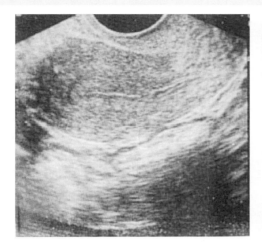
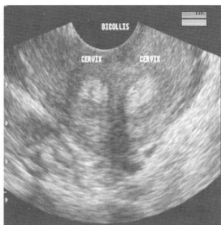

FIGURE 2.5: Normal cervix

We advocate a transvaginal scan at the very first visit of the couple by the infertility specialist himself/herself just after a p/s exam, this will enable the clinician to come to a diagnosis on the very first visit regarding problems in vagina, cervix, uterus, endometrium, endometrial cavity, tubes, adnexa, ovaries and general pelvis as a whole. Such an examination helps to decide the further treatment line and actively manage infertility by a single day evaluation test and active management protocol (Rajan, Malhotra) (2000).[7,8]

Vaginal and Cervical Factor Infertility Evaluation

Vagina and the cervix is the first obstacle that the spermatozoa have to negotiate on their way to reach the oocyte. Vaginal septae, stenosis, vaginismus and coital difficulties are best assessed by a per speculum examination, however TVS helps to locate vaginal cysts and vaginal infiltrations.

Cervix is composed of cervical glands which secrete mucus in response to estrogens stimulation and this secretion assists passage of sperms. About 5-10 percent of causes of infertility are due to cervical factors, which may be anatomical or functional abnormalities.

Transvaginal ultrasound can very accurately assess both anatomical and functional problems of the cervix.

Assessment of cervicitis, nabothian cysts at internal OS, poor cervical mucus, cervical

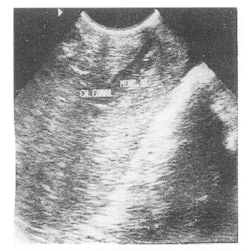

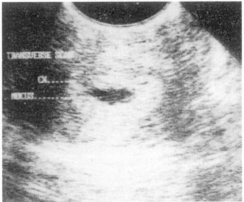

FIGURE 2.6: Cervical mucus

agenesis and cervical stenosis is possible and should be done. Cervical conisation and cervical infections should always be kept in mind and assessed for clinically before a TVS scan.

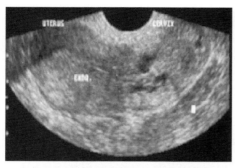

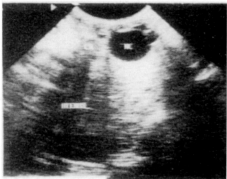

FIGURE 2.7: Nabothian cysts

Uterine Factor Assessment and Evaluation

Uterus is the place for embryo implantation and pregnancy continuation. The normal adult uterus is a muscular organ 6-10 cm in length and 3-5 cm in width and has a unique capacity to grow and expand to hold a full term fetus during pregnancy.

Problems of uterus may lie in the musculature (Fibroids, Adenomyosis, etc.) in the uterine cavity (congenital uterine malformations, adhesions, uterine cavity polyps, etc.) or problems in the endometrial lining, i.e. inappropriate endometrial growth and secretory transformations in response to progesterone from corpus luteum.

TVS can accurately assess the uterine factors and with addition of fluid (saline) by sonohysterography the cavity can be accurately studied, with addition of color flow imaging, color doppler studies of uterine artery, power angio; the spiral artery and endometrial vascularization can be evaluated to score the uterus for favourability of implantation (uterine scoring system for Reproduction) (Applebaum, Dalal, Malhotra).

The Uterus

Transvaginal ultrasound examination of the body of uterus is done to observe detailed view of the myometrium and any anomalies, leiomyomas are one of the most common benign neoplasms in women and have been reported to occur in up to 40 percent of women over the age of 35. A leiomyoma may be suggested by generalized enlargement of the uterus, irregularities in the surface contour, distortion of the endometrial echo, or as areas of hyper or hypoechogenicity compared with the surrounding normal myometrium. Since leiomyomas are composed of smooth muscle cells with acoustic characteristics similar to the surrounding normal uterine tissue they may not be imaged as a separate entity. Uterine leiomyomas do not have a true capsule and there may not be an acoustic interface and therefore no echo resulting from a structural boundary. A submucosal myoma within the uterine cavity may be imaged as an area of increased echogenicity and may be mistaken initially for blood, mucus or a polyp in the uterine cavity (Figure 2.8).

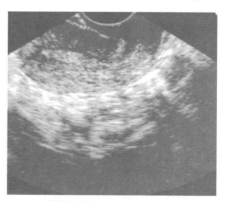

FIGURE 2.8: Normal uterus

Endometriosis

Endometriosis is a condition where there is ectopic menstruating endometrium leading to adhesions and/or cysts called as the chocolate cysts. Minor degrees of endometriosis cannot be diagnosed by sonography. The endometrioma cyst wall is generally shaggy and irregular, sometimes with septations. These cysts are homogenous with a low level echo pattern with good through transmission. They have fine stippling pattern filling the whole of the cyst.

Fibroids

Fibroids can cause infertility by blocking the cervical canal or by blocking the fallopian tubes mechanically. Fibroids press over the endometrial cavity and this diminishes the available endometrium for implantation and also interferes with the transport of sperms and oocytes. Intramural myomas also increase the uterine irritability and are implicated in causing implantation failures or early pregnancy losses (Figure 2.9).

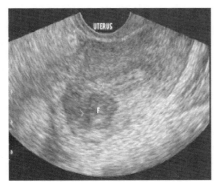

FIGURE 2.9: Fibroid uterus

Transvaginal ultrasound is the most useful tool for screening for fibroids. The uterus is enlarged, and may have contour deformity (Figure 2.10) and focal masses with different echogenocities (Hypoechoic usually, hyperechoic when calcified and may be isoechoic also).

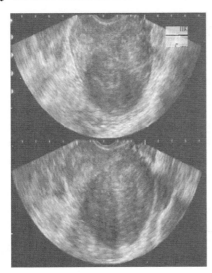

FIGURE 2.10: Fibroid causing contour problem

Congenital Anomalies

Congenital anomalies of the uterus occur in about 0.1-0.4 percent of general population of women and are due to the embryological problems in Mullerian system. Congenital anomalies of the uterus cause infertility and also is a significant cause of Recurrent pregnancy loss.[9, 10] About 80 percent of women with congenitally abnormal uterus may have no problems in conceiving but anomalies are responsible for almost 20 percent of recurrent pregnancy loss and hence should be carefully looked for and treated whenever encountered during infertility evaluation (Figures 2.11A and B).

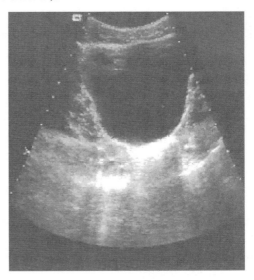

FIGURE 2.11A: Bicornuate uterus: TAS

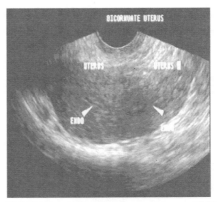

FIGURE 2.11B: Bicornuate uterus: TVS

Uterine congenital anomalies can be diagnosed by HSG, TVS, contrast sonohysterography, hysteroscopy and laparoscopy and by a MRI 3D HSG and TVS without saline contrast are the commonest methods. The anomalies which can be diagnosed are bicornuate uterus, unicornuate uterus, intrauterine septa (complete, incomplete or arcuate) (Figure 2.12).[11]

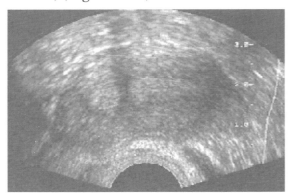

FIGURE 2.12: Septate uterus

Sonohysterography

Instillation of sterile saline into the uterine cavity under ultrasound guidance (TVS) will let us study the uterine cavity without any radiation exposure and without exposure to contrast media (Figure 2.13). The saline distended cavity is anechoic surrounded by symmetric endometrial lining. Sonohysterography will enable the diagnosis of Asherman's syndrome or intrauterine adhesions, polyps, submucous fibroids and uterine septa (Figures 2.14 and 2.15).[12] HYCOSY or contrast hysterosalpingo sonography involves the use of a sonography contrast media (Echovist) (Figures 2.16A and B). In the future in the better understanding this may replace the more invasive HSG as a first time investigation of the infertile female.

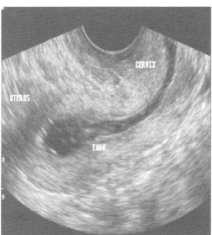

FIGURE 2.13: Saline contrast sonography

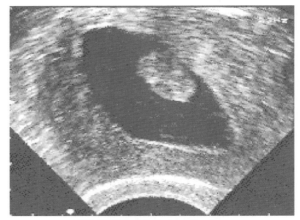

FIGURE 2.14: Polyp fibroid

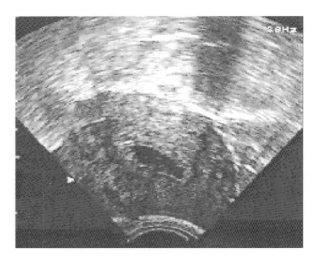

FIGURE 2.15: Asherman syndrome

Adenomyosis

Endometriosis is a disease in which typically the endometriotic implants are scattered in various extrauterine locations. However, sometimes the ectopic endometrium goes into the myometrium and causes adenomyosis. This endometrial tissue starts to proliferate inside the myometrium and tends to bleed on progesterone withdrawal during the menstrual cycle thus giving the uterus a typically speckled appearance resembling 'Salt' and 'Pepper' (Hyperechoic areas and hypoechoic areas). Depending on the extent of lesion and the severity of disease the uterus will appear enlarged and sometimes all of the adenomyosis areas may together look like a fibroid (Adenomyoma) (Figure 2.17).

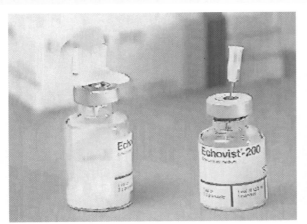

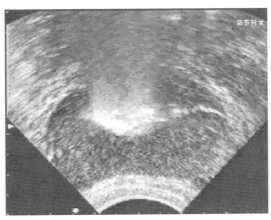

FIGURES 2.16A and B: Echovist

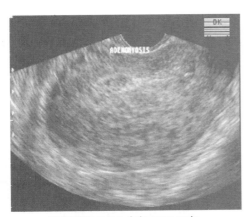

FIGURE 2.17: Adenomyosis

Color Doppler imaging (Figure 2.18) helps as the blood flow in these lesions resemble spiral arterial endometrial blood flow pattern while that of the fibroid is single vessel on the periphery. Also the identification of capsule around the mass is seen in leiomyomas while adenomyomas have no capsules.

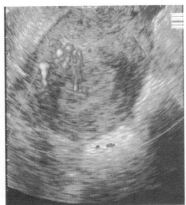

FIGURE 2.18: Color Doppler in adenomyosis

Evaluation of Endometrial Growth

Endometrium is the inner lining of the uterus and has receptors for ovarian hormones and in response to the Estradiol from the ovaries (or exogenous), the endometrial lining grows in a typical pattern which is recognisable by TVS. After ovulation (36-48 hr. later) the corpus luteum starts producing progesterone and the endometrial cells and endometrium will now start exhibiting secretory changes which is also well identified by TVS and color Doppler. Endometrial growth correlates well with ovarian hormone levels. For ultrasound evaluation of the endometrium, we need to look at endometrial thickness, endometrial pattern and color flow in spiral arteries and endometrial receptivity scoring.

Endometrial thickness is the maximum distance between the echogenic interfaces of the myometrium and the endometrium, measured in a plane through the central longitudinal axis of the uterus. Very easy to obtain the plane and very easy and reproducible to measure (Figure 2.19).

The basal study of endometrial thickness should be started from day 2 or day 3 of menstrual cycle to look for proper shedding. The endometrium on this day should appear as a thin bright echogenic line or the cavity shows some blood with debris. A thick endometrium on basal scan (Day 2) indicates improper endometrium shedding (Figure 2.20).

The endometrium grows at the rate of 0.5 mm/day in the proliferative phase and 0.1 mm/day in the luteal phase. A thickness of more than 7 mm

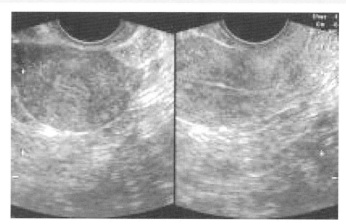

FIGURE 2.19: Endometrial measure

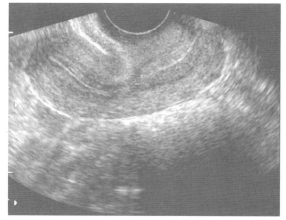

FIGURE 2.21: Day 9 endometrium

in the preovulatory period is associated with higher pregnancy rates.[13]

Endometrial pattern is the relative echogenecity of the endometrium and the myometrium as seen on a longitudinal TV scan. In a typical 3 layer pattern of proliferative phase (Figure 2.21), the central line represents the uterine cavity and the outer lines represent the basal layer. Outside this is a hypoechoic interface in between endometrium and myometrium (sometimes described as 5 line endometrium) (Figure 2.22). The hypoechoic area in between the two bright lines represents functional layer of the endometrium.[14] Endometrium growth and pattern can be graded and classified.

Four patterns have been described from a fully echogenic endometrium (Grade A) to a distinct black region surrounding the midline.[15]

Smith's Grading

Grade A : Bright endometrium represents post ovulation or the luteal phase

Grade B : Endometrial reflectivity is similar to the myometrium. This characterizes late follicular phase.

Grade C : A solid area of reduced reflectivity appears as a darker area next to the lighter myometrium. This is the pattern of mid follicular phase.

Grade D : Echoes are absent in the endometrium, but a bright central echo is seen, described as the triple line.

Late follicular phase endometrial pattern Grade B on the day of hCG is more associated with pregnancy (Smith *et al*).[15]

Post ovulatory the endometrial echogenicity changes with loss of layers but spiral flow increases (Figure 2.25).

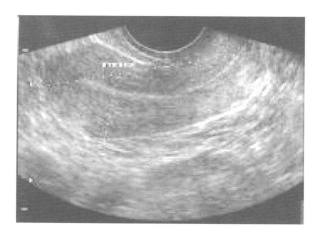

FIGURE 2.20: Day 2/3 endometrium

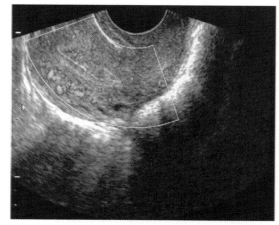

FIGURE 2.22: Periovulatory endometrium

Endometrial Thickness and Menstrual Cycle

Phase	Appearance
Menses (day 1-5)	Hypoechoic area is blood. Myometrial contractions are frequent. Thickness < 4 mm
Early follicular phase (day 6-10)	Distinct 'triple-line' pattern. Hypoechogenic endometrium. Thickness 7-9 mm.
Late follicular phase (day 11 ovulation)	Endometrial appearance similar to myometrium. Thickness 9-12 mm at ovulation
Luteal phase	Bright, fluffy appearance. Absence of triple line. Thickness 10-14 mm

Nowadays the endometrium pattern is simply described as multilayered or non-multilayered. Serafini[16] has shown that a multilayered pattern to be more predictive of implantation than any other parameter measured.

Color flow Doppler of endometrium and uterine arteries[17] have been extensively studied by Steer et al and they have found that no pregnancy occurred if the PI of uterine artery was > 3 and there was no spiral artery blood flow in the endometrial zones.

Color Doppler Addition of color Doppler studies in evaluations of endometrial blood flow patterns and uterine artery flow pattern enabled us to evaluate the physiology of the endometrium. Various scoring systems have been proposed for prediction of implantation by color Doppler. The most popular is Appelbaum's USSR.[18] Estrogen produces a vasodilatory effect on the uterine arteries. It has been seen that RI, PI of uterine artery drops with increasing estradiol levels. (Figure 2.23).

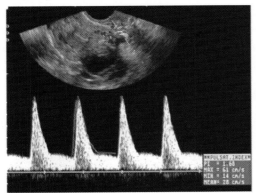

FIGURE 2.23: Uterine A

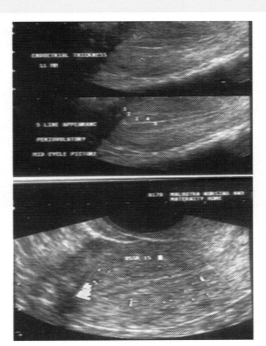

FIGURE 2.24: Uterine zones

Depending on the vascularization of the endometrial layers the late proliferative triple line endometrium is divided into four zones (Figure 2.24).[19]

Zones

1. 2 mm thick area surrounding zone 2.
2. Hyperechoic outer layer.
3. Hypoechoic inner layer.
4. Endometrial cavity

Applebaum's Uterine Scoring System for Reproduction (USSR)

Ultrasound and the UBP [18]

Ultrasound offers a simple, reliable, reproducible, quick and non-invasive method of assessing the female pelvic region, especially follicular and endometrial growth.

The qualities of the uterus–i.e. the UBP–can be determined using transvaginal color Doppler sonography (TV-CDS). According to Applebaum, certain sonographic qualities of the uterus are noted during the normal mid-cycle. These include:

• Endometrial thickness ≥ 7 mm in greatest anterior-posterior (A-P) dimension (full thickness measured from the myometrial endo-

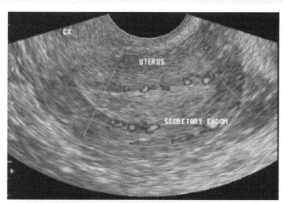

FIGURE 2.25

metrial junction to the endometrial myometrial junction).

- Triple layered ('5-line') endometrial appearance.
- Myometrial contractions causing a 'wave like' motion of the endometrium.
- Homogenous myometrial echogenicity.
- Uterine artery blood flow < 3.0, as measured by pulsatility index (PI) on Doppler.
- Blood flow within zone 3 (hypoechoic inner layer; see Table 2.1) of the endometrium on color Doppler.
- Myometrial blood flow internal to the arcuate vessels (seen on gray scale examination).

Care to be taken while eliciting recording uterine biophysical profile by ultrasound.

Ultrasound and the UBP[18]

Special care is needed in determining the UBP with ultrasound and color Doppler imaging; the following guidelines are recommended:

1. If necessary, use both transabdominal ultrasound and TVS to determine the presence of a '5-line' endometrial appearance. Depending on uterine position, a 5-line appearance may be seen on one and not the other (and vice versa).
2. Do not 'rush' the color Doppler study. Endometrial blood flow is of low velocity; if the sweep through the endometrium is too rapid, flow may not be seen. Additionally, endometrial blood flow is somewhat 'mercurial'–it may seem to 'come and go', and appear in some areas and not in others.
3. Try to make the endometrium as specular (reflective) as possible, using the techniques

TABLE 2.1: Appelbaum's uterine scoring system for reproduction (USSR)

Parameter	Determination	Score
Endometrial thickness (mm)	< 7	0
	7-9	2
	10-14	3
	> 14	1
Endometrial layering	No layering	0
	Hazy 5-line appearance	1
	Distinct 5-line appearance	3
Endometrial motion [no. of myometrial contractions in 2 minutes (real time)]	< 3	0
	≥ 3	3
Myometrial echogenicity	Course, inhomogenous	1
	Relatively homogenous	2
Uterine artery Doppler flow (PI)	2.99-3.0	0
	2.49	1
	< 2	2
Endometrial blood flow in zone 3	Absent	0
	Present, but sparse	2
	Present multifocally	5
Myometrial blood flow (Gray scale)	Absent	0
	Present	2

Values assume a technically adequate ultrasound examination with no abnormalities of uterine shape or development, no other gross uterine abnormalities (e.g. significant masses), and a normal ovarian cycle (e.g. without evidence of ovarian uterine dyscoordination).[1]

of manual manipulation of the anatomy and probe pressure to achieve this.

4. Scan endovaginally both coronally and sagittally–there may be a difference in how well the blood flow is imaged.
5. When measuring the endometrium in the A-P dimension, endeavor to do so in the absence of contractions, as these may affect the result. Also whenever possible, obtain the measurement in a standard plane such as when both the endometrial and cervical canals appear continuous.

Tubal Evaluation

Normal tubes are isoechoic and are not usually visualized by TVS unless there is fluid contrast. The use of fluid contrast for evaluation of tubes has been described in literature as **Sion Test** from Mumbai or as **Sion Procedure** of sonosalpingography.

Sonosalpingography

Endosonography as a tool for checking the patency of fallopian tubes was an expected development with great strides taken within the field of gynecology. Sonosalpingography also known as Sion Test, used transvaginal sonography to confirm the tubal patency by visualizing the spill of fluid from the fimbrial end of fallopian tubes. Fallopian tubes are isoechoic and cannot be normally seen on Ultrasound unless pathological or fluid surrounds the tubes. We propose to perform this test not as a substitute for Hysterosalpingography or laparoscopy but as an noninvasive, cheap outdoor screening procedure in patients of infertility.

No. 8 Fr. Foley's catheter is put inside the uterus. The bulb is inflated with 2 ml of distilled water. Prior to procedure the patient is asked to evacuate the bladder and base line vaginal scan is performed. 20-60 ml of solution containing ciplox, hylase and dexamethasone is taken in 50 ml catheter tip syringe and pushed via Foley's catheter and spill is studied from the fimbrial end (Figures 2.26 and 2.27).

The Foley's bulb is then deflated and some saline is pushed slowly to evaluate the uterine cavity as sonohysterography (Figure 2.28).

We have done the *Sion procedure* in the patients of suspected pelvic factors. In this we have flooded the pelvis using the same fluid about 200-300 ml, pushed via Foley catheter and visualized the fallopian tubes.

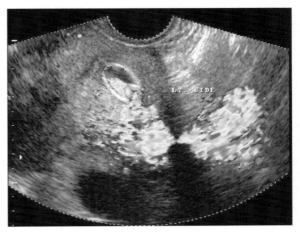

FIGURE 2.27

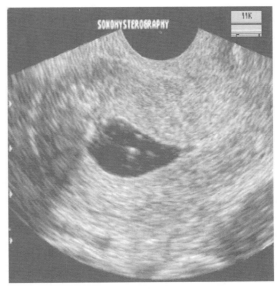

FIGURE 2.28

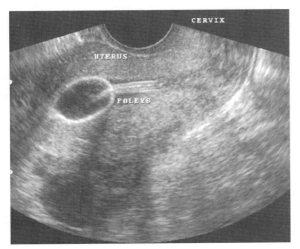

FIGURE 2.26

Sonosalpingography is a good noninvasive screening test for evaluating tubal patency. Sonosalpingography however does not replace the good old Hysterosalpingography in certain specific indications.

Laparoscopy has its additional advantage of having a therapeutic value also.

Sion procedure has an additional advantage of visualising pelvic adhesions and tubo-ovarian mobility.

Hy-Co-Sy The use of positive contrast media offers much more information rather than the use of sterile saline as negative contrast.[19]

TABLE 2.2: Comparison of 3 procedures			
Factors to be assessed	*HSG*	*Laparoscopy*	*Sonography*
Cervix			
Cong. Abnormalities	+	–	+
Cervicities	–	–	+
Uterus			
Cong. Abnormalities	+	Hysteroscopy	+
Myometrium	–	–	++
Endometrium	–	–	++
Tubes			
Morphology	+	+	+
Mobility	–	+	+
Patency	+	+	+ SSG
Ovaries			
Morphology	–	+	+
Follicles	–	+	++
Adhesions	–	++	+
Pouch of Douglas	–	+	+
Cost/Time	++	+++	+
Radiation/GA	+	+	–
Therapeutic value	–	++	+

Echovist (SHU 45-4; Sherring AG, Berlin) is an ultrasound contrast medium consisting of a suspension of monosaccharide microparticles (50% galactose, 2 µ in diameter) in a 20 percent aqueous solution of galatose. Whenever this immediately reconstituted media is injected in the uterus through a Foley's catheter (No. 8) or a plastic HSG cannula under TV scan, the tubal patency[20, 21] and uterine cavity can be accurately studied (Figure 2.29).

Transvaginal Hy-Co-Sy is a diagnostic technique for the investigations and DD of uterine cavity and tubal patency.

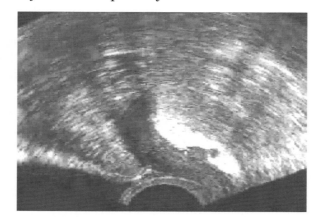

FIGURE 2.29: Hy-Co-Sy

Ovarian Evaluation by Ultrasound

Ovary probably is the most frequently scanned organ by ultrasound in an infertile woman determining of ovarian status and follicle monitoring are one of the first steps in the evaluation of an infertile woman. It should be kept in mind that a detailed history including menstrual history is very essential for correlating findings of TVS.

Ovarian Study

By ultrasound the ovary is fairly easily recognized usually lying in the ovarian fossa and recognized in front of the iliac vessels when the TV probe is panned to the vaginal fornices. Sometimes a bimanual examination improves the image by bringing the ovary nearer to the probe (Figure 2.30).

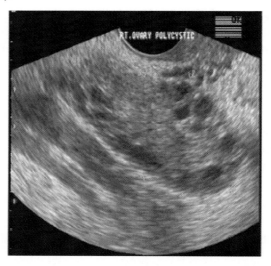

FIGURE 2.30: Normal ovary in front of iliac vessels

The ovary is imaged for its morphology (Normal, Polycystic or Multicystic) for its abnormalities (cysts, dermoids, endometriomas, tumors, etc.) for its follicular growth in ovulation monitoring and for evidence of ovulation and corpus luteum formation and function.

Follicular Development

There are often a few follicles (less than 10 mm in diameter) that can be imaged throughout the menstrual cycle and even during menstruation and these preantral follicles are too small to be imaged. Under the influence of follicle stimulation hormone (FSH) released by the anterior pituitary gland in response to pulsatile GnRH during the early part of the menstrual cycle, a few follicles will undergo progressive development. Granulosa cells in developing follicles will secrete increasing amounts of estrogen and follicular fluid, and the follicles will increase in size. As follicular stimulation progresses, one or occasionally two follicles will continue to develop into the dominant follicle(s). Many of the developing follicles will not pass the development stage of 10 to 14 mm diameter before they degenerate. Hackeloer et al[22] noted a linear increase in the size of the dominant follicle through a normal menstrual cycle. Developing follicles destined to ovulate, increase in size 1 to 2 µm/day and reach a maximum diameter of 16 to 33 mm before ovulation. Selection of the dominant follicle is thought to occur by cycle days 5 to 7 but is not apparent sonographically until cycle days 8 to 12. Other antral follicles of the developing cohort will generally undergo atresia and will not exceed 14 mm in diameter. However in 5 to 11 percent of natural cycles, two dominant follicles may develop, but they are generally in opposite ovaries. Potential ovulatory follicles will have a diameter of 10.5 mm or greater (Figures 2.31 and 2.32).

Prediction of Ovulation

A small echogenic mass that is thought to represent the cumulus oophorus may sometimes

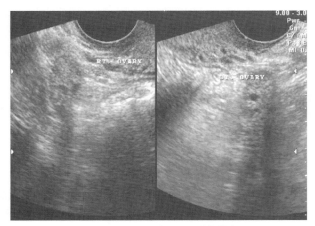

FIGURE 2.31: Preantral follicles

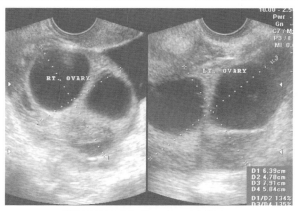

FIGURE 2.32: Dominant follicle

be noted projecting into the follicle. Visualization of the cumulus oophorus has been reported in 80 percent of follicles greater than 17 mm in diameter. Ovulation is reported to be within 36 hours of seeing the cumulus. However Zandt-Stastny[23] have challenged this view and have noted that the cumulus is only 100 to 150 µ size and would not be expected to be visualized by sonography. Zandt Stansky et al have suggested that structures imaged in follicles thought to represent the cumulus are artifacts. After the LH surge, the theca tissue becomes hypervascular and edematous and the granulosa cell layer begins to separate from the theca layer. This is appreciated sonographically as a line of decreased reflectivity around the follicle. Picker et al[24] in 1987 suggested that this sonographic sign means impending ovulation within 24 hours. Jaffe and Ben-Aderet[25] in 1984 described the same sign, which they called a ôdouble contourö and suggested that this is occurs a few hours before ovulation. Within 6 to 10 hours before ovulation separation and folding of the granulosa cell layer produces a crenation or irregularity of the lining of the follicle. This has also been suggested as sign of impending ovulation. Unfortunately, despite the fact that there are a number of sonographic signs that have been described to precede ovulation, there is currently no sonography sign that predicts exactly when ovulation will occur, the signs only give evidence that the time of ovulation is nearing. The mean peak diameter before ovulation reported by Kerin et al[26] was 23.6 + 0.4 mm. However there is considerable differences in the same.

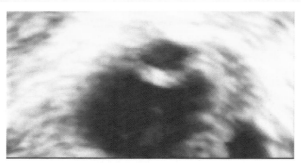

FIGURE 2.33: Dominant follicle showing cumulus

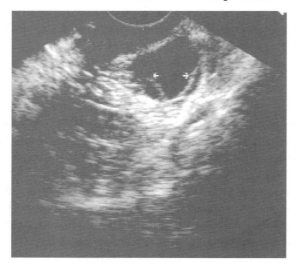

FIGURE 2.34: Double contour

Hence the potential signs of Impending Ovulation are:
- Presence of a dominant follicle (usually more than 16 to 18 mm)
- Anechoic area, double contour, around the follicle (possible ovulation within 24 hours)
- Separation and folding of the follicle lining (ovulation within 6 to 10 hours)
- Thickened proliferative endometrium (described later).

Confirming Ovulation

Sonography does appear to be very reliable in confirming ovulation once ovulation has occurred. Disappearance of the follicle is noted in 91 percent of cases after ovulation and a decrease in follicle size occurs in another 9 percent. Other signs suggesting that ovulation has occurred are the appearance of cul-de-sac fluid, particularly when it was not present in a previous scan, or the development of intrafollicular echoes suggesting the formation of a hemorrhagic corpus luteum.

Ovary in Anovulatory Cycles

In an anovulatory cycle, ultrasound imaging of the ovaries will reveal either a lack of any follicular development, particularly in the hypogonadotropic hypogonadal patient with type I or a few non-ovulatory (less than 11 mm) follicles. A dominant follicle larger than 16 mm in diameter will not develop. A cyst may also be associated with anovulation. Anovulation with PCOD will often have enlarged ovaries greater than 8 cm^3 in volume with multiple small subcapsular follicles less than 10 mm in diameter. However, normal sized ovaries do not rule out PCOD. Anovulation can be diagnosed when serial scans do not show development of a follicle. A mature corpus luteum is noted sonographically in about 50 percent of patients after ovulation. If pregnancy does not occur the corpus luteum generally degenerates and disappears just before menstruation. Corpus luteum cysts may be 4 to 6 cm in diameter and occasionally even large but are more commonly 2.5 to 3 cm in diameter. They may persist for 4 to 12 weeks and may be responsible for suppressing normal follicular development until they resolve (Figure 2.35).

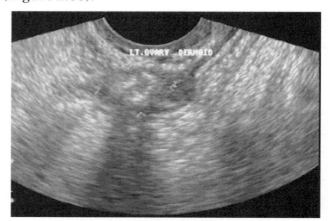

FIGURE 2.35: Ovary lacking any follicles

In PCOD the ovaries are increased in size. The mean volume of the ovary is 12.5 cm^3 with a range from 6 to 30 cm. The classical anatomic criteria are not present in all patients with clinical or endocrine findings suggestive of PCOD. Therefore,

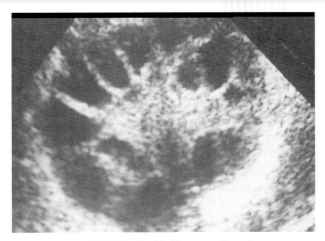

FIGURE 2.36: Multiple small cysts

an ultrasound showing ovarian enlargement can help make the diagnosis, but a normal ultrasound examination with normal size ovaries does not rule out PCOD if the clinical or biochemical abnormalities characteristic of the syndrome are present. Ultrasound may also suggest the diagnosis of PCOD in a patient with normal sized ovaries and the clinical and or endocrine criteria of PCOD by confirming anovulation:

• Enlarged ovary (more than 8 cm)
• Multiple small cysts (0.2-0.6) (Figure 2.36)
• Anovulation (lack of follicular development) (Figure 2.35)
• Resting of follicular endometrium (Figure 2.20).

Endometrium

The endometrial cavity should be visualizable as a separate entity within the uterus in virtually all menstruating patients. The endometrial cavity is generally centrally located in the uterus. The cyclic histologic changes and changes in thickening of the endometrium with hormonal stimulation are well known. This cyclic changes of the endometrium can be imaged using transvaginal ultrasound during the different phases of the menstrual cycle. The hormonal and ovulatory status of the patients can be assessed by evaluating the endometrial patterns.

Sakamoto[6] described the characteristic sonographic imaged noted through the menstrual cycle in 1985. The proliferative endometrium is characterized by (a) the presence of a well-defined three line sign, (b) a hypoechogenic functional layer, and (c) a minimal or absent posterior acoustic enhancement. The three line sign is formed by the central hyperechoic reflection representing the endometrial cavity and the additional hyperechoic reflection representing the thin developing layer of endometrium. There is also a surrounding hypoechoic halo. During the luteal phase, the endometrium is hyperechoic, with posterior enhancement and absence of the three line sign and halo.

Early Proliferative Phase

The anechoic central echo noted during early menses is replaced by a hyperechoic central line and the endometrium begins to thicken, forming the three line sign. The general hypoechogenic character of the functional layer of the proliferative endometrium is thought to be related to the simple configuration of the glands and blood vessels. The outer lines represent the endometrium and the interface between the endometrium and myometrium. These otuer lines may thicken as the estrogen stimulation increases and the follicular phase progresses and blends into a thickened hyperechoic endometrium during the secretory phase. In the follicular phase, the halo which is about 2 mm thick and surrounds the endometrium, is present. There is no posterior enhancement. A follicular phase endometrium greater than 6 mm thick has been associated with a serum estradiol level over 200 pg/ml and a developing follicular greater in diameter.

Late Proliferative Phase

There is continued thickening of the endometrial echo complex in the late proliferative phase. The halo is still present. The endometrial complex is still imaged as three parallel lines, but the outer lines may begin to thicken. The total endometrial thickness increases and may reach 10 mm or greater in total thickness. There is no posterior enhancement. Cervical mucus may occasionally be imaged as hypoechoic density in the endocervix near the time of ovulation.

Luteal Phase

In the luteal phase the endometrium is thickened and is imaged as a homogenous hyperechoic density with posterior enhancement and loss of the surrounding halo. The three line sign is gone. The rate of increase of thickness slows and the endometrial echo complex soon achieves its greater anterior posterior dimension. The echogenicity of the endometrium becomes hyperechoic after coiling and lengthening of the endometrial glands and the production of mucus and increased tortuousity of the glands and blood vessels. Interestingly, acoustic enhancement is usually associated with cystic or fluid-filled structure that are hypoechoic, yet is characteristically seen posterior to the luteinized endometrium. Acoustic enhancement occurring posterior to a hyperechoic structure is unusual and is thought to be related to the increased vascularity of the endometrium. Posterior enhancement is assessed in the anterior posterior pelvic (AP-Pelvic) image plane, since some posterior enhancement may be noted in a transpelvic (T-Pelvic) plane even during mid to late follicular phases. Although it is not known why enhancement is noted in the T-Pelvic plane, one explanation is that small anechoic areas may be noted in the endometrium. These probably represent areas of hemorrhage into the endometrium with endometrial degeneration and herald onset of vaginal bleeding.

Minimally Stimulated or Single Line Endometrium

Patients with low estrogen or excess androgen have generally a single line endometrium similar to a late menstrual endometrium. Care must be taken when interpreting or reporting such measurements as to whether full thickness of both layers of endometrium or only one layer is being used. Since it is generally simpler just to measure the full endometrial thickness this is usually the measurement reported. The average thickness of the proliferative endometrium to be 8.4 mm + 2.2 mm whole the secretory endometrium is 9.6 mm + 3.4 mm.

Endometrial Motion

The endometrium can be seen to move during real time ultrasonographic imaging. This movement can be quite impressive when first seen.

ROLE OF TRANSVAGINAL COLOR DOPPLER IN INFERTILITY

The advent of transvaginal color Doppler Sonography has added a new dimension to the diagnosis and treatment of infertile female. Color Doppler innovation is a unique non-invasive technology to investigate the circulation with organs like uterus and ovaries. Dynamic changes occur almost everyday of the menstrual cycle in a reproductively active female. These events are picked up very well by transvaginal color Doppler and definite conclusions can be drawn regarding the diagnosis, prognosis and treatment of infertile patients. As the vaginal probe lies close to the organs of interest various vessels supplying these structures can be studied in detail like the uterine artery, ovarian artery and their branches.

Study of Menstrual Cycle by Color Doppler

It is very important to study the whole of the menstrual cycle by transvaginal color Doppler during the evaluation of infertility. It provides vital information about follicular dynamics like blood flow to the growing follicle, the vascular supply of the endometrium and corpus luteum vascularization which are very important for a successful outcome in terms of pregnancy.

Changes in the Ovary

The ovaries are situated on either side of the uterus and measure about 2.2 to 5.5 cms in length, 1.5 to 2.0 cms in width and 1.5 to 3.0 cms in depth and are recognized by the presence of follicle of different sizes. The blood is supplied by ovarian artery via the infundibulopelvic ligament and ovarian branch of the uterine artery. There is anasthamosis between the two sources of blood supply. The primary and secondary branches of the ovarian artery grow along with the development of the follicle. Dominant follicle within the ovary can be recognized by transvaginal color

Doppler by day 8th or 10th of the cycle by a ring of angiogenesis around it, when compared to the subordinate follicles which do not demonstrate this. These vessels become more abundant and prominent as the follicle grows to about 20-24 mm in size.

The Phases are as Follows

Early follicular (Day 5-7), late follicular (Day 11-13), Early luteal (Day 15-17) and late luteal (Day 26-28). In general the index values are high in the early part of menstrual cycle and fall as ovulation approaches. According to Kurjak *et al* the RI in the early proliferative phase is 0.54 +/− 0.04 and declines the day before ovulation when it is about 0.44 +/− 0.04.[9]

This is the best time for administration of surrogate HCG. A marked increase in peak systolic velocity with a relatively constant RI of 0.44 +/− 0.04 in the proliferative phase and starts decreasing as ovulation approaches. It starts to fall a day before ovulation and the lowest value of 0.84 +/− 0.04 is seen on the day 18 of the menstrual cycle that is around the time of the implantation window (Figure 2.37).

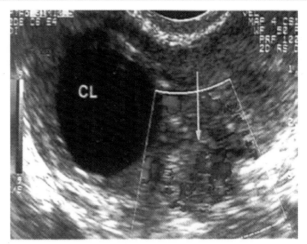

FIGURE 2.38: RI in luteal phase

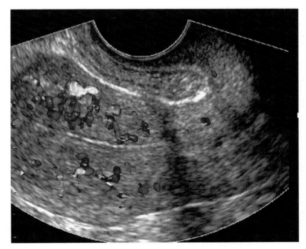

FIGURE 2.39: Vascularity of endometrium

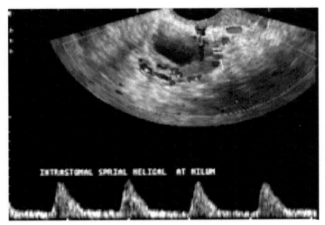

FIGURE 2.37: R. I. of ovarian artery

Luteal Phase Changes in Ovarian Vascularity

The functional capacity of the corpus luteum is assessed by the low impedance flow and the abundance of vessels around it. Mature corpus luteum is a highly vascularized structure with a low RI of 0.44 +/− 0.04. In patients with corpus luteum deficiency the vascularity is not optimal and the RI is raised to around 0.59, with decreased diastolic flow. If pregnancy occurs then low RI of 0.50 continues (Figure 2.38).

Secretory Changes in the Endometrium

Michael Applebaum in his study with transvaginal color Doppler divided the endometrium and periendometrial areas into 4 zones. In the study conducted by him no pregnancy was reported in IVF patients unless vascularity was demonstrated in Zone III or within Zone III or IV prior to transfer (Figure 2.39).

Doppler Assessment of Uterine and Ovarian Flow in Infertility and IVF

Goswamy *et al* found absent diastolic flow in infertility patients and with severe problems and even reversal of diastolic flow.

Role of Transvaginal Color Doppler in other Conditions Associated with Infertility

Luteinized Unruptured Follicle

This condition is recognized by serial ultrasonography to monitor the growth of follicle, with failure to see expected changes at the time of ovulation.

The typical blood flow pattern seen in the corpus luteum is absent.

Luteal Phase Defect

This is due to decreased vascularization of corpus luteum. The three to seven fold increase in blood supply is necessary to deliver, the steroid precursors to ovary and removal of progesterone as shown in experimental animals.

An increasing corpus luteum resistance index indicates less chances of embryo survival specially within first 8 weeks of pregnancy.

Fibroid

To define the borders of fibroid color Doppler is of real help as the vascular supply at the periphery of the leiomyoma can be dilineated very well. Good vascularity denotes a favorable response to GnRH if used before laparoscopic surgery (Figure 2.40).

Endometriosis

On gray scale scan endometrioma is seen as a homogenously echogenic intraovarian mass. Color Doppler may demonstrate the flow around and not within the endometriotic cyst (Figure 2.41).

Tubal Causes

During active phase of PID low impedance blood flow signals are usually detected and after effective antibiotic therapy flow tends to return to normal. In the absence of this change surgery is indicated.

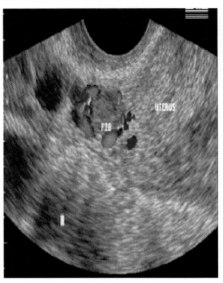

FIGURE 2.40: Vascularity in a fibroid

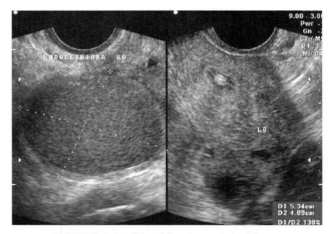

FIGURE 2.41: Blood flow to endometrioma

Polycystic Ovarian Disease (PCOD)

Contrary to the normal ovarian blood flow, which is seen around the growing follicle, PCOD subjects show abundantly vascularized stroma. Waveforms obtained from the ovarian tissue showed a mean resistance index of 0.54 without cyclical change between repeated examinations (Figure 2.42).

Uterine Factor

The possibility of decreased uterine blood flow may be associated with infertility as already discussed in proceeding paragraphs Goswamy *et al* depicted in their study that uterine artery

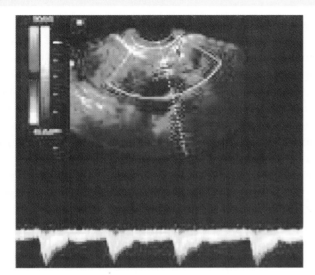

FIGURE 2.42: Blood flow in PCO

indices which were high in failed IVF cases improved after the patients were put on oral estrogen therapy and pregnancy rate improved when compared to those who did not get this treatment.

Color Doppler and its Contribution Towards In Vitro Fertilization

During stimulation protocols color Doppler ultrasound has its greatest contribution in monitoring follicular development and guiding oocyte harvesting procedures. The use of color Doppler ultrasound can occasionally be of help as it avoids accidental puncture of iliac vessels and also vessels on the surface of ovary.

Avoidance of Ovarian Hyper-stimulation Syndrome (OHSS)

In a stimulated cycle resistance of the intra-ovarian vessels measured by transvaginal color Doppler correlates well with number of follicles, that is those with more than 15 mm size. This correlation exists even during the early follicular phase, when follicular recruitment and development have just started. This suggest that vascularization of the follicles may play a role in their maturation from early follicular phase onwards. This study in the early follicular phase can prevent OHSS.

Optimal Conditions for Embryo Transfer

As shown in a recent work by Campbell it is possible to calculate the probability of pregnancy by using PI values of uterine artery on the day Embryo Transfer. Highest probability of pregnancy was predicted for patients who had medium values for PI. Those with high PI had failure rate upto 35 percent. In other words the lower the PI value more the chance of pregnancy. Steer *et al* have shown that if PI is > 3 before ET no pregnancy results.

ULTRASOUND GUIDED ASSISTED REPRODUCTION TECHNIQUES

Historical Review

The ultrasound guided oocyte aspiration was initially performed transabdominally through the full bladder, or directly, through the anterior abdominal wall. Subsequently, transvesical and perurethral approaches were developed. However, the first description of oocyte collection with transvaginal transducer was described by Wikland in 1985.

VAGINOSONOGRAPHIC FOLLICULAR ASPIRATIONS

Introduction

The impact of transvaginal ultrasound has been tremendous since its inception, as it has enabled the operator to visualize pelvic organ as a "close-up" shot. Also, the high resolutions it offers and the consequent high definition image, allows for better and perfect diagnosis of the pathology, than with the transabdominal ultrasound. Having said this, it is also important to note, at the stage, that the operator has to be well-versed with the orientation and the planes of transvaginal ultrasound to achieve the above.

The ability to diagnose conditions earlier and better than with transabdominal approach has put Vaginosonography in an enviable position for interventional procedures to be carried out on the pelvic organs. Thus, the transvaginal transducer coupled with the biopsy guide, has become of late a crucial weapon in the armamentarium of the interventional ultrasonologist. Transabdominal ultrasound intervention is mainly a free-hand technique, whereas with transvaginal ultrasound, it becomes a guided procedure where in the operator can be confident that the needle will follow the path charted out by the software generated biopsy line on the monitor. Also, unlike the former, transvaginal ultrasound-guided procedures, have the advantage of easy accessibility to the pelvic organs in the needle path.

The dramatic entry of interventional transvaginal sonography was made primarily for the purpose of oocyte retrieval in the assisted reproduction programmes, which was hither to done via laparoscopy. Hence, transvaginal sonography, besides diagnosis, also started playing an important role, in the therapeutic field.

VAGINOSONOGRAPHIC PUNCTURE PROCEDURES

Assisted Reproduction Techniques

- In-vitro fertilization and Embryo transfer (IVF and ET)
- Gamete intrafallopian transfer (GIFT) and SIFT
- Intrafollicular insemination (IFI)
- Direct intraperitoneal insemination (DIPI)
- Peritoneal oocyte sperm transfer (POST).

Patient Preparation

Short general anesthesia with Ketamine or Pentothal is the preferred mode for transvaginal sonography-guided aspiration. Sometimes, when there are few follicles, we administer intravenous analgesia, as the punctures are few and procedure is short.

Procedure

Patient is placed in the lithotomy position. Vagina is cleaned with Betadine solution and this is then rinsed thoroughly with normal saline so that no trace of Betadine remains. Intravenous antibiotic is given intraoperatively.

Transvaginal transducer is cleaned with absolute alcohol solution and then with normal saline. It is then covered with a disposable, sterile plastic sheath, same as that used for the Endo-

scopic video camera. Biopsy guided, which is washed with normal saline, is attached to the transducer. The assembly is introduced within the vagina. The software-generated biopsy guideline on the monitor is lined up with the follicle to be punctured. Gauge 16/17 Biopsy guide is used for these procedures. The Cook's IVF Ovum aspiration needle (Gauge 17) with the tubing and the bung is used for puncture. The bung is introduced into the Falcon test tube, the other end of tubing is connected to suctions apparatus with foot-controlled device. Suction is adjusted at 100 mmHg.

Under ultrasound guidance, the needle is introduced into the follicle and fluid is aspirated by applying the suction. A single channel needle is used, curetting of the follicle is done at the end of the aspiration and when the follicle has completely collapsed, the needle guide is realigned to the next follicle and procedure repeated. All the follicles of one ovary are aspirated with a single puncture. If need be, the needle is flushed with culture medium, on completion of one ovary or when there is a bloody tap. After, all follicles are aspirated, including the intermediate ones, the transducer is removed and the guide detached. The vagina is swabbed with normal saline and bleeding from the puncture site looked for. Then, the vaginal transducer is reintroduced and the pelvic area is scanned for active hemorrhage (Figure 2.43).

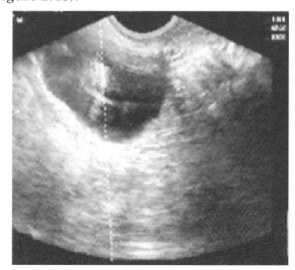

FIGURE 2.43: Ovum pick up

Complications

1. *Vaginal puncture hemorrhage* This may result after the needle is removed. Usually vaginal packing and direct pressure upon the puncture site stems the flow and nothing else seems to be necessary.
2. *Hemorrhage within the pelvis and / or ovarian follicles* This may be detected by post-procedural ultrasound. However, we have not encountered any catastrophic bleeding into the ovary or from its surface. Careful monitoring is essential.
3. *Vascular injuries* Internal iliac vessel puncture is a major complication and laparotomy may have to be done to arrest the hemorrhage.
4. *Pelvic infections* occur even after the administration of antibiotics.

Embryo Transfer

Usually, transcervical embryo transfer is undertaken as a blind procedure. Very rarely, when the cervix is stenosed or tortuous, the embryos are transferred through the myometrium (Surgical Embryo Transfer-Set).

The patient positioning and initial workup is same as was described for oocyte aspiration. The guideline is aligned with the endometrial cavity just below the fundus. A 25 cm 19 gauge needle primed with culture medium is passed through the biopsy guide and then into the uterus. The needle traverses through the myometrium and then it positioned into the cavity. Injected culture medium is seen transiently separating the anterior and posterior surface of the endometrial cavity. A long embryo transfer catheter loaded with the embryos at its tip, is then passed down the needle into the endometrial cavity. The embryos are injected and the catheter and needle withdrawn. In animals, this procedure has been shown to lead to pregnancy in 70 percent cases, but the success in humans is very low.

Direct Intraperitoneal Insemination (DIPI) and Peritoneal Oocyte Sperm Transfer

Direct Intraperitoneal insemination, introduced in 1986, has been used to treat couples with unexplained infertility, cervical mucus hostility, oligospermia, failed donor insemination and women who have ovulated prior to egg collection. The patient is superovulated with CC/HMG or LHRH analogue and HMG. Care is taken develop, however, the cycle is aborted, or the patient is given alternative of oocyte aspiration followed by embryo transfer or GIFT or POST. DIPI is performed 36 hours after administration of hCG. Patient is placed in lithotomy position, vagina is cleaned with Betadine/Normal saline and vaginal probe with biopsy guide is inserted. A pool of free fluid is identified and a gauge 18 needle is passed along the guide and into this pool with a single rapid thrust. The patient is usually sedated intravenously. Aspiration of fluid confirms that needle is in position and then, the washed semen sample is injected. We have had success rate of 15 percent in 25 selected cases for DIPI. But, this procedure does not have a role in the routine treatment of infertility.

Mason and colleagues placed both sperms and oocytes in the pouch of Douglas reasoning that most patients with unexplained infertility will have gamete abnormalities rather than a problem with ovum pick-up by the tubes.

In this technique, peritoneal oocyte and sperm transfer (POST), the patients are superovulated as in IVF cycles. Follicles are aspirated by the transvaginal route and when all follicles have been aspirated, the needle is introduced under Vaginal ultrasound guidance, into the pouch of Douglas which is repeatedly rinsed with the culture medium until the aspirated fluid is clear. A long embryo transfer catheter, loaded with three eggs and 4 million prepared sperms, is passed along the needle and its contents injected into the pouch on Douglas. We have done 10 cases of POST in various set-ups and have had a cumulative pregnancy rate of 30 percent per procedure. This technique is simpler to perform than IVF or GIFT, it has two distinct advantages over DIPI in that the egg release from the follicle is guaranteed and the spare eggs may be inseminated to confirm the fertilising ability, and then transferred.

Direct Intrafollicular Insemination

This procedure was carried out in a Colombian study wherein the follicles were not aspirated, but the prepared sperm sample was injected directly into the unruptured follicle 34-36 hours after administration of hCG. The study includes a limited population and has shown to have no major complication or sequelae. The pregnancy rate was 20 percent in this study. However, the possibility of an ectopic gestation (Ovarian/tubal) is there and we must consider this procedure only as a seldom alternative to IUI or GIFT when the patient does not desire intervention.

Ovarian Hyperstimulation

Ovarian hyperstimulation is more commonly seen in recent times due to the universal prevalence of assisted reproduction treatment. Controlled ovarian stimulation with GnRH and HMG/FSH is desired for IVF/GIFT/IUI cycle. However, sometimes, even with careful and close monitoring these may go haywire and result in the hyperstimulated ovaries. It can be classified into mild, moderate and severe degree, depending upon the associated clinical and sonographic findings. The presence of free fluid/ascites is a common feature with ovaries containing large cysts and measuring 7 cm. in diameter or above. Vaginal sonography is necessary to provide a constant monitoring for these cysts, as well as for free fluid estimation. Vaginosonography-guided aspiration of the free fluid from the pouch of Douglas with the patient in reverse Trendelenburg position is considered as a mode of treatment, and should be carried out in cases of mild to moderate degrees of hyperstimulation. The ovaries are very vascular and should not be touched but treated conservatively. If the cysts persist after 2 or 3 cycles then they may be aspirated under vaginal sonography guidance.

Prevention

When the ovaries are stimulated with ovulation induction hormones in an assisted reproduction cycle monitoring of the follicular growth with hormonal assays is done on a daily basis. If there are multiple intermediate follicles in either or both ovaries and/or if the serum E2 level when 3 or more follicles reach dominant size of 18 mm is and E_2 more than 3500 pg/ml then the hCG

administration is withdrawn. This would prevent the blow-up of these stimulated ovaries and thereby reduce the potential for ovarian hyperstimulation. Alternatively, these follicles could be aspirated without prior hCG administration and the oocytes collected.

Managing ART pregnancies and their complications transvaginal ultrasound is an important tool in the diagnosis of early viable pregnancies and their number and implantation site. Bleeding complication of ART pregnancies are best managed under ultrasound guidance.

Complications like ectopic pregnancy. Hetrotrophic pregnancy and high order multiple pregnancy also essentially need to be diagnosed and closely monitored by transvaginal ultrasound scan.

CONCLUSION

Ultrasound today has revolutionised the practice of infertility. To practise infertility and ART without a transvaginal scan is unthinkable in this modern era of technology. The addition of color Doppler has given us a good insight to the physiology of female insight to the physiology of female pelvis. Color Doppler today helps in prediction of success and complications. The addition of interventional procedures have simplified ART to an out patient procedure and prevented major operations in cases of ectopic pregnancy and ovarian cysts. 3-D has now given us a new dimension of volume estimation and sculpture like images.

REFERENCES

1. American Institute of Ultrasound in Medicine safety considerations for diagnostic ultrasound equipment. Bethesda: AIUM 1985.
2. Mc Ardle CK. Ultrasound in infertility. In: Seibel MM (Ed) Infertility: A Comprehensive Text. Norwalk, CT: Appleten and Lange 1990;285-302.
3. McClure RD, Hricak H. Scrotal ultrasound in the infertile man. J Urol 1986;135:711-15.
4. Krone KD, Carroll BA. Scrotal ultrasound. Radiology Clin North Am 1985;23:123-29.
5. Kim ED, Lipshultz LI. Role of ultrasound in the assessment of male infertility. J Clin Ultrasound 1996;24: 437-53.
6. Kupesic S, Ziegler D de. Ultrasound and Infertility. The Parthenon Publishing Group 2000;1-22.

7. Rajan R. Single day infertility evaluation.
8. Malhotra N, Malhotra J. Active management of infertility: Abstracts world congress of infertility 1999-2000.
9. Golan A, Langer R, Bukovsky I, Cospi E. Congenital anomalies of the mullerian system. Fertil Steril 1989;51:747-55.
10. Hager JH, Archer DF. Marchese SG, Muracca-Clemens M, Gasver KL. Etiology of recurrent pregnancy loses and outcome of subsequent pregnancies. Obstet Gynaecol 1983;62:574-81.
11. Winfield AC, Wentz AC. Diagnostic Imaging of Infertility. Baltimore: William and Wilkins 1937.
12. Gancherand P, Piacenza JM, Salle B, Rudiogoz RC. Sonohysterography of uterine cavity: preliminary investigations. J Clin Ultrasound 1995;23:339-48.
13. Rabinowitz R, Laufer N, Lewin A, Nawot D, Bar I, Margalioth EJ, Schenker JJ. The value of ultrasonographic endometrial measurement in the prediction of pregnancy Fertil Steril 1986;45:824-28.
14. Forrest TS, Elyaderani MK, Muilenburg ML, Bentra C, Kable WT, Sallivan P. Cyclic endometrial changes: ultrasound assessment with histologic correlation. Radiology 1988;167:233-37.
15. Smith B, Porter R, Ahuja K, Craft I. Ultrasonic assessment of endometrial changes. J In vitro Fertil Embryo Transfer 1984;1:233-38.
16. Serafini P, Batzofin J, Nelson J, Olive D. Sonographic uterine predictors of pregnancy in women undergoing ovulation induction for assisted reproductive treatments. Fertil Steril 1994;62:815-22.
17. Steer CV, Campbell S, Pampiglione JS, Kingsland CR, Mason BA, Collins WP. Transvaginal color flow imaging of the uterine arteries during the ovarian and menstrual cycles. Human Reproduction 1990;5:391-95.
18. Applebaum M. The Uterine Biophysical Profile (UBP). In Allahabadia G (Ed.): Endosonography in Obstetrics and Gynaecology. Mumbai Rotunda Medical Technologies Ltd., 1997;343-52.
19. Bonilla-Muscles F, Simon C, Sampais M, Pellicer A. An assessment of hysterosalpingosonography (HSSG) as a diagnostic tool for uterine cavity and tubal patency. J Clinic Ultrasound 1992;20:175-81.
20. Deichert U, Schlief R, Van de Sandt M, Juhnke L. Transvaginal hysterosalpingo contrast sonography (Hy-Clo-Sy) compared with conventional tubal diagnostics. Human Reproduction 1989;4:418-24.
21. Campbell S (Ed.). View points in medicine: Infertility investigations in Europe and the Future role of Hy-Co-Sy. Worthing Combridge Medical Publication.
22. Hackeloer BJ, Fleming R, Robinson HP et al. Correlation of ultrasonic and endocrinologic assessment of human follicular development. Am J Obstet Gynecol 1979;135: 122.
23. Zandt Stastny D, Thorsen MK, Middeton WD et al. Inability of sonography to detect imminent ovulation. AJR 1989;152:91.
24. Picker RH, Smith DH, Tucker MH, Saunders DM. Ultrasonic signs of imminent ovulation. J Clin Ultrasound 1983;11:1.
25. Jaffe R, Ben-Aderet N. Ultrasonic screening in predicting the time of ovulation. Gynecol Obstet Invest 1984;18:303.
26. Kerin JF, Kirby C, Morris D et al. Incidence of the luteinized ruptured follicle phenomenon in cycling women. Fertil Steril 1983;40:620.

• Pankaj Desai • Ashu Gupta

3

Infections and Infertility

Infection is a common cause of infertility. In the 1970s Westrom (1985) found that after three episodes of salpingitis, a woman had 75 percent incidence of tubal occlusion. Improved and newer approaches to infections helped the incidence drop to 54 percent by 1980, which is still a worrisome number. This problem is not confined to some parts of the world. In fact, Borisov in Bulgaria (1999) found that gynecological infections in women of reproductive age are connected with considerable economic losses both for diagnosis and treatment and for temporary disability. There are annually 12,000-15,000 pelvic infections in women of reproductive age in Bulgaria. Late sequelae includes infertility, ectopic pregnancy, and chronic disability. The management of all these complications exceeds considerably the expenses if proper diagnosis and treatment of the pelvic infections has been administrated. About 25 percent of the women who have had salpingitis are expected to be affected by infertility. The most frequent causes for pelvic infections are sexually transmitted pathogens and intrauterine manipulations—dilatation and curettage, lUDs.

Epidemiology

Infertility is presumably underestimated because diagnostic evaluation involves a specialist (Moore D *et al* 1990). A review of the literature reveals that 60 to 80 million couples experience infertility worldwide and by 2 million couples (15%) in the United States wherein infection is the major cause

(Fugate *et al* 1996). Sciarra (1993) summarized that regions with high infection rates with human immunodeficiency virus (HIV) also show a high incidence of post infection infertility. Extrapolation from annual reports suggests an occurrence of 3 million lower genital tract infections yearly in the United States. Continuing the extrapolations, Moore D *et al* (1990) postulated that 30 percent of these infections cause pelvic inflammatory disease (PID) and that at least 20 percent result in infertility. Laparoscopic evaluations showed on an average 11 percent frequency of tubal occlusions after a single episode of salpingitis, increasing to 54.3 percent after three episodes.

Common Features of Infections Producing Infertility

Portals of entry for these infections that are usually STDs include genitalia, urinary meatus, mouth, rectum, and skin (Cohen F 1993).

Infections in Male Infertility

In one study, a STD history in men did not influence sperm quality or pregnancy rates. However, some other works have contested this claim. Bulgarian workers in this field have shown that diagnosis of male genital tract inflammations plays a significant role in andrology. Although genital infections are often silent they can severely impair male infertility (Akush 2000).

This generates a valid controversy. Microorganisms can be isolated from most seminal fluid samples, but the significance of bacteriospermia is uncertain because many males lack symptoms associated with the bacterial infection of the reproductive tract. The data on the influence of urogenital tract infections on fertility are contradictory. In many cases opportunistic microorganisms cause such classical infections of the urogenital tract as epididymitis and prostatitis, as well as subclinical reproductive tract infections.

Some possible pathophysiological mechanisms of the development of infertility linked with infection of the ejaculate are considered: its direct effect on the fertile properties of the seminal fluid due to a decrease in the number of spermatozoa, the suppression of their motility, changes in their morphology and fertilizing capacity, its indirect influence due to the inhibition of spermatogenesis resulting from testicular damage, autoimmune processes induced by inflammation, secretory dysfunction of the male accessory sex glands as a consequence of the infection of the reproductive tract organs, leukocytospermia with its secondary influence of the ejaculate parameters, etc. Acute inflammation may cause transitory disturbances in sperm quality and secretion, yet the full impact of its timing and duration is unclear. Epididymitis secondary to urethritis produces azoospermia by obstruction. As epididymitis progresses, it may result in abscess formation, testicular infarction, and infertility due to extensive scarring similar to that found in PID. Gonococcal infection may produce seminiferous tubule breakage thereby leaking sperms into the interstitium; antibodies to sperm then form impairing sperm motility. The importance of the pathogenic properties of microorganisms for the localization of the inflammatory process in the urogenital tract of males and their role in the pathogenesis of male infertility are, therefore, requiring much greater and carefully designed studies (Zh2000).

Infections and Male Infertility

Inflammatory process in the genital tract of the male partner has an important role to play in infertility. Male accessory gland infections account for about 15 percent of male reproductive tract infections. (Szymanski W 2002). It is associated with increased count of WCs in the semen and elevated levels of pro-inflammatory cytokines in the semen and the testes. It is, therefore, important to consider clinical investigations that help improve evaluation and treatment of male infertility (Diemer T 2003).

Substantial proportion of women treated for *Chlamydia trachomatis* are reinfected by untreated male sex partner and so effective strategies to ensure partner's treatment is needed. Repeated infection can be treated by giving women, doses of erythromycin to deliver to male sex partners (Schillinder JA 2003).

Tuberculosis of male seminal duct can be an important cause of male infertility as a result of multiple epididymal scarring. In these cases testicular sperm extraction is a method of choice for sperm retrieval (Szymanski W 2002).

Thus, partner treatment is essential to avoid reinfection. Condoms protect against HIV, Chlamydia gonorrhea and syphilis. (Szymanski W 2002)

Strategies for preventing the spread of chlamydia and other infections should be to a greater extent directed towards men and should include better accessibility to SD clinics.

However, a STD history in women negatively influenced pregnancy rates. STDs can affect fertility or implantation as pathogens infect the cervix, endometrium, and fallopian tubes.

Furthermore, destruction of the fallopian tubes leads to tubal occlusion and infertility.

It is quite understandable that sexual contacts should be examined and treated appropriately (Gates 1993). Empiric STD treatment for infertility may be emotionally damaging by instilling false hope. It is imperative for health care providers to recognize predictors of PID because most cases are asymptomatic (Fugate KA *et al*, 1996).

At this stage specific infections that produce infertility are discussed in greater details.

PELVIC TUBERCULOSIS

Pelvic tuberculosis in the female is confined principally to the reproductive tracts, particularly the endometrium and fallopian tubes. This disease is still quite rampant in India and the developing countries. Genital tuberculosis would be more frequently diagnosed if strong association between genital tuberculosis and infection were considered in the evaluation of ever-infertile patient in areas where tuberculosis is endemic (Tripathy SN, 2002). Incidence of infertility in genital tuberculosis was 58 percent and the risk factors not conducive to pregnancy were secondary amenorrhea, no endometrium on curettage and negative chromopertubation. Conception rate is low—19.2 percent, live birth rate being still low. The outcome of infertility in genital tuberculosis is not optimistic. *In vitro* fertilization and embryo transfer offers some hope to these women (Tripathy SN, 2002).

Pathology of Pelvic Tuberculosis

Infectious agents in the mycobacteria class cause tuberculosis. The mycobacteria are obligate aerobes distinctive for their acid fast staining characteristic. Tuberculosis is usually caused by *Mycobacterium tuberculosis.*

With rare exceptions, tuberculosis of the female pelvis is secondary to a tuberculous infection elsewhere, usually the lungs. Organs of the female reproductive tract are usually infected from a hematogenous miliary spread from a primary pulmonary lesion, from hematogenous spread from a secondary miliary site, from lymphatic spread from a primary pulmonary site to intestinal lymph nodes and then to the pelvis, by direct extension from adjacent abdominal organs (small intestines, appendix, rectum, bladder) that are the site of tuberculous infection. Fistulas between the intestinal tract and the fallopian tubes have been reported with pelvic tuberculosis.

Both fallopian tubes are involved in almost all patients with pelvic tuberculosis. About one half of patients with tuberculosis salpingitis will have tuberculous endometritis. Tuberculosis of the cervix is present in 5 percent of cases. At operation one may find evidence of generalized tuberculous peritonitis with small miliary tubercles covering all peritoneal surfaces and pelvic organs. Unless tubercles are seen, the diagnosis may not be easy

until the pathologist examines microscopic sections. Tubercles form in the lining of the tube.

Clinical Features of Pelvic Tuberculosis

Pelvic tuberculosis occurs most frequently in patients between the ages of 20 and 40. The most common symptoms of pelvic tuberculosis include pelvic pain, general malaise, menstrual irregularity and infertility. A low grade fever than on occasion may produce a fulminating septic course is noted in most cases of active or subacute disease. The failure of fever to subside with high doses of broad-spectrum antibiotics is a classic feature of pelvic tuberculosis. A clinical course that is refractory to antibiotic therapy for the usual pelvic inflammatory disease should always alert the clinician to the possibility of tuberculosis.

On pelvic examination, bilateral adnexal tendency is the rule. The tenderness is usually less marked than with acute gonococcal or streptococcal infection. Occasionally, a large tuberculosis tubo-ovarian mass may be palpated on pelvic examination and even seen through the abdominal wall.

Diagnosis of Pelvic Tuberculosis

More than two thirds of the cases are diagnosed at the time of laparotomy performed for some other indication, or at the time of investigation for infertility or abnormal uterine bleeding. The most common symptom is infertility and the second most common symptom is lower abdominal and pelvic pain. Some patients are completely asymptomatic and are found to have pelvic tuberculosis in connection with investigation for other disorders such as infertility. A dilatation and curettage or endometrial biopsy will be diagnostic in some cases, especially if performed in the late premenstrual phase of the menstrual cycle. In addition to standard microscopic sections, the specimen may be examined by fluorescent antibody technique. Acid-fast staining of tissue or culture of menstrual blood is effective in detecting the organism in approximately 10 percent of cases. Genital tuberculosis is a paucibacillary form of a disease of which smears and cultures are usually negative. However

Polymerase Chain reaction, amplification of *Mycobacterium tuberculosis*. DNA can be used to support clinical and histological diagnosis of a typical case of culture negative female tuberculosis. (Baun SE, 2001). Mantoux test has limited utility in diagnosis of active genital tuberculosis during the childbearing age. However in infertile women with positive Mantoux test laparoscopy may be advocated early (Raut VS, 2001).

Treatment

Tuberculosis treatment is guided by two most important factors:

1. History of previous treatment (untreated case)
2. Status of microbiologic positivity for acid-fast bacilli (AFB), i.e. sputum smear examination

Based on these two factors, a patient can be classified into category I, II or III. Treatment involves two phases (1) intensive phase of 1 to 3 months and (2) continuation phase of 3 to 8 months.

- *New cases (Category I)* It includes the following types of patients:
  1. New cases, i.e. previously untreated with positive smear examination.
  2. New cases with severe forms of tuberculosis such as meningitis, pericarditis, extensive pleurisy, intestinal or genitourinary tuberculosis. Smear examination for AFB may be negative. Diagnosis of tuberculosis is made on the presence of histological evidence.

- *Relapses and treatment failure (Category II)*

  Relapse is defined by the presence of smear positive tuberculosis in a patient who has been declared cured in the past by a physician.

  Treatment failure is diagnosed if the smear examination remains positive in a newly diagnosed patient even after 3 months or more after start of chemotherapy. It is also diagnosed if the sputum smear is positive for AFB in a patient who has interrupted treatment for more than 2 months upto 5 months after start of chemotherapy.

- *Smear negative and extrapulmonary tuberculosis (Category III)*

  The category includes patients with limited parenchymal involvement, most children, primary tuberculosis, pleural effusion with negative smear examination. Standard antituberculous therapy is an initial three-drug regimen for 2 months, continuing with two drugs for a further 7 months, totaling 9 months of treatment. Recently a 2-month four-drug regime, continuing with two drugs to total just 6 months, is also highly effective and many physicians now omit the fourth drug even in these ultra-short course treatment.

The two drugs used throughout the treatment period are usually rifampicin (10 mg/kg/day, not to exceed 600 mg daily) and isoniazid (5 mg/kg/day not to exceed 300 mg). In the past the third drug used during the initial 2-4 months was usually ethambutol (5-25 mg/day not to exceed 2.5 gm daily), but more physicians now prefer pyrazinamide (15-30 mg/kg/day, not to exceed 2.5 gm/day), which does not have the problems of ocular toxicity seen with ethambutol and clinical improvement is faster. Earlier workers suggested avoiding rifampicin if possible during pregnancy because of teratogenic effects in animals, but there is no evidence of teratogenicity in humans and the drug is now widely regarded as safe (Snider *et al*, 1980).

Rifampicin is a bactericidal and potent sterilizing drug against mycobacteria. It is rapidly absorbed and distributed in both intra- and extra-cellular fluid. Side effects include hepatitis, nausea, vomiting, hypersensitivity skin reactions, purpura, thrombocytopenia and febrile reaction.

Ethambutol is also readily absorbed and is fairly nontoxic and has a bacteriostatic effect. A major problem is the development of optic neuritis resulting in impairment of visual acuity and color perception and should be monitored periodically.

Pyrazinamide, a orally administered well-absorbed drug is weakly bactericidal. It is particularly useful in the first two months. Pyrazinamide is hepatotoxic and causes nongouty polyarthralgia. Davidson recommended its use in pregnancy, citing the need for effective drugs in this era of increasing drug resistance and non-compliance (Davidson *et al* 1990).

Category I

These cases should be treated on the highest priority.

Intensive phase Two months of 4 primary drugs consist of Isoniazid 300 mg, Rifampicin 450 mg, pyrazinamide 1500 mg and ethambutol 1200 mg.

Continuation phase 4 to 6 months of daily INH and rifampicin in the same dosage as above or according to sputum susceptibility report. In cases where rifampicin cannot be continued, it may be replaced by ethambutol for at least 6 months after the initial intensive phase.

Category II

In these patients resistant to one or more drugs should be suspected. If feasible sputum specimen should be sent for culture and susceptibility testing.

Intensive phase Three months of 4 primary drugs as in category I should be given as supervised treatment. If the sputum smeares negative for AFB at 3 months, the continuation phase is started. If the sputum smear is positive at 3 months, the 4 oral drugs are continued for another month.

Continuation phase Consists of 5 months of isoniazid, rifampicin, after completion of the continuation phase; she is no longer eligible for re-treatment regimen. The patient is managed as a chronic case.

Category III

New cases of AFB smear negative pulmonary and extrapulmonary TB who are not very serious, thus priority is low.

Intensive phase Treatment can be instituted with three drugs, i.e. isoniazid, rifampicin and pyrazinamide for 2 months.

Continuation phase Treatment can be completed with two drugs, i.e. isoniazid and rifampicin for 4 months or INH and thiacetazone or ethambutol for 6 months.

Surgery

Surgery in the management of patients with pelvic tuberculosis producing infertility should be reserved for specific indications. In general, surgery is reserved for those patients who have failed to respond to an adequate trial of medical therapy. These include:

1. Persistence or enlargement of an adnexal mass after 4-6 months of antituberculous antibiotic therapy. The rare possibility of an ovarian tumor must always be considered, even though pelvic tuberculosis is also present. Pelvic ultrasonography should be useful in following the response of adnexal masses to treatment.

2. Primary unresponsiveness of the tuberculous infection to antibiotic therapy, as evidenced by persistent spiking temperature, leukocyte sis, elevated sedimentation rate, and evidence on biopsy of continued endometrial infection.

3. Difficulty in obtaining patient cooperation for continued long-term therapy. In these cases, some workers are accustom to giving brief course of streptomycin. 0.5 g/12 hr. intra-muscularly for 1 week prior to surgery, to perform definitive surgery, and then give 0.5 g/24 hr. in the postoperative period for 2 weeks. A persistent effort should be made to obtain the patient's cooperation for continued antituberculous therapy postoperatively. It is advisable to continue treatment for a year or longer. Isoniazid and rifampicin should be used if possible. A common reason for failure of treatment is a tendency to discontinue drugs after only a few months because the patient appears well (Thompson JD *et al*, 1992).

For young patients who are anxious to child-bearing, conservative adenectomy should be tried out only if it is possible to do so after carefully evaluating the extent of the adnexal disease and finding is minimal. It is unwise for the surgeon to be committed to a specific operative procedure prior to the time of surgery, since conservative pelvic surgery for tuberculosis may constitute poor surgical judgment, once the operative findings are known. The patient should be forewarned that conservative surgery and such surgery are considered medically advisable.

However, with the advent of ART one more method of treating these cases have become a reality albeit with limited success.

CHLAMYDIA

Chlamydia trachomatis is the most common sexually transmitted bacterium worldwide. Genital chlamydia infection affects people of all social classes. Generally, chlamydial infection presents less overtly than other STDs, persists longer and carries more serious consequences (Walker CK 1994). *C trachomatis* the causative organism is spread primarily through sexual contact. It has a long latent period (Driscoll, 1991). About 20 percent of all chlamydia infected women suffer from partial or complete tubal occlusion (Clad A, 2002) In western studies, upto ninety percent of infertile women with tubal impairments have elevated antibody titers to chlamydia (Czerwanka, 1994). Unfortunately chlamydial infection customarily is asymptomatic and atypical as compared with other STDs. Also complicating the diagnosis is the fact that lower genital tract culture results may be negative.

It is, however, quite sad that though the medical world has since understood the importance of this condition so well but the laity hardly knows anything about it. This can have a direct bearing on the control and cure of this condition especially in infertile patients. Devonshire P *et al* (1999) showed that barely half the participants in their study had heard of chlamydia and gonorrhea. Further knowledge of either infection was very poor. This can have serious implications for public health. The reasons for this are unclear and require exploration before targeted health promotion. Doctors and the popular media are acceptable, and potentially effective, sources of information. Acquisition of knowledge is important, both to reduce sexual risk taking behavior and its consequences, and to allow for informed consent for chlamydia screening programs.

Impact on Fertility

Chlamydia is a major cause of PID (Czerwanka K, 1994; Driscoll, 1991). Infection with this organism includes an inflammatory response that causes necrosis of secretory cells and subsequent scarring, ascending upward to destroy ciliated cells, kinking tubal mucosa, causing endometritis.

The passage of ova or sperm is inhibited, and implantation is prevented. Although total tubal obstruction is not found, the presence of chlamydia does prevent pregnancy: 60 to 70 percent of tubal sterility is traced to chlamydia (Grodstein F, 1993; Moore *et al,* 1990).

Recently Nalbanski *et al* (1999) reported an interesting study regarding tubal patency and chlamydial infection. The study was carried out on 162 infertile women (110 with primary and 52 with secondary infertility), patients of the University Clinic of Gynecologic Endocrinology and Infertility, Sofia. This study was designed to estimate the effect of chlamydial infection as a cause of tubal pathology in infertile women. Evidence of past chlamydial infection was determined by the presence of antichlamydial IgG antibodies by commercial ELISA test. 101 of the patients examined were positive for antichlamydial IgG antibodies (62.3%). 76 women were examined for tubal patency by means of hysterosalpingography and/or laparoscopy. 38 women had patent tubes and 38 women had tubal occlusion (20 had bilateral and 18 unilateral occlusion). 29 of these women with unilateral or bilateral tubal occlusion had a presence of IgG antichlamydial antibodies in their sera (76.3%) compared to 17 of the women with patient tubes (44.7%). The risk for tubal obstruction in women with positive serology for Chlamydia is 3.22 compared to 0.85 risk in the women with negative serology for chlamydia. The results of the present study indicate that women with evidence of past chlamydial infection are 4 times more likely to have obstructed fallopian tubes compared to women who had no such evidence.

Diagnosis

Diagnosis and identification of chlamydia may be hampered by lack of rapid, easy, sensitive and specific methods (Mouton, 2002). Systemic and local antibodies regularly develop in genital infection caused by *Chlamydia trachomatis*. Such antibodies may often persist for years after the infection and may not be a sign of parent infection. Chlamydia antibodies have been useful for demonstrating association between *Chlamydia trachomatis* and tubal factors in infertility (Persson K, 2002). Antibodies to Chlamydia heat shocked protein 60 predict a presence of tubal scarring. It is mandatory to examine the patient for chlamydial serology at the beginning of the diagnostic protocol in order to ensure adequate management prior to more invasive procedures such as hysterosalpingography or laparoscopy.

Genotyping is a powerful epidemiological tool but is not yet ready for routine clinical use. However, resistant strains causing treatment failures with problem of emerging antibiotic resistant strains cannot be neglected (Persson K, 2002).

Rezokova J *et al* in 1999 studied the effect of chlamydia on male infertility and found that IgA antichlamydial antibodies in the ejaculate proved in 62 percent of the examined men with an abnormal spermiogram a useful indicator of infection in the genital tract. With the increasing number of sexual partners the number of pathospermias increased.

Treatment Approaches

Erythromycin, tetracycline, or doxycycline has shown clinical efficacy. Penicillin is ineffective. Chlamydia may not actually be eradicated after treatment despite apparently negative culture results. Clindamycin may be used if other treatments are ineffective.

GONORRHEA

Gonorrhea is caused by the bacteria *N. gonorrhoeae*, which evokes a pyogenic, inflammatory reaction characterized by purulent exudates (Cook D L et al, 1986). As the organism replicates, the oxidation-reduction potential of the environment diminish, allowing polymicrobial disease: this explains why it is common to discover co-existing pathogens (Monif GRG et al, 1990).

Symptomatology comprises of dysuria, urinary frequency, dyspareunia, pelvic pain, lower abdominal pain, purulent and fowl smelling vaginal discharge, unusual vaginal bleeding, fever, and cervical tenderness. Culture on Thayer-Martin medium is the preferred method of diagnosis because Gram stains may not always be reliable. Gonorrhea is significantly different from chlamydial infection in as much as most men and 50 percent of women are symptomatic, prompting patients to seek earlier diagnosis and treatment.

Impact on Fertility

Gonorrhea damages the reproductive tract by traveling upwards along the mucosa, through the cervix to the adnexa, causing a reduction in ciliary activity and the induction of sloughing (Walker CK, 1994). Subsequent episodes of infection augment the risk of PID induced infertility, possibly causing tubo-ovarian abscess. Gonorrhea also leads to splinting of the fallopian tubes and altering the tubo-ovarian disposition. *N. gonorrhea* is a major cause of PID, ectopic pregnancy and infertility and can facilitate HIV infections also. (MMWR morb. Mortal weekly, 2002).

Treatment Approaches

Gonorrhea seems to be an acute infection, responding readily to treatment. Penicillin/probenecid is the regimen of choice. Tetracycline, doxycycline, and erythromycin can be substituted for penicillin-allergic or penicillin resistant cases (Jensen, 1985; Monif, 1990). Fluoroquinolones are used widely because they are less expensive, orally administrable and can be given in a single dose therapy. Ceftriaxone and cefixime is recommended as an alternative to penicillin in areas with a high prevalence of penicillinase producing *N. gonorrhoeae* (PPNG). Combination treatment to address concomitant chlamydial infection also should be considered (also refer Table 3.1).

Stigmata or sequelae of the infection in the form of abscess or adhesions requires surgical intervention. Microsurgical intervention in cases of open surgeries and endoscopic adhesiolysis for closed surgeries is recommended.

TRICHOMONIASIS

Clinical Presentation

The prevalence of trichomonas has been reported to be approximately 32 percent of all gynec patients. *Trichomonas vaginalis*, a parasitic

TABLE 3.1: Some current (1989)
CDC recommendations for antibiotic treatment

1. Uncomplicated ureteral, endocervical, or rectal infections with N. gonorrhoeae in non-pregnant adult females	Ceftriazone 250 mg IM once. Doxycycline 100 mg orally bid × 7 days
2. Uncomplicated ureteral, endocervical or recent infections with C. trachomatis in non-pregnant adult females	Doxycycline 100 mg orally bid × 7 days Or Tetracycline 500 mg orally qid × 7 days
3. Pelvic inflammatory disease	a. Ambulatory management: Cefoxitin 2 g IM Plus Probenecid 1 g orally Plus Doxycycline 100 mg orally bid × 10-14 days. Or Tetracycline 500 mg orally qid × 10-14 days.

(Patients who do not respond to therapy within 72 hours should be hospitalized for parenteral therapy).

b. In-patient management

1. Recommend Regimen

Cefoxitin 2 g q 6 hr.
Or
Cefotetan IV 2 gq l2 hr.
Plus
Doxycycline 100 mg 1 12 mg q 12hr. orally or IV

(The preceding regimen is given for at least 48 hours after patient clinically improves).

- After discharge, continue doxycycline 100 mg orally b.i.d. × 10-14 days.

2. Recommend Regimen-B

Clindamycin IV 900 mg × 8 hr.
Plus
Gentamycin loading dose IV or IM (2 mg/kg)
followed by a maintenance dose (1.5 mg/kg) × 8 hr.

(The preceding regimen is given for at least 48 hours after the patient clinically improves).

- After discharge, continue doxycycline 100 mg daily b.i.d. × 10-14 days.

(Centers for Disease Control, MMWR, 1989. Sexually Transmitted Diseases; Treatment Guidelines 38.21,1989.)

protozoan, can be harbored in the genital tract until a time when an imbalance allows proliferation (Cook DL, 1986). Classic symptoms include frothy malodorous greenish-white vaginal discharge, itching, irritation, spotty edema, and reddening of the cervix called *strawberry mucosa* (Cook DL, 1986). Such infection may also be identified by edema of the vulva, dyspareunia, dysuria, and frequency. It is easily identified during a routine wet film smear.

Impact on Fertility

Trichomonas attaches to vaginal mucosa, ingests bacteria and leukocytes, and acts as a carrier for other pathogens. Its role has been under-recognized as a trigger for infertility. Subsequent infections also extend the hazard of infertility by

further compromising the environment, allowing multiple pathogens to cause additional tissue damage (Grodstein F *et al,* 1993).

Treatment Approaches

Metronidazole is the drug of choice. Newer drugs like secnidazole and tinidazole are equally effective but better tolerated due to easier dosage schedules. Attention to personal hygiene must be emphasized.

PELVIC INFLAMMATORY DISEASE

Pelvic inflammatory disease is an inflammation of the epithelial surfaces of the fallopian tubes, usually caused by one or more STDs that ascend the mucosa from the cervix to the endometrium, the salpinx, and in some cases, the peritoneum.

The generally accepted theory pontifies that anything that alters the vaginal environment and facilitates the propelling of pathogens upward increases the susceptibility to PID (Fugate KA, 1996). Risk factors have been identified and include age (adolescence or greater than 30 years old), smoking, the number of sexual partners, i.e., more than two), use of an intrauterine device (IUD), multiple STDs, douching, cocaine use, and co-infection with HIV, (Cates W, 1993; Grodstein, 1993; Korn AP, 1995; Walker CK, 1994). The clinical course is altered in women co-infected with HIV: pathogenic organisms may ascend more easily because of decreased mucosal and immune functioning (Korn AP, 1995).

Asymptomatic PID, accounting for approximately 80 percent of PID diagnoses, is of greater concern than overt PID (Cates W, 1993). Only 60 percent of women diagnosed with PID show evidence on laparoscopy (Moore DE, 1990).

Recently, Russian workers in Olenberg studied the contribution of non-enteric Escherichia infections (NEI) to the formation of male and female infertility. They found a negative influence of NEI on infertility besides other conditions (ZH, 2000).

Impact on Fertility

Lower genital tract infections gain access to the uterus, fallopian tubes, and ovaries by ascending through the normally protective cervical barrier (Cook DL, 1986). During menstruation, the endocervical canal is slightly dilated; allowing pathogens easier access to pelvic structures; the sloughing of the endometrium is a favorable environment for pathogenicity (Cook DL, 1986). Adnexal adhesions and masses result when salpingitis involves the bowel and bladder (Levin S, 1987). The effects of PID are numerous-tubal infertility, ectopic pregnancy, tubo-ovarian abscess, and endometritis (Czerwenka K, 1994). When mistakenly identified as appendicitis, ruptured cyst, ectopic pregnancy, or endometriosis, untreated PID can continue to damage the upper genital tract (Walker CK, 1994).

Treatment Approaches

The goals of treatment are to alleviate symptoms, interrupt pathogenicity, and minimize sequelae by providing hydration, antibiotics, and pain relief. Although early intervention improves the chances of limiting the sequelae of PID, major complications can still occur in women receiving appropriate treatment. A combination of broad-spectrum antibiotics is recommended, given the polymicrobial nature of PID. The type of antibiotic used in treating symptomatic PID has minimal effect on fertility outcome; in fact, the antibiotic treatment used to cure PID does not reverse preexisting tubal damage (Moore DE, 1990). The CDC guidelines outline several treatment regimens. Ambulatory patients not responding to treatment within 48 to 72 hours should be hospitalized. Two inpatient combinations serve as the gold standard regimen cefoxin/doxycycline and clindamycin/tobramycin. Treatment of the sexual partner with ceftriazone/doxycycline is recommended, regardless of symptomatology. Likewise, fluoroquinolones have been advocated as single agent treatment. The removal of lUDs after treatment is recommended because recovery is delayed if they are left in place (Levin S, 1987). Bed rest in Fowler's position head and knees elevated may be suggested to assist in pelvic drainage. Drainage of localized abscess if any should be prompt and complete. However, the adhesions resulting in infertility following such a fulminant PID are hardly preventable (also refer Table 3.1).

MYCOPLASMA

Impact on Fertility

Existing data are not definitive regarding a causal relationship between a subclinical mycoplasma infection and infertility. One hypothesis is that endometrial tissue infected with *M. hominis* may inhibit sperm migration by inducing changes in the ciliated cells that line fallopian tubes (Monif GRG, 1990). Some strains of *U. urealyticum* isolated from infertile women can produce a neuroaminidase like substance that may interfere with sperm implantation. It is microbiologic environment that controls these two organisms, both of which grow best in microaerophilic environments. Therefore, a preexisting or concurrent condition that elicits a local inflammatory response tends to enhance the probability of mycoplasma colonization. Although most women with acute salpingitis show antibodies to *M. hominis,* its cytopathic effect on the fallopian tubes remains to be demonstrated fully (Walker CK, 1994). *In vitro,* there has been no correlation between mycoplasma growth and tubal damage; it can lead to a self-limiting salpingitis, but it is unclear whether it is a causative factor or a secondary invader (Cassell GH, 1994).

The role of mycoplasma in infertility is, therefore, controversial. Most likely, they are opportunists. Some researchers believe that genital tract mycoplasma have a greater role in recurrent miscarriages and pelvic infections than in precipitating acute salpingitis and consequent infertility. Other studies clarify the impact of mycoplasma on tubal damage. Kundsin and co-workers (1986) studied middle and upper income women in Boston to determine the incidence of STDs among 99 patients seeking second opinions regarding their failure to conceive. Only 15 of the subjects were negative for mycoplasma by either culture or endometrial biopsy histology.

Treatment Approaches

After appropriate antibiotic therapy (as indicated by sensitivity testing), there were 43 pregnancies in the Boston group within the first year: 28 healthy babies were delivered. Similarly, in a French investigation, mycoplasmal cultures were obtained in all women with reproductive abnormalities, and anti-mycoplasmal treatment led to recovery in the cases in which mycoplasma was the only infection (Jahier J, 1985).

In contrast, Upadhyaya and coworkers (1983) found that whereas *U. urealyticum* was present in a significantly higher proportion of infertile (versus fertile) women, eradication of the organism had little effect on pregnancy rates. Monif (1990) also cites studies that show no improved conception rates after eradication of mycoplasma. Wallach (1995) encourages that samples be obtained for ureaplasma culture from a patient with unexplained infertility. If positive, he suggests treating both partners. *U. urealyticum* are resistant to the sulfonamides, trimethoprim, rifampicin, and all anti-microbial agents that inhibit cell wall synthesis. For the 20 to 40 percent of clinical isolates of *M. hominis* and the 15 percent of *U. urealyticum* that are resistant to the tetracyclines, the use of clindamycin and erythromycin, respectively, can be effective.

A key question is whether mycoplasma is a risk factor for infertility or simply a concurrent infection. Although the studies to date are contradictory and inconclusive, most researchers agree that if the mycoplasma does have a role in infertility, it probably is not a significant one.

Predisposing Factors to Tubal Occlusion

Moore and Cates (1990) identified the following risk factors that predispose women to tubal occlusion resulting from PID.

1. *PID history* Each new episode of acute salpingitis roughly doubles postsalpingitis infertility rates.
2. *Age* Women aged more than 24 years have salpingitis-related tubal damage more frequently than those aged 15 to 24 years.
3. *Severity of pelvic inflammation,* as assessed by diagnostic laparoscopy—the more severe the inflammatory changes, the more likely is tubal infertility.
4. *IUD history* Users of the Dalkon shield and other devices run a higher than average risk of tubal infertility. Barrier based contraception, including diaphragms and condoms (especially) with spermicides) can offer protection from infection. More research is required to learn whether oral contraceptives can provide protection from acute PID.
5. *Smoking history* Smoking decreases humoral-mediated and cell mediated immunity (*in vitro*) and increases the risk of tubal infertility. The presence of an IUD exacerbates the risk.

The influence of these factors is key in designing a nursing care and patient education plan.

SUMMARY

Before the advent of antibiotics, tubal infertility was identified as related to *N. gonorrhoea* infections and PID. In the 1960s, Westrom and colleagues confirmed the impact of STD-induced salpingitis on subsequent tubal infertility. In the 1970s, the role of *C. trachomatis* as a major cause of PID (in addition to gonococcal infections) became increasingly clear. The mycoplasmas have been suspected as potential contributors to STD-based infertility; additional data are needed to guide the practitioner more definitively in this area. More recently, the close relationships among behaviors associated with STD and HIV infection have been better understood.

Sexually transmitted diseases affect human fertility primarily by infecting the upper genital tract of women, rarely do they produce infertility in men. Fallopian tube damage is dependent on the causative organism, the duration of infection, the type of exposure, the phase of the menstrual cycle, the presence of intrauterine contraception devices, the use of barrier method contraception, and previous genital tract injury.

BIBLIOGRAPHY

1. Akush Ginekol (Sofiia). No title available: 2000;39(1):18-20.
2. Baun SE, Dooely DP, Wright J, Kost ER, Storey DF. J Reprod. Med 2001;46(10):929-32.
3. Borisov I. Inflammatory gynecological diseases as a social problem in women of reproductive age: Akush Ginekol (Sofiia) 1999;38(4):33-35.
4. Cassell GH, Waites KV. Genital mycoplasma infections. In Hoerprich PD: Infectious Diseases 5th. edn. Philadelphia: JB. Lippincott 1994;664.
5. Cates WR, Joesoef MR, Golman MB. Atypical PID: Can we identify clinical predictors? Am J Obst. Gynecol 169:341, 1993.
6. Christiansen G, Birkelund S. Is vaccine for Chlamydia a Reality; Best Pract Res Clin Obstet Gynaecol 2003;16(6):889-900.
7. Clad A. The Umsch 2003;59(9):459-63.
8. Cohen F: Clinical manifestations and treatment of HIV infections and AIDS in women in Cohen FL, Durham JD (Eds): Women, Children, and HIV/AIDS: 1st edn. New York: Springer, 1993;83.
9. Cook DL, Porth CM. Sexually transmitted diseases. In Porth CM (Ed): Pathophysiology: Concepts of Altered States, 2nd edn. Philadelphia: JB Lippincott, 1986;581.
10. Czerwenka K, Louss F, Hosmann J, et al. Salpingitis caused by Chlamydia trachomatis and its significance for infertility. Acta Obstet Gynecol Scand 1994;73:771.
11. Davidson PT. Treating tuberculosis: What drugs, for how long? Ann. Intern Med 1990;112:393-94.
12. Devonshire P, Hillman R, Capewell S, Clark BJ. Knowledge of Chlamydia trachomatis genital infection and its consequences in people attending a genitourinary medicine clinic Sex Transm Infect. 1999;75(6):409-11.
13. Diemer T, Hales DB, Weidner W. Andrologia 2003;35(1):55-63.
14. Driscoll GL, Dodd J, Tyler JPP, et al: Positive chlamydia serology and its effect on factors influencing outcome of its in vitro fertilization treatment. Aust NZ J Obstet Gynecol 1991;32:145.
15. Greendale GA, Haas ST, Holbrook K, et al. The relationship of Chlamydia trachomatis infection and male infertility. Am J Public Health 1993;83:996.
16. Grodstein F, Goldman MB, Cramer DW. Relation of tubal infertility to history of sexually transmitted diseases. Am J Epidemiol 1993;137:577.
17. Jensen MD, Bobak IM. Maternity and Gynecologic Care: The Nurse and the Family, 3rd edn. St. Louis: CV Mosby, 1985.
18. Korn AP, Landers DV. Gynecologic disease in women infected with human immunodeficiency virus type I. J Acquir Immune Defic Syndr 1995;9:361.
19. Levin S. Pelvic inflammatory disease. In sexually Transmitted Disease, St. Louis: Year Book Medical Publishers, 1987.
20. MMWR Morb Mortal Wkly; Rep 2002;22:51(46):1041-44.
21. Monif GRG. Infections. In Sievel MM (Ed.) Infertility: A Comprehensive Text. East Norwalk, CT. Appleton and Lange, 1990;235.
22. Moore DE, Cates W Jr. Sexually transmitted diseases and infertility. In Holmes K, Cates W, Lemon S, et al (Eds): Sexually Transmitted Disease. New York: McGraw-Hill, Incl. 1990;763.
23. Mouton JW, Peters MF, Van Rissort, VOS JH, Verkooyen RP: Int J STD AIDS 2002;13(Suppl-2):26-29.
24. Nalbanski B, Borisov I, Slavkova V, Filipov E. The effect of chlamydial infection on tubal patency: Akush Ginekol (Sofiia) 1999;38(3):22-24.
25. Persson K. The role of serology, antibiotic susceptibility testing & serological determination in genital chlamydial infection; Best Pract Res Clin Obst & Gynecol 2002;16(6):801-14.
26. Raut VS, Mahashm AA, Sheth SS. Int J Gynaecol Obstet 2001;72(2):165-69.
27. Schillinger JA, Kissinger P, Calvet H. Sex transm disease 2003;30(1):49-56.
28. Sciarra JJ. Pelvic infections and infertility. Eur J Obstet Gynecol Reprod. Biol 1993;19:19.
29. Sciarra JJ. Reproductive health: A global prospective. Am J Obstet Gynecol 1993;168:1549.
30. Snider DE, Layde PM, Johnson MW, Lyle HA. Treatment of tuberculosis during pregnancy. Am Rev Respir Dis 1980;122:65-78.
31. Szymanski W, Ludwikowski G, Sobcinski Z, Kotzbach R, Grabiee M. Evaluation of co-existence of symptoms and antispeatozoal antibodies in sperms of men treated for infertility. Ginekol 2002;73:583-87.

32. Thompson JD, Spence MR. Pelvic Inflammatory disease in Te Linde's Operative Gynecology. 17th edn. Philadelphia: JB Lippincott Company, 1992;593.
33. Tripathy SN. In J Gynaecol Obstet 2003;76(2);159-63.
34. Walker CK, Landers DK. Pelvic inflammatory disease. In Pastrek JG: Obstetric and Gynecologic Infectious Disease. New York: Reven Press, 1994;111.
35. Wallach EE. Unexplained infertility. In Wallach EE, Zacur HA: Reproductive Medicine and Surgery, 1st edn. St. Louis: Mosby, 1995;459.
36. Watson EJ, Templeton A, Russell I, Paavonen, J Mardw PA, Stray A, Pederson BS; The accuracy and efficacy of screening test for Chlamydia trachomatis: A systematic review; Jr. Med Microbial; 2002;7(12):1021-31.
37. Westrom L. Pelvic inflammatory disease: Bacteriology and sequelae. Contraception 1987;36:111.
38. Zh Mikrobiol Epidemiol Immunobiol No title available: 2000;2:106-10.

• Kamala Selvaraj

4

Immunology in Infertility

Recently more and more studies have reported relationship between immune system alterations and infertility. Improved technologies such as monoclonal antibodies and enzyme-linked immunosorbent assay (ELISA) have greatly contributed to this progress (Micheal R Caudle, 1988).[1] It has been proved beyond doubt that presence of antisperm antibodies in either partner can lead to infertility and fetal wastage. Fetal wastage could be in the form of chemical pregnancy, preclinical pregnancy, empty sac syndrome, missed abortion, IUD, or premature rupture of membranes. Therefore, it depends on the clinician's discretion to decide which couples need to undergo further investigation.

INTRODUCTION

Nearly 100 years ago, both Metchinkoff and Metalnikoff demonstrated the antigenicity of sperm from both experimental animal and from humans. However, it was not until 1954 that both Rumpke and Wilson each separately reported that the formation of antisperm antibodies could be a cause of infertility in the male.[2, 3]

Koji Nakagawa and Shyuji Yamano were the first to demonstrate that sperm- immobilizing antibodies blocked *in vitro* sperm penetration through human zona pellucida and that the inhibition was reversible.[4]

Sperm antibodies in the form of autoantibodies in male and alloantibodies in female patients directed against sperm antigens may prevent fertilization of the oocyte into the female genital tract and are, therefore, one of the major reasons for an immunologically induced infertility. Fertility disorders of unknown etiology of male as well as female patients result to a considerable amount (up to 20%) from antisperm antibodies.

In the male, the sperm agglutinating or sperm immobilizing factors cause infertility and affect early embryonic development. In the female, there are antioocyte antibodies which impede fertilization.

Etiology

Specific antigens appear on the sperm surface from the beginning of spermatogenesis at puberty. It still remains unclear how these self-antigens can be tolerated and stay unrecognized by the immune system (Acosto *et al*, 1996).[5] Meanwhile, although women are inoculated intravaginally with spermatozoa during coitus, it will not usually result in the development of antisperm antibodies. Suppressor T cells may play an important role in preventing the development of autoimmunity to sperms.

Antibodies are secreted into the fluids of the accessory glands, specifically the prostate and seminal vesicles. At the time of ejaculation, the fluids from these glands contribute to the seminal plasma. They then come into contact with the sperm and may cause them to clump (Silverburg and Turner).[6]

In women, the sperm in the genital tract following intercourse does not seem to be a factor in the production of ASAB. However, events that induce trauma, or introduce sperm to the mucous membrane outside of the reproductive tract, can induce antibody formation. Proposed examples of such events include trauma to the vaginal mucosa during intercourse or the deposition of sperm into the gastrointestinal tract by way of oral or anal intercourse (Golumb *et al*).[7]

Certain factors may cause the development of antisperm antibodies:

a. Testicular trauma or orchitis
b. Genitourinary tract infection
c. Vasectomy/vaso-vasostomy and genital tract obstruction
d. Spinal cord injury
e. Female sexual practices
f. Homosexuality
g. Intrauterine insemination

Testicular Trauma or Orchitis

Testicular trauma and orchitis may cause the breaching of blood-testis barrier.

Genitourinary Tract Infection

Seminal antisperm antibody activities are increased in cases with genital tract infections with Mycoplasma and Chlamydia.

Vasectomy/Vaso-vasostomy Genital Tract Obstruction

There are reports stating the presence of serum antisperm antibodies present in 50-80 percent of men who have undergone vasectomy with or without subsequent vasovasostomy. This is probably due to the release of sperm antigens from the epididymis after spermatozoa degradation.

Spinal Cord Injury

Long-term ejaculation and sperm retention results in the development of antisperm antibodies in nearly 80 percent of the cases.

Female Sexual Practices

Approximately 40-45 percent of prostitutes test positive for antisperm antibodies and the percentage increases with those who have never used contraceptive methods. Hypothetically, this may be explained by repeated inoculations with different sperms antigens and microorganisms.

Homosexuality

Homosexual men have head-directed antibodies of the IgM class in their serum. Tail directed IgG antibodies are more frequently detected in the serum of heterosexuals.

INTRA UTERINE INSEMINATION

For The Male

a. Immunology of semen-Semen possesses both antigenic and immunosuppressive properties. Two types of antisperm antibodies can be identified:
   – Immobilising antibodies
   – Agglutinating antibodies (JMG Hollanders, 1996)[8]

As the sperm cell matures, the spermatozoa acquire the antigens gradually. The antigen sites of the sperm are:
   – Acrosome
   – Postacrosome
   – Equatorial region
   – Mid-piece
   – Tip of the tail (Alexander and Anderson, 1988)[9]

Majority of the antigens are situated at the surface. While some get exposed only after the outer membranes of the acrosome are broken down, some antigens can be identified even in the embryo (Solter and Schachner, 1976),[10] ovary (Menge and Fleming, 1978)[11] and placenta (Berkotwiz *et al* 1985).[12]

The development of the sperm antigens occurs at puberty, but these do not provoke an immune response in the adult male because of the blood-testis barrier. This barrier prevents the spermatic material from entering the circulatory system and prevents the lymphocytes, immunoglobulins and complement from entering the testis (Gilula *et al*, 1976).[13]

The local immunoregulatory mechanism also exists in the testis and epididymis which prevents the antibody formation (Ritchie *et al*, 1984).[14]

Seminal plasma inhibits T-cells, B-cells, natural killer cells, macrophages, polymorphonuclear leukocytes and the action of complements. This extensive system prevents auto-immunity developing in the male, both humoral and cellular.

For The Female

The antisperm antibodies in the female possibly adversely affects fertilization, embryo quality and pregnancy rates.

Cervical hostility includes a variety of disorders including anatomical, hormonal and immunological conditions. In most cases it is diagnosed by the PCT (Post Coital Test).

Cervical mucus can become hostile to spermatozoa and impair sperm ascent in the uterus. Mucus is said to be hostile if the *spinnbarkeit* appearance is abnormal during the infertility work-up. Mucous secretion and viscosity may be reduced during prolonged estrogen deficiency, or with infections caused by Trichomonas and Chlamydia.

Immune Responses in the Female Reproductive Tract

IgM antibodies do not transude into, but secretory IgA are located in the female genital tract. IgG antibodies in the circulation also transude into the female reproductive tract and impair reproductive function. The primary indication for testing antisperm antibodies is an abnormal PCT.

The female genital tract is immunologically well protected. Both IgG and IgA immunoglobulins are secreted locally in the genital tract and are detectable in the vaginal secretions. The concentrations of these are high in the follicular phase and low in the mid cycle. This pattern is reversed in the uterine secretions. Antisperm antibodies secreted locally in response to the deposition of the sperms in the female genital tract do not reflect the level found in the serum. antibodies can impair sperm motility and function by causing:

• Agglutination
• Reduced or total loss of motility
• Impaired cervical mucus penetration

• Alterations in capacitation and acrosomal reaction
• Inefficient sperm-egg fusion.

ASAB AND IVF OUTCOME

Contrary to the expressed concern, that antisperm antibodies (ASAB) inhibit nidation or fetal growth, high implantation and pregnancy rates were reported upon IVF-ET treatment of immunologic infertile women. Similar results were also reported by Shibara *et al* but they concluded that the observed high pregnancy rate in the ASAB positive group was probably due to fewer associated infertility problems (Demirol *et al*).[15]

When should the antisperm antibodies test be done?
1. When there is a history of infection
2. Local injury of the testis
3. Seminal analysis revealing sperm agglutination or poor PCT
4. Very early pregnancy wastage

At our center, we perform this test routinely in the initial work-up of the infertility couple.

DIAGNOSIS

– Plasma titers of antibodies found during infertility work-up
– IgA and IgG anti-sperm antibodies in the cervical mucus
– Non-progressive motility of spermatozoa in cervical mucus
– Poor PCT
– Huhner test or Kremer test
– In vitro sperm penetration test.

CLINICAL EFFECTS OF ANTISPERM ANTIBODIES

• Interference with sperm production.
• Restriction of sperm penetration and survival.
• Reduction of sperm motility
• Damage of the integrity of sperm plasma membrane.
• Interference with the sperm capacitation and / or acrosome reaction.
• Interference with sperm/zona pellucida binding and /or penetration.

- Inhibition of sperm–oolemma fusion.
- Inhibition of early cleavage of fertilized eggs.
- Suppression in the development of the embryo.
- Interference with the implantation process (WR Yeh et al, 1996).[16]

Laboratory Tests for Antisperm Antibodies

Antisperm antibodies of IgA and IgG have been implicated in subfertility by reducing the progression of sperm through cervical and/or interfering with sperm binding at the zona pellucida. Their levels can be measured in the seminal plasma, or serum of either the male or female using either the MAR or immunobead tests (Gulekli et al).[17] In our hospital, we test for antisperm antibody for each and every couple who come with history of infertility and BOH.

1. Sperm Mucus Contact Test (SCMC)–(Kremer and Jager)[18]
2. Franklin and Duke's test
3. Kibricks' gelatin agglutination test (GAT) [19]
4. Tray agglutination test (TAT)
5. Mixed agglutination reaction (MAR)
6. Radio labeled antiglobulin assay
7. Panning procedure
8. Immunobead test (IBT)
9. Indirect IBT
10. Enzyme-linked immunosorbent assay (ELISA)
11. Anti-sperm antibody latex agglutination test
12. Anti-sperm antibody latex agglutination test–Ig typing
13. Anti-sperm antibody hemagglutination test; Flow cytometry (FCM)
14. Immunofluorescence test.

Sperm Mucus Contact Test (SCMC)

A drop of mucus is placed on glass slide and a drop of semen is added, mixed with the mucus, and covered with a cover slip. The slides are then placed in a moist petri dish at room temperature and then examined.

SCMC test is done in various combinations
- Patient sperm and patient mucus
- Donor sperm and donor mucus
- Patient sperm and donor mucus
- Donor sperm and patient mucus

Significance of the Test

The non-progressive shaking movements of the spermatozoa in the cervical mucus is due to the interaction between the antisperm antibody coated spermatozoa and the glycoprotein micelles in cervical mucus.

The interaction is explained as follows:
- Progressively moving spermatozoa coated with sperm antibody stick to the network of long glycoprotein micelles in normal cervical mucus.
- The same shaking motility appears when anti sperm antibodies are present in the cervical mucus.
- A positive SCMC test is caused by IgA in cervical mucus and on the sperm surface, although it can also be caused by IgG on the spermatozoal surface.

The Interpretation of the Test

The samples are examined at magnification of 400 X (phase contrast microscope)
To know the shaking percentage:
- Percentage of progressively motile spermatozoa (%PM)
- Percentage of locally motile spermatozoa with quick shaking moments (%LM)

$$\text{Shaking percentage (\%S)} = \frac{\% LM}{\% PM + \% LM} \times 100$$

The whole slide is screened and all the percentages are estimated as multiples of 10. The test is read after 15 to 30 minutes and is considered to be positive when the percentage is more than 30, but is thought to be of clinical importance only when the percentage is more than 75.

Franklin and Duke's Test

This is a Tube Slide Agglutination Test (TSAT). Here a mixture of donor semen and complement-inactivated patients' serum is incubated at 37° C for 60 minutes. An aliquot is placed on a slide and observed for head to head type agglutination.

Kibricks' Gelatin Agglutination Test

Kibricks' gelatin agglutination test (GAT) is performed by suspending semen from a donor without ASAB with the complement-inactivated serum of the patient in a gelatin mixture in a small glass tube at 37°C for 60 minutes. The formation of large agglutinated clumps of sperm at the bottom of the tube indicates presence of ASAB.

Tray Agglutination Test (TAT)

Friberg[20] introduced this test by using micro liter volumes of reagents. Here donor sperm and patient serum are incubated in a flat-bottom tissue-typing tray and agglutination is observed using an inverted microscope. The TAT is more sensitive than GAT as it detects head to head agglutination and tail-to-tail agglutination.

Mixed Agglutination Reaction (MAR)

- Uses antiserum to IgG to bridge the gap between the antibody-coated sperms and latex particle that have been conjugated with human IgG.
- End point is the presence of clumping.

This test is used to identify autoantibodies produced by men and adsorbed to sperm in the ejaculate (Direct Test), or can be used to demonstrate ASAB in body fluids such as serum, cervical mucus and seminal plasma (Indirect Test). In this procedure Red blood cells (RBCs) are coated with IgA or IgG. These treated red cells are now mixed with anti-IgA or anti-IgG. Red Blood cells treated this way are now incubated with the sperms to be investigated. If the sperms are coated with ASAB of the IgA or IgG, they will adhere to the red cells.

The results can be quantified according to the percentage of the sperms which are adherent to the RBCs. It is reliable, but time-consuming and needs a good laboratory facility.

Radio Labeled Antiglobulin Assay

In this test, Xenogenix radio-iodinated antiglobulins are used to trace quantitatively the presence of ASAB.

Panning

This procedure is done by adding mouse anti-rabbit sperm serum to the sperms, which have been coated with immunoglobulins and agglutination is detected microscopically.

Immunobead Test (IBT)

This test uses beads labeled with anti-IgG, anti-IgA, or anti-IgM antibodies and provides the class of antibodies seen on the sperm. The sites on the sperm where the beads are adherent can also be noted. Anti-IgA antibody is localized to the tail of sperm and anti-IgG to the head. Antibodies localized to the tip of the tail are not very important whereas antibodies on the rest of the tail can interfere with the sperm motility. Antibodies on the head of the sperm can cause failure of sperm-egg interaction.

The immunobead test uses rabbit anti-human immunoglobulin. 1 drop of immunobead suspension is mixed with one drop of sperm suspension on a slide. A cover slip is placed over it and incubated for 30 minutes. Sperm-immunobead complexes can be observed. The percent of motile sperms, localization of bead attachment [head,

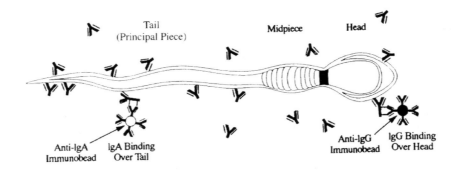

FIGURE 4.1: Schematic drawing (Acosta et al)[21] of the immunobead test. Anti-IgA or Anti-IgG covalently linked in poly acrylamide beads binds to IgA or IgG bound to the sperm surface

tail, tail-tip] and number beads bound per sperm is recorded.

This test is highly specific, sensitive and reproducible.

Indirect IBT

Here ASAB are detected in serum, follicular fluid, cervical mucus and seminal plasma. Aliquots of the sample are incubated with donor sperm, which has been proven negative by the direct IBT. ASAB, if present in the test sample, will bind to the donor sperm, which then interact with immunobeads.

Enzyme-linked Immunosorbent Assay (ELISA)

This test was first described in 1971. It is used to detect and quantify sperm autoimmunity. ELISA uses anti-human immunoglobulin with covalently linked enzymes to detect the presence of antibodies in body fluids. In ELISA procedure, antigen is immobilized by passive adsorption to solid phase (Silicone rubber, glass) and test sera are incubated with this antigen to allow for Ag-Ab binding. The serum is then washed and is exposed to enzyme (alkaline phosphatase, glucose oxidase) coupled anti-human immunoglobulin. Following another wash, a substrate (p-nitrophenyl phosphate) is added. The degree of color change following degradation of the substrate is directly proportional to the antibody concentration.

Antisperm Antibody Latex Agglutination Test

By means of the sperm-antibody latex agglutination test even smallest amounts of sample material like serum, seminal plasma and follicular fluid can be examined. Only if antibodies directed against sperm antigens are present in sample material, latex particles coated with this antigen will agglutinate within 1-2 minutes. The test is carried out on special slides delivered with the kit.

Antisperm Antibody Latex Agglutination Test–IgTyping

With this typing test immunoglobulins detected in sample materials are classified as IgG, IgM and IgA. Analysis is done only in sample, which have previously been shown to contain sperm antibodies of a determined titer.

Diluted samples (cervical mucus, uterine lavage and seminal fluid) are pre-incubated with the corresponding anti-class antibody (anti-IgA, anti-IgG, anti-IgM). In the second step, samples are mixed with latex particles coated with sperm antigen. Non-appearance of agglutination within 1-2 minutes indicates the immunoglobulin class added to the sample at the beginning.

Antisperm Antibody Hemagglutination Test

This test is based upon specially pretreated and sensitized red blood cells (SRBC) coated with sperm antigen. Antibodies in the sample agglutinate with coated SRBC within 120 min.

FCM Test

Flow cytometry (FCM) analysis of live antibody-coated spermatozoa subjected to immunofluorescence staining is considered an objective method for the quantitative detection of ASAB. But the cross-linking of cell surface antigen (Ag) with bivalent antibodies and/or antigen-antibody (Ag–Ab) complexes with second antibodies may induce the reorganization of surface components (patching and capping) and result in their shedding from the sperm surface.

Immunofluorescence Test

This test utilizes fluorescent–conjugated antiglobulins to detect sperm bound antibodies. It has a high false-positive rate.

TREATMENT FOR ANTISPERM ANTIBODY

At this point there is still no unique way to improve the sperm performance and/or promote the fecundity of those who suffer from ASAB.

Therapeutic modalities include
1. Occlusion therapy
2. Condom therapy
3. Enzyme therapy
4. Immunosuppression
5. Immunization with partners lymphocytes
6. In vitro sperm processing
7. Intrauterine insemination (IUI)

8. *In vitro* fertilization and embryo transfer (IVF and ET)
9. Gamete intrafallopian tube transfer (GIFT)
10. Artificial reproductive techniques (ART)

Occlusion Therapy

Occlusion therapy was apparently proposed by Franklin and Dukes (1964)[22] It was supposed that if the semen does not come into contact with the tissue of the female genital tract for an extended period of time, the female partner's ASAB level would subside. The first unprotected intercourse must be timed to occur at the time of ovulation, to prevent a booster antigenic stimulation.

Condom Therapy

Women with high titers of ASAB may respond to condom therapy. Condom use must be absolute to prevent further exposure of the female immune system to sperm antigens. Serum should be tested regularly at three months intervals.

Enzyme Therapy

Some authors have tried adding protease culture medium in an attempt to disagglutinate the spermatozoa. Sephadex has been used to separate antibody-free spermatozoa.

Immunosuppression

Corticosteroid Therapy

96 mg of prednisolone is administered during the last week of the female's menstrual cycle for three alternate cycles. Either a high dose short-course regimen (96mg methylprednisolone orally taken daily for 7 days) or a low- dose long course regimen (2 mg dexamethasone acetate IM injected daily for 13 weeks) has been reported to be effective in decreasing the titer of ASAB. The apparent pregnancy rates were reported to be about 22 percent where only the men were treated, and about 14 percent when only women were treated. The decreased antibody levels were probably due to increased Ig catabolism and decreased synthesis after steroid administration. To minimize side effects of the steroids, local corticosone was tried in infertile women with ASAB. The initial results revealed that this local treatment seemed to be promising.

Low dose therapy can be administered as follows:
i. Prednisone, 15 mg/day for a minimum of 3 months.
ii. Prednisone – 60 mg per day for 7-21 days.
iii. Dexamethasone–2-3 mg per day for 9-13 weeks.
   i.e. 20 mg BD from days 1–10–of their partners cycle followed by 5 mg on day 11 and day 12 (Hendry et al 1990).[23]

Steroids should be reserved for patients with long-term infertility and significant titers, after they are counseled regarding the risks of such treatment. Donor insemination is a clear option in severe or refractory cases of male ASAB.

Cyclosporin

Only a limited number of reports are available. None are placebo controlled.

Immunization with the Partner's Lymphocytes

A recent study has revealed that immunization by intradermal injection with 4×10^7 paternal lymphocytes collected from 30 mL of heparinized paternal whole blood separated on a Ficoll–Hypaque gradient, into the forearms of each patient four times at intervals of 2 to 4 weeks could significantly reduce the ASAB titers (Sugi, et al, 1993).[24] The mechanism of action may be partly explained by the increased concentration of suppressor T-cells and decreased levels of cytotoxic T-cells and B cells after immunotherapy. The clinical applications of this modality, however, require further elucidation.

In Vitro Sperm Processing

In vitro sperm processing consists of:
• Rapid dilution and washing of sperm
• Immunobinding on Mage's plate
• Immunomagnetic separation
• Addition of albumin to semen collection wells
• In vitro sperm capacitation

Diagnosis of Different Sperm-mucus Interaction

Disturbances

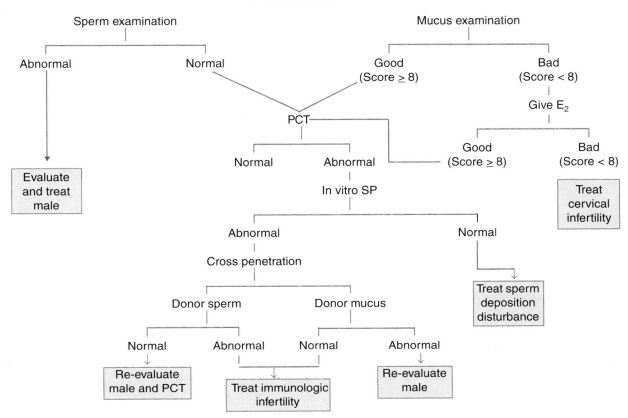

In vitro processing of semen to remove the antisperm antibodies is advocated on the presumption that spermatozoa become coated, with antibodies at the time of ejaculation.

Rapid dilution and washing of semen result in a variable decrease in IgG and/or IgA binding.

Immuno binding to Mage's plate is reported to be quite effective in increasing the proportion of antibody-free motile spermatozoa. An efficient selection of antibody-free spermatozoa can be achieved prior to "swim-up" migration by immuno-binding in polystyrene petri-dishes coated with purified anti-human Ig antibodies (Mage's plate). The obtained non-adherent sperm populations are depleted of 27-100 percent of IgG and IgA antibodies.

Immunomagnetic separation by incubation of semen with immunoglobulin–linked magnetic microspheres (Magnetic protaspheres,

Boehringer) helps to separate antibody-free sperm from antibody- coated sperm (Vigano P *et al*, 1991).[25] However, preliminary reports demonstrated that it worked only partially in the separation of IgA-bound spermatozoa, and failed to separate IgG coated spermatozoa. An immuno-column separation technique was developed to pass the diluted ejaculate through a column of dextran beads to allow the subsequent separation of antibody free sperm from antisperm antibodies coated sperm. The result of column processing revealed that not only did it increase sperm motility, but also significantly enhanced hamster egg penetration.

Adding 50 percent serum to semen sample collection wells, followed by rapid washing of the specimen, was suggested to increase the proportion of antibody free spermatozoa in the sample. A retrospective study has demonstrated that the addition of the serum to the collection device significantly improves both the oocyte fertilization and subsequent conception rate.

In vitro capacitation was carried out by incubating sperm in Tyrode's medium with 0.5 percent human serum albumin as the capacitation medium (Lenzi et al, 1992).[26]

Intrauterine Insemination (IUI)

Infertile women with cervical immunity to sperm can benefit from IUI. The pregnancy rates vary from 23 to 40 percent. If sperm autoimmunity is the only factor found, there is a nearly 80 percent chance that pregnancy will occur within the first two insemination attempts. Theoretically, although IUI overcomes the barrier of antibodies from cervical mucus, it cannot circumvent the damage that may be caused by antibodies in the uterine and tubal fluids.

In Vitro Fertilization and Embryo Transfer (IVF and ET)

IVF could be considered as a useful treatment for couples with immunological infertility. The sperm autoantibodies can interfere with fertilization, particularly when more than 80 percent of motile spermatozoa are antibody bound. Data suggest that IgA class antibodies may exert more deleterious effects on oocyte fertilization than IgG antibodies (Clarke et al, 1985). [27]

Gamete Intrafallopian Transfer (GIFT)

Vander Merwe [28] reported that by using the GIFT procedures with rapidly washed spermatozoa, pregnancy rate of 24.1 percent per cycle (7 of 29) can be achieved. GIFT brings the ova into direct contact with free-swimming spermatozoa, thereby excluding all the immunological barriers from the cervical mucus upwards.

Artificial Reproductive Techniques (ARTs)

In assisted fertilization, micromanipulation techniques have been gradually accepted in the treatment of patients with severe male factor and/ or low fertilization potential. Although the results of ASAB treated by these procedures are yet to be reported, the beneficial effects of bypassing the zona pellucida can be foreseen.

Treatment in GG Hospital

In our hospital, if the husband has even few sperms in the semen, we do not perform testicular biopsy as it can trigger the production of ASAB. When the wife suffers from ASAB we advise the couple to use barrier contraception (condom), except on the day of the ovulation, during when the couples are advised to have direct contact. Wymesone/Decdak (42 numbers of 0.5 mg tablets) is prescribed to be taken along with meals and not on empty stomach, and preferably with an antacid. They are taken as one tablet thrice a day for the first 7 days, and one tablet twice a day for the next 7 days and one tablet once a day for the next 7 days (total of 21 days) with one-week gap before the next course can start.

Husband is advised to start the tablets on the 21st day of the wife's menstrual cycle and the wife to start on the first day of the menstrual cycle.

Results and Discussion

		No of cases	Percentage
Peter R Brinsden	Bourn Hall Clinic	6000	25
Kamala Selvaraj et al	GG Hospital, Chennai	1000	15.6

It was also observed that ASAB were found to be the highest in the age group of 31 to 40 years (21%) in males and 20 to 30 years (17.8%) in females.

Correlation of ASAB and the Years of Married Life

SI	No. of years after marriage	No. of cases done	Percentage
1	1	2	–
2	2	6	16.6
3	3	7	14.3
4	4	38	21.0
5	5	38	13.0
6	6	32	6.3
7	7	28	10.7
8	8	44	18.2
9	9	47	23.4
10	10	45	26.7
11	Above 10	213	16.9

The percentage of positive cases starts increasing from four years and above of married life and doubles after eight years and above. This reveals that number of years of marriage also contributes for high titer of antisperm antibodies.

In our experience, prevalence of infertility is more in couples with the same blood groups, especially O&O, B&B and O&B. ASAB was also more marked in the couples with the same blood groups.

CONCLUSION

Immunological Infertility is a relatively new concept. The disorders discussed herein are the most common infertility conditions with known immunologic factors. It is now clear that this has a considerable role in the investigation and treatment of infertility. In this chapter we have tried to provide an indication of the laboratory tests which may be required and what treatment may help the infertile couples. With the increasing advent in scientific advances, more sophisticated tests will come into existence, thus helping us overcome all these problems.

Antisperm antibodies have been detected in the sera of infertile couples and their presence is reported to correlate with poor fertility rates. However, antisperm antibodies may also occur in proven fertile men. Thus, the clinical significance and predictive value of antisperm antibodies in infertility remains unclear.

REFERENCES

1. Micheal R Caudle. Current Therapy of Infertility, Reproductive Immunology 1988;3:46.
2. Rumpke P. The presence of sperm antibodies in the serum of two patients with oligozoospermia. Vox Sang (Basel) 1954;4:135-40.
3. Wilson L. Spermagglutinins in human semen and blood. Proceedings of the society of experimental biology and medicine 1954;85:652-55.
4. Koji Nakagawa, Shyuji Yamano. Quality of embryo does not affect the implantation rate of IVF-ET in infertile women with antisperm antibodies. Fert and ster, 1999;72:1055.
5. Anibal A Acosta, WR Yeh, Van Der Merwe. Ch. Antisperm Antibodies 2: Clinical aspects. Human Spermatozoa in Assisted Reproduction 1996;13:154.
6. Kaylen M Silverberg, Tom Turner. Ch. Evaluation of sperm. Textbook of assisted reproductive technologies David K Gardner et al (Eds.) 2001;69.
7. Golumb J, Vardinon N, Hommonai ZT et. al. Demonstration of antispermatozoal antibodies in variocele-related infertility with an enzyme linked immunosorbent assay (ELISA). Fertil steril 1986;45:397-405.
8. JMG Hollanders, JA Carver-Ward, KA Joroudi, E Meuleman, UV Sieck, SA Took. Male Infertility from A to Z, A concise encyclopedia, 1996;4(Aa):15-17.
9. Nancy J Alexander, Deborah J Anderson. Ch Immunology of Semen, Modern trends in infertility and conception control 1988;4(28):447.
10. Solter D, Schachner M. Brain and sperm cell surface antigen (NS-4) on pre-implantation mouse embryos. Dev Biol 1976;52:98.
11. Menge AC, Fleming CH. Detection of sperm antigens on mouse ova and early embryos. Dev Biol 1978;63:111.
12. Berkowitz RS, Alexander NJ, Goldstein DP, Anderson DJ. Reactivity of anti-human sperm monoclonal antibodies with normal placenta, hydatidiform mole and gestational choriocarcinoma. Gynecol Oncol 1985;22:334.
13. Gilula NB, Fawcett DW, Aoki A. The Sertoli cell occluding junctions and gap junctions in mature and developing mammalian testis. Dev Biol 1976;50:142.
14. Ritchie AWS, Hargreave TB, James K, Chisolm GD. Intraepithelial lymphocytes in the normal epididymis: A mechanism for tolerance to sperm auto-antigens? Br J Urol 1984;56:79.
15. Aygul Demirol, Erdal Aktan, Timur Gurgan. Ch. Current immunological assays. The ART and Science of ART. Gautam Allahbadia (Ed): 2003;295.
16. Yeh WR, Acosta AA, Van Der Merwe. Ch. Antisperm antibodies 2: Clinical aspects. Human spermatozoa in assisted reproduction. Anibal A Acosta, Thinus F Kruger (Eds): 1996;13(Table I and II):151-53.
17. Bulent Gulekli, Tim J Child, Seang Lin Tan. Ch Initial investigation of the patient. Textbook of assisted reproductive technologies. David K Gardner et al (Eds.) 2001;410.
18. Kremer J, Jager S. The sperm cervical mucus contact test: A preliminary report. Fertil Steril 1976;27:335-40.
19. Kibricks, Belding DL, Merrill B. Methods for the detection of antibodies against mammalian spermatozoa: Gelatin agglutination test. Fertil Steril 1952;3:419-38.
20. Friberg. A simple and sensitive micromethod for demonstration of sperm agglutinating activity in serum from infertile men and women. Acta obsterica gynaecologica scanlinavica 1974;36:21-29.
21. Anibal A Acosta, Thinus F Kruger. Ch. Antisperm antibodies 2: Clinical aspects. Human spermatozoa in

assisted reproduction (2nd edn.) (Figure 2, Table 4), 1996;152, 156, 157.

22. Franklin RR, Dukes CD. Antispermatozoal activity and unexplained infertility. Amer jour of obs and gyn 1964; 89:6-9.

23. Hendry WF, Hughes L, Scammell G, Pryor JP, Hargreave TB. Comparison of prednisolone and placebo in subfertile men with antibodies to spermatozoa. Lancet 1990;335:85.

24. Sugi T, Makino T, Maruyama T, Nozawa S, Iizuka R: Influence of immunotherapy on antisperm antibody titer in unexplained recurrent aborters. Am F Reprod Immunol 1993;29:95-99.

25. Vigano P, Fusi FM, Brigante C, Busacca M, Vignali M. Immunomagnetic separation of antibody-labelled from antibody-free human spermatozoa as a treatment for immunologic infertility. A preliminary report. Andrologia 1991;23:367-71.

26. Lenzi A, Gandini L, Lombardo F, Micara G, Culasso F, Dondero F. In vitro sperm capacitation to treat Antisperm antibodies bound to the sperm surface. Am F reprod. Immunol 1992;28:51-55.

27. Clarke GN, Lopata A, MC Bain JC, Baker HWG, Johnston WIH. Effect of sperm antibodies in males on human in vitro fertilization. Am F reprod Immunol 1985;8:62-66.

28. Van Der Merwe JP, Hulme VA, Kruger TF, Menkveld R, Windt ML. Treatment of male sperm autoimmunity by using the gamete intrafallopian transfer procedure with washed spermatozoa. Fertil Steril 1990;53: 682-87.

• Pratap Kumar

5

Unexplained Infertility

INTRODUCTION

The term "unexplained infertility" may be applied to a couple that has failed to establish a pregnancy despite an evaluation uncovering no obvious reason for infertility, or after correction of the factors identified as probably responsible for the infertility.[1] Unexplained infertility should be diagnosed only when ovulation has been established, tubes are patent, adequate sperm-cervical mucus interaction has been shown, with no evidence of endometriosis, adnexal adhesions or intrauterine pathology and the male partner has demonstrated normal sperm production.[2] It is commonly accepted that approximately 15 percent of couples will be determined to have unexplained infertility.

Four principles should be considered in developing a systematic approach to unexplained infertility.[1]

- Determination of whether the preceding evaluation of the couple with unexplained infertility was complete with reference to current diagnostic standards
- Re-evaluation of the results of all preceding diagnostic studies and observations to determine whether they were appropriately interpreted
- Awareness that any given factor considered normal and compatible with fertility at the onset of the diagnostic evaluation may change during the course of the work-up

- A realization that many of the processes necessary for conception are inaccessible for evaluation.

Chances of Conception and Age

With increasing awareness in the population that many types of infertility are amenable to treatment, there is a tendency for couples with short-term infertility to seek medical intervention at an earlier stage. Before labeling a couple as infertile, and accepting that any pregnancy achieved subsequent to their presentation at the clinic is due to treatment, it is essential to acknowledge that couples with unexplained infertility of one year's duration have a high chance of a spontaneous pregnancy over the next 12 months. It has been reported that pregnancy rates in normal couples with one year's infertility show an interesting variation in the percentage who achieved pregnancy which is related to age.[3]

A 20-year-old woman with one year infertility has a 76 percent chance of conceiving in the next 12 months. This chance of pregnancy decreases to 57 percent for a 30-year-old woman, is further reduced for a 40-year-old, but remains within the range of 40 percent in these older women.

Testing for Unexplained Infertility

The investigations required to make a diagnosis of unexplained infertility include ultrasound, ovulation confirmation, hysterosalpingogram or laparoscopy and a semen analysis. If no explanation for a couple's infertility is discovered after a standard evaluation, additional testing may be beneficial.

Semen Analysis and Fertilizing Capacity

Semen analysis does not provide adequate measurement of more subtle sperm functions. Unfortunately, further tests of sperm function are not widely available and their validity has been questioned, like that of the Hamster egg penetration test. Investigations have found no correlation between the Hamster egg penetration assays and fertilization or pregnancy rates following IVF.[4]

Recent guidelines published by the Royal College of Obstetricians and Gynecologists (RCOG) recommend that the essential investigations consist of semen analysis, midluteal serum progesterone levels and tubal patency test by hysterosalpingogram or laparoscopy.[5] The RCOG also recommends that there is no need for endometrial biopsy, postcoital tests, sperm function tests, detection of antisperm antibodies and hysteroscopy in routine investigation (Table 5.1). Although many of these investigations have been used in the management of infertility in the past, there is no definite evidence that they help to improve pregnancy rates in infertile couples. Therefore, cost-effective management of infertility precludes their use.

Embryo Development and Genetic Control

During the first two cleavage divisions, the embryo relies on the maternal mRNA produced during oogenesis. The new embryonic transcripts are thought to be activated during the 4-cell stage of development. This mechanism may, however, fail and be one of the factors for not achieving pregnancy.

Uterine Receptivity and Unexplained Infertility

A prospective controlled study[7] of 87 nulliparous women with unexplained infertility and 32 fertile and infertile parous controls was analyzed. Immunohistochemical staining was done for alpha 1, 4 and beta 3 integrin subunits in endometrial biopsies obtained during the window of implantation (days 20-24). All endometrial biopsies from parous controls contained positive immunostaining for the alpha 1 and beta 3 integrin subunits in glandular epithelium. In contrast, compared with parous controls, biopsies from women with unexplained infertility had significantly reduced beta 3 expression, with similar expression of alpha 1 and alpha 4 subunits. These findings suggest that defective uterine receptivity may be an unrecognized cause of infertility.

Blastocysts send signals to the mother which exert profound effects on maternal endocrinology and physiology. Human blastocysts secrete hCG *in vitro*, especially after hatching. Multiple factors are involved in initiating hCG secretion from blastocyst by day 7 to 8 *in vitro*, including insulin and platelet-derived growth factor.[8] Blastocysts can be divided as producers and nonproducers. Producers stimulate the uterine epithelium to produce integrin and nonproducers do not.[9] The absence/non-occurrence of these factors may contribute to unexplained infertility.

Molecular Control of the Implantation Window

The human endometrium is the end organ of the hypothalamo-pituitary-ovarian axis. Therefore, it

TABLE 5.1: Investigations for infertility—correlation with pregnancy rates[6]		
Established correlation with pregnancy	*Not consistently correlated with pregnancy*	*Not correlated dating with pregnancy*
1. Semen analysis	1. Postcoital test	1. Endometrial dating
2. Tubal patency via HSG/laparoscopy	2. Zona-free Hamster penetration test	2. Varicocele assessment
3. Midluteal serum progesterone	3. Cervical mucous penetration test	3. *Chlamydia* testing
	4. Hysteroscopy antisperm antibody assays	4. Falloposcopy

is susceptible to the changes during infertility treatment that originate from disturbances in the normal functioning of this axis. In addition, some cases of unexplained infertility may be due to altered endometrial function. This disturbed endometrial function may originate from lesions in the molecular repertoire that are crucial to implantation. The human endometrium becomes receptive to implantation by the blastocyst within a defined period during the menstrual cycle. The duration of this so-called "endometrial receptivity" or "implantation period" seems to span from few days after ovulation to several days prior to menstruation.[10] The members of the molecular repertoire that make endometrium receptive to implantation are gradually being recognized. Among these are the cytokines, integrins, heat shock proteins, and trophinin. In addition, the expression of a second set of genes including the tumor necrosis factor-alpha (TNF-alpha) may be the appropriate signal for the closure of the implantation window to make the endometrium refractory to implantation and to prepare it for menstrual shedding.

Finding markers of the receptive time in a woman's cycle understandably has become a priority. Numerous studies have indicated that the timing of implantation appears to extend from cycle day 20 through day 24. The use of integrins as markers of uterine receptivity has been further supported by the finding of aberrant B_3 expression in women with LPD and mild endometriosis.[11] Integrin expression in the uterus is highly regulated during implantation. The appearance and disappearance of two of the heterodimeric molecules frame the "implantation window." Alpha VB_3 (the vitronectin receptor) appears abruptly and reliably on day 6 postovulation. Alpha VB_1 (a fibronectin receptor) appears just after ovulation and persists until day 10. A defective expression of alpha VB_3 may be associated with infertility. A loss of VB_3 called type I infertility involves out-of-phase endometrium. Hence B_1 is active at ovulation and switched off at midcycle and B_3 is active at implantation.[12] This may also contribute to unexplained infertility. However, deficiency of any of these factors may cause unexplained infertility.

TREATMENT

The therapeutic approaches to unexplained infertility have ranged from simple reassurance to inspired empiricism. Anecdotal evidence is available that each form of therapy, conservative or aggressive is associated with some success but the beneficial effects claimed for investigations or treatments take little or no note of the possibility that the pregnancy might have occurred by chance.

In general terms, there are two approaches to the treatment of a couple with unexplained infertility:
- Increase the availability of gametes, e.g. ovulation induction
- Increase the proximity of gametes, e.g. IUI, IVF.

The principal treatments for unexplained infertility include expectant observation with superovulation, IUI (intrauterine insemination) and IVF (*in vitro* fertilization). One relatively inexpensive empirical therapy is IUI with washed sperm.

Expectant Management

The likelihood of pregnancy without treatment among couples with unexplained infertility is less than that of normal fertile couples but greater than zero.[13]

Role of Ovulation Induction

Ovulation induction is performed in patients with unexplained infertility as a dynamic test of ovarian reserve as well as concomitant treatment.

Clomiphene Citrate

The rationale behind giving clomiphene citrate to women with unexplained infertility is to overcome a subtle but as yet unknown defect or to increase the number of follicles available per cycle to augment the chances of conception. Treatment of apparently ovulating women with clomiphene citrate may result in the improvement of a subtle or unidentified defect in folliculogenesis or ovulation. The empiric use of clomiphene citrate has been evaluated in various studies. These studies involve comparisons of clomiphene citrate with placebo. A consistent doubling of pregnancy rates is seen in patients with unexplained infertility when clomiphene citrate and hMG is used.[14] The cost of therapy is much lower than with gonadotropins alone. Generally a 4 to 6 months trial of clomiphene citrate with IUI is justified in most patients with unexplained infertility.

Gonadotropins

In patients who have failed clomiphene citrate therapy or in older patients, human menopausal gonadotropin (hMG) is preferred to clomiphene citrate for superovulation because it promotes the development of a greater number of follicles.

Superovulation and IUI

In the past 10 to 15 years, there has been a marked increase in the use of superovulation with or without IUI, for the treatment of unexplained infertility. Both clomiphene citrate (CC) and human menopausal gonadotropin (hMG) have been used for superovulation. A randomized study of 21 couples with unexplained infertility attempted to assess the efficacy of IUI therapy.[15] The overall pregnancy rate after IUI was 11.9 percent per cycle or 20 percent per couple compared with only one pregnancy in 65 cycles using timed intercourse.

With respect to ovarian stimulation there are two explanations: (i) it may overcome a subtle defect in ovulatory function undiscovered by conventional testing and/or (ii) it may enhance the likelihood of pregnancy by increasing the number of eggs available for fertilization. According to the latter rationale, ovarian stimulation might improve the monthly pregnancy rate by simply increasing the number of oocytes available for fertilization and implantation. Along similar lines, increasing the density of motile sperm available to these eggs might further enhance the monthly probability of a pregnancy.

In couples who have failed with an adequate trial (usually 3 cycles) of CC and IUI, then hMG may be added. The use of hMG increases the number of preovulatory follicles over that in spontaneous cycles while avoiding the potentially antiestrogenic actions of clomiphene on the endometrium and cervical mucus. A retrospective analysis of 85 couples treated empirically with hMG/IUI therapy, included 22 percent with unexplained infertility and 65 percent with previously treated endometriosis.[16] After hMG stimulation, IUI was performed 36 to 40 hours after hCG was given. The cycle fecundity rate for idiopathic infertility was 19 percent. While comparing the results of IUI alone versus hMG with IUI, it was seen that the cycle fecundity rate was 19.3 percent with IUI versus 2.4 percent without it.[17]

In a meta-analysis[18] it was shown that the common odds ratio of achieving a pregnancy with the use of FSH and IUI was 2.37 (95% confidence interval (CI) 1.43 to 3.90) which was significantly better than with FSH and timed intercourse. Using a stepwise logistic regression analysis of the data from 5214 cycles in 22 trials in the same study, it was reported that the odds ratio for pregnancy with FSH use was 2.85 (95% CI, 2.18-3.66).

Clearly, IUI offers a significant advantage in the treatment of these patients. In a large randomized prospective controlled trial,[19] 932 study couples with unexplained infertility were analyzed in four groups: (i) intracervical insemination, (ii) IUI, (iii) superovulation and intracervical insemination and (iv) superovulation and IUI. The pregnancy rates in the four groups were 10 percent, 18 percent, 19 percent and 33 percent respectively. It was concluded that couples treated with superovulation and IUI were 3.2 times more likely to become pregnant when compared to couples in the intracervical insemination group (95% CI, 2.0-5.3). The couples treated with either IUI alone or with superovulation and intracervical insemination had nearly twice the pregnancy rates reported in the intracervical insemination only group.

In Vitro Fertilization and GIFT

A meta-analysis[20] concluded that the cycle fecundity rate was better with IVF (26%) when compared to controlled ovarian hyperstimulation with IUI (15%).

The most complex and expensive empiric therapies for unexplained infertility are IVF and

GIFT. IVF has an additional advantage when compared to GIFT of assessing fertilization as an additional test of unexplained infertility. In approximately 25 percent of patients with unexplained infertility, fertilization does not occur. Identification of these couples may allow other alternatives for therapy including the use of donor sperm, donor eggs or the use of zona drilling (assisted hatching) and microinjection techniques. Despite this high percentage of patients with fertilization problems, the overall pregnancy rate with IVF in couples with unexplained infertility is comparable to other diagnostic groups undergoing IVF. Pregnancy rates of 14 to 32 percent per cycle have been reported in couples with unexplained infertility.[21] Gamete Intra-fallopian Transfer (GIFT) has also been used in couples with unexplained infertility. However, in modern technology GIFT is losing its importance.

CONCLUSION

Unexplained infertility should be a diagnosis of exclusion. An adequate work-up of the infertile couple should be completed, though many biochemical events cannot be proved. Empirical therapy of a couple with unexplained infertility should progress through the least expensive and least invasive therapies to the more complex therapies. A trial of 3 to 4 cycles of ovulation induction and IUI with washed sperms, and finally IVF is a reasonable advice.

REFERENCES

1. Wallach EE, Moghissi K S. Unexplained infertility. In Behrman SJ, Kistner RW, Patton GW (Eds): Progress in Infertility (3rd edn), Little Brown and Co: Boston 799-819.
2. Williams SR. In Hammond MG, Talbert LM (Eds): Empiric Therapy of Unexplained Infertility: A Practical Guide for the Physician (3rd edn) Blackwell scientific: Oxford 211-20.
3. Wood C, Baker G, and Trounson A. Current status and future projects. In Wood C, Trounson A (Eds): Clinical In Vitro Fertilization, Springler—Verlag: Berlin 11-26.
4. Kuzan FB, Muller CH et al. Human sperm penetration assay as an indicator of sperm function in human in vitro fertilization. Fertil Steril 1987;48: 282.
5. Royal College of Obstetrician and Gynecologists. The Initial Investigation and Management of the infertile couple—Evidence based Clinical Guidelines 1998;2.
6. Crosignani PG, Collins J, Cooke ID et al. Unexplained infertility—the recommendation of the ESHRE workshop. Hum Repord 1993;8:977.
7. Lessey BA, Castelbaum AJ, Sawin SW et al. Integrin as markers of uterine receptivity in women with primary unexplained infertility. Fertil Steril 1995;63(3): 535-42.
8. Lopatea A, Oliva K. Chorionic gonadotropin secretion by human blastocysts. Hum Reprod 1993;8(6):932-38.
9. Edwards RG. New concepts in embryonic growth and implantation. Hum Reprod 1998;13(3):279.
10. Tabibzadeh S. Pattern of expression of integrins molecules in human endometrium throughout the menstrual cycle. Hum Reprod 1992;7:876-82.
11. Ilesanmi AO, Hawkins DA, Lessey BA. Immunohistochemical markers of uterine receptivity in the human endometrium. Microsc Res Tech 1993;25: 208-22.
12. Lessey BA, Castelbaum AJ, Saurin SJ et al. Aberrant integrin expression in the endometrium integrin expression in the endometrium of women with endometriosis. J Clin Endocrinol Metab 1994;79: 643-49.
13. Guzick DS, Sullivan MW, Adamson GD et al. Efficacy of treatment for unexplained infertility. Fertil Steril 1998;70(2):207-13.
14. Daftary G, Taylor HS. The use of ovulation induction in the treatment of unexplained infertility. Infertil Repro 2000;11(3):385-98.
15. Martinex AR, Bernardus RE. Intrauterine insemination does not clomiphene does not improve fecundity in couples with infertility due to male or idiopathic factors—a prospective randomized, controlled study. Fertil Steril 1990;53:847.
16. Dodson WC, Whitesides DB, Hughes CL et al. Superovulation with intrauterine in the treatment of infertility—a possible alternative to gamete intrafallopian transfer and in vitro fertilization. Fertil Steril 1987;48:441.
17. Nulsen JC, Walsh S, Dumez S et al. A randomized and longitudinal study of human menopausal gonadotropin with intrauterine insemination in the treatment of infertility. Obstet Gynecol 1993;82:780.
18. Hughes EG. The effectiveness of ovulation induction and intrauterine insemination in the treatment of persistent infertility—a meta-analysis. Hum Reprod 1997;12:1865.
19. Guzick DS, Carson SA, Coutifaris C et al. Efficacy of superovulation and intrauterine insemination in the treatment of infertility. N Engl J Med 1999;340:177.
20. Peterson CM, Hatasaka HH, Jones et al. Ovulation induction with gonadotropins and intrauterine insemination compared with in vitro fertilization and no therapy—a prospective non-randomized cohort study and meta-analysis. Fertil Steril 1994;62:535.
21. Audibert F, Hendon B et al. Results of IVF attempts in patients with unexplained infertility. Human Reprod 1989;4:766.

• Jatin P Shah

6

Declining Fertility

The past decade has seen numerous reports in literature implying a significant deterioration of semen quality in the form of reduced sperm concentration, impaired motility and increased abnormal forms of spermatozoa. Extensive coverage of these reports in both medical, as well as lay literature has sparked off what is probably the controversy of the century. The issue is of vital importance because if proven to be true, it threatens the very existence and continuation of the human species. A preliminary review of literature in the fields of medicine, chemical and pharmaceutical industry and environmental science indicates that this deterioration is probably a genuine occurrence and may have alarming implications for the human race.

It was Carlson[1] in 1992, who first reported his study showing evidence of decreasing semen quality in the past 50 years. Linear regression of data weighted by number of men in each study showed a significant decrease in mean sperm count from 113 million/mL in 1940 to 66 million/mL in 1990 (p < 0.0001) and in seminal volume from 3.4 to 2.75 mL (p 0.027), indicating an even more pronounced decrease in sperm production than expressed by decline in sperm density. The biological significance of these changes in emphasized by a concomitant increase in the incidence of genitourinary abnormalities such as testicular cancer and possibly also cryptorchidism and hypospadias, suggesting a growing impact of factors with serious effects on male gonadal

function. This was followed by McLeod's[2] 10 years study in the USA published in 1979, which had reported no such change. The group from Copenhagen postulated that the remarkable increase in frequency of testicular abnormalities over a relatively short period of time might be due to environmental rather than genetic factors. There is an epidemiological link between the occurrences of different testicular abnormalities. Therefore, common prenatal influences may also have a deleterious effect on male fertility. Carlsen's report received extensive coverage in the international press and issue captured popular imagination. Although subsequent studies[3-9] from Europe corroborated Carlsen's findings, a large study from the USA by Fisch *et al*[10] in 1996, from three prominent semen banks showed no decline in sperm counts over a 25 years period in 1,283 men. Similarly, Benshushan from Israel in 1997 showed that during the past 15 years there has actually been an increase in total motile sperm count, secondary to an increase in semen volume, and a decline in normal morphology that is independent of the age and duration of abstinence in fertile men. Others in the field, without quoting actual data criticized the popular reports of semen deterioration on statistical grounds claiming that the quadratic and spline-fit models would fit the data better than the linear regression model used by Carlsen's group.[11] Variations in methodology of semen collection, counting and differences in the duration of abstinence were other reasons quoted for the alarming results.[12] The Indian reports, both from the Institute for Research in Reproduction, Mumbai and from Mehta *et al*,[13] Bangalore seem to agree with this declining trend of semen quality over the years. ART experts from urban centers also find an overall decline in male fertility over the past two decades. The implications are serious and urgent measures, both investigative and corrective are required to tackle this problem, which could threaten our very existence.

Investigators far unanimously agree that this decline is due to an increased estrogenic influence in our day-to-day life. Sharpe and Skakkeback[14] have gone on record to state that modern day humans now live in a virtual sea of estrogens. Dietary fads and fashions, increased consumption of dairy produce and Soya all promote increased enterohepatic circulation of estrogens resulting in increased endogenous estrogens. Synthetic estrogens may have increased through use of oral contraceptives by women and orally active anabolic steroids in the livestock. Also, the increasing prevalence of obesity, implying greater extragonadal conversion of androgens into estrogens might contribute to this pool of endogenous estrogen.[15] Chemicals and pesticides such as organophosphorus compounds, combustion end products and biodegradation resistant chemicals such as dichlorodiphenyltrichloroethane and polychlorinated biphenyls invariably present in the food chain contribute to the pool of exogenous estrogens.[14] Besides these exogenous and endogenous estrogens, the fast pace of modern life, stress, smoking, sexually transmitted diseases and contraceptives have all contributed to this deterioration.

The epidemiological aspect of this decreasing trend in sperm counts has to be studied worldwide. Even within various centers there are reports of geographical variations within regions. The implications of these geographical variations with regard to etiology are worth exploring. Some workers have attributed these variations to environmental nutrition and other causes. Others have attributed it to difference in protocol of analysis and yet others have stated that these differences may be inherent. The need of the day is to initiate large scale prospective studies using standardized analytical methods, unbiassed selection accounting for differences in race, age, socioeconomic status, urbanization, ethnicity, medical and reproductive history, lifestyle patterns and occupation to establish prima facie that the problem is real. Possible environmental factors and dietary changes need to be investigated and corrected. Estrogenic influences, both exogenous and endogenous need to be reduced. This would imply large-scale research in the fields of agriculture, chemical and pesticide industries and nutrition. Most of the etiologies regarding this decline in sperm counts have remained at a stage of hypothesis. There is a need to verify numerous postulates. This will include pharmacokinetic studies in xenobiotics, study of the effects of various synthetic estrogens like hormonal contraceptives on human and use of anabolic steroids on the livestock. Study of dietary estrogenic influences like obesity, low fiber diet and phytoestrogens on fertility should be undertaken. This will also include a thorough review of veterinary medicine for the effect of global environmental factors on animal fertility.

Until such time that corrective measures are implemented on a large-scale basis, assisted reproduction continues to offer renewed hope to many infertile men. Recent advances in the field of *in vitro* fertilization and embryo transfer (IVF-ET) and intracytoplasmic sperm injection (ICSI) make certain that the propagation of the species continues in spite of the decline in sperm quality. Today, ICSI remains the last and often first resort for most cases of severe male infertility. Successful pregnancies and live births have been reported with ICSI using ejaculated sperm, sperm retrieved from the epididymis (MESA), sperm retrieved from the testes (TESA), sperm obtained by electroejaculation and more recently even late spermatids. On the horizon we have the prospects of germ cell injection into a mature oocyte for obtaining a pregnancy.

REFERENCES

1. Carlsen E, Givercman A, Keiding N et al. Evidence for decreasing quality of semen during past 50 years. Br Med J 1992;305:609-13.

2. McCleod J, Wang Y. Male fertility potential in terms of semen quality—a review of the past, as study of the present. Fertil Steril 1979;31:103.
3. James WH. Secular trend in reported sperm counts. Andrologia 1980;12:381.
4. Leto S, Frensilli FJ. Changing parameters of donor semen. Fertil Steril 1981;36:766.
5. Farrow S. Falling sperm quality—fact or fiction? Br Med J 1994;309:1.
6. Ginsburg J, Okolo S, Prelevic G et al. Residence in the London area and sperm density. Lancet 1994;343:230.
7. Irwine DS. Falling sperm quality (letter). Br Med J 1994;309:476.
8. Van Waeleghem K, De Clereq M, Vermeulen L, Schoonjans F et al. Deterioration of semen quality in young Belgian men during recent decades (Abstract) Hum Reprod 1994;9(Suppl 4):73.
9. Givercman A. Declining semen quality and increasing incidence of abnormalities of male reproductive organs—fact or fiction? Hum Reprod 1995;10(Suppl 1):158.
10. Fisch H, Goluboff ET, Olson JH et al. Semen analyses in 1283 men from the United States over a 25 years period: No decline in quality. Fertil Steril 1995;63:887.
11. Olsen GW, Bodner KM, Ramlow JM et al. Have sperm counts been reduced 50 per cent in fifty years? A statistical model revisited. Fertil Steril 1995;63:887.
12. Bromwich P, Cohen J, Stewart I et al. Decline in sperm counts: An artefact of changed reference range of "normal"? BMJ 1994;309:19.
13. Mehta RH, Anand Kumar TC. Declining semen quality in Bangaloreans: A preliminary report. Curr Sci 1997;72:621.
14. Sharpe RM, Skakkebaek NE. Are estrogens involved in falling sperm counts and disorders of the male reproductive tract? Lancet 1993;341:1392.
15. Verdeal K, Ryan DS. Naturally occurring estrogens in plant foodstuffs—a review. J Food Prot 1979;7:577.

Section 2

Endocrinological Disorders of Infertility

• Kamini A Rao • Arati R Rao

7

Hyperprolactinemia and Thyroid Disorders

HYPERPROLACTINEMIA

PROLACTIN—THE HORMONE

Since it was first identified in 1971, much information has been gathered about prolactin–its physiology, functions and the control of its synthesis and release.[1]

Chemical Composition

Prolactin is a protein (197–199 amino acids) product of the anterior pituitary. Chemically similar to growth hormone and human placental lactogen; it has a molecular weight of 24000 Daltons.

A single gene located on Chromosome 5 encodes it for prolactin synthesis and function.

Three types of prolactin have been identified based on differences in size and structural modifications that are the result of glycosylation, phosphorylation, additions and deletions–little, big and big big prolactin (Figure 7.1) The importance of this is that the varying forms are associated with different bioactivity and immunoactivity–e.g. little prolactin has more biological activity than the bigger forms.

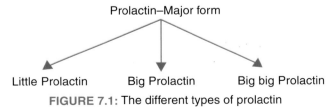

Prolactin–Major form

Little Prolactin   Big Prolactin   Big big Prolactin
FIGURE 7.1: The different types of prolactin

Sites of Secretion

Prolactin is secreted by the acidophils of the anterior pituitary. A glycosylated form of the hormone is secreted by the endometrium in the luteal phase and by the decidua of pregnancy.[2-4]

Ectopic secretion though rarely seen, has been found to be associated with pituitary tissue in the pharynx, bronchogenic carcinoma, renal cell carcinoma, gonadoblastomas and ovarian dermoid tumors.[5, 6]

Control of Secretion

This is the only pituitary hormone whose control is mainly inhibitory; the main factor involved is Dopamine–released by the hypothalamus into the portal system. Prolactin secretion is inhibited and stimulated by the association and dissociation of dopamine from its receptors (D2) on the acidophils.[7]

Estrogen increases prolactin synthesis, while Serotonin and Thyrotropin Releasing Hormone [TRH] stimulate prolactin release. Other factors involved include angiotensin II, vasopressin, growth factors, Vasoactive Intestinal Peptide (VIP), etc.

Pattern of Secretion

Prolactin secretion follows a circadian rhythm, with the maximum secretion 5 to 8 hrs after the onset of sleep. At all times though, the release is pulsatile; with the frequency of pulses becoming maximum midcycle, and then declining in the luteal phase.

Functions

The primary function of Prolactin is to enhance breast development in pregnancy, and to induce lactation after delivery. In addition, by binding to specific receptors in the gonads, lymphoid cells and liver–it affects fertility, immunity and liver functions.

Normal Values

Normal serum Prolactin is generally less than 30 ng/ml; though there may be individual inter-laboratory variations.

Hyperprolactinemia

Hyperprolactinemia, a condition characterized by elevated serum Prolactin levels, is the most common endocrine disorder of the hypothalamo-pituitary axis. It could result from a variety of conditions both physiological and pathological. The prevalence varies from less than 1 percent of the general population, to almost 17 percent in women with reproductive disorders.[8]

TABLE 7.1: Etiology of hyperprolactinemia

Physiological	Pathological
REM sleep	Tumors-prolactinoma
Pregnancy	Hypothalamic/pituitary lesions
Nipple stimulation	Idiopathic
Stress	Polycystic ovarian disease
Coitus	Hypothyroidism
	Chest wall injury
	Renal failure
	Liver failure
	Drugs-dopamine analogs
	Phenothiazines
	Estrogens
	Opiates
	Cimetidine
	Methyldopa
	Reserpine

Effect on Female Reproductive Function

Prolactin has a significant effect on the female reproductive function by acting on the hypo-thalamo-pituitary-ovarian axis. In addition, it has a direct action on the ovaries, which is supposed to be responsible for the menstrual irregularities associated with hyperprolactinemia; probably regulating ovarian steroidogenesis by its actions on the aromatase enzyme.[9]

It is interesting to note that the action of prolactin on the ovaries varies in the different phases of the menstrual cycle.[10]

In the follicular phase, elevated prolactin levels can disrupt normal follicular development, cause atresia of the dominant follicle and inhibit ovulation.[11,12] On the other hand, the role of prolactin in the luteal phase is not very clear, as it is supposed to both stimulate (by inducing LH receptor formation) and inhibit corpus luteal function (by inhibiting corpus luteal steroido-genesis).[13,14] Animal experiments have found that elevated prolactin levels can induce the develop-ment of adenomyosis—a condition characterized by the implantation or extension of the endometrial glands into the myometrium.[15] This could be another mechanism, apart from ovulatory dysfunction that could cause the infertility associated with hyperprolactinemia.

TABLE 7.2: Effect of hyperprolactinemia on female reproductive function

1. Disrupts normal follicular development
2. Atresia of the dominant follicle
3. Inhibits aromatase enzyme
4. Inhibits progesterone synthesis by the corpus luteum
5. Premature destruction of the corpus luteum
6. Induces uterine adenomyosis

Effect on Male Reproductive Function

As in the female, prolactin has a significant effect on male reproductive function too. By acting on the hypothalamo-pituitary-gonadal axis, it affects

TABLE 7.3: Effect of hyperprolactinemia on male reproductive function

1. Inhibits pulsatile LH release by the anterior pituitary
2. Reduces testosterone synthesis
3. Inhibits 5-alpha reductase activity
4. Structural changes in the testes–Germ cell exfoliation
    Disorganization of seminpherous tubules
    Increased tubule wall thickness
    Lipid accumulation in Leydig cells

not only gonadal and accessory reproductive glands functions, but sexual behavior too.

Hyperprolactinemia is associated with reduced testosterone levels—by inhibiting the pulsatile release of LH from the anterior pituitary and by inhibiting 5-alpha reductase adversely affects spermatogenesis, apart from causing structural changes in the testes.[16-18]

Prolactin related infertility has been classified into primary and secondary disorders (Table 7.4).

Primary disorders are those associated with a basic defect in prolactin metabolism—such as excess synthesis as seen in prolactin secreting tumors. The hyperprolactinemia in these cases is primarily responsible for the associated infertility.

Secondary disorders include conditions such as the polycystic ovarian disease and primary hypothyroidism. Here, the hyperprolactinemia is incidental and not the cause of the infertility.[19, 20]

TABLE 7.4: Classification of prolactin related infertility

Primary	Secondary
Prolactinomas	Polycystic ovarian disease
Empty Sella Syndrome	Primary hypothyroidism
Functional	Drug induced
Idiopathic	

Prolactinomas and Infertility

Prolactinomas are the commonest pituitary adenomas; arbitarily classified into microadenomas—size less than 10mm and macroadenomas-size more than 10 mm.

Infertility in a patient with a prolactinoma is generally due to the accompanying hyperprolactinemia rather than to the tumor size—except in massive lesions.

Diagnosis

As Prolactin is a dynamic hormone that responds readily to a variety of stimuli, caution must be exercised during diagnosis.

Women typically present with a history of amenorrhea, oligomenorrhea or infertility. Occasionally galactorrhea may be the only presenting symptom.

Men typically present with complaints of sexual dysfunction, decreased libido, impotence, gynecomastia and infertility.

Both sexes may present with visual field defects and headaches—if associated with a pituitary tumor.[21]

TABLE 7.5: Common presenting symptoms in prolactin related disorders

1. Amenorrhea
2. Oligomenorrhea
3. Galactorrhea
4. Unexplained infertility
5. Headache
6. Visual field defects
7. Symptoms of hypothyroidism
8. Drug intake
9. Decreased libido

The physical finding most commonly encountered with hyperprolactinemia is galactorrhea. Occasionally visual field defects may be detected.

Typically, a definitive diagnosis can only be made with laboratory studies.

While making the diagnosis of hyperprolactinemia (as indicated by serum prolactin levels more than 30 ng/ml), is relatively easy; the difficulty lies in identifying the underlying cause.

Patients with modest prolactin elevations should have multiple serum assays in order to minimize the potential for detecting only transient/physiological increases in prolactin. A detailed medication history is essential, and the presence of hypothyroidism, renal failure, or hepatic dysfunction should be evaluated. If the cause of hyperprolactinemia remains ambiguous, a computed tomography (CT) scan or magnetic resonance imaging (MRI) study should be performed to determine the presence of a pituitary tumor. If an underlying cause of elevated prolactin serum concentration is not determined, the hyperprolactinemia is considered to be idiopathic.

TABLE 7.6: Adjuvant investigations in a case of hyperprolactinemia

1. Serum TSH
2. Blood urea nitrogen
3. Serum creatinine
4. Liver function tests
5. Visual field testing
6. CT
7. MRI

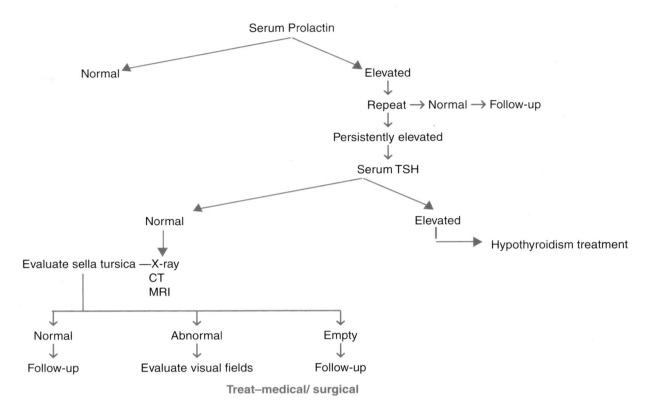

FIGURE 7.2: Flow chart for the assessment of hyperprolactinemia

Serum prolactin is usually measured in the morning, after an overnight or at least 8 to 10 hrs of fasting, as the concentration can be affected by food intake.

A single elevated reading should be reconfirmed because of the known erratic pattern of secretion of this hormone.

Once the diagnosis of hyperprolactinemia has been made, the sella tursica and pituitary and thyroid gland functions should be evaluated.

However, there is no consensus on when radiological investigations should be done.[22] Some recommend that a CT or MRI should be done in all patients diagnosed to have hyperprolactinemia, while others suggest that these investigations need be done only when serum Prolactin exceeds 100 ng/ml or there are definite symptoms and signs of an intracranial space-occupying lesion. This is based on studies, which have shown that serum concentrations of more than 100 ng/ml are almost diagnostic of a pituitary microadenoma; lower concentrations (< 100 ng/ml) have only a 20 percent risk of having a tumor.[23]

Treatment

The treatment of hyperprolactinemia depends upon the underlying cause.

In cases of drug-induced hyperprolactinemia, the offending drug should be discontinued and appropriate therapeutic alternatives should be instituted. In case alternatives do not exist, then medical therapy with dopamine agonists may be warranted.

An associated or underlying primary hypothyroidism should be corrected by the replacement of thyroid hormone.

Prolactinomas on the other hand can be managed by observation, medical therapy, irradiation or surgery.

Medical Therapy

Medical therapy with dopamine agonists has proven to be very effective in normalizing serum Prolactin levels, restoring menstruation and fertility and reducing tumor size in 70 to 90 percent of patients within 3 to 6 months of initiating treatment.

TABLE 7.7: Drugs used in the treatment of hyperprolactinemia			
Drug	*Route*	*Dosage*	*Frequency*
Bromocriptine	Oral	2.5 to 10 mg	8th hrly
Bromocriptine (slow release)	Oral	5 to 15 mg	Daily
Bromocriptine (long acting)	IM	50 to 75 mg	Monthly
Pergolide	Oral	50 to 100 microgms	Daily
Cabergoline	Oral	400 to 3000 microgms	Weekly

Serum prolactin levels should be assessed once in 3 to 4 weeks of initiating therapy. This would not only indicate efficacy, but also help to appropriately titrate the medication dosage. In addition, symptoms such as headache, visual defects, menstruation and sexual function in males should be evaluated to assess clinical response to treatment. Once serum prolactin levels have normalized, evaluation may be done once in 6 to 12 months.

Bromocriptine–is the first dopamine receptor agonist introduced for the treatment of hyperprolactinemia; it is a strong D2 receptor agonist with a partial affinity to D1 receptors. Therapy with bromocriptine normalizes prolactin serum concentrations, restores gonadotropin production, and shrinks tumor size in approximately 90 percent of patients with prolactinomas.

Treatment is typically initiated at 1.25 to 2.5 mg once daily at bedtime to minimize adverse effects. The dose can be gradually increased by 1.25 mg increments every week to obtain desirable serum prolactin concentrations. Usual therapeutic doses of bromocriptine range from 2.5 to 15 mg per day, although some patients may require doses as high as 40 mg per day. Bromocriptine is usually administered in two or three divided doses, but once-daily dosing has also been shown to be effective.

The most common adverse effects associated with bromocriptine therapy include central nervous system symptoms such as headache, lightheadedness, dizziness, nervousness, and fatigue. Gastrointestinal effects such as nausea, abdominal pain, and diarrhea are also common.

An important aspect is the use of bromocriptine in pregnancy, although, it does not appear to be teratogenic,[24] some clinicians discontinue therapy as soon as pregnancy is detected because the effects of in-utero exposure to bromocriptine on gonadal function and fertility of the offspring remains to be determined. More recent studies have shown a beneficial effect of bromocriptine in the management of recurrent miscarriages. In some patients with macroprolactinomas undergoing rapid tumor expansion, bromocriptine therapy must be continued throughout pregnancy.

Bromocriptine should be administered with food to reduce the incidence of adverse gastrointestinal effects. Although most of these adverse effects diminish with continued treatment, about 12 percent of patients will not tolerate the adverse effects associated with bromocriptine therapy.

New extended-release dosage forms of bromocriptine are being investigated to improve tolerability and compliance. These include a long-acting injectable form of bromocriptine, which can be administered as monthly intramuscular injections in doses of 50 to 75 mg, and a slow-release oral formulation that is given as a single daily dose of 5 to 15 mg. Vaginal preparations of bromocriptine are also being studied in an effort to decrease the incidence of adverse effects associated with oral dosage forms.

Pergolide is a dopamine receptor agonist with an affinity for both D1 and D2 receptors.

Pergolide therapy is initiated at a dose of 25 to 50 µg given once daily at bedtime.

The adverse effects of pergolide are similar to those of bromocriptine and include nausea, headache, vomiting, and dizziness in about 30 percent of patients.

The use of pergolide during pregnancy has not been evaluated as extensively as with bromocriptine and should be avoided until additional data become available.

Cabergoline: is a long acting dopamine receptor agonist with high specificity and affinity for the

D2 receptors. It has been shown to effectively reduce serum prolactin concentrations in 80-90 percent of hyperprolactinemic patients. This drug is often used when patients cannot tolerate the side effects or are non-responsive to bromo-criptine.

The initial dose of cabergoline for the treatment of hyperprolactinemia is 0.5 mg once weekly or in divided doses twice weekly. This dose may be increased by increments of 0.5 at 4-week intervals based on serum prolactin concentrations. The usual dose is 1-2 mg weekly; however, doses as high as 4.5 mg weekly have been used.

The most common adverse effects reported with the use of cabergoline are nausea, vomiting, headache, and dizziness–these are similar to those seen with bromocriptine only the incidence is about 3 percent when compared to the 12 percent associated with bromocriptine therapy. Other side effects include drowsiness, fatigue, paresthesias, dyspnea, suffocation sensation, epistaxis and orthostatic hypotension.

The use of cabergoline in pregnancy has not been extensively studied. However, several case reports of women who received cabergoline therapy during the first and second trimesters of pregnancy have not documented an increased risk of spontaneous abortion, congenital abnor-malities, or tubal pregnancy. However, due to the long half-life and limited data on cabergoline use in pregnancy, most clinicians recommend that women receiving cabergoline therapy who plan to become pregnant should discontinue the medication one month before planned conception.

Surgery

Trans-sphenoidal surgical resection is one of the earliest known modalities of treatment for pituitary adenomas.

Complications of surgery are few and mortality is rare, however, long-term studies have shown that there will be a substantial risk or recurrence of the hyperprolactinemia and occasionally of the tumor itself.[25]

General indications for pituitary surgery include patient drug intolerance, tumors resistant to medical therapy, patients who have persistent visual defects despite adequate medical treatment and those with large cystic or hemorrhagic tumors or who experience pituitary apoplexy.[26]

Radiotherapy

Irradiation by means of external (linear cobalt or proton beam therapy) and internal (yttrium as pituitary implants) modalities has been used in the management of prolactinomas. Probably the only indication for radiotherapy today is the presence of persistent disease following surgery and in rapidly growing tumors; the benefits do not outweigh the risks in routine treatment.

The main disadvantage apart from poor, delayed and inconsistent results is the risk of damaging the surrounding structures and the potential to cause hypopituitarism.

Treatment of Prolactinomas

Options available for the treatment of Prolac-tinomas include observation, medical and surgical modalities.

Medical therapy is the initial treatment of choice–with bromocriptine being used as the first line drug. This is probably due to its efficacy and safety profile.[27] Some studies have described the benefit of Cabergoline over Bromocriptine in terms of biochemical response, tumor shrinkage and the occurrence of side effects.[28]

Surgery may be required especially for macro-adenomas and microadenomas which are not responsive to medical therapy

Hyperprolactinemia is a frequent cause of anovulatory sterility, although spontaneous pregnancy may occur occasionally. Available treatment options for this disorder include medical therapy with dopamine agonists, radiation therapy, and transphenoidal surgery. In most cases, medical therapy is considered the most effective treatment, and bromocriptine has been the mainstay of therapy. Cabergoline, a new dopamine agonist, appears to be better tolerated than bromocriptine and is at least as effective if not more effective than bromocriptine. This form of treatment is highly effective for both idiopathic and tumoral hyperprolactinemia. If the only cause of infertility is chronic anovulation due to hyperprolactinemia, a 60-80 percent pregnancy rate can be achieved with medical therapy alone.

REFERENCES

1. Moult PJ, Besser G. Prolactin and gonadal function. IPPF Med Bull 1981;15(4):3-4.
2. Malsar IA, Riddick DH. Prolactin production by human endometrium during the normal menstrual cycle. Am J Obstet Gynecol 1979;135:751.
3. Malsar IA, Ansbacher R. Effects of Progesterone on decidual prolactin production by organ cultures of human endometrium. Endocrinology 1986;118:2102.
4. Daly DC et al. Evidence of short loop inhibition of decidual prolactin synthesis by decidual proteins. Parts I and II, Am J Obstet Gynecol 1986;155:358-63.
5. Lloyd RV, Chandlre WF et al. Ectopic pituitary adenomas with normal anterior pituitary glands. Am J Surg Path 1986;10:56.
6. Palmer PE et al. Prolactinoma in the wall of an ovarian dermoid cyst with hyperprolactinemia. Obstet Gynecol 1990;75:540.
7. Martinez de la Escalera G, Weiner RI et al. Dissociation of dopamine from its receptors as a signal in the pleiotropic hypothalamic regulation of prolactin secretion. Endocrinol Review 1992;13:241.
8. Biller BM, Luciano A, Crosignani PG, Molitch M, Olive D, Rebar R, Sanfilippo J, Webster J, Zacur H. Guidelines for the diagnosis and treatment of hyperprolactinemia. J Reprod Med 1999;44(12 Suppl):1075-84.
9. Martikainen H et al. Prolactin suppression by bromocryptine stimulates the aromatization of testosterone to Estradiol in women. Fertil Steril, 1989.
10. Kaupilla A et al. Hyperprolactinemia and ovarian function. Fertil Steril 1988;49:437.
11. Siebel MM et al. Periovulatory follicular fluid hormone levels in spontaneous human cycles. J Clin Endocrinol Metab 1989;68:1073.
12. Mc Natty KP et al. The relationship between plasma prolactin and the endocrine microenvironment of the developing human antral follicle. Fertil Steril 1979;32:43.
13. Wang C et al. Prolactin inhibition of Estrogen production by cultured rat granulose cells. Mol Cel Endocrinol 1980;20:136.
14. Tan G J S et al. Effects of prolactin on steroid production by human luteal cells in vitro. J Endocrinol 1983;96:499.
15. Mori T et al. Animal model of uterine adenomyosis–is prolactin a potent inducer of adenomyosis in mice? Am J Obstet Gynecol 1991;165:232.
16. Murray FT et al. Return of gonadal function in men with prolactin secreting pituitary tumors. J Clin Endocrinol Metab. 1984;59:79.
17. Bartke A et al. Influence of prolactin and pituitary isografts on spermatogenesis in dwarf mice and hypophysectomised rats. J Endocrinol 1982;46:321.
18. Katovich MT et al. Alterations of testicular functions induced by hyperprolactinemia in rats. J Androl 1985;6:179.
19. Keye WR et al. Prolactin secreting pituitary adenomas, similar frequency and diagnosis of menorrhoea-galactorrhoea. JAMA 1980;244:1329.
20. Blackwell RE et al. Report of the National Symposium on the clinical management of prolactin related reproductive disorders. Fertil Steril 1986;45:606.
21. Luciano AA. Clinical presentation of hyperprolactinemia. J Reprod Med 1999;44(12 Suppl):1085-90.
22. Molitch M et al. Evaluation and treatment of the patient with pituitary incindentaloma. J Clin Endocrinol Metab 1995;80:3.
23. Blackwell RE et al. Assessment of pituitary function in patients with serum prolactin > 100 ng/ml. Fertil Steril 1979;32:177.
24. Turklaj T et al. Surveillance of bromocriptine in pregnancy. JAMA 1982;247:1599.
25. Serri O et al. Recurrence of hyperprolactinemia after selective trans-sphenoidal adenomectomy in women with prolactinomas. NJEM 1983;209:280.
26. Biller BM. Diagnostic evaluation of hyperprolactinemia. J Reprod Med 1999;44(12 Suppl):1095-99.
27. Molitch ME. Medical management of prolactin-secreting pituitary adenomas. Pituitary 2002;5(2):55-65.
28. Colao A et al. Dopamine receptor agonists for treating prolactinomas. Expert Opin Investig Drugs 2002;11(6):787-800.

THYROID DISORDERS
IN INFERTILITY

Thyroid disorders–both hypo- and hyperthyroidism are known to have a profound effect on pregnancy and reproduction.

HYPERTHYROIDISM

The effect of severe hyperthyroidism on the fertility potential of an individual is well documented, but the effects of the mild and moderate forms of this disorder are not very clear.[1]

The etiology of hyperthyroidism could be due to a variety of causes, some are listed in the Table 7.8 below.

TABLE 7.8: Etiology of hyperthyroidism
1. Graves disease
2. Solitary toxic nodule
3. Toxic multi nodular goiter
4. Acute thyroiditis–Viral
a. Autoimmune
b. Post-radiotherapy
5. Thyrotoxicosis facititia
6. Exogenous iodine administration
7. Metastatic differentiated thyroid carcinoma
8. TSH secreting tumors
9. HCG secreting tumors
10. Hyperfunctioning ovarian teratomas

Hyperthyroidism and Female Fertility

Elevated thyroxine concentrations lead to increased levels of the sex hormone binding globulin (SHBG). This, in turn, accounts for the raised concentrations of Estradiol and Testosterone in the blood. Apart from this, the follicular phase baseline serum FSH and LH concentrations are also increased with an attenuated mid-cycle LH surge. Consequently, oligovulatory or anovulatory cycles with a wide range of menstrual disorders (ranging from amenorrhea to menometrorrhagia) may be seen.

Hyperthyroidism and Male Fertility

As in the female, the elevated thyroxin concentrations is responsible for increased levels of sex hormone binding globulin, which in turn accounts for the higher serum estradiol and testosterone concentrations. As the estradiol is less "bound" to the SHBG, the bio-availability is higher–resulting in a relatively hyper-estrogenic state in these men; manifested by gynecomastia, spider angiomas, decreased libido and impaired sperm parameters–mainly sperm motility.[2,3]

Diagnosis

The diagnosis of hyperthyroidism is based upon clinical findings and serological assays.

Assessment of the clinical manifestations (Table 7.9) would give a reasonable indication to the presence of the disorder, which could then be confirmed by serum hormonal assay.

TABLE 7.9: Clinical manifestations of hyperthyroidism	
Symptoms	*Signs*
Weight loss	Irritability
Increased appetite	Psychosis
Irritability	Hyperkinesis*
Restlessness	Exophthalmos*
Malaise	Lid lag
Muscle weakness	Conjunctival edema
Tremors	Ophthalmoplegia
Choreoathetosis	Goiter
Breathlessness	Systolic hypertension
Palpitations	Tachycardia
Heat intolerance	Atrial fibrillation*
Vomiting/diarrhea	Weight loss
Eye complaints	Fine tremors
Neck swelling	Warm peripheries
Oligomenorrhea	Proximal muscle wasting
Loss of libido	Proximal myopathy
Gynecomastia	Palmar erythema
Tall stature	Pretibial myxoedema
Myolysis	
*Signs of greater discrimination	

The best screening tool, however, is the serum TSH assay. This is based on the fact that as the levels of the serum T3 and T4 rise, the concentration of TSH will fall exponentially, giving an accurate estimation of the severity of the condition.

Once the diagnosis is established, further tests to identify a possible cause may be carried out—ultrasound, radioactive iodine uptake, anti thyroid antibody titers etc. (Table 7.10).[4,5]

TABLE 7.10: Investigations in hyperthyroidism
1. Serum TSH
2. Serum T4
3. Serum T3
4. Radioactive Iodine uptake
5. Ultrasound
6. Antithyroid antibodies

Treatment

Once an infertile patient is found to be hyper-thyroid, immediate therapy to restore a euthyroid state is recommended.

The benefit of treating patients with sub-clinical hyperthyroidism is not proven. However, in the presence of ovulatory dysfunction where no other cause can be determined, empirical therapy may be attempted to establish a biochemically euthyroid state.

Hyperthyroidism can be treated medically, surgically or by irradiation, depending on the etiology.

In the infertile patient, desirous of conception, medical therapy would be the best option. The drugs used to inhibit the formation of thyroid hormones are Carbimazole and Propylthiouracil (Table 7.11).

TABLE 7.11: Drugs used in the treatment of hyperthyroidism		
Name	*Dosage*	*Adverse effects*
Antithyroid drugs		
Carbimazole	10–20 mg 8th hrly	Rash, nausea, fever Vomiting, Arthralgia Agranulocytosis Jaundice Immunosuppression
Methimazole	10–15 mg 8th hrly	
Propylthiouracil	100-200 mg 8th hrly	Rash, Nausea, Vomiting Agranulocytosis
Beta blockers for symptomatic relief		
Propanolol	40–60 mg 6th hrly	Avoid in asthma, cardiac failure
Nadolol	40-240 mg daily	

Symptomatic relief may require beta-blockers such as propanolol and nadolol.

Treatment is given for 4 to 6 weeks before review of the serum parameters and clinical response. Beta-blockers may be given only till the patient becomes euthyroid. The dosage of the anti-thyroid drugs is to be titrated and gradually reduced to the minimum dose of 5 mg daily. Treatment may be discontinued once the patient is euthyroid on 5 mg Carbimazole per day.

Following medical treatment about 50 percent will relapse—usually within the next 2 years. This may necessitate the use of long-term antithyroid therapy.

There are few indications where the patient would benefit from surgical intervention (Table 7.12). It must be remembered that surgery is not without complications—which could include H. hypothyroidism, hypoparathyroidism (transient in 10%, permanent in less than 1%) recurrent laryngeal nerve palsy (1%), etc.

Subtotal thyroidectomy should be carried out only after establishing a euthyroid state. Antithyroid drugs are generally withdrawn about 2 weeks before surgery, and Potassium Iodide is supplemented to reduce the vascularity of the gland.

TABLE 7.12: Indications for surgical intervention in hyperthyroidism
1. Large goiter
2. Persistent drug side effects
3. Poor compliance with medication
4. Recurrent hypothyroidism
5. Patient's choice

Irradiation is unacceptable in the young infertile patient. However, Radioactive Iodine (I-131) in the empirical dose (18–40 × 10 10 Bq) used to destroy the thyroid gland has been determined not to affect fecundity[6] but its use is still viewed with trepidation.

HYPOTHYROIDISM

Hypothyroidism is characterized by a spectrum of clinical manifestations that are directly or indirectly related to the deficiency of the thyroid hormones.

Moderate and severe degrees of hypothyroidism have a detrimental effect on the reproductive potential of both men and women, but the same cannot be said of the mild and sub-clinical forms.

Primary hypothyroidism is due to thyroid gland failure, while secondary hypothyroidism occurs due to disorders of the hypothalamo-pituitary axis, which results in the inadequate production of bio-active TSH.

Etiological factors are listed in the Table 7.13.

TABLE 7.13: Etiology of hypothyroidism
Primary
1. Congenital–Agenesis
Ectopic thyroid remnants
2. Defect in synthesis–Iodine deficiency
Dyshormonogenesis
Antithyroid drugs
3. Autoimmune–Hashimoto's thyroiditis
4. Atrophic
5. Infective
6. Post-surgery
7. Post-radiotherapy
8. Peripheral resistance to thyroid hormones
Secondary
1. Hypopituitarism
2. Isolated TSH deficiency

Hypothyroidism and Female Fertility

The effect of hypothyroidism on the reproductive potential has been well documented in women– probably due to the fact that this disorder is more often seen in females.[7]

Menstrual irregularities, spontaneous first trimester miscarriages, premature deliveries, unexplained stillbirths and infertility are some of the manifestations.[8]

Almost 70 percent of infertility in hypothyroid females is due to anovulation.[9]

Hypothyroidism is also common in women with unexplained infertility, and not often seen in women with tubal factor.[10]

Menstrual irregularities are seen in approximately 23 to 25 percent. Oligomenorrhea is probably the most common clinical manifestation.[11]

Menorrhagia, sometimes seen in these women is due to a combination of anovulation, poor uterine muscle tone and platelet dysfunction.[12]

Hypothyroidism and Male Fertility

Hypothyroidism in the male has a less clear cut effect on the reproductive system. Apart from the non-specific findings of decreased libido, it has been claimed that hypothyroidism in males is associated with testicular dysfunction.[13]

However, other studies have shown that the seminal alterations caused by hypothyroidism are not sufficiently intense to induce male infertility.[14]

Diagnosis

Hypothyroidism has some protean clinical manifestations, which could indicate the presence of this disorder (Table 7.14).

TABLE 7.14: Clinical manifestations of hypothyroidism	
Symptoms	*Signs*
Tiredness/malaise	Mental slowness*
Unexplained weight gain	Psychosis/dementia
Anorexia	Poverty of movement
Cold intolerance	"Peaches and cream" complexion
Poor memory	Loss of eyebrows
Change in appearance	Periorbital edema
Depression	Dry thin hair*
Psychosis	Macroglossia
Coma	Deafness
Deafness	Deep voice
Poor libido	Anemia
Goiter	Hypertension
Puffy eyes	Hypothermia
Dry brittle hair	Bradycardia*
Arthralgia	Dry skin
Myalgia	Obesity
Constipation	Cold peripheries
Menstrual disturbances	Carpal tunnel Syndrome
Symptoms of other	Proximal myopathy
Autoimmune disorders	Myotonia
	Muscle hypertrophy*
	Slow relaxing reflexes
	Edema

*Indicates sign of greater discrimination

Confirmation of the diagnosis is by serological assay, which would demonstrate a deficiency of the thyroid hormones (Table 7.15).

TABLE 7.15: Thyroid function tests		
Test	*Use*	*Misleading*
Total T4	Hypothyroidism	Pregnancy
Free T4	Thyrotoxicosis	Estrogen therapy
	Hypothalamo–pit	NSAID therapy
Total T3	Thyrotoxicosis screening	
TSH	Neonatal hypothyroidism	
	Thyrotoxicosis	
	Hypothalamo pit disease	
TRH test	? Use	

Once the diagnosis is established, the presence of autoimmune disorders must be looked for. Assay of antimicrosomal antibodies and anti thyroglobulin antibodies are useful indicators of the risk of progression.

Screening for hypothyroidism is best done using a sensitive TSH assay. However, this may not be very accurate in conditions that do not produce enough bioactive TSH–as seen in recent onset hypothyroidism and in hypothalamo-pituitary disorders. In these cases it would be better to assay free T4 along with the TSH.

Treatment

With established hypothyroidism, there is no doubt about the benefit of hormone therapy.

Thyroxin extract is used to replenish the depleted hormones.

One study, conducted by Oravec S *et al* on the benefit of thyroxin replacement in infertile women with hypothyroidism and ovulatory dysfunction, indicated pregnancy rates of upto 64 percent following treatment.[15]

The treatment of sub-clinical hypothyroidism is still very controversial. Some authors' (propogate) the empirical use of thyroxin in these women, on the basis of the lack of any significant negative effect, improved sense of well being, and enhanced fertility; others insist on the benefit of treatment only in the setting of documented hormone deficiency.

Another debatable situation arises in the anovulatory, but euthyroid woman. While there is insufficient evidence on this subject, it must not be forgotten that one could be overlooking a phase of early or incipient hypothyroidism in these women. This could become manifest in any situation that increases the thyroid demand–pregnancy, gonadotrophin drugs, etc.[16]

Given the theoretical benefit of Thyroxin, it may be worthwhile to supplement very low doses of the hormone while attempting conception. Long-term randomized multicentric studies are required to document the efficacy of this approach.

REFERENCES

1. Becks GP et al. Thyroid disease and pregnancy. Med Clin North Am 1991;75:121.
2. Clyde HR et al. Elevated plasma Testosterone and gonadotrophin levels in infertile males with Hyperthyroidism. Fertil Steril 1976;27:662.
3. Krassas GE, Pontikides N, Deligianni V, Miras K. A prospective controlled study of the impact of hyperthyroidism on reproductive function in males. J Clin Endocrinol Metab. 2002;87(8):3667-71.
4. Kidd GS et al. The hypothalamo-piyuitiary-testicular axis in thyrotoxicosis. J Clin Endocrinol Metab 1979;48:798.
5. O'Brian AD et al Reversible male subfertility due to hyperthyroidism. BMJ 1982;285:691.
6. Krassas GE. Thyroid disease and female reproduction. Fertil Steri. 2000;74(6):1063-70.
7. Choux E, Crequat J, Madelenat P. Thyroid ultrasonography and infertility. Contracep Fertil Sex. 1995; 23(11):694-950.
8. Davis LE et al. Hypothyroidism complicating pregnancy. Obstet Gynecol 1988;72:108.
9. Goldsmith R E et al. The menstrual pattern of thyroid disease. J Clin Endocrinol Metab 1962;12:846.
10. Arojoki M, Jokimaa V, Juuti A, Koskinen P, Irjala K, Anttila L. Hypothyroidism among infertile women in Finland. Gynecol Endocrinol 2000;14(2):127-31.
11. Gynecol Endocrinol. 2000 Apr;14(2):127-31 Thyroid disease and female reproduction. Fertil Steril 2000 Dec;74(6):1063-70.
12. Edson TR et al. Low platelet adhesiveness and other hemostatic abnormalities in hypothyroidism. An Int Med 1975;82:324.
13. Wortsman J et al. Abnormal testicular function in men with primary hypothyroidism. Am J Med 1987;82;207.
14. Corrales Hernandez JJ, Miralles Garcia JM, Garcia Diez LC. Primary hypothyroidism and human spermatogenesis. Arch Androl 1990;25(1):21-27.
15. Oravec S, Hlavacka S. Disorders of thyroid function and fertility disorders. Ceska Gynekol 2000;65(1):53-57.
16. Mandel SJ et al. Thyroid function during gonadotrophin therapy (abstract). Presented at the 10th International Congress of Endocrinology. The Endocrine Society, San Francisco, 1996.

• Shreyas Padgaonkar

8

Luteal Phase Defect

Luteal phase defect is a controversial entity But evaluation of luteal phase and treatment of luteal phase defect is a wide spread practice. Luteal phase detect is associated with infertility and randomised trials have demonstrated improvements in terms of conceptions or normal endometrial histology.[1]

The classical method of evaluation of luteal phase is endometrial dating using Noyes criteria. Other methods used are plasma progesterone estimation, Basal body temperature, ultrasonography, endometrial proteins measurements. Endometrial biopsy at about day LH + 5 with histological dating > 2 days behind the corresponding chronological date is a widely used criteria. A single mid luteal progesterone level ~ 0 nmol/l is considered as a threshold value by many investigators

PATHOPHYSIOLOGY

Corpus Luteum Function

Corpus luteum (CL) is a two cell organ consisting of granulosa and theca cells which are luteinized with the LH surge. These two cell populations behave in different fashions during the life of CL. Luteinized granulosa cells have FSH induced LH receptors which respond to the LH surge and secrete progesterone (P) for 10 days after which the steroidogenesis stops. These cells are unable to respond to LH pulses or hCG stimulation. These cells do not undergo mitotic division.

Luteinized theca cells have endogenous LH receptors and respond to LH pulses by P and Estradiol (E_2) synthesis. These cells multiply and are capable of responding to hCG stimulation from the pregnancy.

Progesterone secreted by the CL transforms the endometrium to a secretory form. It induces specific endometrial proteins through P4 receptor action allowing implantation. Follicular phase E_2 induces P4 receptors on the endometrial cells. Excessive or inadequate E_2 can induce too early or delayed induction of endometrial proteins. Abnormality of CL function can result from:

1. Aberrant follicular phase
2. Subnormal P production
   - Follicle aspiration
   - Hyperprolactinemia
   - Hypothalamo-pituitary dysfunction
     (Down regulation, Gonadotrophin stimulation, extremes of weight, extremes of reproductive life, stress)
3. Abnormal endometrial response
4. Other causes
   - Clomiphene citrate
   - Luteinized unruptured follicle

TREATMENT OF LUTEAL PHASE DEFECT

Various agents are used in the treatment of luteal phase defect (LPD). Clomiphene citrate and gonadotropins are used to improve the follicular phase aberrations. Progesterone is used by intramuscular, vaginal or oral route. Human chorionic gonadotropin (hCG) administered in two to three doses is known to increase P production and prolong luteal phase Due to lack of consensus in diagnosis, placebo-response randomized placebo-controlled trials are required to compare efficacy of various therapeutic regimens which are rare.[1] At present the therapy aimed to improve defects in endometrial response to P are lacking. But luteal phase support seems to be a mandatory part of superovulation strategies for assisted reproductive technologies.

LUTEAL PHASE SUPPORT IN ASSISTED REPRODUCTION

Over the years improvements in stimulation protocols for ART mainly centred around obtaining oocytes of better quality and numbers. Improvements in culture conditions can improve embryo quality. But implantation also involves endometrial preparation partly controlled by estrogen in follicular phase, which is closely monitored by hormone assays and sonography. The luteal transformation and supplementation is still largely empirical.

Need of Luteal Support

The luteal insufficiency can arise in ART cycles from the agents used in stimulation protocols. Aspiration of granulosa cells during oocyte recovery can also be partly responsible.

Different stimulation protocols have different effects on the luteal function Pulsatile LH secretion in the luteal phase is essential for corpus luteal function. Supraphysiological levels of estrogen and progesterone will reduce the frequency of LH secretion by acting on the hypothalamus. Use of GnRH analogs will block the pituitary secretion of LH. Meta-analysis of eighteen randomised trials of luteal support in GnRH analog cycles showed improvement in pregnancy rates with hCG and progesterone.

Granulosa cells have specific receptors for GnRH. When granulosa cell from women treated with GnRH analogs are cultured in vitro the progesterone (P4) production in response to hCG is lower than those treated with a combination of clomiphene citrate and gonadotropins and the peak of progesterone production is delayed by 2 days in the GnRH-analog treated group.[4] When cultured in the absence of hCG, these granulosa cells demonstrated a rapid decline in both the spontaneous P4 secretion rate and the ability to secrete P4 in response to hCG. Presence of hCG in culture prevents these alterations'.[5] Different analogs and duration of their use may affect the granulosa cells in different ways. Buserelin has shown to inhibit P4 production more than Leuprolide and the effect is more evident in the long protocol.[6]

Granulosa cells isolated from GnRH analog cycles showed a blunted progesterone production when stimulated with hCG as compared to cells from GnRH antagonist cycle. It is suggested that GnRH analog but not antagonist affect the expression and/or activation of LH receptors in the granulose cells.[7]

Accidental GnRH analog administration and failure to use HRT by oocyte recipients with uneventful pregnancies can indicate that the need for luteal support may be over stressed. Tavaniotou et al[8] compared LH concentrations in IVF cycles using hMG with or without GnRH antagonist. They suggested a possible central action of exogenously administered hCG via a short loop mechanism as an additional factor inhibiting LH secretion.

- Clomiphene citrate (CC) occupies the hypothalamic estrogen receptor over a prolonged period of time. This might be responsible for higher luteal LH concentration in CC cycles. CC antagonist cycles also demonstrate higher LH levels compared to gonadotropin cycles.[9] These observations may suggest that luteal phase supplementations may not be essential for CC stimulated cycles.[10]

Luteal Support Protocols

The main protocols used to supplement luteal phase are progesterone supplementation or hCG stimulation.

Following are the commonest drugs used:
- Human chorionic gonadotropin
- Intramuscular progesterone
- Intravaginal progesterone

- Oral progesterone
- Progesterone gel
- Estradiol valerate with progesterone

Human Chorionic Gonadotropin (hCG)

Usually 1500 to 2000 IU hCG is administered every three days 3 to 4 times. Ovarian hyperstimulation syndrome can occur in about 5 percent of patients. Its use is avoided if serum E_2 levels are above 2500 pg/ml or number of follicles exceeds ten.

Progesterone

Intramuscular progesterone is used daily in the dose of 25 to 50 mg. It achieves serum progesterone values that are within the range of luteal phase and results in sufficient secretory transformation of the endometrium and satisfactory pregnancy rates. These are oil-based injections and can be painful.

Orally micronised progesterone is administered in a dose of 300 to 600 mg in three divided doses. Oral progesterone and IM progesterone result in comparable levels of circulating progesterone. However, oral progesterone results in a reduced implantation rate per embryo.[11,12] Orally administered progesterone is rapidly metabolised in the gastrointestinal tract and can show inter- and intraindividual variability. Metabolites of orally ingested progesterone can have hypnotic effects.

Vaginally progesterone is used in 600 to 800 mg dose in two or three divided doses. Serum levels of progesterone achieved after vaginal progesterone application are lower than those after IM administration[13] but can achieve adequate endometrial secretory transformation. Some studies have shown it to be superior to IM progesterone.[14]

Vaginally administered progesterone seems to have better bioavailability in the uterus because of first uterine pass effect.

A recent meta-analysis[1] concluded that IM progesterone or hCG improved the treatment outcome. Both were equally effective. Intramuscular progesterone was superior to vaginal or oral use.

Progesterone is also available as 8 percent gel used once a day in 90 mg dose. It is shown to be equally effective as IM progesterone.[16] But some studies have shown a lower implantation and ongoing pregnancy rates after its use.[17,18]

Estradiol Supplementation

Role of oestradiol in luteal phase is still unclear. Superiority of hCG over progesterone supplementation may be due to higher E_2 levels achieved. Studies in past failed to demonstrate advantage of adding E_2 to the luteal support.[19,20] One study claimed adverse effect of elevated E_2 on implantation when hCG was added to vaginal progesterone supplementation.[21] Estradiol may be beneficial when stimulation protocol results in low levels of E_2 such as utilizing depot GnRH analogs.[22]

Duration of Luteal Support

Luteal support is usually continued till placental steroidogenesis is adequate by 12-13 weeks of gestation. But recently these practices have been questioned. IVF pregnancies show greater levels of progesterone than normal pregnancies, with higher luteal contribution in form of 17 alpha-hydroxyprogesterone upto 8 weeks.[23] Stoval et al[24] showed that early discontinuation of luteal support in women with serum progesterone level > or = 60 ng/ml did not affect delivery rates. A prospective randomised trial demonstrated that delivery rates remained unchanged when the luteal support was discontinued after positive hCG test.[25]

Luteal supplement is an essential part of assisted reproductive technologies. But these therapies lack definite goals and monitoring methods Better understanding of physiological processes and randomised trials are required to improve the regimes for luteal support.

<u>REFERENCES</u>

1. Baalasch J, Vanrella JA, Marquez M, Burzaco I, Gonzalez-Meerlo J. Dydrogestrone versus vaginal progesterone in the treatment of endometrial luteal phase deficiency. Fertil Steril 1982;37:751-54.
2. Jonse GS, Aksel S, Wentz AC. Serum progesterone values in the luteal phase defects, effect of chorionic gonadotropin. Obstet Gynecol 1974;44:26-34.
3. Soliman S, Daya S, Collins J, Hughes EG. The role of luteal phase support in infertility treatment: A

metaanalysis of randomized trials. Fertil Steril 1994;61(6): 1068-76.

4. Pellicer A, Miro F. Steroidogenesis in vitro of human granulosa-luteal cells pre-treated in vivo with gonadotropin-releasing hormone analogs. Fertil Steril 1990;54(4):590-96.

5. Edgar DH, Whalley KM, Gemmell JA, James GB, Mills JA. Effects of in-vitro exposure to hCG on subsequent hCG-responsiveness of human granulosa cells obtained following treatment with GnRH analogue and gonadotrophins: An in-vitro model for luteal phase support. Hum Reprod 1991;6(2):198-202.

6. Miro F, Sampaio MC, Tarin JJ, Pellicer A. Steroidogenesis in vitro of human granulosa-luteal cells pre-treated in vivo with two gonadotropin releasing hormone analogs employing different protocols. Gynecol Endocrinol 1992;6(2):77-84.

7. Mitwally MF, Casper RF. J Assist Reprod Genet 2002;19(8):384-89.

8. Tavaniotou A, Albano C, Smitz J, Devroey P. Comparison of LH concentrations in the early and mid-luteal phase in 1VF cycles after treatment with HMG alone or in association with the GnRH antagonist Cetrorelix. Hum Reprod 2001;16(4):663-67.

9. Tavaniotou A, Albano C, Smitz J, Devroey P. Effect of clomiphene citrate on follicular and luteal phase luteinizing hormone concentrations in in vitro fertilization cycles stimulated with gonadotropins and gonadotropin-releasing hormone antagonist. Fertil Steril 2002;77(4):733-37.

10. Van Steirteghem AC, Smitz J, Camus M, Van Waesberghe, Deschacht J, Khan L, Staessen C, Wisanto A, Bourgain C, Devroey P. The luteal phase after in-vitro fertilization and related procedures. Hum Reprod 1988;3(2) 161-64.

11. Licciardi FL, Kwiatkowski A, Noyes NL, Berkeley AS, Krey LL, Grifo JA. Oral versus intramuscular progesterone for in vitro fertilization, a prospective randomized study. Fenil Steril 1999;71(4):614-18.

12. Tavaniotou A, Smitz J, Bourgain C, Devroey P. Comparison between different routes of progesterone administration as luteal phase support in infertility treatments. Hum Reprod Update 2000;6(2):139-48.

13. Smitz J, Devroey P, Faguer B, Bourgain C, Camus M, Van Steirteghem AC. A randomized prospective study comparing supplementation of the luteal phase and early pregnancy by natural progesterone administered by intramuscular or vaginal route. Rev Fr Gynecol Obstet 1992;87(10):507-16.

14. Smitz J, Devroey P, Faguer B, Bourgain C, Camus M, Van Steirteghem AC. A prospective randomized comparison of intramuscular or intravaginal natural progesterone as a luteal phase and early pregnancy supplement. Hum Reprod 1992;7(2):168-75.

15. Pritts EA, Atwood AK. Luteal phase support in infertility treatment: A meta-analysis of the randomized trials. Hum Reprod 2002;17(9) 2287-99.

16. Schoolcraft WB, Hesla JS, Gee MJ. Experience with progesterone gel for luteal support in a highly successful IVF programme. Hum Reprod 2000;l5(6):1284-88.

17. Abate A, Perino M, Abate FG, Brigandi A, Costabile L, Manti F. Intramuscular versus vaginal administration of progesterone for luteal phase support after in vitro fertilization and embryo transfer. A comparative randomized study. Clin Exp Obstet Gynecol 1999;26(3-4): 203-06.

18. Damario MA, Goudas VT, Session DR, Hammitt DG, Dumesic DA Crinone 8% vaginal progesterone gel results in lower embryonic implantation efficiency after in vitro fertilization-embryo transfer. Fertil Steril 1999;72(5):830-36.

19. Smitz J, Bourgain C, Van Waesberghe L, Camus M, Devroey P, Van Steirteghem AC. A prospective randomized study on oestradiol valerate supplementation in addition to intravaginal micronised progesterone in buserelin and HMG induced superovulation. Hum Reprod 1993;8(l):40-45.

20. Lewin A, Benshushan A, Mezker E, Yanai N, Schenker JG, Goshen R. The role of estrogen support during the luteal phase of in vitro fertilization-embryo transplant cycles: A comparative study between progesterone alone and estrogen and progesterone support. Fertil Steril 1994;62(l):121-25.

21. Mochtar MH, Hogerzeil HV, Mol BW. Progesterone alone versus progesterone combined with HCG as luteal support in GnRHa/HMG induced 1VT cycles: A randomized clinical trial. Hum Reprod 1996;l1(8):1602-05.

22. Farhi J, Weissman A, Steinfeld Z, Shorer M, Nahum H, Levran D. Estradiol supplementation during the luteal phase may improve the pregnancy rate in patients undergoing in vitro fertilization—embryo transfer cycles. Fertil Steril 2000;73(4):761-66.

23. Abate A, Brigandi A, Abate FG, Manti F, Unfer V, Perino M. Luteal phase support with I7alpha-hydroxyprogesterone versus unsupported cycles in in vitro fertilization: A comparative randomized study Gynecol Obstet Invest 1999;48(2):78-80.

24. Stovall DW, Van Voorhis BJ, Sparks AE, Adams LM, Syrop CH. Selective early elimination of luteal support in assisted reproduction cycles using a gonadotropin-releasing hormone agonist during ovarian stimulation. Fertil Steril 1998;70(6):1056-62.

25. Nyboe Andersen A, Popovic-Todorovic B, Schmidt KT, Loft A, Lindhard A, Hojgaard A et al. Progesterone supplementation during early gestations after IVF or ICSl has no effect on the delivery rates: A randomized controlled trial. Hum Reprod 2002;17(2):357-61.

• PK Sekharan

9

Polycystic Ovarian Syndrome

INTRODUCTION

Ever since Stein and Leventhal[1] reported on seven women with polycystic ovaries and amenorrhea in 1935, continued research has led to the better understanding of the pathophysiology of the syndrome with promising therapeutic options. The polycystic ovary syndrome (PCOS) is one of the most common endocrine disorders, affecting 4-6 percent of unselected women of reproductive age.[2] In addition to the endocrine abnormalities leading to menstrual disorders, hyperandrogenism and anovulatory infertility, many women with PCOS demonstrate metabolic aberrations, most importantly the association of insulin resistance. The endocrine and metabolic abnormalities associated with PCOS leads to far reaching long-term health hazards to these women, like glucose intolerance and type II diabetes, increased risk factors for CHD, adverse lipid profile, hypertension, hyperinsulinemia and obesity.

Pathophysiology

The primary abnormality in polycystic ovary syndrome could reside within the ovaries or the ovarian abnormalities could be secondary to extra ovarian disturbances.[3-6] One of the most intriguing but yet unanswered questions is whether PCOS is an inborn error or an acquired disease. It is possible that a multitude of endocrine, paracrine and metabolic factors are involved. Anyhow, PCOS starts with puberty and definitely

ends with menopause. The essential endocrine feature of PCOS is an increased production of androgens. The main source of hyperandrogenism is the ovary. The ovary contains a large number of subcortical antral follicles which are lined by a few layers of granulosa cells while the surrounding theca cells and the underlying stroma are abundant. The presence of a large number of follicles of size varying from 6-10 mm arranged in the periphery in a necklace pattern and the increase in ovarian volume largely due to an increase in stroma is the classical finding on ultrasonography. The multiple antral follicles are *not atretic,* but follicular *maturation* and progression to *ovulation is arrested.*

It is now clear that many patients with PCOS have compensatory hyperinsulinemia due to some degree of insulin resistance. Insulin and insulin-like growth factor-I (IGF-I) augments the effect of LH on ovarian steroidogenic activity and on the GnRH pulse generator. Obesity seen in at least half of PCO subjects has an addictive effect on insulin resistance. The upper body obesity, seen in PCOS increases the androgen production and free testosterone levels. Both obese and nonobese PCOS women display marked impairment of catecholamine-induced lipolysis. As a result of catecholamine resistance, a compensatory increase in sympathetic activity may also induce insulin resistance. Androgens are converted by peripheral aromatization to estrogens which stimulate synthesis of LH but suppress the secretion of FSH. Chronic stimulation with LH supports the production of androgens by theca cells. The peripheral pool of androgens is supplemented by an activated adrenal production of androgens. Due to the low FSH levels, the intra-ovarian conversion of androgens to estrogens is partially inhibited keeping the ovaries in a hyperandrogenic state with arrest of follicular maturation. Many factors concur to establish and perpetuate PCOS. Their vital role is evident by the fact that different therapeutic interventions can restore ovulation or interrupt the perpetuating cycle.

The Hypothalamic Connection

One of the main characteristics of PCOS is the abnormal LH/FSH ratio. Compared to the gonado-trophin levels in the early follicular phase of ovulatory cycle, LH secretion is increased while FSH levels remain subnormal and constant. This inappropriate secretion of gonadotrophins is the key issue in the continuation of the anovulatory state of PCOS subjects. Although the intraovarian regulation of steroidogenesis is a complex matter, simplified it can be proposed that increased LH levels induces increased androgen steroidogenesis by the theca cells and stroma, which are in abundance, and that a reduced FSH secretion is responsible for the decreased conversion of the androgens to estrogens in the granulosa. However, it is not clear, whether the inappropriate gonado-trophin secretion is the result of normal feedback mechanisms at the pituitary level while the hypothalamus is only playing a permissive role by providing an intermittent but steady production of GnRH; or does the hypothalamic control of the pituitary function play a primary role in the genesis and continuation of PCO syndrome.

The GnRH Pulse Generator

LH secretion in PCO patients is characterized both by an increased pulse frequency and amplitude. The gonadotrophin pattern of high LH and low FSH can be due to an increased frequency of GnRH pulsatile secretion.[6] Chronically elevated estrogen levels can affect pituitary sensitivity to GnRH both by direct action on LH synthesis and by up-regulating GnRH receptors causing an increased response of LH. The selective negative feedback effect of estrogens on the FSH on the other hand mitigates the response of FSH. The enhanced pulsatile secretion of GnRH is attributed to a reduction in hypothalamic opioid inhibition because of the chronic absence of progesterone. High-frequency GnRH pulses up-regulate the synthesis of the LH β-subunit and down-regulate β-subunit of FSH resulting in relatively greater synthesis and secretion of LH than FSH. One explanation for the accelerated GnRH pulse frequency is a possible link between the neuro-endocrine and metabolic changes in PCOS. Receptors for insulin, IGF-I and IGF-II as well as α and β estrogen receptors are expressed in GnRH neuronal cell lines. Activation of IGF-I receptor induces cell proliferation and GnRH gene expression and secretion. Thus, the GnRH neuron is a target for functional regulation both by steroids and by insulin and the IGFs. Through this pathway, a primary metabolic derangement could lead to activation of the GnRH pulse generator.

Insulin Resistance and Molecular Defects in Insulin Signaling

Approximately 50-60 percent of PCOS patients suffer from insulin resistance compared to the prevalence of insulin resistance in the general population of 10-25 percent.[7-9] Insulin resistance in PCOS leads to compensatory hyperinsulinemia which seems to play a major role in the patho-genesis of hyperandrogenism of PCOS. Hyper-insulinemia stimulates androgen secretion by the ovarian theca, excess growth of the basal cells of the skin resulting in acanthosis nigricans, and abnormal hepatic and peripheral lipid metabolism. Insulin resistance and hyperinsulinemia cause many features of PCOS, is supported by the fact that the various insulin sensitizing agents like diazoxide, metformin, troglitazone and d-*chiro*-inositol has been found to improve clinical features.

Dunaif *et al* (1989) determined *in vivo* insulin action on peripheral glucose utilization and found that insulin resistance was present in both "lean" and "obese" women with PCOS, but they noted that the resistance was greater in obese subjects.[7] A postreceptor defect has been suggested by Dunaif *et al* as a cause of insulin resistance in PCOS.[10] It has been shown that insulin receptor autophosphorylation and tyrosine kinase activity are necessary for the cellular response to insulin. The final effector system involved in glucose uptake into the cell involves the insulin regulatable glucose transporter (GLUT4). Serine phosphorylation has been shown to impair insulin receptor tyrosine kinase activity, and excessive serine phosphorylation has been demonstrated in insulin receptors of skeletal muscle and fibroblasts from insulin resistant patients with polycystic ovary syndrome [10] Enlarged adipocytes from obese individuals overproduce tumor necrosis factor alpha (TNFα) and result in increased serine phosphorylation of the insulin receptor: and further aggravates the insulin resistance in obese PCO subjects.[11, 12]

Stimulation of Ovarian Cytochrome P450c17α by Insulin

P450c17α is a key enzyme in the biosynthesis of ovarian androgens, and is a bifunctional enzyme that possesses both 17α-hydroxylase and 17, 20-lyase activities. In the theca cell of the ovary, P450c17α converts progesterone to 17α-hydroxyprogesterone via its 17α-hydroxylase activity, and then converts 17α-hydroxyprogestrone to androstenedione via its 17, 20-layse action. Androstenedione is converted into testosterone by the enzyme 17β-reductase. Many women with PCOS manifest increased P450c17α activity and the recent evidence suggest that it is due to the hyperinsulinemia and is partially reversible with metformin.[13-15]

Hyperinsulinemia Leads to Hyperandrogenemia

Hyperandrogenemia seen in PCOS is as a result of the insulin stimulation of the ovarian androgen production. The possible mechanisms for hyperandrogenemia in polycystic ovary syndrome is the stimulation of CytochromeP450c17α activity in the theca cells by insulin, effect of insulin to increase the pulse and amplitude of LH secretion, and decrease in the production of serum sex hormone binding globulin (SHBG). Hyperinsulinemia can reduce serum SHBG levels in obese women with PCOS independently of any effect on serum sex steroids. Hyperandrogenemia is also due to the adrenal androgen excess as a result of a genetic trait or due to the increased serine phosphorylation of CP450c17α leading to increased production of DHEAS, a mechanism which is activated by hyperinsulinemia. Adrenal hyperandrogenism occurs in about 50 percent of PCOS patients, concurrently with ovarian hyperandrogenism, the indicator is an elevated level of DHEAS.

Hyperprolactinemia in PCOS

The review of the recent evidence suggests that PCOS and hyperprolactinemia are independent disorders with unrelated causes.[16] Diagnostic approach should be directed to exclude physical stress, medication, hypothyroidism and pituitary lesions. The addition of a dopamine agonist (bromocriptine or cabergoline) to a regimen of clomiphene citrate may be considered as ovulation induction options in PCO subjects with hyperprolactinemia.

Leptin

Leptin is a protein hormone synthesized and secreted by adipocytes.[17] It is a product of the *ob* gene that signals the amount of energy stores to the brain and has been implicated in the regulation of food intake and energy balance. The observation that leptin levels were significantly elevated in approximately 30 percent of lean and obese women with PCOS suggests that Leptin may have a role in the pathogenesis of PCOS.[18] The development of new leptin analogues with high penetrating capacity to cross the blood-brain barrier and the investigation of other approaches to overcome the leptin resistance at the level of hypothalamus are awaited.

Clinical Presentation and Diagnosis

Clinically, PCOS encompasses a spectrum of findings from hyperandrogenism in lean, normally menstruating women to obese women with severe hirsutism and oligomenorrhea or amenorrhea, as originally described by Stein and Leventhal. The accepted definition of PCOS is a state of chronic anovulation accompanied by hyperandrogenism, with clinical manifestations including hirsutism, acne, elevated testosterone and androstenedione, androgen-dependent alopecia, and frequently, not always, obesity.

Menstrual symptoms, often with perimenarchial onset, are the most common complaints among women with PCOS. Amenorrhea was reported in 47-66 percent of cases while 16-30 percent of patients will have regular periods. As many as 60 percent of patients will have hirsutism, but virilization is uncommon. Acne has been described in 25 to 35 percent of patients in large series. Up to 50 percent of patients presenting with infertility will have PCOS and are more common in women with recurrent pregnancy loss. Manifestation of unopposed estrogenic stimulation, including menorrhagia, endometrial hyperplasia, and endometrial carcinoma, occur in a significant proportion of patients.

Obesity, defined as a body mass index (BMI) greater than 25, is found in 35 to 50 percent of women with PCOS. Obese women with PCOS are more likely to be hirsute and infertile. In one study, the incidence of infertility were 40 percent higher among PCOS women with a BMI greater than 30 kg/m^2 when compared with women whose BMI was less than 30.[19] Acanthosis nigricans associated with hyperandrogenism and insulin resistance (HAIR-AN) is seen in many obese patients.

Family history is an important clinical feature of PCOS. The pattern of inheritance was thought to be autosomal dominant with decreased penetrance. The phenotype also includes hyperandrogenism, early balding in men, and glucose intolerance.

Ultrasonographic appearance: As per Adams et al,[20] the typical polycystic pattern was defined by the presence of 10 or more cysts measuring 2 to 18 mm in diameter in a single plane arranged peripherally around an increased amount of central stroma is diagnostic of PCOS. The subcapsular arrangement of the multiple cysts gives the appearance of "necklace" distribution. Transvaginal ultrasonography will show small multiple echo free cysts of 2 to 8 mm in diameter, arranged around a prominent highly echogenic stroma. An increase in the amount and echogenicity of the ovarian stroma distinguishes the PCO from multifollicular ovary seen in normal puberty and hypothalamic anovulation.

Endocrine Screening

Prolactin and TSH levels are tested to rule out pituitary or thyroid disease as an etiology of anovulation. LH and FSH may be analyzed and they are usually seen in a ratio of > 2.5 to 3. However, a normal LH/FSH ratio does not exclude the possibility of PCOS. An FSH level will also help rule out premature ovarian failure in women with amenorrhea. Total testosterone and DHEAS are evaluated to rule out androgen-producing neoplasm. Total testosterone level of 200 ng/dL is suggestive of a virilizing tumor. A virilizing tumor of adrenal may be suspected if the value of DHEAS greater than 800 mcg/dL. A level of 17 hydroxyprogesterone more than 5 ng/ml is diagnostic of late onset congenital adrenal hyperplasia.

Glucose Tolerance Test

The incidence of impaired glucose tolerance amongst PCO subjects is 35 to 45 percent and about 7 to 10 percent of them will have type II diabetes mellitus. A fasting glucose to fasting insulin ratio less than 4.5 is predictive of insulin resistance. Values on the 2 hr glucose tolerance test are as follows: < 140 mg/dL (normal), 140-199 mg/dL (impaired glucose tolerance), and > 200 mg/dL (type 2 diabetes).

Overall, the clinical presentation is critical to the diagnosis of PCOS, which has been defined as ovulatory dysfunction and hyperandrogenism in the absence of other causes. Most ovulatory dysfunction can be suspected based on history, with targeted hormonal testing. Physical findings suggestive of hyperandrogenism provide the next important step in the diagnosis. An assessment of obesity and fat distribution should be part of the clinical examination.

Approach to Infertility in PCOS

Since anovulatory cycles are the cause of infertility in PCOS, the goal in managing these patients is induction of ovulation. The approach should be to use progressively more aggressive treatment strategies until ovulation is established and pregnancy can be achieved. The patient must be made aware of the side effects of the drugs to be used and the potential risks of treatment, including multiple gestation and ovarian hyperstimulation syndrome (OHSS). Ensuring patient safety may require using less aggressive treatment modalities, but with lower pregnancy rates.

Weight Reduction

Obesity affects at least 50 percent of women with PCOS and may independently affect the adverse health consequences of the syndrome. In obese women, weight reduction alone may lead to spontaneous ovulation and pregnancy. Obese women will require a higher dose of clomiphene citrate and/or gonadotrophins perhaps because they are more likely to be hyperinsulinemic. They may also have worse outcomes in terms of ovulation rates and pregnancy loss. Jakubowicz and Nestler[21] have reported a decrease in insulin and in total and free testosterone levels and an increase in SHBC in PCO subjects with caloric restriction. Because of all these reasons, weight reduction should be the first step in the management of PCOS.

Clomiphene Citrate

Even though, for most patients with PCOS, the pharmacological agent of choice to induce ovulation is clomiphene citrate, the pregnancy rate is less than 40 percent of the ovulation rate and the early pregnancy loss is high. It is prudent to start Metformin initially for patients with obesity, hyperandrogenism and/or hyperinsulinemia for 6-8 weeks along with caloric restriction before the clomiphene therapy. Metformin

therapy results in resumption of normal cycles in amenorrheic women with PCOS leading to spontaneous ovulation and pregnancy.[22, 23] Even non-obese women with PCOS demonstrate an intrinsic form of insulin resistance and will be benefited by metformin therapy.

Those who do not ovulate with weight reduction/metformin therapy may be started on clomiphene therapy. The starting dose is 50 mg/day for 5 days from 5th day of the spontaneous or progesterone withdrawal bleeding. Monitoring of ovulation is better done by transvaginal ultrasonography 5 to 7 days after the last dose of clomiphene citrate. When the follicular size reaches 18-20 mm, injection human chorionic gonadotropin (hCG) is given in a dose of 5000 to 10,000 IU. Maximum success with clomiphene is within the first 3 to 4 months and there is no point in continuing with clomiphene citrate for more than 6 cycles and increasing the dose to more than 150 mg/day. There are also reports of association of ovarian cancer with clomiphene citrate use of more than 12 cycles.[24]

Strategies to improve outcome in clomiphene treatment cycles: In cases of adrenal hyperandrogenism associated with PCOS, as evidenced by a DHEAS level of more than 200 µg/dL, dexamethasone in a dose of 0.25 mg/day is given at bed time with better results. To counter the antiestrogenic effect of clomiphene citrate on the endometrium, ethenylestradiol is started after the last day of clomiphene with improved results.[25]

Gonadotropins

Use of gonadotropins for induction in clomiphene resistant cases is a more aggressive approach to ovulation induction in PCOS. To reduce the risk of multiple gestation and ovarian hyperstimulation syndrome, low-dose, "step-up" regimens are employed. The starting dose is 75 IU or less of FSH from the 3rd day with transvaginal ultrasound follicular study to achieve monofollicular development. The dose increment is limited to 37.5 IU/day and is made no more frequently than every 7 days. The ovulatory hCG trigger 5000-10000 IU is given once the lead follicle is 18 mm and above. The hCG trigger is withheld if there are more than three follicles of 16 mm and above with estradiol levels greater than 2500 pg/ml. Low-dose "step-down" regimen, where the dose reduced once the lead follicle reaches 10 mm, mimics the normal menstrual cycle and gives even better results.[26] The availability of recombinant preparations may have greater bioavailability and lower total dose requirements.

GnRH Agonists and Antagonists

The elevated baseline or midfollicular LH levels in PCO subjects leads to higher rates of anovulation, ovulation without conception, and early pregnancy loss than controls. Down regulation with GnRH analogue and then induction with gonadotropin will avoid the premature LH surge and improve treatment outcome. Availability of GnRH antagonists has become the better therapeutic option to avoid premature LH surge in PCOS. Unlike GnRH agonists, which act on chronic administration through down regulation, the antagonists lead to an immediate block of gonadotropin secretion. Concurrent ganirelix and follitropinbeta therapy is an effective and safe regimen for ovulation induction in women with polycystic ovary syndrome.[27]

Letrozole

Letrozole is an aromatase inhibitor which blocks the negative feedback of estrogen on the pituitary by reducing the estrogen levels and pituitary will increase the gonadotropin output and may lead to ovulation. Since the half-life is shorter than that of clomiphene citrate, Letrozole may not produce the adverse endometrial effects as with clomiphene citrate. The dose is 2.5 mg/day for 5 days from 5th day. The ovulation rate is comparable to clomiphene citrate.

Insulin Sensitizing Agents

Given the central role of hyperinsulinemia and insulin resistance in the pathophysiology of PCOS, insulin sensitizing agents have the potential to ameliorate insulin resistance and alleviate the spectrum of endocrine, metabolic and reproductive abnormalities in women with PCOS.

The drugs available are metformin, a biguanide, the thiazolidinedione group of drugs like troglitazone, rosiglitazone, pioglitazone and englitazone, and phosphoglycan D-chiro-inositol.

Metformin

The action of metformin is on multiple metabolic pathways, reduces the absorption of glucose, suppress hepatic glucose output and gluconeogenesis.[28] It also improves the action of insulin at the cellular level by enhancing glucose uptake by fat and muscle cells and by increasing insulin receptor binding.[29] Reduction in free fatty acid release from adipose tissue further enhances insulin sensitivity.[30] Importantly, the actions of metformin are not associated with an increase in insulin secretion and hence hypoglycemia is not a risk. Metformin is a safe, cost-effective drug with a good safety profile. To reduce the mild gastrointestinal side effects, it is given with meals. Lactic acidosis is a major complication, but rare, seen if given to patients with hepatic or renal impairment. The drug is started at a smaller dose of 500 mg daily for one week, 500 mg twice a week for the next week and then 500 mg three times a day. For very obese patients, metformin may be given at a dose of 850 mg twice a week.

A significant reduction in circulating concentrations of androgens has been observed after metformin therapy, which appears to correlate with improved insulin sensitivity. The amelioration of insulin resistance obviate the suppressive effect of insulin on hepatic SHBG and IGFBP-I production resulting in decreased bioavailability of testosterone. Improvement in insulin sensitivity would be expected to have a favorable effect on cardiovascular risk factors. Improvement in ovulatory profile occurs after short-term metformin therapy, and appears to be independent of weight loss, duration of treatment and dosage used.[22] When used alone, or in conjunction with other ovulation induction agents, metformin play an important role in anovulatory infertility associated with PCOS. Pregnancy rates of 39 percent when used alone and 89 percent when combined with clomiphene citrate[31] have been reported. It may also be effective when used as pretreatment in ovulation regimens with Gonadotropins, and it may correct disordered folliculogesis, decreasing the incidence of cycle cancellation.[32]

Continuing Metformin during Pregnancy

In a pilot study conducted by Gluck *et al* (2001), it was concluded that metformin therapy throughout pregnancy in women with PCOS decreases the otherwise high rate of first-trimester spontaneous abortion observed among women not receiving metformin. Metformin does not seem to have teratogenic effects.[33] In the treated group, the incidence of spontaneous abortion was 10 percent compared to the 73 percent incidence in the control. The beneficial effect of reducing the level of PAI-I by metformin is thought to be improving the pregnancy outcome.[34]

Hyperinsulinemia in PCOS and Effect of Metformin

Glucose stimulated insulin level was studied by the author in 75 patients with PCOS diagnosed by clinical features, hormonal pattern and ultrasound criteria and in 25 controls matched for weight.

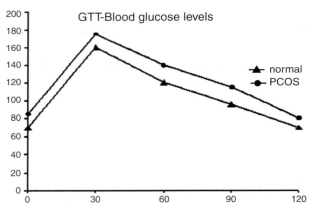

FIGURE 9.1: Blood glucose level with 75 gm oral GTT in normal and PCO subjects.

In both the controls and PCO subjects, the blood glucose levels were within normal limits. In order to maintain this normal blood sugar levels, the PCO subjects were to release three to four-fold amount of insulin as it is shown in the Figure 9.2 (Hyperinsulinemia).

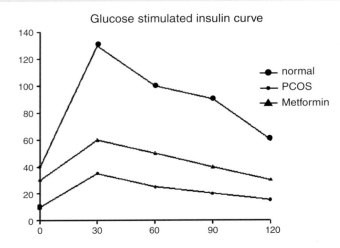

FIGURE 9.2: Insulin levels after GTT (75 gm) in normal, PCOS, and after metformin therapy in micro IU/ml

These patients were started on metformin 500 mg twice a day for one week and then 500 mg three times a day for another seven weeks. Glucose stimulated insulin levels was studied after 8 weeks of metformin therapy by giving 75 gms oral glucose. The insulin level was almost near normal after metformin therapy.

Thiazolidinedione Group of Drugs

Insulin sensitizing agents of the thiazolidinedione group have more pronounced effects on insulin sensitivity, endocrine profile, menstrual and ovulatory function in women with PCOS.[35] These drugs bind to peroxisome proliferator-activated receptor gamma (pparγ) in adipose tissue, which then binds to the retinoid X receptor, which in turn promotes the transcription of the genes involved in glucose metabolism. However, troglitazone, the most commonly known member of the group was withdrawn because of hepatotoxicity, and experience with the newer derivatives like rosiglitazone and pioglitazone is limited. In a recent randomized controlled trial, short-term rosiglitazone therapy enhances both spontaneous and clomiphene-induced ovulation in overweight and obese women with PCOS. Rosiglitazone therapy improves insulin sensitivity and decreases hyperandrogenemia primarily through increase in SHBG.[36] In another study, it was observed that combined rosiglitazone and clomiphene was an effective therapeutic regimen for correcting insulin resistance in patients with PCOS, possibly by reducing IGF-1 bioavailability to the ovaries, thus modifying the hyperandrogenic intrafollicular milieu that occurs in PCOS. In addition, the clinical and hormonal responses were better than clomiphene alone.[37]

D-chiro-inositol

Inositol phosphoglycans act as mediators of post receptor signaling of the activated insulin receptor. Administration of D-chiro-inositol may serve as a precursor for inositolglycan mediators of insulin signal transduction, and found to lower circulating insulin and improve insulin action in primates. In a placebo-controlled trial, D-chiro-inositol given to women with PCOS, found to reduce insulin secretion during GTT and increases plasma SHBG with spontaneous ovulation.[38] As with metformin therapy D-chiro-inositol also does not cause hypoglycemia.

Surgical Induction of Ovulation

For many years, ovarian wedge resection through laparotomy was standard treatment for infertile women with PCOS. Even though a high ovulation rate was claimed, the pregnancy rate was low and in many cases, postoperative adhesions replaced hormonal infertility with mechanical infertility.[39] With the advances in understanding the pathophysiology of PCOS, medical treatments replaced surgery for PCOS-induced infertility. It was replaced by medical ovulation induction with clomiphene and gonadotropins. However patients with PCOS treated with gonadotropins often have a polyfollicular response and are exposed to the risks of ovarian hyperstimulation syndrome (OHSS) and multiple pregnancies. With the availability of laparoscopic and microsurgical techniques, minimally invasive laparoscopic procedures as a potentially permanent treatment for PCOS restored interest in surgical options. Laparoscopic "ovarian drilling" with cautery or laser vaporization on one or both ovaries have been used to restore ovulation and with advantage of avoiding OHSS and multiple pregnancies.[40] Ovarian drilling with minilaparoscopy under local anesthesia is equally effective with a short hospital stay.[41] Use of harmonic scalpel for ovarian drilling is a new development. Ultrasonographic puncture of the follicles is reported to give comparable success rate to that of laparoscopic ovarian drilling in PCOS.[42] In a recent report, minipalarotomy and ovarian wedge resection observing microsurgical technique has given very good results, 78 percent pregnancy rate within 6 months and 90 percent pregnancy in two years, in women with PCOS who failed to respond to clomiphene citrate and gonadotropins.[43]

Although surgical approach is not considered as the first line of therapy in patients with PCOS, in those who failed to respond to clomiphene citrate and gonadotropins, operative management may be a viable option.

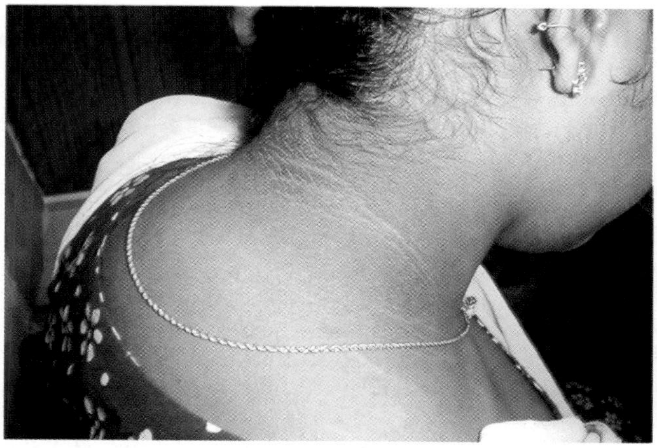

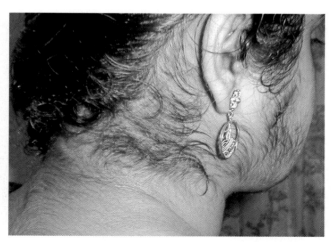

FIGURE 9.3: Acanthosis Nigricans in an unmarried girl with PCOS (PKS)

FIGURE 9.4: Hirsutism in an unmarried girl with PCOS (PKS)

CONCLUSION

PCOS is a multifactorial disorder principally characterized by ovarian hyperandrogenism and anovulation. Hyperinsulinemia appears to play a key pathogenic role in the hyperandrogenism in many women with PCOS, regardless of whether they are obese or lean. Hyperinsulinemic insulin resistance may act at several levels to contribute to the anovulation and infertility of PCOS. Pharmacologic treatment that improves insulin sensitivity and lowers circulating insulin levels may allow for spontaneous ovulation or for greater success of standard induction protocols. Women with PCOS are at increased risk for the development of impaired glucose tolerance or type 2 diabetes mellitus, dyslipidemia, hypertension, and atherosclerosis. Some of these potential complications are likely related to the hyperinsulinemia and insulin resistance. Therefore, the use of insulin-sensitizing drugs may be indicated for the prevention or treatment of these associated disorders.

REFERENCES

1. Stein IF, Leventhal ML. Amenorrhea associated with bilateral polycystic ovaries. Am J Obstet Gynecol 1935;29:181-91.
2. Redo Azziz. Polycystic ovary syndrome, insulin resistance, and molecular defects in insulin signaling. J Clin Endocrinol Metab 2002;87(9):4085-87.
3. Mc KemmaTJ. Pathogenesis and treatment of polycystic ovary syndrome. N Engl J Med 1988;318:558-62.
4. Franks S. Polycystic ovary syndrome changing prospective. Clin Endocrinol 1989;31(87):120.
5. Barnes R, Rosenfield RL. Polycystic ovary syndrome pathogenesis and treatment. Ann Intern Med 1989;102: 386-99.
6. Rebar RW: Gonadotrophin secretion in PCO Seminars Repord Endocrinol 1984;2:223.
7. Dunaif A, Segal KR, Futterweit W, Dobrjansky A. Profound insulin resistance, independent of obesity in polycystic ovary syndrome. Diabetes 1989;38:1165-74.
8. Legro RS, Fingood D, Dunaif A. A fasting glucose to insulin ratio is a useful measure of insulin sensitivity in women with polycystic ovary syndrome. J Clin Endocrinol Metab 1998;83:2694-98.
9. Bonora E, Kiechl S, Willeit J, et al. Prevalence of insulin resistance in metabolic disorders. The Bruneck study. Diabetes 1998;47;1643-49.
10. Dunaif A, Xia J, Book C et al. Excessive insulin receptor serine phosphorelation in cultured fibroblasts and in skeletal muscle; a potential mechanism for insulin resistance in the polycystic ovary syndrome. J Clin Invest 1995;96:801-10.
11. Kern PA, Saghizadeh M, Capp E et al. The expression of tumor necrosis factor alpha in human adipose tissue J Clin Invest 1995;95:2111-19.
12. Hotamisiligil GS, Peraldi P, Budavari A et al. IRS-I mediated inhibition of insulin receptor tyrosine kinase activity in TNFα and obesity induced insulin resistance. Science 1996;271:665-68.
13. Velazquez EM, Mendoza SG, Hamer T et al. Metformin therapy in polycystic ovary syndrome reduces hyperinsulinemia, insulin resistance, hyperandrogenemia and systolic blood pressure, while facilitating normal menses and pregnancy. Metabolism 1994;43:647-54.
14. Velazquez EM, Acosta A, Mendosa SG et al. Menstrual cyclicity after metformin therapy in polycystic ovary syndrome. Obstet Gynecol 1997;90:392-95.
15. Velazquez EM, Mendosa SG, Wang P, Glueck CJ. Metformin therapy is associated with a decrease in plasma plasminogen activator inhibitor-I, lipoprotein(a), and immunoreactive insulin levels in patients with polycystic ovary syndrome. Metabolism 1997;46: 454-57.
16. Bracero N, Zacur HA. Polycystic ovary syndrome and hyperprolactinemia. Obst Gynecol Clin North Am 2001;28:77-84.
17. Zhang Y, Proenca R, Maffei M et al. Positional cloning of the mouse obese gene and its human homologue. Nature 1994;373:425.
18. Kalro BN, Loucks TL, Berga SL. Neuromodulation in polycystic ovary syndrome. Obst gynecol Clin North Am 2001;28:35-62.
19. Balan AH, Conway GS, Kaltsas G et al. Polycystic ovary syndrome: The spectrum of the disorder in 1741 patients. Hum Reprod 1995;10:2107-11.
20. Adams J, Franks S, Polson DW et al. Multifollicular ovaries, Clinical and endocrine features and response to pulsatile gonadotrophin releasing hormone. Lancet 1985;(ii):1375.
21. Jakubowicz DA, Nestler IE. 17alfa hydroxyprogesterone responses to leuprolide and serum androgens in obese women with and without polycystic ovary syndrome after weight loss. J Clin Endocrinol Metab 1997;82: 556-60.
22. Velazquez E, Acosta A, Mendosa SG. Menstrual cyclicity after metformin therapy in polycystic ovary syndrome. Obstet Gynecol 1997;90:392-95.
23. Valazquez EM, Mendosa S, Hamer T, Sosa F, Glueck CJ. Metformin therapy in polycystic ovary syndrome reduces hyperinsulinemia, insulin resistance, hyperandrogenemia, and systolic blood pressure while facilitating normal menses and pregnancy. Metabolism 1994;43(5):647-54.
24. Whittemore AS, Harris R, Itnyre J et al. Characteristics relating to ovarian cancer risk collaborative analysis Am J epidemiol 1992;136:1184-1203.

25. Gerli S, Gholami H, Manna C et al. Use of ethinyl estradiol to reverse the antiestrogenic effects of clomiphene citrate in patients undergoing intrauterine insemination. Fertil Steril 2000;73:85-89, erratum Fertil Steril 2000;74:424.

26. Homber R, Howles CM. Low-dose FSH therapy for anovulatory infertility associated with polycystic ovary syndrome:Hum Reprod Update 1999;5:493-99.

27. Elkind-Hirsch KE, Webster BW, Brown CP, Vernon MW. Concurrent ganirelix and follitropin beta therapy is an effective and safe regimen for ovulation induction in women with polycystic ovary syndrome. Fertil Steril, 2003;79(3):603-07.

28. Bailey CJ. Metformin; an update. Gen pharmacol 1993;24:1299-1309.

29. Matthaei S, Hamann A, Klein HH et al. Association of metformin's effect to increase insulin stimulated glucose transport with potentiation of insulin induced translocation of glucose transporters from intracellular pool to plasma membrane in rat adipocytes. Diabetes, 1991;40:850-57.

30. Abbasi F, Kamath V, Rizvi AA. Results of a placebo controlled study of the metabolic effect of the addition of metformin to sulfonyl urea treated patients. Evidence for a central role of adipose tissue. Diabetes care. 1997;20:1863-69.

31. Nestler JE, Jakubowicz DJ, Evans WS, et al. Effects of metformin on spontaneous and clomiphene induced ovulation in the polycystic ovary syndrome. N Eng J Med 1998;338:1876-80.

32. De L, La M, Ditto A et al. Effects of metformin on gonadotrophin induced ovulation in women with polycystic syndrome. Fertil Steril 1999;72:282-85.

33. Glueck CJ, Phillips H, Cameron D et al. Continuing metformin throughout pregnancy in women with polycystic ovary syndrome appears to safely reduce first–trimester spontaneous abortion: A pilot study. Fertil Steril 2001;75:46-52.

34. Gleuck CJ, Wang P, Fontaine RN et al. Plasminogen activator inhibitor activity. Metabolism 1999;48; 1589-95.

35. Dunaif A, Scott D, Finegood D et al. The insulin sensitising agent troglitazone improves metabolic and reproductive abnormalities in the polycystic ovary syndrome. J Clin Endocrinol Metab. 1996;81:3299-3306.

36. Ghazeeri G, Kutteh WH, Bryer-Ash M, Haas D, Ke RW. Effect of rosiglitazone on spontaneous and clomiphene citrate induced ovulation in women with polycystic ovary syndrome. Fertil Steril 2003;79(3):562-66.

37. Shobokshi A, Shaarawy M. Correction of insulin resistance and hyperandrogenism in polycystic ovary syndrome by combined rosiglitazone and clomiphene citrate therapy.J Soc Gynecol Investig 2003;10(2): 99-104.

38. Nestler JE, Jakubowicz D, Reamer P et al. Ovulatory and metabolic effects of D-chiro-inositol in the polysystic ovary syndrome. N Engl J Med 1999;340:1314-20.

39. Toaff R, Toaff ME, Peyser MR. Infertility following wedge resection of the ovaries. Am J Obstet Gynecol. 1976;1:124(1):92-96.

40. Campo S. Ovulatory cycles, pregnancy outcome and complications after surgical treatment of polycystic ovary syndrome. Obstet Gynecol Surv 1998;53:297.

41. Zullo F, Pellicano M, Zupi E, Guida M, Mastrantonio P, Nappi C. Minilaparoscopic ovarian drilling under local anesthesia in patients with polycystic ovary syndrome. Fertil Steril 2000;74(2):376-79.

42. Domitrz J, Szamatowicz J, Swiatecka J, Grygoruk C, Wolczynski S, Szamatowicz M. Two treatment methods of infertility associated with polycystic ovarian syndrome Ginekol Pol 2002;73(10):835-40.

43. Yildirim M, Noyan V, Bulent Tiras M, Yildiz A, Guner H. Ovarian wedge resection by minilaparatomy in infertile patients with polycystic ovarian syndrome: A new technique. Eur J Obstet Gynecol Reprod Biol 2003;26:107(1):85-87.

• Radha Reddy

10

Hirsutism

Hirsutism is the development of androgen dependent terminal body hair in a woman in areas in which terminal body hair is not found.[1] Terminal body hair is stiff and pigmented, normally seen in men on the face, chest, abdomen and back and which are not normal in women.

Virilization refers to the concurrent presentation of hirsutism with a broad range of signs suggestive of androgen excess, such as acne, frontotemporal balding, deepening of voice, decrease in breast size, clitoral hypertrophy, increased muscle mass, and amenorrhea or oligomenorrhea. Virilization is seen less frequently than hirsutism and may reflect a severe underlying pathological condition, such as malignancy or androgen secreting tumors. Thus, hirsutism may be the initial manifestation of virilization.

Conditions with generalized hair growth that do not represent true hirsutism include:
- Lanugo—soft vellus unpigmented hair that is androgen independent and covers the whole body. This type of hair is seen in infants.
- Hypertrichosis—diffuse increased total body vellus hair. This condition can be caused by drugs (minoxidil, diazoxide, cyclosporine) and systemic illnesses like hypothyroidism, anorexia, and malignancy.

EPIDEMIOLOGY

The overall prevalence of hirsutism is unknown, though approximately 5–10 percent of all women demonstrate some form of this condition.[2] The race, ethnicity and women's own perception of normal must be considered when defining this condition. Most Caucasian, Native American and Oriental women have little body hair, whereas Mediterranean, African American and South Asian women have moderately heavy body hair; serum androgens being similar in all groups.[3]

Whatever the women's background, one must initiate evaluation for hirsutism if the pattern of hair growth has changed or rate of growth has increased.[4] Historically, hair has served as an organ of beauty for men and women. Being in an era of hairless female beauty, the psychological consequences of hirsutism can be more devastating to the patient than the underlying physiologic concerns.[5]

BASICS OF HAIR

Several facts about hair are relevant to the management of hirsutism.[6,7] Hair grows from individual follicles that form part of a pilosebaceous gland unit. The number of hair follicles is set at birth and is same for both sexes, but the degree of differentiation varies between the sexes. In humans, hair growth is continuous, but in various stages of development in a given area, resulting in a static number of hair. Disorders causing high level of synchrony of growth can lead to excess hair. Length of life cycle of the hair determines the length of the hair—scalp hair having the longest cycle of 2-6 years. The length of the life cycle also helps determine the duration required to see the effectiveness of any treatment modality used to modify hair growth, i.e. may need 3-6 months of treatment before effectiveness of therapy for hirsutism can be determined.

The growth cycle of the hair consists of three phases[8] —anagen, catagen and telogen. Anagen comprises 80-90 percent of the cycle and is the growth phase. It is influenced by various therapeutic modalities. Catagen is the involution phase and telogen the quiescent phase, both of which account for 10-15 percent of the cycle.

The three hair types include:
• Lanugo—body hair seen in the infant and newborn.
• Vellus—fine hair covering the adult body
• Terminal hair—thick, pigmented hair seen on the scalp, eyebrows, eyelashes before puberty and secondary sexual sites after puberty. This hair develops from vellus hair.

Hormonal Control of Hair

Areas of the body dependent on androgen input include the face, neck, chest, abdomen, axilla, upper arms, inner thighs and pubic regions. Part of the scalp is also androgen sensitive. Androgen stimulation of the pilosebaceous unit in these areas leads to conversion of the vellus to terminal hair by the interaction of testosterone with the androgen receptor as well as intracellular conversion of testosterone to the more potent dihydrotestosterone by the enzyme 5 alpha-reductase (Figure 10.1).[9] Whereas there are two types of 5 alpha reductase isoenzymes–Type 1 and 2, the activity of these in the facial or abdominal skin of hirsute women remains to be determined

Skin is a major site of testosterone formation in women, in whom half of the testosterone production is derived from peripheral conversion of 17ketosteroids such as DHEA, DHEA—sulfate and androstenidione.[10] Skin is not capable of de novo synthesis of androgens but it has all the

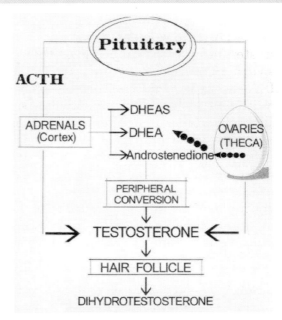

FIGURE 10.1: Conversion of vellus to terminal hair. DHEA = dehydroepiandrosterone; DHEAS= dehydroepiandrosterone sulfate

enzymes required for conversion of the prohormones into testosterone and the most potent androgen dihydrotestosterone (Figure 10.2).[11]

Estrogen tends to shorten the telogen or the quiescent phase, increase the synchrony of hair growth and lead to finer, less pigmented and slower growing hair. This effect is best seen in pregnancy, when the anagen phase is increased to 90 percent with growth of hair. In the postpartum state, hair returns to telogen phase with resultant shedding of the hair.[12]

HIRSUTISM

Hirsutism is caused by either:
• Increased androgen production by the ovary
• Increased androgen production by the adrenals
• Rarely, increased target organ production of androgen.

Sources of androgen secretion in normal women are shown in Table 10.1.

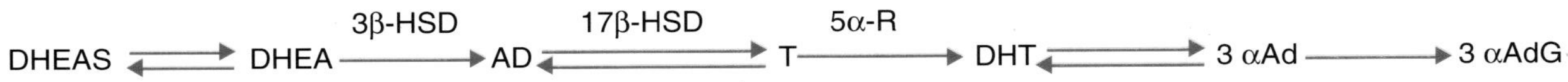

$$DHEAS \rightleftharpoons DHEA \xrightarrow{3\beta\text{-HSD}} AD \xrightleftharpoons{17\beta\text{-HSD}} T \xrightarrow{5\alpha\text{-R}} DHT \rightleftharpoons 3\,\alpha Ad \longrightarrow 3\,\alpha AdG$$

FIGURE 10.2: A schematic representation of androgen metabolism in the skin. The skin metabolizes weak androgens such as DHEA-sulfate (DHEAS) to the more potent ones, such as DHT. The enzymes are 3ß-hydroxysteroid dehydrogenase

Several different androgens may be secreted in excess in hirsute women:
- Testosterone excess is usually of ovarian origin
- Dehydroepiandrosterone sulfate (DHEA-S)/ DHEA excess is of adrenal origin—they have very little intrinsic androgenic activity. Both are mainly converted to androstenedione and testosterone in the adrenal gland and peripheral tissues.
- Androstenedione excess can be of adrenal or ovarian origin.

The commonest cause of hirsutism in women is anovulation causing excessive androgen secretion (both testosterone and androstenidione) by the ovary. Adrenal causes are relatively rare.

TABLE 10.1: Sources of serum androgens in normal females

Androgen	Ovary	Adrenal	Peripheral conversion
DHA	10%	10%	0
DHEA-S	< 5%	> 95%	0
Androstenedione (A)	50%	50%	0
Testosterone (T)	25%	25%	50%
Dihydrotestosterone (DHT)	0	0	100% (from A &T)
3-Androstenediol glucoronide	0	0	100% (from DHT)

Androgens circulate in a bound and unbound fashion. In normal women, 80 percent of testosterone is bound to sex hormone-binding globulin (SHBG), 19 percent is bound to albumin, and 1 percent circulates free in the blood stream. In hirsute women free testosterone is higher at 2 percent and in men it is 3 percent. This clinical correlation confirms that androgenicity depends mainly on unbound testosterone. In addition, the androgen effect depends on the level of SHBG. It is possible for hirsute women to have normal levels of testosterone with a suppression of SHBG or increased activity of 5 alpha-reductase and subsequently elevated DHT.

ETIOLOGY OF HIRSUTISM

The most common cause of hirsutism is PCOS, accounting for nearly 60 percent of all cases of hirsutism. Idiopathic hirsutism accounts for 20-30 percent of all women with hirsutism,

remaining 10 percent or less being due to other rarer endocrine causes (Table 10.2).

TABLE 10.2: Causes of hirsutism in women

Common
- Idiopathic hirsutism
- PCOS

Rare
- Hyperprolactinemia
- Drugs
  Danazol
  OCP—containing androgenic progestins
- Congenital adrenal hyperplasia, mostly 21-hydroxylase deficiency
- Hyperthecosis
- Ovarian tumors
  Sertoli-Leydig cell tumors
  Granulosa-theca cell tumors
  Hilus cell tumors
- Adrenal tumors
- Severe insulin resistance syndromes

Idiopathic Hirsutism (IH)

Idiopathic hirsutism (IH) is a diagnosis of exclusion. Its strict definition includes a hirsute woman with normal ovulatory function and normal androgen levels.[13] Using this definition, the prevalence of IH is very low, less than 20 percent. Exaggerated 5 alpha reductase activity, androgen receptor polymorphisms and abnormal androgen metabolism are all thought to be plausible mechanisms. Serum total and free testosterone, DHEAS, 17OHP are all usually normal in IH. Routine measurements of 3 alpha androstenediol glucoronide are not recommended in clinical practice, though elevated, it is not specific for IH.[14] The onset of IH is generally after puberty, gradually progressive and associated with a family history of hirsutism.

Polycystic Ovary Syndrome (PCOS)

Polycystic ovary syndrome (PCOS) is the most common cause of hirsutism in women. Minimal criteria for diagnosis include:
- Menstrual irregularity
- Hyperandrogenism–clinical (hirsutism, balding) or biochemical (increased androgens–testosterone/DHEAS)
- Exclusion of other causes of hirsutism like CAH/ androgen secreting tumors/androgen ingestion, etc.

Thus, ultrasound of the ovaries or other biochemical parameters (except those to exclude other causes) are not mandatory for the diagnosis of PCOS.[15, 16] Hirsutism begins gradually at puberty and is usually associated with menstrual irregularity and features of insulin resistance like acanthosis nigricans, obesity, etc.

Hyperprolactinemia

Hyperprolactinemia with occasional mild increase in DHEAS has been noted in women with hirsutism. Whether hyperprolactinemia *per se* can cause hirsutism is unknown. However, the underlying problem in most of these women is probably PCOS.[4]

Congenital Adrenal Hyperplasia (CAH)

Congenital adrenal hyperplasia (CAH) accounts for 5 percent of cases with hirsutism. It is almost always due to 21 hydroxylase deficiency, which leads to increased 17 hydroxy progesterone and androstenedione, without associated cortisol deficiency. It is usually late onset, with hirsutism and menstrual irregularities beginning at puberty.

Ovarian Tumors

Ovarian tumors androgen secreting tumors account for only 5 percent of ovarian tumors. They are generally associated with rapidly progressive hirsutism. Serum testosterone levels is generally over 150-200 ng/dL and tumors are detected on vaginal ultrasound.

Adrenal Tumors

Adrenal tumors are a rare cause of hirsutism. Adenomas generally secrete testosterone, but carcinomas of the adrenal gland secrete DHEA/DHEAS and cortisol. Occasional carcinomas lose the ability to sulfate DHEA, so normal DHEAS does not rule out the possibility of tumor.[17] Nevertheless, an unequivocally elevated DHEAS is suggestive of adrenal malignancy.

EVALUATION OF HIRSUTISM

As majority of women with hirsutism have IH or PCOS, evaluation of the patient entails ensuring that the patient does not have some of the rarer, more serious causes of hirsutism like adrenal or ovarian tumors. Features that suggest rare causes of hirsutism include:

- Abrupt onset, short duration and progressive nature of hirsutism
- Older age of onset of hirsutism, rather than near puberty
- Signs of virilization
- Moderate to severe increase in androgen levels, like S.testosterone > 150 ng/dL, free testosterone > 2 ng/dL, serum DHEAS > 500 µg/dL in young women.[18]

History and Physical Examination

History and physical examination help determine the cause of hirsutism.

History should include:
- Menstrual history-age at menarche, regularity of menses, pregnancies, use of OCP, and ovulatory symptoms. Women with regular menstrual cycles and ovulatory symptoms are unlikely to have hyperandrogenism.
- History of hirsutism, acne, balding.
- Time of onset and rate of progression of hirsutism.
- Weight—obese patients are more hyperandrogenic
- Medications—ingestion of Danazol and androgenic oral contraceptives like levonorgesterol.
- Family history—hirsutism, acne, obesity, menstrual irregularities, infertility all suggest a family history of PCOS. Work up for CAH should be considered if there is positive family history for the same.
- Current hair removal techniques or medications tried for hirsutism.

Physical exam to determine the extent and cause of hirsutism
- Identify between
  - Hirsutism–terminal hair in androgen dependent areas like upperlip, chin, chest, etc
  - Hypertrichosis–vellus hair all over the body
- Determine the extent of hirsutism using the modified Ferriman Gallwey scoring system. Nine sites are assessed and graded between Grade 1–mild hirsutism, to Grade 4-frank

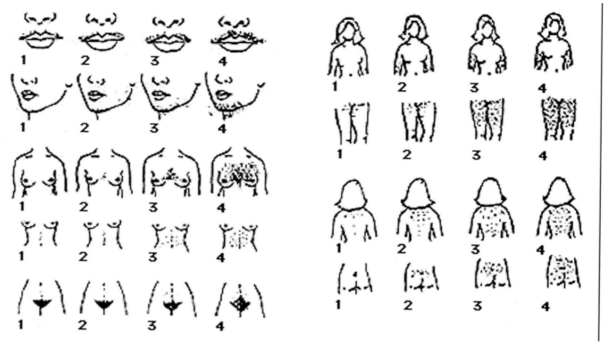

FIGURE 10.3: Hirsutism grading

virilization. A score of 8 or more indicates hirsutism and only 5 percent of women qualify by this criteria (Figure 10.3).[19]
- Signs of androgen excess-acne, seborrhea, temporal balding.
- Features of Cushing's-body fat distribution, striae, thin skin, etc.
- Insulin resistance–acanthosis nigricans
- Virilization–deepening of voice, clitoromegaly, frontal or crown balding, increased muscle mass.
- Galactorrhea–for hyperprolactinemia
- Abdominal and pelvic exam for androgen producing tumor.
- Weight, BP, etc.

Lab Evaluation

Lab evaluation is generally not required for a woman with long-standing, slowly progressive, mild hirsutism with regular menses. Unless the history and examination point to a particular condition, serum testosterone, which is mainly produced by the ovary, and serum DHEAS, mainly produced by the adrenals, are the most useful screening tests.
- Blood glucose, lipid profile in PCOS

- *S Testosterone*–is the single best estimate of androgen production in the hirsute women. S Testosterone values below 150 ng/dL exclude most ovarian and adrenal androgen secreting tumors as well as ovarian hyperthecosis.[17, 20, 21] In women with androgen excess, due to decreased sex hormone binding globulin (SHBG),[22] serum free testosterone is a more sensitive indicator of androgen excess than total testosterone. But serum free testosterone is not routinely indicated as serum total testosterone provides an adequate estimate of androgen excess and readily identifies those who need additional workup.[4] Hirsute women with markedly elevated testosterone and normal ovulatory cycles should be worked up for adrenal tumors.
- *S Prolactin* should be measured in women with irregular menses. S Prolactin may be marginally elevated in women with PCOS. S Prolactin over 150 ng/dL is suggestive of a prolactinoma, whereas levels over 50 ng/dL can be due to stalk compression and warrant an MRI to rule out a tumor.
- *S DHEAS* should be monitored in women with progressive hirsutism or virilization to rule out

adrenal tumors. Values are age specific, and values greater than 500 µg/dL suggest an adrenal tumor.

- *S FSH* is to be measured in women with irregular menses to rule out menopause. Hirsutism occurs due to decrease in estradiol causing decrease in SHBG and increased free testosterone.
- *S LH* is high in women with PCOS with alteration in FSH:LH ratio. This is not mandatory for the diagnosis of PCOS.
- *S.17 hydroxy progesterone*–a fasting 8.00 AM sample during the follicular phase, if greater than 200 ng/dL is suggestive of LOCAH. LOCAH is confirmed if the S.17OHP is greater than 1000 ng/dL, 60 minutes post Synacthen 250 µg IM.
- Overnight 1 mg *dexamethasone suppression* test or a 24 hour urine free cortisol should be done if Cushing's syndrome is suspected.
- *S 3 alpha androstanediol glucoronide* is a metabolite of dihydrotestosterone and adds little useful information to the management of hirsutism.[23, 24]
- *Pelvic USG* is useful in identification of ovarian tumors or PCOS. Current high resolution scans with vaginal probes can identify tumors/cysts as small as 3-5mm.Large cysts, solid masses, complex cysts that do resolve by 2-4 weeks are suspicious for tumors. In PCOS, the ovaries are enlarged, with a rim of peripheral small cysts, no more than 8 mm in size, with dense central stroma. Pelvis USG is not mandatory for the diagnosis of PCOS. Up to 30 percent of normal women may have cysts in the ovary. Polycystic ovaries may also be seen in women with CAH and adrenal tumors.
- *Abdominal CT or MRI* is indicated if S DHEAS is very high or other hormone secreting adrenal tumor is suspected. Routine imaging of adrenal gland is not recommended because of the high prevalence of incidentalomas of the adrenal gland.
- *Laparotomy or laparoscopy*–should be considered in women with irregular menses, serum testosterone > 200 ng/dL, negative CT/MRI adrenals and USG pelvis, as a small ovarian tumor may have been missed.

- *Ovarian or adrenal vein sampling*–is seldom useful, and highly dependent on the skill of the radiologist.

Hence the diagnostic approach to hirsutism should be as follows:[4]

- Women with long-standing mild to moderate hirsutism, with a positive family history and regular menstrual cycles need no work up.
- Women with mild to moderate hirsutism should have a serum testosterone level. S Prolactin should be done if menstrual cycle is irregular.
- Women with rapidly progressive hirsutism, irregular menses and features of virilization should have a serum DHEAS level in addition to serum testosterone.
- Other tests should be done only as clinically indicated.

TREATMENT OF HIRSUTISM

Hirsutism is only a minor cosmetic problem in a fair number of patient's, requiring only reassurance. In individuals, in whom hirsutism is severe enough to cause psychological problems, or is associated with a medical condition, treatment includes mechanical removal of hair, drugs that reduce androgen secretion, androgen action or both, as well as treatment of the cause. Goals of therapy include not only slowing or stopping hair growth but also treatment of associated menstrual irregularity and infertility. [25]

Nonpharmacological Treatment of Hirsutism

This is a safe and effective method for treatment of hirsutism. It should be encouraged in all women either alone or in combination with drug therapy. A common misconception is that mechanical hair removal, especially shaving, cause hair to grow more rapidly.

- Depilation—(shaving) is partial removal of hair close to the skin surface. It is safe and effective.
- Epilation—evulsion of hair from the hair follicle by plucking or waxing. Contrary to popular beliefs, neither the rate of hair growth nor the diameter of the hair is increased.
- Chemical depilatories and bleaching is effective, but can cause skin rashes.
- Electrolysis—involves electrocoagulation of the hair follicles using thermolysis and direct

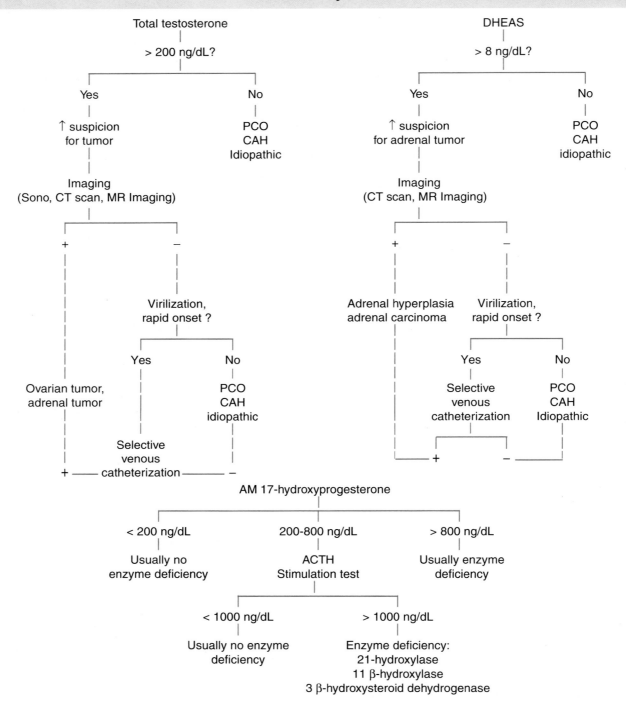

FIGURE 10.4: How to investigate and treat hirsutism

current. Although considered permanent, it can cause regrowth of hair in 25-50 percent of women depending on the severity of hirsutism. Excessive electrolysis can cause skin thickening and scarring. It is also expensive and time consuming.

• Laser treatment—involves damage to hair follicles by direct photothermolysis. It is quick and effective, but very expensive. It can lead to permanent hair loss in many women. It is most effective in women with lightly pigmented skin with dark terminal hair. It can lead to pigmentation and scarring in some.

- Eflornithine hydrochloride 13.9 percent is a topical cream that is approved for use as a hair remover. It is an inhibitor of hair growth by inhibiting protein keratin synthesis. It is not a depilatory and must be used indefinitely.[26, 27]
- Weight loss in obese women reduces androgen production, and thereby reduces hair growth and regularizes menses.

Pharmacological Treatment of Hirsutism

In clinical practice, the modified Ferriman Gallwey score is used to access response to therapy along with history of lengthening of intervals between mechanical therapy sessions. No hormone measurements are required. When in doubt, testosterone levels are adequate to ensure that the condition is not worsening. But in clinical trials, weight of the shaved hair and measurement of shaft diameter are more accurate parameters. Patients need to be informed that response time to therapy is at least 3-6 months as half-life of the hair follicles is 6 months. Generally, treatment for hirsutism due to the two most conditions, i.e. PCOS and IH, is indefinite, as increased androgen production and sensitivity is life long. In 80 percent of the women, hirsutism recurs 6 months after discontinuation of treatment.[28] All medications for hirsutism need to be stopped when a pregnancy is desired.

Oral Contraceptives (OCP)

Oral contraceptives (OCP) are considered first line of therapy for hirsutism, and slow hair growth in 60-100 percent of women.[29] OCP's work by reducing LH dependent ovarian androgen production, increasing SHBG and thereby reducing free testosterone, and reduction of adrenal androgens.

Therapy should begin with low dose estrogen and nonandrogenic progesterone such as desogestrel and norgestimate. Norgestrel and levonorgestrel should be avoided because of their androgenic properties. Usual starting dose is Ethinyl estradiol (EE) 35 mg and 0.5 mg norethindrone for lean women and EE 35 mg and 1 mg norethindrone for obese women. If there is break

through bleeding, higher estrogenic OCP with Ethinyl estradiol (EE) 35 mg and 1 mg ethinodiol diacetate should be used. OCP containing 0.15 mg of desogestrel was found to be comparable to OCP with 2 mg of cyproterone acetate (Diane 35) in improvement of serum androgen levels and FG scores.[30]

Insulin Sensitizers in PCOS

Insulin sensitizers in PCOS–few small studies have looked at Metformin and Glitazones in the treatment of hirsutism in PCOS patients, and have found them to be effective, but not as effective as OCP.[31-35] Therefore, these agents may be used as adjuncts in combination with OCP's.

Antiandrogen Therapy

The antiandrogens that are available for the treatment of hirsutism are Spironolactone, Flutamide, Finasteride and Cyproterone acetate (CPA). All these drugs are teratogenic and should be used with OCP's in women during their reproductive years. The combination of antiandrogens and OCP's, works better for severe hirsutism than either drug alone.

Spironolactone

Spironolactone is an aldosterone antagonist structurally related to progesterone. It reduces the LH/FSH ratio, inhibits 5 alpha reductase, and competes with DHT for binding to the androgen receptor and SHBG. Hirsutism scores improve in 60-70 percent of women. Usual dose is 100 mg/day, and dose range is 50-200 mg/day.[36, 37] Main side effects are hyperkalemia, GI and menstrual irregularities. Spironolactone is used in combination with OCP as primary therapy, when one drug is ineffective and also to prevent menstrual irregularity.[38-40]

Flutamide

Flutamide inhibits binding of testosterone to its receptor and is more potent than spironolactone in the treatment of hirsutism.[41,42] It is hepatotoxic, and associated with death, therefore generally not used in the treatment of hirsutism.[43]

Usual dose is 250 mg/day, although up to 250 mg BD may be used.

Finasteride

Finasteride inhibits the conversion of testosterone to dihydrotestosterone by blocking the enzyme type 2-5 alpha-reductase in the prostate. Type 1-5 alpha-reductase is responsible for this reaction in the skin. Finasteride is less effective than spironolactone in the treatment of hirsutism, and generally works better when used in combination with OCP's.[44, 45] Daily dose is 5 mg/day.

Cyproterone Acetate (CPA)

Cyproterone acetate (CPA) is a progestin with antiandrogen action. It inhibits the androgen receptor, reduces 5 alpha reductase activity in the skin, as well as increases hepatic clearance of testosterone. It may be used alone or in combination with OCP's in the treatment of hirsutism, and is effective in 70 percent of women. Daily dose is 2 mg/day or between 12.5-100 mg for 10 days of the month. It is best used with estrogen to prevent bone loss.[46] In a prospective randomized control trial of 40 hirsute women treated with Diane 35 alone or in combination with finasteride 5 mg/day for one year, the combination group had better hirsutism reduction scores.[47]

Comparative Studies of Antiandrogens in Hirsutism

Very few studies exist comparing efficacies and safety of the various antiandrogens.[48] One study by Venturoli *et al* compared flutamide (250 mg), finasteride (5 mg), ketoconazole (300 mg) and ethinyl estradiol with cyproterone acetate (12.5 mg, 10 days of the month) in 66 women with hirsutism.[49] At the end of one year, the Ferriman Gallwey scores improved by 60 percent in the ethinyl estradiol–CPA group, 55 percent in the flutamide group, 53 percent in the ketoconazole group and 40 percent in the finasteride group. Maximum side effects were with ketoconazole.

Another study compared spironolactone 100 mg, flutamide 250 mg, finasteride 5 mg with placebo in 44 women with hirsutism for 6 months.[50] The FG score and hair diameter was reduced to a similar degree in all the treatment groups compared to placebo.

Gonadotropin-releasing Hormone Agonist

Gonadotropin-releasing hormone agonist inhibits gonadotropins and thereby ovarian androgen synthesis and reduction in hirsutism. As it also causes estrogen deficiency, it is generally used with OCP. However, the combination of GnRH agonist with OCP was found to be less effective than OCP's in combination with flutamide or cyproterone.[51] Therefore, the cost of GnRH therapy does not justify its use in the treatment of hirsutism.

Treatment of Other Causes of Hirsutism

Hyperprolactinemia

Hyperprolactinemia is treated with Bromocriptine or cabergoline, if due to a prolactinoma. If mild increased prolactin is due to PCOS, generally no treatment is required.

CAH

CAH-hirsutism responds better to antiandrogen therapy than glucocorticoids. But, glucocorticoids are required for restoration of ovulation and fertility.[52]

Ovarian and Adrenal Tumors

Ovarian and adrenal tumors are treated with surgical resection.

CONCLUSION

Hirsutism is more a cosmetic problem with psychosocial consequences rather than a physiological disease. The rare woman with underlying serious medical disorder needs to be identified and treated appropriately. The rest need reassurance or a combination of mechanical hair removal and medical therapy which offers a speedier improvement than medications alone. Once the androgen mediated transition from vellus to terminal hair occurs, the change is permanent, thereby necessitating indefinite therapy.

REFERENCES

1. Ferriman D, Gallwey JD. Clinical assessment of body hair growth in women. JCEM 1961;21:1440.
2. Redmend GP, Bugfield WF. Treatment of androgenic disorders in women. Cleveland Clinic Med J 1990;S7:423-32.
3. Carmina E, Koyama T, Chang L, et al. Does ethnicity influence the prevalence of adrenal hyperandrogenism and insulin resistance in PCOS? Am J of Obstret Gyn 1992;167:1807.
4. Taylor AE, Barbieri RL. Pathogenesis and causes of hirsutism. Clin Endo Uptodate 2002.
5. Hoch DL, Seifer DB. New treatment of hyperandrogenism and hirsutism. Obstret Gyn Clinics 2000;27:3.
6. Ebling FJ. The biology of hair. Derm Clin 1987;5:467-81.
7. Habif TP. Hair diseases in clinical dermatology, 2nd edn., St. Louis, CV Mosby 1990;598-615.
8. Pans R. Principles of hair cycle control. J Derm 1998;25:793-802.
9. Plouffe Jr L. Disorders of excessive hair growth in the adolescent. Obstret Gyn Clinics 2000;27:79-99.
10. Rosenfield RL, Lucky AW. Acne, hirsutism and alopecia in adolescent girls. Clinical expression of androgen excess. Endo Clin of North Am 1993;22:507-32.
11. Deplewski D, Rosenfeld RL. Role of hormones in pilosebaceous unit development. Endo Reviews 2000;21(4):363-92.
12. Lynfield YL. Effect of pregnancy on the human hair cycle. J Invest Derm 1960;35:323-27.
13. Azziz R, Carmina E, Sawaya ME. Idiopathic hirsutism. Endo Reviews 2000;21(4):347-62.
14. Paulson RJ, Serafini PC, Catalino JA, Lobo RA. Measurement of 3a, 17b androstenediol glucoronide in the serum and urine and correlation with skin 5 a reductase activity. Fertil Steril 1996;46:222-26.
15. Zawadzki JK, Dunaif A. Diagnostic criteria for PCOS: Towards a rational approach. In: PCOS. Dunaif A, Givens JR, Haseltine FP, Merriam GR (Eds): Blackwell Scientific publications, 1992:377.
16. Taponen S, Martikainen H, Ruokonen A, et al. Hormonal profile in women with self-reported symptoms of oligomenorrhea and or hirsutism. North Finland Birth Cohort 1966 Study. JCEM 2003;88:141-47.
17. Dereksen J, Nagesser SK, Meinders AE, et al. Identification of virilizing adrenal tumors in hirsute women. NEJM 1994;331:968.
18. Zumoff B, Rosenfeld RS, Strain GW, et al. Sex differentiation in 24hr. mean plasma concentration of DHA and DHEAS and DHA and DHEAS ratio in normal adults. JCEM 1980;51:330.
19. Hatch R, Rosenfeld RS, Kim MH, Tredway D. Am J Ob and Gyn 1981;140:815.
20. O'Drisoll JB, Manitora H, Higginsion J, et al. A prospective study of the prevalence of clear-cut endocrine disorders and PCOS in 350 patients presenting with hirsutism or androgenic alopecia. Clin Endocrin 1994;41:231.
21. Friedman CI, Schmidt GE, Kim MH, Powell J. Serum testosterone concentration in the evaluation of androgen producing tumors. Am J of Obs and Gyn 1985;153:44.
22. Nestler JE, Jakubowicz DJ. Decreases in ovarian c P450, 17 a activity, and serum free testosterone after reduction of insulin secretion in PCOS. NEJM 1996;335:617.
23. Horton R, Hawks D, Lobo R. 3a, 17b androstenediol glucoronide in plasma: A marker of androgen action in IH. J Clin Invest 1982;69:1203.
24. Pang S, Wang M, Jefferies S, Riddick L, Clark A, Estrada E. Normal and elevated 3a, 17b androstenediol glucoronide concentration in women with various causes of hirsutism and its correlation with degree of hirsutism and androgen levels. JCEM 1992;75:243-48.
25. Rittmaster RS. Medical treatment of androgen dependent hirsutism. JCEM 1995;80:2559-63.
26. "The Pink Sheet" 2000;62:7.
27. Coyne Jr PE. The eflornithine story. J of Am Acad of Derm 2001;45:784-86.
28. Kokaly W, McKenna TJ. Relapse of hirsutism following long-term successful treatment with estrogen progesterone combination. Clin Endo 2000;52:379.
29. Burkman RT Jr. The role of oral contraceptive in the treatment of hyperandrogenic disorders. Am J Med 1995;98:1305
30. Mastorakos G, Koliopoulos C, Creatas G. Androgen and lipid profiles in adolescents with PCOS who were treated with two forms of combined OCP. Fertil Steril 2002;77:919.
31. Azziz R, Ehrman D, Legna DS, Whitcomb RW, et al. Troglitazones improve ovulation and hirsutism in PCOS. A multicenter, placebo controlled trial. JCEM 2001;86:1626-32.
32. Eltver K, Imir G, Dormusoglu F. Clinical endocrine and metabolic effects of metformin added to ethinyl estradiol-CPA in non-obese women with PCOS: A randomized controlled study. Human Reproduction 2002;17:1729-31.
33. Morin Paprinen LC, Jaipaninen JS et al. Endocrine and metabolic effects of Metformin and ethinyl estradiol-CPA in obese women with PCOS. A randomized study. JCEM 2000:85:3161-68.
34. Ibanez L, Valls C, Zegher FD et al. Additive effects of insulin sensitizer and antiandrogen treatment in young nonobese women with hyperinsulinemia, hyperandrogenism, dyslipidemia and anovulation. JCEM 2002;87:2870-74.
35. Morin Paprinen L, Vaukponen I, Tapnainen JS et al. Metformin versus ethinyl estradiol–CPA in treatment of nonobese women with PCOS. A randomized study. JCEM 2003;88:148-56.
36. Cuming DC, Yang JC, Reban RW, Yen SSC. Treatment of hirsutism with spironolactone. JAMA 1982;247:129S.

37. Lobo RA, Shenpe D, Serafini P, et al. The effect of two doses of spironolactone on serum androgens and anagen hair in hirsute women. Fertil Steril 1985;43:200.

38. Pittaway DE, Maxson WS, Wentz AC. Spironolactone in combination drug treatment for unresponsive hirsutism. Fertil Steril 1985;43:878.

39. Board JA, Rosenberg SM, Smeltzer SS. Spironolactone and estrogen progesterone therapy for hirsutism. South Med J.1987;80:43.

40. Farquhar C, Lee O, Toomath R, Jepson R. Spironolactone versus placebo or in combination with steroids hirsutism and or acne. (Cochrane review). The Cochrane library, Issue 2002.

41. Cusan L, Dupont A, Gomez JL, et al. Comparison of flutamide and spironolactone in treatment of hirsutism. A randomized control clinical trial. Fertil Steril 1994;61:281.

42. Giotta L, Cianci A, Marletta A et al. Treatment of hirsutism with flutamide and low dose OCP in PCOS. Fertil Steril 1994;62:1129.

43. Wysowski DK, Freiman JP, Tourtelot JB, Horton ML. Fatal and nonfatal hepatotoxicity associated with flutamide. Am Int Med 1993;119:1150

44. Wong IL, Morris RS, Chang L, et al. A prospective randomized trial comparing finasteride to spironolactone in the treatment of hirsute women. JCEM 1995;80:227.

45. Falsia E, Filliponi S, Mancini V, et al. Effect of finasteride in IH. J Endo Invest. 1998;21:694.

46. Castelo-Branco C, Martinez de Osaba MJ, Pons F, et al. GnRH analog plus OCP containing desogestrel in women with severe hirsutism. Effect on hair, bone, and hormone profile after one year of use. Metab 1997; 46:437.

47. Sahin Y, Dilber S, Kelestimur F. Comparison of Diane 35 and Diane 35 plus finasteride in the treatment of hirsutism. Fertil Steril 2001;75:496.

48. Fruzzetti F, Bersi C, Parrini D, Ricci C, Genazzani AR. Treatment of hirsutism: Comparison between different antiandrogens with central and peripheral effects. Fertil Steril 1999;71:445-451.

49. Venturoli S, Maraschelci O, Colombo FM, et al. A prospective randomized controlled trial comparing low dose flutamide, finasteride, ketoconozole and CPA-estrogen regimens in the treatment of hirsutism. JCEM 1999;84:1304.

50. Moghetti P, Tosi F, Toshi A, et al. Comparison of spironolactone, flutamide and finasteride efficacy in the treatment of hirsutism. A randomized double blind placebo controlled trial. JCEM 2000;85:89.

51. Pazos F, Escobar-Morreale HF, Balsa J. A prospective randomized controlled trial comparing the long acting GnRH agonist triptorelin, flutamide and CPA used in combination with OCPs in the treatment of hirsutism. Fertil Steril 1999;71:122.

52. Speiser PW. CAH owing to 21-hydroxylase deficiency. Endo and Metab Clinics 2001;30.

• **Meenakshi Bharath**

11

Fertility Treatment in Primary and Secondary Amenorrhea

PRIMARY AMENORRHEA

INTRODUCTION

Menstruation is the endpoint of a cascade of events that begins in the hypothalamus and ends in the uterus. This mechanism is the fundamental basis of reproduction and menstruation represents the failure to achieve such reproductive success in the timeframe of the menstrual cycle. Amenorrhea will ensue if any part of this either fails to function endocrinologically, or, if there is a developmental deficiency.[1]

Primary amenorrhea is defined as the absence of menstruation by the age of 14 years, in the absence of growth or development of secondary sexual characteristics, or of no menstruation by the age of 16 years, regardless of normal growth and development of secondary sexual characteristics.[2]

The normal development of the hypothalamo-pituitary-ovarian-uterine axis along with an intact outflow tract that connects the internal genital source of flow with the outside is a prerequisite for normal menstruation. Thus, the easiest way to analyze amenorrhea is to look for defects at each level and then look for a solution to this problem.

• *Compartment 1*—disorders of the uterus and lower genital tract
• *Compartment 2*—disorders of ovarian function
• *Compartment 3*—disorders of the anterior pituitary
• *Compartment 4*—disorders of the hypothalamus.

CLINICAL EVALUATION

A careful history and physical examination is mandatory. The history may elicit psychological dysfunction or emotional stress, eating disorder. presence of genetic anomalies in the family and also of other siblings having similar problems. On clinical examination, the patient may be found to be underweight, may have loss of sense of smell, show iso-or heterosexual characteristics, have the physical stigmata of Turner's syndrome and other signs of abnormal growth or development. There may be evidence of systemic disease. The presence of a normal reproductive tract or the absence of any part of it is most significant. The art of effective diagnosis, besides clinical examination is one that relies to a considerable degree on the use of ultrasound.[3] With the ultrasound (US) machines constantly improving in resolution and the use of vaginal probes—the anatomy of the uterus, its abnormalities, the endometrium, and the adnexal structures especially the ovaries and their morphology are clearly visualized.[4] An ultrasonographic assessment would therefore help to make a proper clinical diagnosis. The biochemical investigations should include assessment of circulating levels of sex hormones and gonadotropins, which will give us the maximum information to be able to localize the site of abnormality. Other biochemical tests are optional.

Compartment 1

Mullerian Anomalies

Segmental disruptions of the outflow tract include imperforate hymen, transverse vaginal septum at any level, absent vagina and noncanalization of the cervix. Less common is the presence of the uterus, but with an absent cavity or the presence of a cavity with a congenitally absent endometrium. These patients come with the classical history of cyclical abdominal pain and on examination a mass arising from the pelvis may be present. An abdominoperineal ultrasonography will give us a good idea of the lesion.[5] The treatment is surgical decompression of the mass. The best results are obtained when it is in the hematocolpos stage. Hematometra and hematosalpinx have a poorer prognosis due to the destruction of the endometrium from compression and inflammation and also due to the occurrence of endometriosis. These patients if treated early may not need any fertility treatment at all.

Mayer-Rokitansky–Küster-Hauser Syndrome

These patients have a completely absent or hypoplastic vagina and variable presence of the remaining Mullerian segments. However, ovarian function is normal therefore, they can biologically mother a child. Such patients will need the aid of a surrogate to have a baby, as most often they have associated severe mullerian agenesis.[6] Conditions in which the genetic complement of the patient is not 46XX is not given consideration here.

Tuberculosis

Tuberculosis is a common disease of the childhood in India and this may affect the pelvis, with resultant tubercular endometritis. Primary amenorrhea may present if the endometrium is badly damaged with intrauterine adhesions. The size of the uterus is reduced,[7] though the gonadal function is normal—possibly due to a deficiency of estrogen receptors in the endometrium and myometrium. Uterine synechiae can be detected by ultrasonography, hysterography or hysteroscopy and treated by lysis, followed by priming of the endometrium with estrogens for 3 to 6 months.[8] But results of this treatment are not very encouraging. Rarely will a patient become pregnant after having been diagnosed as having tubercular endometritis. If pregnant then she can have antitubercular treatment after the 14th week of pregnancy without any detrimental effects to the fetus.[9] However it is difficult to achieve a pregnancy and tubercular endometritis precludes the use of IVF (the traditional treatment for pelvic tuberculosis). If so, then her only recourse may be to resort to being a genetic mother—with her oocytes being fertilized by her husband's sperm and then being placed into a surrogate carrier.

Compartment 2

Turner's Syndrome

Turner's syndrome is a genetic abnormality in which there is loss of one X chromosome resulting in gonadal dysgenesis. Women with Turner's syndrome have normal ovarian development till about 20 weeks of intrauterine life (IUL). Thereafter, there is a failure of the oocyte to undergo further maturation, (which requires the influence of both the X chromosomes). The oocytes then undergo a process of accelerated atresia and at the time of menarche there are none or very few oocytes present. The ovary in these cases consists mainly of stroma and therefore is unable to produce estrogen. However, there is normal female organ development, as the absence of a Y-chromosome results in the normal development of the mullerian ducts and therefore the presence of a normal uterus, tubes and a vagina. In the case of Turner mosaics—a few of the patients may exhibit estrogenic activity with the associated development of secondary sexual characteristics and have occassionally conceived also. In the majority of these patients who would like to conceive, the only method of assisted conception is to go in for estrogenic priming of the uterus followed by utilization of donor oocytes.[10]

Resistant Ovarian Syndrome

These women have elevated levels of gonadotropins in the presence of apparently normal ovarian tissue. It is believed that these women may have an absence of FSH receptors in the ovarian follicles and are therefore unable to respond to FSH.[11] Pregnancies have been reported in these patients usually after a period of estrogen administration but occasionally spontaneously, suggesting that the receptor resistance to gonadotropins is sometimes reversible.[12] In many ways, these females behave like those with premature ovarian failure. If ovulation induction does not succeed, then they would need to resort to donor oocytes.

Radiation and chemotherapy Radiotherapy when given to women prior to menopause and especially before the completion of the family should be always done after shielding the pelvis. When the radiation field excludes the pelvis there is no risk of premature ovarian failure. If the pelvis is radiated, the effect of radiation is dependent upon the age of the patient and the dosage of radiation. Younger women show a resistance to complete castration due to the higher number of oocytes present in the ovaries. If the radiation received by the ovaries is more than 500 rads, the patient may incur 60 to 70 percent sterilization. If she receives more than 800 rads to the ovaries, there is permanent (100%) sterilization. The steroid levels begin to fall and the gonadotropins levels begin to rise within 2 weeks of receiving radiation to the ovaries. This may result in immediate amenorrhea or appear later as premature ovarian failure.

Thus, elective transposition of the ovaries (by laparoscopy) out of the pelvis, prior to irradiation provides a good prospect for future fertility.[13,14] Harvesting and cryopreservation of oocytes prior to radiation, or the more recent freezing of ovarian tissue to be returned after the completion of the radiation therapy, is still in the experimental stages.

Alkylating agents and multiple cytotoxic drug therapy (given in breast cancer) are also very toxic to the ovaries. As with radiation, there is an inverse relationship between the doses required for ovarian failure and age at the start of the therapy.

Resumption of menstruation and pregnancy may occur, but there is no knowing who will reacquire ovulatory function, and who will not.

Compartment 3

Hyperprolactinemia

Serum prolactin assay is a part of the routine blood tests done for amenorrheic patients. The amenorrhea associated with elevated prolactin levels is due to the prolactin induced inhibition of the pulsatile secretion of GnRH, resulting in the suppression of LH, interference with ovarian steroid production, abnormalities in the luteal phase, progesterone synthesis, and the prevention of the positive feedback of estradiol on the LH surge.

When a prolactin level of more than 100 ng/mL is found in a patient, she must have a coned-down radiograph of the sella tursica to detect presence of an adenoma. If this shows some abnormalities, then the patient needs to have an MRI, which will give more information.

If the investigation shows a microadenoma which is less than 10 mm in size then no surgical intervention is necessary—only dopamine agonistic drugs will be necessary to bring the prolactin level down to normal and correct the amenorrhea. If it is a macroadenoma (> 10 mm size) then it may require surgical removal especially since it can produce optical problems.

The best dopamine agonist drug available is bromocriptine. Only 10 percent of patients cannot tolerate this orally, getting nausea, headache and faintness as the initial problems. Side effects can be minimized by slowly building tolerance towards the usual dose, 2.5 mg bid. Newer dopamine-agonistic drugs are available—like cabergoline with a weekly dosage schedule and lower rate of side effects.

Approximately 80 percent of hyperprolactinemic women achieve pregnancy after dopamine-agonistic treatment.

Hypothyroidism

Only a few patients presenting with amenorrhea will have hypothyroidism, which is not clinically apparent. It is not good enough to check their thyroxine levels—these may be normal because of highly of TSH secretion. Therefore, it is only correct to check and see if the TSH levels are also within the normal range. If the level is high, that means there is subclinical hypothyroidism which, when treated, will promptly result in correction of the amenorrhea.

Compartment 4

Hypogonadotropic Hypogonadism

Primary amenorrhea can be due to deficiency in GnRH pulsatile secretion, with the resultant low levels of FSH and LH and estradiol, comparable with or lower than those in the normal early follicular phase. This is why these patients have short stature and lack secondary sexual characteristics. On examination of the uterus and ovaries on vaginal ultrasonography—it is characteristically seen that both uterus and the ovaries are smaller in size than normal with little or no development of the endometrium. To develop good secondary sexual characteristics, these girls will have to be started on low doses of oral estrogens, which are gradually increased over a 2 years period. It is only after a 12 to 18 months period of this estrogen therapy that cyclical progesterone therapy is started. Patients with anosmia (Kallmann's syndrome) and hypogonadotropic hypogonadism fall into this category.

As for fertility treatment, these women need ovulation induction with gonadotropins only, as clomiphene citrate is ineffective here. As they have low levels of gonadotropins, they will have to be started with injections of gonadotropins—usually HMG (both FSH and LH) commencing with a dosage of 150 IU from the 3rd day of the periods (induced withdrawal bleed) and then increasing after a week of injections if there is no ovarian response. Sometimes it may take up to 3 weeks of stimulation before a good response can be elicited. It may be also necessary to increase the dosage of gonadotropins if there is an inadequate follicular response. There should be no hesitation to increase the dosage. Once you have decided to make the patient ovulate—pursue it to the end. Another practical tip is that many a times the ovaries are not visible and only begin to be seen when the follicles start growing. The endometrium may not keep in pace with the follicular growth—and occasionally one may need to wait a day or two for the endometrium to reach 10 mm even when the follicles are of the right size (18-20 mm). In these patients the injection of hCG 10,000 units has to be given to make them ovulate, since they have no endogenous secretion of LH. Postovulatory progesterone support will be required if they become pregnant, then it should be continued till 12 weeks of gestation.

Anorexia Nervosa/Exercise Induced Amenorrhea

Anorexia nervosa is the most common functional disorder affecting adolescent girls causing amenorrhea. Here the girls are underweight and this is of psychological origin—as they do not want to eat. The 10th percentile of body fat at age 13 years is equivalent to 17 percent body fat—the minimum required for attaining menarche—or a girl needs to attain an approximate weight of 45 kg before she attains menarche. If she is chronically underweight either due to poor eating or due to excessive exercise, (as in the case of athletes—who have begun training young or in ballet dancers) then they suffer from primary amenorrhea. This is because they have persistent low levels of gonadotropins due to decrease in the pulsatility of the secretion of GnRH from the hypothalamus. Thus, an increase in the weight of the patient along with an increase in the fat percentage will result in the return of the GnRH pulses and consequently the secretion of the gonadotropins. This results in the starting of the menstruation. Once this is done then fertility is rarely a problem.

SECONDARY AMENORRHEA

Secondary amenorrhea is defined as absence of periods in a previously menstruating woman for a length of time equivalent to a total of at least 3 of her previous cycle intervals or 6 months of amenorrhea.

Sometimes cases of primary amenorrhea can also present as secondary amenorrhea. There are women with primary amenorrhea who have had drug-induced bleeding. Therefore, accurate history of whether the initial bleeding episodes were spontaneous or drug induced must be elicited.

Here we will discuss those causes of secondary amenorrhea that have not been discussed under primary amenorrhea.

A good history of the pattern of menstruation after menarche and the rate of onset of amenorrhea is mandatory. A general physical examination will help us to have an idea as to where the problem lies, with emphasis on weight gain or loss, nutritional status, hair distribution, signs of hypothyroidism or hyperthyroidism and galactorrhea.

Abdominal examination is important to detect any ovarian tumors or abdominal masses. A pervaginal examination is done to assess the status of the ovaries, uterus, cervix and vagina. Vaginal ultrasonography will give invaluable information of what is the cause of the secondary amenorrhea—for the structure of the ovaries can be clearly visualized and so is the uterus with the status of the endometrium (estrogenized or not). This will indicate to us what exactly we are dealing with.

Compartment 1

Asherman's Syndrome

Asherman's syndrome, the cause of secondary amenorrhea or hypomenorrhea following destruction of the endometrium, is mainly due to a rigorous curettage resulting in intrauterine scarring. The curettage usually follows:
• Septic abortion or hydatidiform mole

• Overzealous dilatation and curettage done for any cause
• Curettage performed for secondary PPH, especially due to adherent placenta

It can also occur following uterine surgery including cesarean section, myomectomy, or metroplasty.

At hysterography, the typical patterns of multiple synechiae is seen. This can also be seen on ultrasonography. The endometrial thickness seems to have a prognostic implication in the treatment. If the endometrium is found to be 6 mm or more then treatment would have a good result. But if the endometrium is less than this, then the prognosis for treatment is not as good.[15] Diagnosis is more accurate by hysteroscopy which will detect minimal adhesions that are not seen on hysterogram.

Prior to the advent of hysteroscopy—Asherman's syndrome was treated with dilatation and curettage—as a blind procedure and it was often not curative. With hysteroscopy and direct visualization, lysis of the adhesions can be done by cutting, cautery or laser producing better results. Following the operation, the walls of the uterine cavity have to be prevented from adhering to each other. Previously an intrauterine device (IUD) was utilized for this purpose; but the pediatric Foley's catheter appears to be a better option—the bulb being filled with 3 mL of fluid and removed after 7 days. This is done under antibiotic cover and prostaglandin synthetase inhibitors to reduce infection and uterine cramping. Another device which can be used, is the "March intrauterine balloon"—whose shape is the same as the normal endometrial cavity. The thin short tubing does not protrude from the vagina and is therefore a great convenience to the patient.[16] The patient is treated with high doses of estrogens (2.5 mg conjugated estrogens daily for 3 of 4 weeks with medroxyprogesterone acetate 10 mg being added in the 3rd week) for the development of the endometrium. Occasionally the procedure may have to be repeated to regain reproductive potential. Approximately 70 to 80 percent of patients treated in this manner will achieve pregnancy spontaneously.

Tuberculous endometritis may produce secondary amenorrhea—this has already been discussed before.

Compartment 2

Polycystic Ovarian Syndrome

Polycystic ovarian syndrome (PCOS) has become a major area of research. As the awareness of this disorder increases, more cases will be diagnosed. About 30-40 percent of the population have this condition but not all of them are aware of it.

This syndrome is associated with hyperandrogenism and anovulation, which may not be evident when the patients are in their teens, but with weight gain the signs and symptoms of PCOS begin to manifest. They would suffer fewer symptoms if they were underweight rather than overweight .

Diagnosing ovaries which show the polycystic condition is made easy by vaginal ultrasonography with the appearance of a larger than normal sized ovary, the "string of pearls" appearance and a hyperechogenic stroma. This modality of diagnosis sometimes far more accurate than an estimate of serum gonadotropins (reversal of the FSH/LH ratio).

Fertility treatment for those who suffer anovulation due to PCOS can consist of ovulation induction with clomiphene citrate only or in combination with gonadotropins. With the advent of GnRH-a the treatment of PCOD has been revolutionized. The subsequent discovery that these women have varying degrees of insulin resistance, has resulted in administration of drugs like glucophage which increase insulin sensitivity and help in the restoration of ovulation, or, if not, attaining a better response to CC therapy.[17] This subject of PCOD is being dealt with in greater detail in another chapter.

Premature Ovarian Failure

Premature ovarian failure affects approximately 1 percent of all women under the age of 40 years.

In most cases, a definitive etiology cannot be established.

Genetic disorders like ovarian dysgenesis is the cause in early onset POF, while autoimmune diseases are the common cause of POF at a later age. Mumps is the most common infection associated with POF. Its effect is maximal during the fetal and pubertal periods, when even a subclinical infection can result in ovarian failure. The diagnosis of POF is based on a triad of amenorrhea, elevated gonadotropins levels, and symptoms of estrogen deficiency. Serum FSH levels of 15 miu/mL is certainly in the perimenopausal range but may be associated with sporadic ovarian activity. Those with FSH levels above 40 miu/mL will invariably have no ovarian activity at all.[11, 18] The probability of success with fertility treatment of POF is very low indeed. Induction of ovulation using a sequential combination of oral estrogen and progesterone therapy followed by a course of HMG has given good results.[12] This is because estradiol therapy results in a temporary suppression of serum FSH and a consequent redevelopment of FSH receptors in the ovaries. Many a time, the dosage of gonadotropins given are very high, or the patients may be put on the flare protocols of ovulation induction. If conception cannot be achieved with one's own eggs then the patient may have to resort to donor oocytes. Once a person has been found to have POF, other siblings should take care as they may also have the same, therefore the earlier they have their children, the better for them. Ovarian and adrenal tumors are not dealt with here.

Compartment 3

Hyperprolactinemia has already been discussed.

Sheehan's Syndrome

Women who have severe postpartum hemorrhage usually develop pituitary necrosis, and this leads to hypogonadotropic amenorrhea. The treatment for this is the same as outlined before.

CONCLUSION

The varied etiologies of primary and secondary amenorrhea make it a very difficult topic to discuss. Only those causes of amenorrhea which are amenable for fertility treatment have been mentioned here. If the cause of the amenorrhea is correctly diagnosed then fertility treatment can be instituted in most instances with varying degrees of success.

REFERENCES

1. Edmonds DK. Primary amenorrhoea. Progress in Obstetrics and Gynaecology 10:281-96.
2. Speroff L, Glass RH, Kase NG. Clinical Gynaecologic Endocrinology and Infertility (6th edn) Williams and Wilkins: Baltimore 1999;421-85.
3. Pratap Kumar et al. Imaging in Obstetrics and Gynaecology (2nd edn). FOGSI publication, Jayapee Brothers: New Delhi, 1998.
4. Tan SL, Jacobs HS. Recent advances in the management of patients with amenorrhoea. Clinics in Obstetrics and Gynaecology 1985;12(3).
5. William RM, McCoy MC, Fritz MA. Combined abdominal-perineal sonography to assist in the diagnosis of transverse vaginal septum. Obstet Gynecol 1995;85:882-84.
6. Batzer FR, Corson SL, Gocial B, et al. Genetic offspring in patients with vaginal agenesis—specific medical and legal issues. Am J Obstet Gynecol 1992;167:1288.
7. Nogales-Ortiz F, Tarancon I, Nogales FF. The pathology of female genital tuberculosis. Obstet Gynecol 1979;53:422-28.
8. Parikh FR, Nadkarni SG, Kamat SA, et al. Genital tuberculosis—a major pelvic factor causing infertility in Indian women. Fertil Steril 1997;67(3):497-500.
9. Yip SK, Wong SP, Fung TY et al. Unassisted conception with a normal pregnancy outcome in a woman with active Mycobacterium tuberculosis infection of the endometrium. J Reproduc Medi 1999;44(11):974-76.
10. Press F, Sharipo HM, Cowell CA, et al. Outcome of ovum donation in Turner's syndrome patients. Fertil Steril 1995;64(5):995-98.
11. Baber R, Abdalla H, Studd J. The premature menopause. Progress in Obstetrics and Gynaecology 9:209-23,
12. Check JH, Case JS. Ovulation induction in hypergonadotropic amenorrhoea with oestrogen and human menopausal gonadotropin therapy. Fertil Steril 1984;42:919-22.
13. Treissman MJ, Miller D, McComb PF. Laparoscopic lateral ovarian transposition. Fertil Steril 1996;65(6):1229-31.
14. TulandiT, Al-Took S. Laparoscopic ovarian suspension before irradiation. Fertil Steril 1998;70(2):381-83.
15. Schlaff WD, Hurst BS. Preoperative sonographic measurement of endometrial pattern predicts outcome of surgical repair in patients with severe Asherman's syndrome. Fertil Steril 1995;63(2):410-13.
16. Hurt RB. Text and Atlas of Female Infertility Surgery (3rd edn) CV Mosby: St. Louis.
17. Acbay O, Gundogdu S. Can Metformin reduce insulin resistance in polycystic ovary syndrome? Fertil Steril 1996;65:946.
18. Anasti JN. Premature ovarian failure: An update. Fertile Steril 1998;70(1):1-15.

12

Obesity in Infertility Practice

Obesity is a serious nutrition dependant pathology, with far reaching health consequences–especially on reproductive function. Body fat has an important role in the initiation and maintenance of reproductive functions in both men and women. An optimal body mass is required for the successful functioning of the same. This is evidenced by the fact that almost 12 percent of the cases of primary infertility are overweight!.[1]

Being overweight is when the body weight is in excess of the standard ideal weight for height, while obesity is the presence of excess body fat.[2]

Some of the methods in use for assessing body fat include skin fold thickness, underwater weighing, MRI, Infrared spectroscopy and dexa densitometry; however all of these are not really applicable in routine practice, the Body Mass Index or the Quetlet Index is used routinely.[3]

The Body Mass Index (BMI) is calculated by a formula using the height of the person in meters and the weight in kilograms. The BMI in an average adult is expected to be about 25 kg/mt squared (Table 12.1). While a BMI of 28 kg/m^2 warrants treatment, obesity is defined as the BMI

being 30 kg/m^2 or more. This would indicate the presence of approximately 30 percent excess body weight.

The quantity of fat is not as significant as the distribution or location of fat. Independent of weight, abdominal fat appears to have a more deleterious effect on fertility than fat deposition elsewhere in the body.[4] The coexistence of upper body obesity, hyperandrogenism, polycystic ovaries and infertility, and the fact that any increase in weight will exacerbate the hormonal and ovulatory dysfunction accompanying these conditions is evidence enough for the role of adipose tissue in reproductive function. While it has been seen that upto 70 percent of infertile overweight women will conceive spontaneously following weight loss, often obesity evaluation and treatment is overlooked in any infertility management programme.[5]

Types of Obesity

Different types of human obesity have been recognized based on the phenotype or the distribution of the body fat.
- Type I—excess of total body fat without any particular defined distribution pattern (global obesity)
- Type II—Excess of subcutaneous fat especially on the trunk and abdomen (android obesity)
- Type III—Excess of fat in the abdominal viscera (abdominal visceral obesity)
- Type IV—Excess of fat in the gluteo-femoral region (Gynoid obesity).

TABLE 12.1: The implications of the body mass index
The Body Mass Index = $\dfrac{\text{weight in kgs}}{\text{height in metres squared}}$
• Underweight– < 19 kg/m^2 • Normal Weight–19.1 to 24.9 kg/m^2 • Overweight–25 to 29.9 kg/m^2 • Obese– > 30 kg/m^2

TABLE 12.2: Types of obesity			
Type I	*Type II*	*Type III*	*Type IV*
Global	Android	Abdomino-visceral	Gynoid
Random fat distribution	subcutaneous deposition	abdominal-visceral deposition	gluteo-femoral deposition
	waist–hip ratio = > 0.8		waist-hip ratio = < 0.8

The distribution of the adipose tissue is important, as different hormonal and metabolic changes have been identified with fat deposition at different sites. While the normal tendency of the female is the gynoid type of fat deposition–where fat is mainly deposited in the gluteofemoral region, it has been seen that the central type (abdomino visceral) of obesity has the most deleterious effects in terms of both hormonal levels and fertility outcome. This would not only mean a higher incidence of menstrual abnormalities, infertility, miscarriages, but also higher concentrations of Luteinizing hormone, androgens, estrone, insulin, triglycerides, VLDL, and a reduced concentration of HDL.[6,7]

Obesity and the Reproductive Function

The interplay between adipose tissue and hormonal secretion/function/metabolism indicates the close association of the two.

Just as fat can bring about changes in the reproductive system, manipulation of the hypothalmo-pituitary-gonadal axis will instigate change in food intake, body weight and fat distribution.

For instance, Cortisol and Insulin increase fat deposition by stimulating the enzyme lipoprotein lipase, while estrogens, testosterone and growth hormone bring about lipolysis by inhibiting the same enzyme. The effect of progesterone is still inconclusive (Table 12. 3).

Adipose tissue is also an important site of steroid hormone metabolism. It is able to convert the androgens-testosterone and androstenedione to estrogens–Estradiol and estrone respectively by means of the enzyme aromatase found in the periadipocyte vascular stroma.Estradiol is further metabolized to estrone, and dehydroepian-drosterone to androstenediol (Table 12.4). This is probably why most obese persons are hyper-estrogenic.

TABLE 12.4: Role of adipose tissue as an endocrine organ
Metabolism of Estrogens to less active forms
Conversion of Androgens to Estrogens
Storage of steroid hormones
Effect on Insulin secretion by pancreas–affects SHBG levels

In females this may manifest as early menarche, menstrual disorders, infertility, poor pregnancy outcome including miscarriage and impaired fetal well-being. Infact, the incidence of menstrual disorders that is about 2.6 in women with a normal BMI, is increased to about 8.4 in women who are 75 percent above ideal body weight for height.[8] Males with obesity may be present with reduced testosterone levels and infertility. The effect of obesity on the gonadal functions has been enlisted in Table 12.5.

TABLE 12.5: Effect of obesity on gonadal function		
Parameter	*Testes*	*Ovaries*
Normal	Size	Increased-? Hyalinization
Reduced	SHBG	Reduced
Normal	Basal s.FSH & LH	Normal
Normal	Response to LHRH	Normal
Raised	Estrone & Estriol	Raised
Normal	Response to Clomiphene	Impaired? higher dose
Reduced	s.Androgens	Raised

Delayed consequences in both men and women include diabetes mellitus, arteriosclerosis, coronary artery disease, cerebrovascular disease,

TABLE 12.3: Interplay between hormones and fat deposition

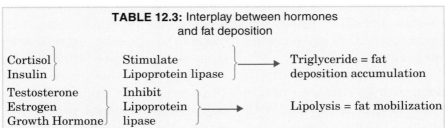

hypertension, and a higher prevalence of malignancy.[9] While the fact that overweight conditions may lead to infertility by altering both secretion and metabolism of sex steroids has already been established, current evidence indicates that leptin could form the physiological link between obesity and infertility.[10]

The Role of Leptin in Infertility

Leptin or the Ob-Protein is a protein hormone synthesized and secreted by mature adipocytes. This not only serves as an indicator of the fat stores to the brain, but also stimulates areas of the hypothalamus involved in energy homeostasis, which leads to increased basal metabolism and reduced appetite.[11] Apart from these two major functions, Leptin has been found to have a direct effect on the ovary. In fact, leptin receptors are present on both the granulosa and the theca cells, and the concentration of this hormone in follicular fluid mimics serum levels.

By inhibiting the Insulin like Growth Factor 1 (IGF 1), leptin acts by blocking the FSH stimulated estradiol production. It also inhibits the synthesis of progesterone and pregnanolone, which may be due to the reduced expression of the enzyme adrenodoxin,[12] or by acting as a cofactor along with insulin.[13]

Though it has been suggested that leptin levels are elevated in women with PCOD, there is no apparent effect of weight loss, insulin sensitizers, or pituitary downregulation on the leptin levels in these women.[14-16] Despite innumerable reports, the conflicting results show that the exact role of leptin in ovarian function is not known yet.[17]

Management of Obesity in Infertility

Though obese persons are very likely to accept the impact of obesity on their reproductive function, they often regard the weight loss program as a waste of time and effort. Education, counseling and constant motivation will form the basis of managing these couples.

The routine baseline investigations for infertility must be done, along with specific tests to rule out other disorders that may be associated with obesity–hypothyroidism, Cushing's disease, etc.

(Table 12.6). The most important clinical assessment is the evaluation of the body mass index.

TABLE 12.6: Unusual causes of obesity

Genetic—associated with hypogonadism
       E.g: Prader-Willi syndrome, Lawerence-Moon
       Biedel syndrome

Cushing's syndrome
Hypothyroidism
Stein-Levinthal syndrome
Hypothalamic disease—trauma, tumor

Weight loss and appropriate lifestyle changes must be promoted as the first line of therapy to these couples. However, the most effective way of achieving and maintaining weight loss is still unclear. Sensible eating with regular exercise, cognitive behavioral therapy and a supportive group environment will probably produce the best results.

Restriction of calories is the foundation of any weight loss program. An ideal diet would contain 50 percent carbohydrates, 15 to 20 percent proteins and less than 30 percent fat.

Low calorie diets (less than 1200 k cal/day) can help an obese individual lose upto 450 gms every week, which can be further improved upon if regular exercise is undertaken too.

Anorectics should be used with caution as they are habit forming-especially amphetamine. Some of the less stimulatory drugs (diethylproprion, fenfluramine) may be used as short-term measure to help overcome hunger, especially in the initial stages of a diet program.

Morbid obesity may require surgery. In these cases, currently the most accepted procedure is gastric plication–where stapling across the walls of the stomach creates a smaller stomach pouch.

Along with the diet, the patient must be enrolled into a regular exercise program. The best time for exercise is before or at least 2 hr after a meal. However, the patient should be given the freedom to adjust her exercise schedule to one that is most appropriate for her lifestyle.

Data suggest that modest weight losses of upto 10 percent of the original weight are effective in improving hormonal profiles, menstrual regularity, and ovulation and pregnancy rates.

Ovulation induction in obese women poses a special challenge. Most studies have shown that an increasing BMI is associated with an increasing dosage of both clomiphene citrate as well as gonadotrophins[18,19] needed to induce ovulation. This has been attributed to the sequestration of these drugs in the adipose tissue. In fact, Shepard has reported that the average dose of clomiphene required to induce ovulation in an overweight woman is about 200 mg.[20] There, however, does not appear to be any correlation between the body mass index and conception rates,[18] though poorer pregnancy outcomes have been reported by several authors, indicating the probable coexistence of some subtle endocrine abnormality,[21] or the presence of oocytes with poor fertilization and implantation potential.[22]

Insulin sensitizers (metformin, rosiglitazone) have an important role to play especially in the obese female with polycystic ovarian disease to reduce the associated insulin resistance, hyperandrogenism and the BMI.[23,24]

The role of adipose tissue in reproduction has been established beyond doubt. Excess or deficiency of body fat can both lead to reproductive failure. It is important that this condition be recognized, treated and given the importance that it deserves. These couples require constant motivation and understanding in helping them cope with their condition. All patients attending an infertility clinic should have their BMI assessed at the initial visit and appropriate measures instituted as required.

POINTS TO BE REMEMBERED

1. Overweight and obesity in women have significant consequences in terms of morbidity and mortality.
2. Central and Android forms of obesity have a more detrimental effect on reproductive function than the other types.
3. While infertility may actually be due to some other cause, achievement of an optimal or near optimal body mass index will produce the best results of treatment.
4. Body Mass Index should be assessed at the initial visit.

5. All overweight and obese women should have a blood sugar and a lipid profile done to look for glucose intolerance and hyperlipidemia.
6. Low Calorie Diet along with exercise forms the basis of treatment. Along with this appropriate lifestyle changes must be included and the provision should be made for continued support system to instill the necessary confidence and motivation

REFERENCES

1. Green BB, Weiss NS et al. Risk of ovulatory infertility in relation to body weight Fertil Steril. 1988;50:721.
2. Ravussin E, Swinburn BA. Pathophysiology of obesity. Lancet 1992;340-404.
3. Pasquali R, Cassimirri F. the impact of obesity on hyperandrogenism and polycystic ovarian syndrome in premenopausal women. Clin Endocrinol Oxf 1993;39:1-16.
4. Moran LJ, Norman RJ. The obese patient with infertility: A practical approach to diagnosis and treatment. Nutr Clin Care 2002;5(6):290-97.
5. Bates GW, Whitworth NS. Effect of body weight reduction on plasma androgens in obese infertile women Fertil Steril. 1982;38:406.
6. Norman RJ, Masters S et al. Ethnic differences in insulin and glucose response to glucose between White and Indian women with polycystic ovarian syndrome. Fertil Steril. 1995;63:58-62.
7. Kaye SA, Folsom AR et al. The association of body fat distribution with lifestyle and reproductive factors in a population study of postmenopausal women. Int J Obes1990;14:583-91.
8. Norman RJ, Clark AM. Reprod Fertil Dev. 1998;10:55-63.
9. Bouchard C. Physical Activity Sciences Lab, Laval University, Quebec, Canada.
10. Aggarwal SK et al. J. Clin. Endocrinol Metab 1999;84(3):1072-76.
11. Ahima RS Dushay J, et al. Leptin accelerates the onset of puberty in normal female mice. J Clin Invest 1997;99:391-95.
12. Barkan D: Jia Dantes Endocrinology 140 1999;(4):1731-38.
13. Brannian JD, Zaho Y et al. Hum Reprod. 1999;14(6):1445-48.
14. Brzechffa PR Jakimuik AJ et al. Serum immuno reactive leptin in women with polycystic ovarian syndrome. J Clin Endocrinol Metab 1996;81:4166-69.
15. Mantzoros CS Dunaif A et al. Leptin concentrations in the polycystic ovary syndrome. J Clin Endocrinol Metab 1997;82:1687-91.
16. Nader S et al The effect of a desogesterol containing oral contraceptive on glucose tolerance and leptin concentrations in hyperandrogenic women, J Clin Endocrinol Metab 1997;82:3074-77.

17. Duggal PS, et al. The invivo and invitro effects of exogenous leptin on ovulation in rats. Endocrinology 1976;141:1971-76.

18. Dickey RP, Taylor SN et al. Relationship of clomiphene dose and patient weight to successful treatment. Hum Reprod. 1997;12:449-53.

19. McClure N, Mc Quinn B et al. Body weight, body mass index and age:predictors of menotropin dose and cycle outcome in polycystic ovarian syndrome. Fertil steril 1992;58:622-24.

20. Shepard MK et al. Relationship of weight to successful induction of ovulationwith clomiphene citrate. Fertil Steril 1979;32-641.

21. Wang X, Davies M et al. Body mass and probability of pregnancy during assisted reproduction treatment. Retrospective study. BMJ. 2000;321:1320-21.

22. Krizanovska K, Ulcova-Gallova Z, Bouse V, Rokyta Z. Obesity and reproductive disorders Sb Lek 2002;103(4):517-26.

23. Kazerooni T et al. Effects of Metformin on hyperandrogenism in women with polycystic ovarian syndrome. Gynecol Endocrinol. 2003;17(1):51-56.

24. Haas DA, Carr BR, Attia GR. Effects of metformin on body mass index, menstrual cyclicity, and ovulation induction in women with polycystic ovary syndrome Fertil Steril. 2003;79(3):469-81.

Section **3**

Male Factor Infertility

• K Prabhakara • A Radharama Devi

13

Cytogenetics of Male Infertility

INTRODUCTION

Reproduction and genetics have always been interlinked. The introduction of assisted reproductive technologies (ARTs), opened many interplays between these disciplines and several clinical topics. These include the link between genetics and infertility, especially male infertility. The findings on cytogenetics and molecular genetics in male factor infertility are two such topics in the forefront of infertility research.

As early as 1957, Ferguson and Smith *et al* suspected the existence of chromosomal abnor-malities in patients attending infertility clinics.[1] They found the Barr body in 10 of the 91 males studied for azoospermia or severe oligozoo-spermia. Later in 1959, Jacobs and Strong showed that men with Klinefelter syndrome had a 47,XXY chromosomal constitution.[2] Since then, several surveys have been conducted to study the chromosomal abnormalities in male factor infertility prior to the introduction of chromosome banding techniques.[3-11] This chapter reviews studies of cytogenetic investigations related to male infertility, and their application in the management and counseling of such couples.

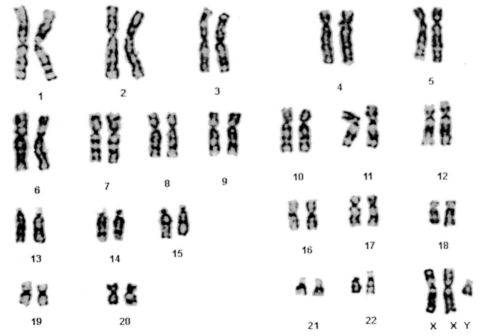

FIGURE 13.1: GTG-banded karyotype showing 47,XXY karyotype observed in Klinefelter's syndrome patients

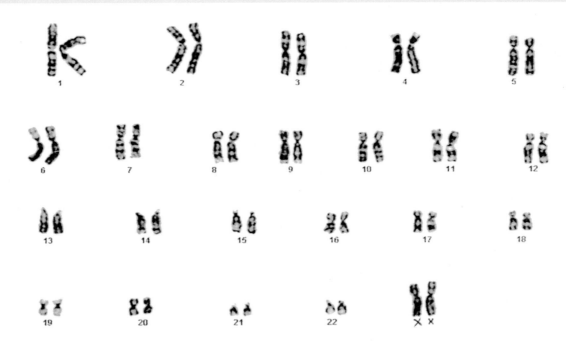

FIGURE 13.2: GTG-banded karyotype from 46,XX phenotypic male

Cytogenetic abnormalities include numerical, structural and microdeletions involving auto-somes and sex chromosomes.

SEX CHROMOSOMAL ABNORMALITIES AND MALE INFERTILITY

Numerical Abnormalities

The sex chromosomal abnormalities are the most common chromosomal abnormalities found in infertile males. The single sex chromosomal abnormality of 47,XXY (Figure 13.1) and mosaics of 46,XY/47,XXY are a relatively common event and more likely to be seen in azoospermic and severe oligozoospermic males.

The gonadal defect in XXY men seems to be related to germ cell survival and sex chromosome constitution.[12] The testicular atrophy seen in Klinefelter's syndrome is caused by a maturation breakdown of the germ cells containing two X chromosomes. Spermatogenesis in these males ranges from severe impairment to apparently normal.

46,XX Males

The 46,XX maleness is characterized by testicular development despite the lack of normal Y chromosome. The frequency of XX males (Figure 13.2) in the general population is very low (1 in 10,000), whereas they are found most frequently in azoospermic men. Several etiologies have been proposed to explain XX maleness: translocation of the testis determining region factor (TDF), equated more recently with the sex determining region Y gene (SRY), from Y chromosome to the distal part of the short arm of the X chromosome during meiosis;[13] mutation in an autosomal or X chromosome gene which permits testicular determination in the absence of TDF;[14] undetected 46,XX/47,XXY mosaics or other mosaics with the Y bearing cell line.

Structural Abnormalities of Y Chromosome

Structural abnormalities involving Y chromosome are found to be higher in infertile males and more so in azoospermic males. Structural abnormalities like dicentric Y, a ring Y chromosome[15] and the pericentric inversion of the Y chromosome (Figure 13.3) are reported to be associated with sperma-togenic failure. However, pericentric inversion of the Y chromosome is considered to be normal heteromorphism.[16] Meiotic studies by above authors have shown that the X and Y short arms

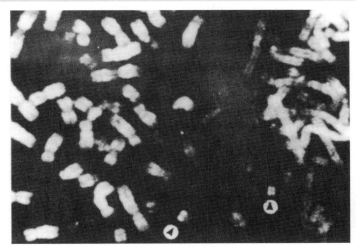

FIGURE 13.3: Two partial metaphases showing pericentric inversion of Y chromosome observed in infertile males (inverted Y chromosomes are shown by arrows)

could not pair at meiosis, because the short arm pairing region of the Y chromosome was present in the center of the abnormal chromosome and not available for end-to-end association with the X chromosome. Therefore, the pairing failure between the XY bivalent at metaphase could cause spermatogenic breakdown.

Reciprocal Translocations Involving Sex Chromosomes

Cytogenetic surveys of infertile men have reported reciprocal translocation between sex chromosome and an autosome.[8,17] In a study of nine male carriers of X-autosome translocations, Madan (1983) reported that regardless of the position of the breakpoint in the X, these men are likely to suffer from disturbances in spermatogenesis leading to severe infertility.[18]

Y-autosome translocation causes similar testicular changes whenever the breakpoint is located in Yq11 region, where the azoospermia factor is mapped.[19] In patients with reciprocal translocation involving Yp region, the outcome would depend on whether the breakage occurred within the pseudoautosomal region, which could lead to faulty XY pairing and subsequent meiotic breakdown.

Microdeletions on Y Chromosome

Tiepolo and Zuffardi (1976) were the first to suggest an association between deletions on long arm of the Y chromosome and azoospermia.[20]

Since then, the azoospermia factor gene (AZF) has been mapped onto Y chromosome within the band Yq11.23.[21] Recent work on molecular genetics of male infertility has mapped the candidate gene DAZ (deleted in azoospermia) on to the Yq region, which is mutated in azoospermic men.[22]

AUTOSOMAL ANOMALIES AND MALE INFERTILITY

Robertsonian Translocations

In infertile males, Robertsonian translocations are reported in about 0.7 percent, though in oligozoospermics it is more frequently observed (1.6%). The most frequent Robertsonian translocation identified is t(13;14).[5,7-9,19] Although Robertsonian translocations are more commonly found in infertile males, their role in oligozoospermia is not clear. The studies of testicular biopsies from carriers of Robertsonian translocation have showed variable pictures, ranging from severe impairment to near normality.[4]

Meiotic studies of sterile carriers of 13;14 Robertsonian translocation[23] and of sterile carriers of 14;21 translocations[17] have revealed that the spermatogenic impairment is related to an increase in the frequency of the XY bivalent and the Robertsonian trivalent association during the pachytene stage. Hence, there may be a correlation between the increased frequency of XY bivalent, and Robertsonian trivalent association and meiotic impairment.

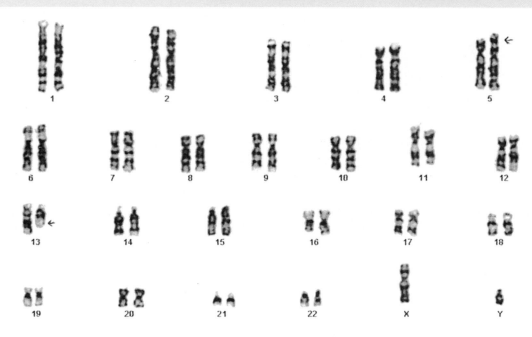

FIGURE 13.4: GTG-banded karyotype showing reciprocal translocation involving chromosomes 5 and 13 observed in a severe oligozoospermic male. Chromosomes 5 and 13 involved in translocation are indicated by arrows

Reciprocal Translocations

Several studies on infertile males suggest that the frequency of reciprocal translocations is about 0.5 percent. When specific semen parameters are considered, 0.9 percent reciprocal translocations were found in azoospermic and 0.8 percent in oligozoospermic men.[9, 24] An example of reciprocal translocation involving chromosomes 5 and 13 is shown in Figure 13.4. The involvement of some reciprocal translocations and abnormalities in spermatogenesis is well reported.[25,26] Some meiotic studies have suggested the mechanism by which autosomal rearrangements might bring about impairment in the spermatogenesis. It was observed that a high frequency of centromere contacts between the translocation configuration and the XY bivalent was formed at the pachytene stage of meiosis I, especially with chain configurations rather than with rings. Such contacts are not frequently seen among the pachytene cells of fertile male translocation carriers. Forejt (1974) suggested that nonrandom associations might produce interference with precocious X chromosome inactivation in the primary spermatocytes which would be required for normal spermatogenesis.[6]

Inversions

Paracentric and pericentric inversions are often reported in infertile males. Inversions of chromosomes 1-3, 5-7 and 9 have been reported.[11] Chandley *et al* carried out meiotic studies on the carriers of inversions in the chromosome 1 and found an extensive disturbance of synapses across the inverted region at metaphase I resulting in a loop formation (Figure 13.5).[24] The infertility effects of chromosome 1 inversion could be due to

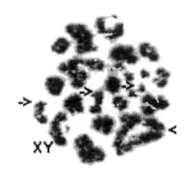

FIGURE 13.5: Meiotic metaphase I from immature germ cells of semen from severe oligozoospermic male showing univalents due to desynapsis (arrows) and quadrivalent configuration formed due to autosomal reciprocal translocation (arrowhead)

germ cell maturation impairment because of the failure of synapses.[27]

Several studies have reported association between the presence of ring chromosomes and extramarker chromosomes associated with male infertility.[3]

Numerical abnormalities of autosomes are not reported in males attending infertility clinics as these abnormalities are not compatible with life except Down syndrome. Fertility in Down syndrome with full trisomy is very rarely reported, whereas fertility in trisomy 21 mosaics is often reported.[28] It has been proposed that the effect of the trisomy 21 condition on spermatogenesis is a consequence of the association of the extra-chromosome 21 with XY bivalents during pachytene.[29]

MEIOTIC STUDIES OF CHROMOSOME ANOMALIES IN MALE INFERTILITY

Abnormal segregation of chromosomes during spermatogenesis may be responsible for male infertility. Testicular biopsies are not routinely performed in infertile men and the investigation of meiotic chromosomes presents a special technical challenge. This has remained a research tool restricted to a few laboratories. There are still several problems in the interpretation of results and comparison of different studies due to application of different techniques and analysis. Blockage or arrest in different stages of spermato-genesis is observed in a number of infertile men with or without chromosome abnormalities in testicular biopsies[27,30-33] and in immature germ cells in the semen.[19,34] These meiotic abnor-malities include complete spermatogenic arrest, low chiasma count, presence of univalents, bivalent fragmentation, asymmetrical bivalents and polyploidy. Meiotic chromosome abnor-malities in different studies varied from 4.3 to 40.4 percent. This variation may be explained by the method of presentation of results by different investigators and the patient profile itself (variation in the interpretation of subfertility, infertility and oligozoospermia). However, it is clear from different studies that meiotic anomalies can explain male infertility.

CYTOGENETIC STUDIES IN SPERMATOZOA OF INFERTILE MEN

It has been established that there is an increase in the frequency of constitutional chromosome abnormalities in the infertile male population, as compared to the general population. In addition to the constitutional chromosome abnormalities, chromosomal instability itself is related to fertility problem. This instability may predispose sperm chromosomes to nondisjunction and/or structural abnormalities. The chromosomal analysis of spermatozoa is possible in two different ways: by allowing human spermatozoa to fertilize zona-free hamster oocytes *in vitro*[25] and by FISH applied directly to sperm nuclei.[35]

Although numerical and structural aberrations of sperm chromosomes can both be investigated by the cross-species fertilization method, this technique is expensive and labor intensive. Only those spermatozoa capable of fusing with hamster oocytes can be assessed. Hence, with this technique chromosomal analysis in pronuclei from germ cells of males with severe infertility is not often reported.

Fluoresent *in situ* hybridization (FISH) allows the analysis of numerical chromosomal abnor-malities in spermatozoa. This is performed using different chromosome specific DNA probes.[35-37] FISH is a highly sensitive and specific method to study a larger number of sperm cells than with the hamster egg penetration test. The FISH technique can be applied on nonmotile and dysmorphic sperms too. The limitation of this method is that only numerical abnormalities for the specific chromosome(s) can be ascertained and no information about other chromosomes can be obtained. Pellestor *et al* (1995) applied the technique of primed *in situ* labeling (PRINS) for the rapid chromosome labeling of spermatozoa.[38] This method provides an interesting alternative to FISH because of the rapidity and simplicity of the protocol, the limited background signal and the high specificity of ologinucleotide primers. The limitation of PRINS is that only one chromosome can be identified in one reaction.

Recently, Ogawa *et al* (2000) described the technique of injection of spermatozoa into mouse oocytes for chromosomal analysis.[39] This method allows the analysis of nonmotile and dysmorphic sperms as the sperms are directly injected into the oocytes. It also yields good G-banding for the detailed chromosomal analysis.

IMPLICATIONS OF CYTOGENETICS OF INFERTILE MEN

Studies of genetic causes of male infertility are important to, not only learn more about the problem of infertility, but also to provide proper genetic counseling for couples implicated with this problem. Assisted reproductive technologies (ARTs) such as intracytoplasmic sperm injection (ICSI) provide the chance of having a child to severe oligozoospermic and azoospermic males. The increased incidence of chromosomal abnormalities in infertile men has raised the concern that the use of chromosomally abnormal sperm from these patients may result in transmission of genetic abnormalities to their offsprings. It is well established that balanced chromosomal rearrangements lead to the increased risk of miscarriages as well as children born with congenital malformations. Hence, screening for genetically determined male factors is very important before enrolment for ICSI. The clinical investigations should include peripheral blood karyotyping, testicular biopsy for the study of spermatogenesis and meiotic studies, an analysis of chromosomal constitution of spermatozoa, DNA analysis of blood and spermatozoa to detect microdeletion on Y chromosomes.

REFERENCES

1. Ferguson-Smith M, Lennox B, Mack WS, et al. Klinefelter syndrome—frequency and testicular morphology in relation to nuclear sex. Lancet ii: 1957;475-76.
2. Jacobs PA, Strong JA. A case of human intersexuality having possible XXY sex determining mechanism. Nature 1959;183:302-03.
3. Kjessler B: Karyotype, meiosis and spermatogenesis in a sample of men attending an infertility clinic. Monographs in Human Genetics S Karger: Basel, Switzerland 1966;2.
4. Chandley AC. Human meiotic studies. In Emery AEH (Ed): Modern Trends in Human Genetics. Butterworths: London 1975;31-82.
5. Hendry WF, Ploani PE, Pugh ACB et al. 200 infertile males: Correlation of chromosomes, histological, endocrine and clinical studies. Br J Urol 1976;47:899-908.
6. Forejt J. Nonrandom association between a specific autosome and the X chromosome in meiosis of the male mouse—possible consequences of homologous centromere separation. Cytogenet Cell Genet 1974;13:241-48.
7. Micic M, Micic S, Diklic V. Chromosomal constitution of infertile men. Clin Genet 1984;25:33-36.
8. Reteif AE, van Zyl JA, Menkveld R et al. Chromosome studies in 496 infertile males with a sperm count below 10 million/ml. Hum Genet 1984;66:162-64.
9. Bourrouillou G, Dastague N, Colombies P. Chromosome studies in 952 infertile males with a sperm count below 10 milloin/ml. Hum Genet 1985;66:366-67.
10. Matsuda T, Nonomura M, Okada K et al. Cytogenetic survey of subfertile males in Japan. Urol Int 1989; 44:194-97.
11. Yoshida A, Tamayama T, Nagao K, et al. A cytogenetic survey of 1007 infertile males. Contracept Fertil Sex 1995;23:103a.
12. De Braekeleer M, Dao TN. Cytogenetic studies of male infertility—a review. Hum Reprod 1991;6:245-50.
13. van der Auwera B, van Roy, De Paepe A et al. Molecular cytogenetic analysis of XX males using Y-specific DNA sequences, including SRY. Hum Genet 1992;89:23-28.
14. Ferguson-Smith MA, Cooke A, Affara N et al. Genotype-phenotype correlations in XX males and the bearing on current theories of sex determination. Hum Genet 1990;84:198-202.
15. Burgoyne PS, Becker T. Meiotic pairing and gametogenetic failure. In Evans CW, Dikinson HG (Eds): Controlling Events in Meiosis Co. of Biologists: Cambridge 1984;349.
16. Kaiser P. Pericentric inversions: Problems and significance for clinical genetics. Hum Genet 1984;68:1-4.
17. Rosenmann A, Wahrman J, Richler C et al. Sperm chromosomes and habitual abortion. Fertil Steril 1985;56:370-72.
18. Madan K. Balanced structural changes involving the human X: Effect on sexual phenotype. Hum Genet 1983;63:216-21.
19. Laurent C, Chandley AC, Dautrilaux B et al. The use of surface spreading in the pachytene analysis of a human t(Y;17) reciprocal translocation. Cytogenet Cell Genet 1982;33:312-18.
20. Tiepolo L, Zuffardi O. Localization of factors controlling spermatogenesis in the nonfluorescent portion of the human Y chromosome long arm. Hum Genet 1976;34:119-24.
21. Ma K, Sharkey A, Kirsch S et al. Towards molecular localization of the AZF locus—mapping of microdeletons in azoospermic men within 14 subintervals of interval 6 of the human Y chromosome. Hum Mol Genet 1992;1:29-33.
22. Reijo AE, Lee T, Salo P, et al. Diverse spermatogenic defects in humans caused by Y chromosome deletion

encompassing a novel RNA-binding protein gene. Nature Genet 1995;10:383-93.

23. Luciani JM, Guichaoua MR, Metti A et al. Pachytene analysis of a man with a 13q;14q translocation and infertility. Cytogenet Cell Genet 1984;38:14-22.

24. Chandley AC, McBeth S, Speed RM. Pericentric inversion in human chromosome 1 and the risk for male sterility. J Med Genet 1987;24:325-34.

25. Martin RH, Hildebrand K, Balkan W, et al. Sperm chromosomal analysis in 9 men heterozygous for a structural chromosomal rearrangement. Genome 1988;30:s252.

26. Chandley AC. The genetics of human reproduction. Experientia 1986;42:1109-17.

27. Lange R, Krause W, Engel W. Analyses of meiotic chromosomes in testicular biopsies of infertile patients. Hum Reprod 1997;12:2154-58.

28. Zuhlke C, Thies U, Braulke I, et al. Down syndrome and male fertility—PCR-derived fingerprinting, serological and andrological investigations. Clin Genet 1994;46:324-26.

29. Johannisson R, Gropp A, Winking H et al. Down syndrome in the male—reproductive pathology and meiotic studies. Hum Genet 1983;63:132-38.

30. Chandley AC, Edmond P. Meiotic studies on a subfertile patient with a ring Y chromosome. Cytogenetics 1971;10:295-04.

31. Egozcue J, Templado C, Vidal F, et al. Meiotic studies in a series of 1100 infertile and sterile males. Hum Genet 1983;65:185-88.

32. Navarro J, Vidal F, Templado C et al. Meiotic chromosome studies and synaptonemal complex by light and electron microscopy in 47 infertile or sterile males. Hum Reprod 1986;1:523-27.

33. Vendrell JM, Garcia F, Viega A, et al. Meiotic abnormalities and spermatogenic parameters in severe oligoasthenozoospermia. Hum Reprod 1999;14:375-78.

34. Prabhakara K, Padman P, Dutta U et al. Meiotic impairment in an oligozoospermic male with translocation t(5;13). Fertil Steril, 2000.

35. Pieters MH, Gereaedts JP, Meyer H et al. Human gametes and zygotes studied by nonradioactive in situ hybridization. Cytogenet Cell Genet 1990;53:15-19.

36. Guttenbach M, Schakowski R, Schmid M. Incidence of chromosome 3,10,11, 17 and X disomy in mature human sperm nuclei as determined by nonradioactive in situ hybridization. Hum Genet 1994;93:7-12.

37. Moosani N, Pattison HA, Carter MD et al. Chromosomal analysis of sperm from men with idiopathic infertility using sperm karyotyping and fluorescence in situ hybridization. Fertil Steril 1995;64:811-17.

38. Pellestor F, Girardet A, Lefort G et al. PRINS as method for rapid chromosomal labelling on human spermatozoa. Mol Reprod Dev 1995;40:333-37.

39. Ogawa S, Araki S, Araki Y, et al. Chromosome analysis of human spermatozoa from an oligoasthenozoospermia carrier for a 13;14 translocation by their injection into mouse oocytes. Hum Reprod 2000;15:1136-39.

• A Henry Sathananthan • WD Ratna Sooriya
• Sulochana Gunasheela • A Trounson

14

The Human Sperm: Its Contribution to Fertilization and Embryogenesis

The sperm cell is a remarkable cell produced by the male human body. It is so very highly specialized for movement to enable it to target the egg cell during fertilization *in vivo* and *in vitro*. Its primary function is to carry the 23 male chromosomes, as well as a minute cell-organelle called the centrosome to the egg at fertilization. The paternal chromosomes together with 23 chromosomes of the egg associate at syngamy, to establish the genetic constitution of the zygote, the first cell of the human baby. The sperm centrosome, on the other hand, provides the machinery for cell division that enables the embryo to cleave repeatedly by mitosis, to develop into the human organism—the essence of activation. This process involves cell division, cell growth and differentiation aided by programmed cell movements, processes regulated by genes to establish the structure of the human body.

Structure of the Sperm Cell

The human sperm cell is paddle-shaped with a rounded head (4-5 microns long and 2-3 microns in width) and a long tail of flagellum about (about 50 microns long) according to WHO statistics. Of course, there are variations in size and form. In fact, the cell is composed of a head, neck, midpiece and tail (Figure 14.1) and is best studied by staining (light microscopy) or by scanning or transmission electron microscopy (SEM & TEM). In sections, most sperm heads present a conical profile rather than a rounded form, which is rare.

However, there is great variation in sperm size, form and internal structure, so much so, that any 2 sperm rarely look alike in fine structure.[1-3] This is in sharp contrast to sperm of bulls and monkeys, where sperm are more uniform in structure. Human sperm present a variety of abnormalities involving all of its constituents, both external and internal, widely documented in the literature (See atlas 1, 25). With respect to the process of fertilization, the important head structures are the outer plasma (cell) membrane (PM), acrosome, postacrosomal region and, of course, the nucleus with highly condensed DNA (Figure 14.1). The neck carries the centrosome, well protected in a 'black box' beneath the basal plate, containing a single functional centriole, which is proximal, whilst the distal is a vestige and reduced in humans.[1-3] The proximal centriole has a distinctive structure composed of 9 triplets of microtubules (MT) resembling a pin-wheel and is surrounded by pericentriolar material (PCM) concealed in a vault of the 'black box'. The centriole (cell centrosome or cell center) seems to be highly protected behind the sperm head, and if it was a precious component and we now know that it is involved in the development of the embryo. The 'black box' is composed of a capitulum and a 9 segmented columns which merge posteriorly with the outer dense fibers of the midpiece and tail. The midpiece and the tail aid in sperm motility and contain an axoneme composed of 9 doublets of MT surrounding a central doublet, assembling a cilium in structure.

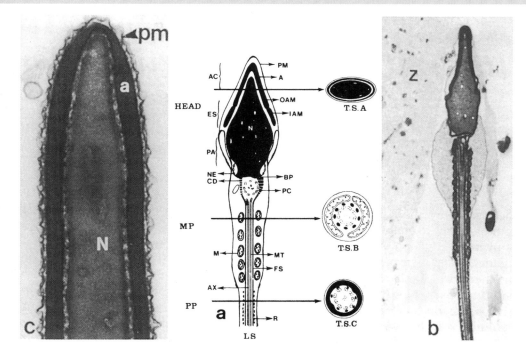

FIGURE 14.1: Sperm structure—(A) Diagram of sperm ultrastructure. A=acrosome (black), AC=acrosome cap, AX=axoneme, BP=basal plate, CD=cytoplasmic droplet, ES=equatorial segment (acrosome), FS=dense fibres, IAM=inner acrosome membrane, M=mitochondria, MP=midpiece, NE=nuclear envelope, OAM=outer acrosome membrane, PA=postacrosomal segment, PC=proximal centriole, PM=plasma membrane, PP=principal piece (tail), R=ribs.

(*Reproduced from Sathananthan et al. 1993*), (B) Whole intact sperm bound by its plasma membrane to the surface of the zona (z). Its structure is self-explanatory. × 15,000. (C) Sperm head showing surface membranes × 70,000

There are other structures–dense fibers and fibrous sheaths surrounding the tail axoneme (Figure 14.1). The PM extends almost to the tip of the tail. The midpiece contains a spiral of mitochondria that provide the energy (ATP) for cellular function and movement. All sperm components are usually incorporated into the oocyte at fertilization. In comparison to sperm, the egg is a drab rounded-cell (about 100-120 microns in diameter) and shows little specialization and retains an abundance of cytoplasm that will eventually sustain the embryo. It is one of the largest cells produced by the human body.

Contributions of the Sperm Head to Fertilization

Fertilization is a spontaneous fusion of 2 cells–sperm and egg.[1, 4-10] The outermost membranes, PM and acrosome (Figures 14.2 and 14.3) are involved in the acrosome reaction (AR) that enables the sperm to penetrate the egg. Sperm capacitation, a physiological process, is a prerequisite for both the AR and hyper-activated motility to enable the sperm to penetrate the egg-vestments. These 2 membranes fuse intermittently to form a shroud of vesicles (vesiculation)

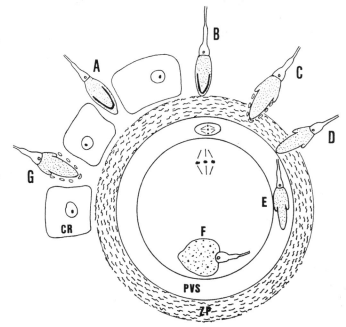

FIGURE 14.2: Diagram of sperm penetration—Sperm penetration through the egg-vestments and sperm incorporation during IVF. A-D and G. Penetration of cumulus and zona pellucida (ZP)—note acrosome reaction (vesiculation). E. Sperm-egg fusion. F. Sperm incorporation. CR=corona cell, PVS=perivitelline space. The egg is at metaphase II of maturation. (*Reproduced from Sathananthan, 1996*)

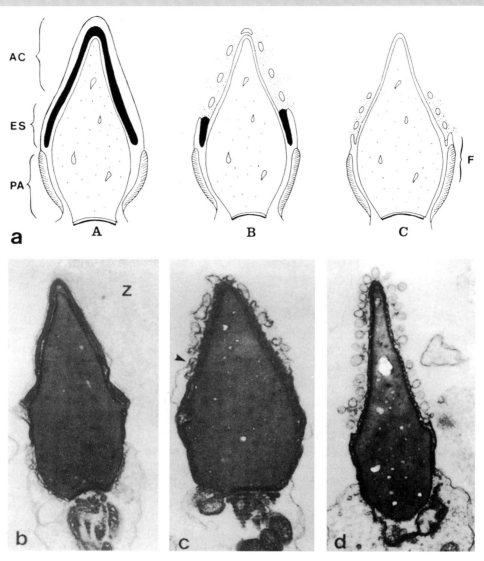

FIGURE 14.3: Sperm acrosome reaction—(A) Diagram of the sperm acrosome reaction: 2 stages. Note vesiculation of surface membranes: fused plasma and outer acrosome membranes. A. acrosome intact. B. acrosome cap reacted. C. Fully acrosome reacted. AC=acrosome cap, ES=equatorial segment, F=fusogenic region, PA=postacrosomal segment. *(Reproduced from Sathananthan et al. 1993).* (B) Acrosome–intact sperm bound to the zona (z) by its plasma membrane × 30,600. (C) Acrosome-reacting sperm (cap region) at the surface of the zona. Note connection between plasma membrane and outer acrosome, where the acrosome has still not reacted (arrow) × 35,700. (D) Acrosome–reacted sperm penetrating the zona. Vesiculation is complete and myriads of vesicles are still attached to the inner acrosome membrane × 25,000. *(B and C Reproduced from Chen and Sathananthan, 1986; D from Sathananthan et al. 1993)*

around the anterior two-thirds of the sperm head releasing enzymes (hyaluronidase and acrosin) for digesting a pathway for penetration through the cumulus and zona pellucida (ZP). This process is akin to cell secretion by exocytosis. Thus, the PM and outer acrosomal membrane (OAM) are lost in the acrosomal region, whilst the inner acrosomal membrane (IAM) remains intact when the sperm reaches the perivitelline space to fuse with the oocyte at fertlization (Figure 14.4). Only acrosome-reacted sperm can penetrate the ZP and fuse with the oocyte. Sperm-oocyte PM fusion (Figure 14.5) occurs between the midsegment (postacrosomal segment) of the sperm and oolemma (egg PM) and the whole sperm is phagocytosed by the egg and incorporated into the

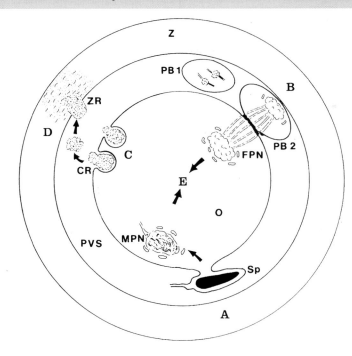

FIGURE 14.4: Diagram of major events at fertilization—(A) Sperm-oocyte membrane fusion. The plasma membrane of the midsegment of the sperm (Sp) in the perivitelline space has fused with the oolemma. The sperm is then incorporated into the ooplasm (O) by phagocytosis (arrow) and begins nuclear DNA decondensation to form a male pronucleus (MPN). (B) Completion of second meiotic maturation (telophase II). The second polar body (PB$_2$) has been abstricted and the female pronucleus (FPN) is developing. PB$_1$=first polar body. (C) Cortical reaction (CR): exocytosis of cortical granules (C). (D) Zona reaction (ZR): dispersed contents of cortical granules interacting with the zona (Z). (E) Association of MPN and FPN occurs eventually (arrows)

ooplasm (egg cytoplasm).[1, 4, 5, 8] The fusogenic zone undergoes molecular changes demonstrable by freeze fracture TEM. Integrins (alpha and beta) on the oolemma of human oocytes and fertilin, a specific sperm receptor in the fusion domain of sperm, have been implicated in sperm-oocyte binding and fusion in mammals.[34] CD9, a protein on the egg membrane, regulates the interaction of fertilin with integrin.

We have now the most compelling evidence that the sperm PM is directly incorporated into the oolemma of the human oocyte[1, 4, 8-10] and this has profound implications after ICSI (see below). The whole of the sperm PM posterior to the acrosome is incorporated into the oolemma in zipper-like fashion and integrated into the zygote membrane to form a mosaic membrane (Figure 14.6). Sperm motility is not required for fusion.[5] The mature oocyte is arrested at metaphase II of meiosis when ovulated and will not develop further until it is fertilized by the sperm and activated to cleave. Meiotic arrest is maintained by maturation promoting factor (MPF), which is regulated by a cytostatic factor (CSF).[32, 34]

Oocyte Activation by Sperm

This is a complex process and involves completion of egg maturation, release of cortical granules (CG) to block polyspermy and more importantly the activation of the sperm centrosome to initiate cell division of the zygote (Figure 14.7). The latter we believe is the essence of activation.[1, 6-10, 23] There are also complex molecular changes that occur within the embryo after fertilization, which is briefly reviewed below (Molecular implications).

Once the sperm is incorporated into the ooplasm its head swells progressively (Figures 14.5 and 14.6), whilst its chromatin decondenses and nuclear envelope expands.[1, 4, 8-10] The IAM is intermittently discarded (Figure 14.6) and a new nuclear envelope is organized by intercalation of flatenned elements of egg smooth endoplasmic reticulum (SER) to accommodate the expanding male pronucleus. Recently, the perinuclear theca has been implicated in mammalian oocyte activation.[34] This is the scanty strip of cytoplasm between the IAM and nuclear envelope (Figures 14.1 and 14.6). Human sperm shows disorganization of the IAM that enables the sperm head to expand exposing the perinuclear theca. It is conceivable that IAM has also a role to play in chromatin decondensation and perhaps oocyte activation, since it is just outside the perinuclear theca. Sperm chromatin decondensation is believed to be influenced by a chromatin decondensing factor contributed by the ooplasm, where DNA-bound protamines are replaced with oocyte histones reducing disulphide bonding. Hence in all these fertilization events, there is interaction and co-operation between sperm and egg components, which can be quite complex and is yet little understood.

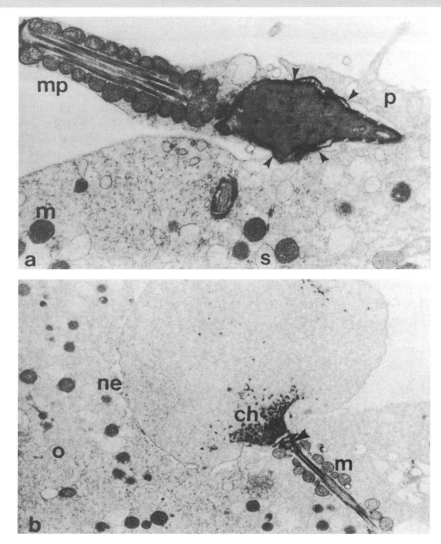

FIGURE 14.5: Sperm-egg fusion and incorporation—(A) Sperm-oocyte membrane fusion: the midsegment of the acrosome–reacted sperm (equatorial vestige and anterior half of the post-acrosomal segment) has fused with the oolemma (between arrows). The egg has extended a phagocytic process (p) that engulfs the head of the sperm. m=mitochondria, mp=midpiece, o=ooplasm, s=smooth endoplasmic reticulum. × 30,600. (B) Normal sperm incorporation in the ooplasm (o): the chromatin has decondensed and the sperm head has expanded to form a MPN. Note centriole (arrow) in the neck region. ch=chromatin, mp=midpiece, ne=nuclear envelope. × 13,200. *(Reproduced from Sathananthan et al. 1986b)*

Other aspects of activation by sperm include the release of CG by the egg, another example of cell secretion by exocytosis.[6-10] This is an instantaneous response by the egg to sperm-egg fusion and is thought to originate from the point of fusion in cascade fashion spreading all around the surface of the egg. This cortical reaction (CR) is necessary to block polyspermy to ensure normal development, since dispermic development is abnormal. The membrane around myriads of these CG are also incorporated into egg PM together with the sperm PM, so much so, that we have now a complex, mosaic membrane on the surface of the zygote, which prevents polyspermy at the level of the oolemma, as well.[11] We reported acrosome reacted sperm in the PVS of eggs after multiple sperm injection. The primary block to polyspermy, however, is the zona, where the contents released by CG interact with the inner zona, chemically hardening that region

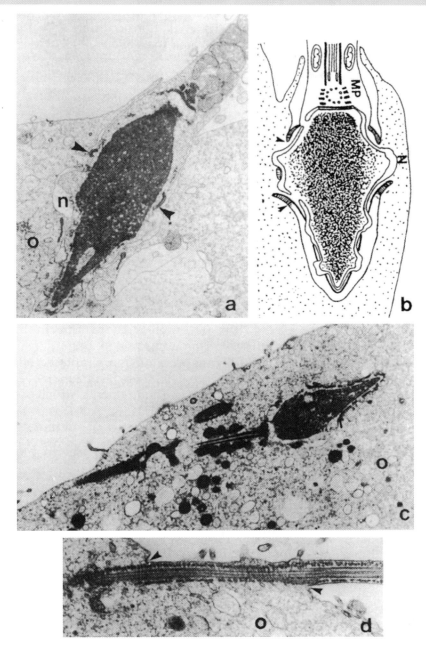

FIGURE 14.6: Sperm membrane incorporation—(A) and (B) Sperm phagocytosis by the egg and incorporation of the sperm plasma membrane into the oolemma. This does not happen in ICSI. The chromatin has begun to decondense and the sperm nuclear envelope (n) is expanding anteriorly. The continuity of the sperm PM and oolemma is evident (large arrows). MP=midpiece, O=ooplasm. (A) × 17,500. (C) Incorporated sperm at egg-surface. Note complete absence of PM × 12,000. (D) Incorporation of the sperm tail PM into the oolemma in zipper-like fashion. Note fusion of sperm PM with oolemma (arrows) × 50,000. *(Reproduced from Sathananthan et al. 1986b)*

(Figure 14.4). The zona has 3 glycoproteins ZP1, ZP2 and ZP3, which have different functions in the gelatinous shell. ZP3 for instance induces the sperm AR. Sperm-egg fusion also triggers the abstriction of the second polar body (PB2) that carries the excess chromosomes to complete meiosis, so that a haploid set remains in the oocyte. This process is also instantaneous and mediated by microfilaments (MF) which constrict the ooplasm to form the polar body. MF are also involved during phagocytosis of sperm soon after gamete fusion, a reaction elicited by the egg cortex. Usually a fertilization bump or cone with MF appears at the point of sperm entry and remains on the surface of the egg for some time after sperm incorporation.[6] There are also thicker filaments in the vicinity of sperm soon after incorporation of unknown function.[5] This is also the time sperm cytosolic factors are released and secondary calcium oscillations occur during activation. Hence, the egg cortex is also activated to accomplish several processes at the time of fertilization.

Contributions of the Sperm Neck (Connecting Piece)

The most important contribution is the sperm centriole, located within the 'black box' (Figure 14.7).[19-23] The point of sperm entry could determine the polarity of the embryo, a new concept in human embryology.[24] The animal-vegetal axis is the first embryonic axis in most animals. However, sperm entry reorganizes the whole ooplasm to form a new axis once the sperm aster is developed in the ooplasm around the sperm centrosome. This sperm mono-aster is a remarkable structure that reorganizes the whole cytoskeleton of the egg by polarising flows of cortical and ooplasmic material.[21-23] The aster grows and occupies the whole of the ooplasm and now consists of myriads of MT radiating from a duplicated sperm centriole (diplosome). The MT actually radiates from pericentriolar material (PCM) that grows around the diplosome by addition of maternal gamma-tubulin derived from the ooplasm to establish a zygote centrosome. Thus, a functional zygote centrosome is formed capable of nucleating MT to form the sperm mono-aster, which later duplicates to form 2 asters which organise the opposite poles of the first mitotic spindle.[21-23] The sperm centriole is associated with specific proteins–centrin, pericentrin, gamma tubulin among other proteins (see molecular dissection of the centrosome by

Schatten).[23] Centrin is a calcium binding protein and is probably involved in the excision of the sperm flagellum from the sperm head to release the centriole from the 'black box'. Mitochondria at the tip of the midpiece are closely associated with the release of the centriole at all stages of sperm head expansion and MPN development in the human (Figures 14.5 and 14.6).[1,4,8] and this could be one of the last functions of the sperm mitochondria in fertilization. The zygote centrosome now resembles normal centrosomes of diploid somatic cells and duplicates at each mitotic cycle during cleavage of the embryo in synchrony with each chromosomal cycle and this process has been traced to the hatching blastocyst in human embryos.[21,22] Thus, the sperm centrosome is inherited, replicated and perpetuated in human embryos and is very likely the ancestor of centrosomes in all fetal and adult somatic cells. Remnants of the 'black box'-capitulum, segmented columns and dense fibers remain associated with the centriole for some time and their fate is unknown. Similarly the fate of the proximal centriolar adjunct (aster of MT) and remnants of the distal centriole is unknown. Does the centriolar adjunct contribute in any way to the formation of the sperm aster?

Contributions of the Sperm Midpiece and Tail

The mitochondria of the midpiece are destined to progressively degenerate, since they carry paternal mDNA, which may be harmful to the embryo. In humans maternal mitochondria remain active as in most mammals and undergo profound changes during early development. Sperm mitochondria appear to progressively degenerate, though they were seen in 8-cell blastomeres associated with the centriole. In bovine embryos, ubiquitin, a proteolytic polypeptide, has been implicated in mitochondrial destruction.[34] Sperm mitochondria in humans become progressively translucent and are easily recognized by their oval shape and association with centrioles and midpiece remnants. We have not seen mitochondria in lysosomes in late

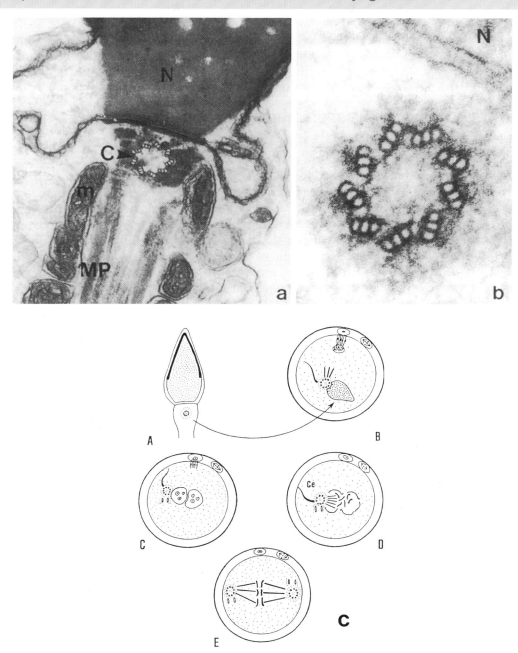

FIGURE 14.7: Inheritance of the sperm centrosome at fertilization—(A) Sperm neck showing proximal centriole (C) composed of 9 triplets of MT within "black box". MP=midpiece, N=nucleus. × 50,000. (B) Descendent of sperm centriole in a 8-cell blastomere. Note classical '9 + 0' organisation of MT associated with PCM. × 150,000. N=nucleus. (C) Diagram of sperm centriolar inheritance. A. Sperm centriole. B. Incorporated sperm showing developing sperm aster. C. Duplicated centriole associated with pronuclei. D. Sperm aster at prometaphase organizing mitotic spindle. E. First mitotic, bipolar spindle showing duplicated centrioles (diplosomes) located at opposite poles and chromosomes at the equator. *(All reproduced from Sathananthan et al. 1996)*

preimplantation embryos. The fate of the flagellar axoneme of MT, dense fibers and fibrous sheaths is unknown. The whole of the sperm flagellum is incorporated into the oocyte at fertilization and is progressively dismantled during development (Figure 14.6).

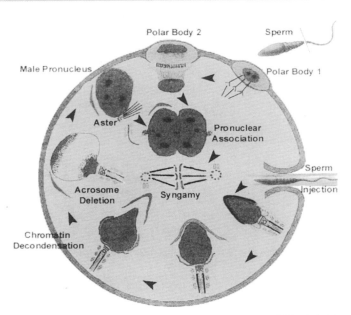

Modified from Kubo (1998) Modern Reprod Med 1:10

FIGURE 14.8: Diagram of fertilization events after ICSI—Sperm injection, sperm incorporation, acrosome deletion, chromatin decondensation, MPN formation, PB2 abstriction, pronuclear association and syngamy are illustrated

Contributions of the Sperm Cell to ICSI

ICSI is an invasive procedure that violates most norms of fertilization (Figure 14.8). Although it is a very successful method of ART, we have some concerns about fertilization and embryo development.[11-14,18] With ICSI fertilization begins with sperm incorporation, since sperm penetration and sperm-egg fusion is bypassed. Also, it is more unnatural than IVF, since there is no selection of sperm either at the egg-vestments or oolemma as the embryologist decides on the single sperm that is injected into the ooplasm. It was originally meant to treat male factor infertility, though now it seems to be often used to treat IVF patients to maximise success rates and some believe it might eventually replace IVF altogether. However, a comparison of ICSI and IVF children by the Belgian group did not show any increased risk of major malformations and neonatal complications after ICSI.[15]

During ICSI the physiological sperm AR is usually prevented and often the acrosome is totally deleted from the head[30] before sperm incorporation (Figure 14.9). If this process is delayed sperm-head expansion could be delayed or even abnormal. One of the most serious concerns in ICSI is that the sperm PM is not incorporated into the oolemma[1,4,12] as during fertilization *in vitro* (Figure 14.6). Whether this membrane is recycled within the ooplasm and later incorporated into the oolemma by 'membrane flux' is not known. The sperm PM, a linear cone of about 50 microns, will eventually end up as a patch on the surface of the zygote PM and end up in one or more blastomeres or some germ layer or even in the germline, which may be critical for future development. Sperm phagocytosis by the egg also does not eventuate with ICSI. Furthermore the point of sperm-entry is predetermined in ICSI and the cytoskeletal organization of the egg is disturbed when the sperm is injected. As in IVF, all the sperm components of the sperm cell are incorporated into the oocyte, including the sperm centrosome, which is so important for embryonic cleavage. Care should be taken not to damage the neck and midpiece when motile sperm are immobilized for ICSI. Similarly it seems advisable to leave the midpiece mitochondria intact.

Oocyte activation seems to follow the IVF process, including molecular events, though it is not triggered by sperm-egg membrane fusion.[31,32] Since fertilization rates are quite high. However, there are some minor concerns about PB2 extrusion and delay in the cortical reaction.[13] The former results in digyny when 2 female pronuclei and 1 male pronucleus are formed and the zygote is triploid, as in dispermy. We found a delay in CG-release, which was observed at the 2-cell stage, which has no consequence in fertilization, since the block to polyspermy is inoperative.

Another major concern of ICSI is the injection of abnormal sperm from male factor patients, which might perpetuate infertility. These sperm could have chromosomal and centrosomal defects, which will result in abnormal embryos.[13, 18] These defects have been documented for IVF too,[1] but could be more prevalent after ICSI. The usual aberrations of embryonic development after IVF-development arrest and retardation of

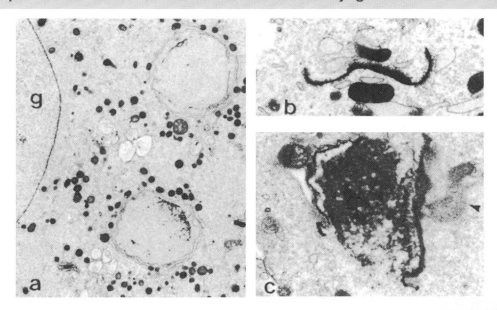

FIGURE 14.9: Sperm incorporation after ICSI—(A) Two developing MPN in a germinal vesicle oocyte showing chromatin decondensation. The surface membranes are absent but new pronuclear envelopes are forming. g=germinal vesicle. × 5,100. (B) Deleted sperm acrosome close to a MPN shown in (a) prior to MPN formation, showing thickened cap and equatorial segment on either side. × 17,500. (C) Depleting acrosome of decondensing abnormal sperm head. Some of its contents have diffused into the ooplasm (arrow). × 17,500. *(Reproduced from Sathananthan,1998a)*

development, irregular cleavage, multinucleation of blastomeres, fragmentation and chromosomal defects are observed after ICSI and this could also be related to stimulation, culture conditions and other factors, as well. Normal, as well as abnormal blastocysts can develop after ICSI.[16] Blastocyst hatching may be aided by opening the zona during the ICSI procedure, but we have identified specialized 'zona-breaker' cells that are involved in the process of hatching in ICSI blastocysts.[17]

We have postulated that bad sperm, particularly those with poor motility could produce poor embryos, a new dimension in the assessment of infertility,[20-22, 25] based on sperm centrosomal structure and function. Sperm with poor motility have a greater incidence of abnormal centrioles, which could compromise embryo development. Abnormal sperm asters, mitotic spindles, micronuclei and multiple nuclei in blastomeres reflecting chromosomal aberrations, may result from centrosomal dysfunction.[13,22,23,28] There is now some clinical evidence to support this theory.[26, 27] There were no pregnancies in 20 cycles of immotile sperm after ICSI. However, successful pregnancies with immotile spermatozoa from

ejaculate, epididymis and testis have been recently reported.[14] Sperm tail nor centriolar defects were reported in these studies.

Molecular Implications: Oocyte Activation

Sperm-oocyte membrane fusion initiates a cascade of events that transform the egg into an embryo. These involve complex morphological, physiological and molecular processes in the egg, primarily induced by the fertilizing sperm cell. Some of the molecular interactions have been documented in the past decade in mammals and may be applicable to humans with caution (See reviews 31-34).

Gamete membrane fusion followed by sperm incorporation (Figure 14.10) opens a gateway for the transduction of specific signals induced by the sperm cell, which occur in a few seconds, minutes or several hours. These trigger the cascade of morphological and physiological events outlined above (Figure 14.4). One of the immediate changes in the human oocyte soon after sperm-egg fusion, demonstrated by confocal laser scanning microscopy, is the release of calcium (Ca^{++} oscillations)

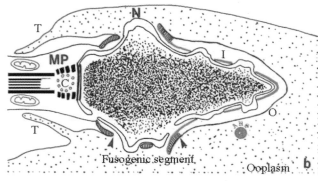

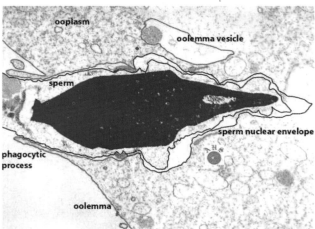

FIGURE 14.10: Sperm incorporation soon after fusion (diagram and TEM)—This sperm (incorporated 3h postinsemination) shows how a pathway opens for molecular interactions between sperm and ooplasm via the fusogenic domain. The sperm factor that activates the egg could originate from the fusogenic, midsegment of the sperm head where sperm-egg membrane fusion occurred (Receptor or cytosolic mediated) or the perinuclear theca between the IAM and nuclear envelope (Cytosolic mediated). C=centriole in black box, I=inner acrosome membrane, MP=midpiece, N= nuclear envelope, O=oolemma, T=phagocytic process of egg. TEM × 35,700 (Modified Sathananthan et al,1986a)[36]

within the oocyte that occurs repetitively in waves and are transient in nature.[29, 30] These oscillations originate from the point of sperm-egg membrane fusion and spread throughout the periphery of the oocyte first before spreading into the central ooplasm (periphery to center propagation). The central oscillations are sustained after the peripherals disappear. Ca^{++} is apparently released from internal stores (presumably SER) within the oocyte. It is mediated by the production of IP3 (inositol 1,4,5-triphosphate) which sensitizes the SER to release Ca^{++}.[31-34] We have demonstrated 2 types of SER in the oocyte—

peripheral aggregates of tubular SER and vesicular elements of SER spread throughout the ooplasm,[6, 8] which could well be involved in these waves of Ca^{++} release. This is possibly the principal function of SER in oocytes. The oscillations occur in about 20 minutes after insemination or is delayed (4 or more hours) after ICSI, possibly due to the mode of sperm incorporation after acrosome deletion in the ooplasm.

Two main theories have been postulated to explain activation of the oocyte at the molecular level.[31-34] (a) Receptor-mediated theory and (b) Cytosolic-soluble sperm factor theory. (a) It postulates a receptor-ligand interaction between the sperm and oocyte plasma membranes which triggers a signaling cascade that culminates in activation. This could be more applicable to IVF where the fusogenic midsegment of the sperm fuses with the oolemma, followed by total incorporation of the sperm plasma membrane into the egg membrane. (b) It postulates the release of a sperm soluble factor into the ooplasm which initiates the Ca^{++} release. This factor called "Oscillin" could originate from either the fusogenic midsegment in humans, since it has been localized in the equatorial region of the sperm acrosome in mammals,[35] or from the perinuclear theca.[34] The cytosolic theory seems to be more acceptable, since it can also explain activation after ICSI (See 32), where no sperm-egg membrane fusion occurs. After both IVF and ICSI, the sperm induced, secondary Ca^{++} signaling cascade has been documented,[29-35] which, in turn, is thought to trigger the early events of fertilization. The events that occur simultaneously with sperm incorporation are sperm aster formation (activation of the sperm centrosome), the cortical reaction preventing polyspermy, completion of egg maturation, sperm DNA decondensation and pronuclear assembly.[1, 8-10, 31] The secondary Ca^{++} release induced by sperm oscillin or other sperm factor could be implicated in all of these processes. However, we must now ask the question whether the sperm centrosome, per se, is also involved in the initiation of oocyte activation, since it clearly initiates mitosis in the human embryo. If all other events of activation eventuate and cleavage of the fertilized egg does not occur, development has failed. It is high time we need to consider all the processes involved in human fertilization—morphological, physiological, biochemical and molecular—to understand the complexities of sperm-egg interaction.

REFERENCES

1. Sathananthan AH (Ed): Visual Atlas of Human Sperm Structure and Function for Assisted Reproductive Technology. National University, Singapore 1996;279.
2. De Kretser DM, Kerr JB. The cytology of the testis. In: Knobil E, Neill J (Eds): The Physiology of Reproduction, 2nd ed. Raven Press, New York. 1994;837-932.
3. Holstein AF, Roosen-Runge EC. Atlas of human spermatogenesis. Grosse Verlag, Berlin 1981.
4. Sathananthan AH, Ng SC, Edirisinghe R et al. Human sperm-egg interaction in vitro. Gamete Res. 1986b; 15:317-26.
5. Sathananthan AH, Chen C. Sperm-oocyte membrane fusion in the human during monospermic fertilisation. Gamete Res 1986;15:177-86.
6. Sathananthan AH, Trounson AO, Wood C. Atlas of fine structure of human sperm penetration, eggs and embryos cultured in vitro. Praeger Scientific, Philadelphia 1986a;279.
7. Yanagimachi R. Mammalian fertilization. In: Knobil E, Neill J (Eds): The Physiology of Reproduction, 2nd edn. Raven Press, New York. 1994;189-317.
8. Sathananthan AH, Ng SC, Bongso A et al. Visual Atlas of Early Human Development for Assisted Technology. National University, Singapore, 1993;209.
9. Sathananthan AH. Human gametes and fertilization. In: S Suzuki (Ed.): Modern Reprod.Med Medical View.Tokyo 1998a;12-21.
10. Sathananthan AH. Ultrastructure of human gametes, fertilization and embryo development. In Trounson AO, Gardner DK (Eds): Handbook of In Vitro Fertilization, 2nd edn., CRC Press, Boca Raton, Florida, 2000;431-64.
11. Sathananthan AH, Ng SC, Trounson AO et al. Human microfertilization by injection of single or multiple sperm: Ultrastructure. Hum. Reprod 1989;4:574-83.
12. Sathananthan AH, Szell A, Ng SC et al. Is the acrosome a prerequisite for sperm incorporation after intracytoplasmic sperm injection (ICSI)? Reprod Fertil Dev 1997;9:703-09.
13. Sathananthan AH, Trounson A. Ultrastructure of ICSI. In: Trounson AO, Gardner DK (Eds): Handbook of In Vitro Fertilization, 2nd edn. CRC Press, Boca Raton, Florida 2000;465-82.
14. Rhouma KB, Miled EB, Attallah K et al. Successful pregnancies after using immotile spermatozoa from ejaculate, epididymis and testis. Eur J Obstet Gynecol Reprod Biol 2003;108:182-85.
15. Bonduelle M, Liebaers I, Deketelaere et al. Neonatal data on a cohort of 2889 infants born after ICSI (1991-1999). Hum.Reprod. 2002;17:671-94.
16. Sathananthan AH, Gunasheela S, Menezes J. Critical evaluation of human blastocysts for assisted reproduction techniques and embryonic stem cell biotechnology. Reprod Biomed Online 2003a;7:219-27.
17. Sathananthan AH, Menezes J, Gunasheela S Mechanics of blastocyst hatching in vitro. Reprod Biomed Online 2003b;7:228-34.
18. Mansour R. Intracytoplasmic sperm injection: A state of the ART technique. Hum Reprod Update 1998;4:43-56.
19. Sathananthan AH, Kola I, Osborne J et al. Centrioles in the beginning of human development. Proc. Natl. Acad. Sci. USA 1991;88:4806-10.
20. Sathananthan AH. Inheritance of paternal centrioles and male infertility. XIIIth World Congress of Obstetrics and Gynaecology, Singapore. Abstr No. 1991;1629.
21. Sathananthan AH, Ratnam SS, Ng SC et al. The sperm centriole: its inheritance, replication and perpetuation in early human embryos. Hum Reprod 1996;11:345-56.
22. Sathananthan AH. Mitosis in the human embryo: The vital role of the sperm centrosome (centriole). Histol Histopathol 1997;12:827-56.
23. Schatten G. The centrosome and its mode of inheritance: The reduction of the centrosome during gametogenesis and its restoration during fertilization. Dev Biol 1994;165:299-335.
24. Edwards RG, Beard HK. Oocyte polarity and cell determination in early mammalian embryos. Mol Hum Reprod 1997;3:863-905.
25. Sathananthan AH. Functional competence of abnormal spermatozoa. In: S Fishel (Ed): Bailliere's Clinical Obstetrics and Gynaecology-Micromanipulation Techniques. Bailliere Tindall, London, 1994;8:141-56.
26. Tournaye H, Joris H, Verheyen G et al. Sperm parameters, globozoospermia, necrospermia and ICSI outcome. In: Filicori M, Flamigni C (Eds): Treatment of Infertility:The New Frontiers, Communications Media for Education, Boca Raton, Florida, 1998; 259-68.
27. Van Steirteghem A, Verheyen G, Joris H et al. ICSI with non-motile and frozen-thawed sperm. In: Filicore M, Flamigni C (Eds): Treatment of infertility: The new Frontiers, Communications Media for Education, Princeton, NJ 1998;243-48.
28. Sathananthan AH. Sperm centrioles and their role in mammalian development. In: Filicore M, Flamigni C (Eds): Treatment of Infertility: The New Frontiers, Communications Media for Education, Princeton, NJ 1998b;229-41.
29. Tesarik J, Sousa M, Mendoza C. Sperm-Induced calcium oscillations of human oocytes show distinct features in oocyte center and periphery. Mol.Reprod.Dev 1995;41:257-63.
30. Sousa M, Barros A, Tesarik J. Developmental changes in calcium dynamics, protein kinase C distribution and

endoplasmic organization in human preimplantation embryos. Mol Hum Reprod 1996;2:967-77.

31. Battaglia DE. Questions about oocyte activation: answers from ICSI? In: Filicore M, Flamigni C (Eds) Treatment of Infertility: The New Frontiers, Communications Media for Education, Princeton, NJ 1998; 249-56.

32. Flaherty SP, Payne D, Mathews CD. Fertilization failures after ICSI. Treatment of Infertility: The New frontiers Communications Media for Education, Princeton, NJ 1998;269-82.

33. Williams CJ. Signalling mechanisms of mammalian oocyte activation. Hum Reprod. Update 2002;8: 313-21.

34. Sutovsky P, Schatten G. Paternal contributions to the mammalian zygote: Fertilization after sperm-egg fusion. Int Rev Cytol 2000;195:1-65.

35. Parrington J, Swann K, Shevchenko VI et al. Calcium oscillations in mammalian eggs trigerred by a soluble sperm protein. Nature 1996;379:364-68.

36. Sathananthan AH. Human Fertilization CD-ROM. Tokyo, Japan, 2003.

• N Pandiyan • Jayant Mehta • A Rajasekaran
• R Jayaganesh • SS Vasan • Nalini Krishnan

15

Male Infertility

SEMEN ANALYSIS AND SPERM PREPARATION

N Pandiyan, Jayant Mehta

INTRODUCTION

Semen analysis remains the single most important test in the evaluation of an infertile male. However, this test is done improperly in most laboratories around the world, leading to erroneous conclusion about a man's fertility. *Here the authors have suggested standardization of procedures for examination and preparation of human semen sample.*

Composition of Semen

Normal semen is a composite mixture of secretions from the testes, epididymes, seminal vesicles, prostate and paraurethral glands.[2] However, these secretions do not mix prior to ejaculation. Each component of semen has distinctive properties and probably distinctive functions.

Constituents of Normal Semen

Semen contains the seminal plasma and the cellular elements. The cellular elements are the spermatozoa, sperm precursors and other cells from the genital tract and a few leukocytes, *which have been collectively referred to as 'round cells'.*

Seminal plasma contains the seminal proteins and other biochemical substances produced by the testes and accessory sex glands.

Normal Semen: Physical Properties

Macroscopic Properties

Color, odor and appearance: *A normal semen sample has an homogeneous* grey and opalescent appearance with a distinctive musty odor. *Opaqueness of the sample depends on the sperm concentration, while presence of red blood cells within the sample gives it a brown color.*

Viscosity The semen is viscous due to the presence of formed elements in the semen.

Liquefaction Semen coagulates just after ejaculation and liquefies within about 30 minutes. Coagulation of semen is due to proteins from the seminal vesicles and liquefaction is due to prostatic secretions. Some normal samples are known to contain jelly-like grains, which do not liquefy and their significance is unknown.

Volume The normal ejaculate has a volume of about 2 to 6 ml. The major contribution to the seminal volume is from the seminal vesicles (70%). Prostate contributes to 20 percent of the seminal volume. Testes and the bulbourethral glands contribute 5 percent each.[4]

Seminal pH Semen is strongly alkaline. The pH ranges from 7.3 to 8.0. The secretions of the seminal vesicles contribute to the alkalinity of the semen. Semen is the strongest buffer in the body. The alkaline semen buffers the acidic environment of the vagina.

Microscopic Properties

Sperm concentration The sperm concentration in a normal ejaculate is 20 million/ml or more. However, the sperm concentration even in a normal fertile individual is notoriously prone for huge variations.[5]

Sperm motility Normal spermatozoa exhibit motility ranging from fast progressive to slow progressive. The spermatozoon moves at a speed of 25 µ/sec or 3 mm/hour. A normal ejaculate has at least 25 percent fast progressive or 50 percent fast and slow progressive spermatozoa.[6]

Sperm morphology A typical spermatozoon has a head, neck, midpiece, principal piece and tail. In a normal ejaculate at least 30 percent of the spermatozoa have a normal morphology.[6]

Cellular elements Some sperm precursors, cells from the other part of the genital tract and a few leukocytes can be seen in a normal ejaculate.

Semen Analysis

Semen analysis remains the single most important test in the evaluation of an infertile male. There are several problems and pitfalls in the evaluation of the semen sample. Proper precautions must be taken in avoiding these pitfalls and care must be taken in evaluating a semen sample.

Patients must be given both written and oral instruction on proper collection of the semen sample in their vernacular or language they understand.

Semen Collection (Container)

Semen collection must be done in a wide mouthed, *sterile* clean, dry, nontoxic container. Test tubes are most unsuitable for semen collection. Attempts at semen collection in a test tube would lead to collection of an incomplete sample, giving rise to erroneous results.

Wet container with water would kill the spermatozoa and would lead to artefactual sperm tail defects. Steam autoclaved containers are not suitable, as, though clean and sterile, they often contain moisture. Plastic containers may be suitable, provided they are of nontoxic grade.

Place of Collection

Most of the laboratories do not provide an exclusive place for semen collection. Bathrooms and toilets are most inappropriate places for semen collection. Ideally semen collection must be done in a separate room, adjoining the laboratory with adequate privacy. Many men may require their wives to be around for semen collection. If, however, a room is not available, semen collection can also be done from the patient's place of residence, but the sample must be brought to the laboratory within half an hour to one hour. During transit, the sample must be kept at body temperature, by keeping it in the shirt pocket or keeping it in the hand. There are some men who have never masturbated and could never collect a sample by masturbation. These men may be encouraged to collect a semen sample by intercourse with a sterile, nontoxic condom.

Method of Collection

Semen sample for analysis should be collected by masturbation. The patients must be encouraged to collect a complete sample. Spillage of any part of the sample would lead to erroneous results. Abstinence: Each laboratory should follow a standard duration of abstinence before semen analysis. We generally advise our patients to follow 4 days abstinence, but anything from 2 to 7 days would suffice. Unduly long abstinence would lead to Asthenozoospermia or unduly short abstinence may lead to oligozoospermia.

Specimen Handling

Semen sample poses a possible biohazard to the laboratory personnel. The container must be labelled with the patients' name and ID number, if any. The specimen must be handled with gloved hands, with extreme care, preferably in a vertical flow laminar cabinet. Semen samples may contain harmful bacteria and viruses and should be disposed off carefully after analysis. Good laboratory practice is fundamental and should not be compromised at any cost.

Semen Variables

Volume

The volume of the semen sample should be accurately estimated by using a graduated cylinder or a pipette or a syringe. The volume can be measured in a graduated syringe large enough to hold the entire volume of semen sample.

Estimation of semen volume by mere inspection would lead to erroneous results and should be discouraged. Semen volume is important to estimate, to establish the total number of spermatozoa in the ejaculate.

Viscosity and Liquefaction

These parameters are assessed by inspection of the sample and by aspiration of the sample into a pipette or syringe. *A normal sample would leave the pipette as small discrete drops, while a very viscous sample would form a thread normally more than 2 cm long.*

Motility

Motility is assessed by evaluation of semen sample after liquefaction. A drop of well mixed semen sample is placed on a clean glass slide and covered with a clean cover slip. Spermatozoa motility is then assessed by evaluation of at least 100 spermatozoa in different fields. Spermatozoa motility is then graded as:
• Rapid linear motility—Grade A
• Slow or sluggish progressive motility—Grade B
• Non progressive motility—Grade C
• Immotile—Grade D

Most laboratories tend to evaluate sperm motility by a cursory inspection or evaluation of a few fields of the semen sample. This is improper and would lead to wrong estimation of sperm motility. It is, therefore, recommended that the motility count should be repeated on two more drops of semen prepared in the same way and the mean of the results reported.

Estimation of Spermatozoa Concentration

There are several methods of estimating sperm concentration in semen sample—the most common and simplest of these is by using the "Hemocytometer". An improved Neubauer counting chamber is widely available and is economical.

Use of this chamber however, requires a dilution factor to be taken into consideration for the final calculation. The semen sample may also have to be diluted in the event of high concentration. It is, therefore, possible to introduce an element of error in calculation of sperm concentration.

The sperm concentration can also be estimated by using Makler or Horwell counting chambers, which do not require dilution factor to be taken into consideration. However, the semen sample with high concentration of cells may require dilution prior to assessment.

These chambers are convenient, but they are far more expensive and their superiority or accuracy over the conventional method remains unproven.

The 80's saw the introduction of the "Computer-assisted semen analysis" (CASA) system which eliminates many of the subjective errors of conventional semen analysis. CASA also, however, requires a technician to focus the proper area.

Morphology

The morphological characteristics of spermatozoa are assessed by preparing a stained semen smear from a fresh specimen of semen. Papanicolaou stain is widely used. One hundred spermatozoa are evaluated to establish a differential count of spermatozoa morphology. Strict criteria should be applied when assessing the morphology and should include defects in head shapes, neck and midpiece, tail and presence of cytoplasmic droplets.

Spermatozoa Viability

The viability of spermatozoa is assessed by using supravital staining techniques. Dead cells with damaged cell membrane take up the stain. Unstained cells are live cells. One hundred spermatozoa are counted and the live/dead ratio is estimated. The technique helps in differentiating live but immotile spermatozoa from dead spermatozoa. The presence of a large number of viable, but nonmotile spermatozoa may indicate "Immotile Cilia Syndrome" and would require "Electron Microscopy" for further elucidation of structural defects.

Normal Semen

It is very difficult to define normal semen. Normal semen by definition is one which when inseminated into a "Normal fertile woman" produces a pregnancy in a reasonable length of time. Several expert committees have gone into this and WHO has recently recommended certain guidelines for establishing a normal semen sample.[6]
- Volume—2.0 ml or more
- Semen pH—7.2 or more
- Spermatozoa concentration—20 million/ml or more
- Total spermatozoa count—40 million per ejaculate or more
- Motility—50 percent or more motile (grade a + grade b) or 25 percent or more with fast progressive motility (Grade a) after liquefaction or within 60 minutes after ejaculation.
- Morphology—at least 30 percent of the spermatozoa should have normal morphology.
- Vitality/Viability—at least 50 percent of the spermatozoa should be viable, i.e. excluding dye-unstained spermatozoa.
- Leukocytes—less than 1 million/cc.

Abnormal Semen Picture

The most common cause of an abnormal semen picture is an artifact. These artifactual errors have already been discussed. The following errors can be noticed in the semen picture.

Color, Odor and Appearance

Reddish color of the semen, suggests the presence of blood in the semen; Hemospermia. This may indicate trauma to the genital tract, inflammation or tumor of the genital tract.

Viscosity

A highly viscous semen sample may cause impaired fertility by interfering with spermatozoa movement.[2] The precise cause of a highly viscous semen sample is not known. When the semen sample has few spermatozoa (Oligozoospermia) or no spermatozoa (azoospermia) the sample may be less viscous.

Liquefaction

Failure of a semen sample to liquefy may lead to entrapment of spermatozoa and cause infertility.[7] This could be due to impairment of prostatic function.

Semen pH

Acidity of a semen sample may indicate infections of accessory sex glands or absence of seminal vesicular secretions.

Volume

Hypospermia is the term used to indicate a very small volume semen—less than 1 ml. This could be due to:
- Bilateral ejaculatory duct obstruction
- Bilateral congenital vasal aplasia
- Inadequate erection and improper mood at semen collection
- Incomplete collection.

The term hyperspermia is used when the semen volume is above 10 ml. It is not clear whether hyperspermia is a cause of infertility. Hyperspermia, however, may affect the sperm concentration by producing "dilutional Oligozoospermia".

Aspermia is the term used to indicate absence of ejaculate. Aspermia could be due to:
- Retrograde ejaculation-where the ejaculate goes back into the bladder
- Anejaculation-where the patient has a problem with ejaculation
- Bilateral ejaculatory duct obstruction-where the ejaculate could be just a drop-secretions from the paraurethral glands.

Sperm Concentration

When the spermatozoa concentration is less than 20 million/ml the condition is referred to as oligozoospermia. It is important to understand that spermatozoa concentration varies widely even amongst normal fertile individuals. Therefore, a man should not be considered oligozoospermic until at least three samples are evaluated at an interval of 3 weeks and 3 months.

Azoospermia is a condition where the semen sample has no spermatozoa in a neat fresh sample or in a centrifuged resuspended sample.

Spermatozoa Motility

When the semen sample has less than 50 percent progressively motile spermatozoa or less than 25 percent fast progressive spermatozoa the semen sample is considered to be "asthenozoospermic". In "total asthenozoospermia" the semen has no motile spermatozoa, but vital staining shows the presence of live, but nonmotile spermatozoa.

Morphology

Presence of more than 70 percent abnormal spermatozoa in the ejaculate is considered as "Teratozoospermia".

Vitality/Viability

If the semen sample shows all dead spermatozoa the sample is considered "necrozoospermic". The *authors are* yet to see a true case of necrozoospermia. The few cases seen were all artifact due to improper collection of semen-unprepared condom collection or collection container impurities.

Computer-assisted Semen Analysis (CASA)

Several automated systems are available for evaluation of spermatozoa parameters with the aid of a computer-aided system. These systems eliminate the subjective errors inherent in the manual system of semen analysis. These are extremely useful research tools, but their superiority over conventional semen analysis done by a well trained sincere technician remains to be proven.[6]

Electron microscopy is not indicated as part of routine semen analysis. However, when the sample shows "total asthenozoosperemia" it is necessary to do an "electron microscopy" to identify "sperm tail defects".

Tests for Antisperm Antibodies

The presence of "Antisperm antibodies" can be surmised by the presence of agglutination in the semen sample. There are two types of tests to further substantiate the presence of "antisperm antibodies": the immuno bead test (IBT) and the mixed agglutination reaction (MAR) test. Antisperm antibodies have never been convincingly shown to be the cause of infertility. Treatment for antisperm antibodies remains largely empirical, mostly of unproven value with a risk of potential toxicity. These tests may, therefore, be indicated in a research laboratory, but they are of no routine clinical significance. Discrimination should be used in choosing couples to be tested for antisperm antibodies.[8]

Biochemical Tests

The only biochemical test of clinical importance is fructose estimation. Absence of fructose in the semen sample may indicate "bilateral congenital absence of the vas deferens" or "ejaculatory duct obstruction".

Computer-aided Sperm Analysis

CASA is a new entrant in the field of semen analysis. The important advantages of the system would be: (i) subjective errors in assessing a semen sample is avoided, (ii) sperm motility can be assessed quantitatively, and (iii) the instrument is capable of handling many samples without undergoing fatigue, which is a common problem in manual assessment.

Sperm Preparation

It is essential for all assisted reproductive techniques. Seminal spermatozoa are incapable of fertilizing the oocyte. Semen serves as a transport media for the spermatozoa. In vivo the spermatozoa, swim out of the seminal plasma soon after ejaculation and liquefaction. The cervical mucus serves as a filter, allowing only the motile spermatozoa to gain access to the uterine cavity. The cervical crypts serve as spermatozoa reservoir.

Principles of Sperm Preparation

Most semen samples contain both motile and non-motile spermatozoa, besides other precursors of spermatozoa and leukocytes. They also contain prostaglandins and other chemicals. Sperm preparation techniques utilize this differential motility of the cells to obtain a sample rich in motile spermatozoa, which can then be used for ARTs. Sperm preparation techniques also help in largely excluding prostaglandins, which if injected into the uterus as in "intrauterine insemination (IUI)" may produce severe uterine cramps and occasional anaphylactic reaction.

Techniques of Sperm Preparation

Many different methods exist for sperm preparation for use in assisted conception techniques. Five alternative methods are described, which authors have used with success. All of these require a physiological culture medium. The commonly used culture medium are: (i) Earle's balanced salt solution (EBSS), (ii) Ham's F-10, (iii) Phosphate buffered salt solution, (iv) Ringer lactate with pH adjusted to 7.4, and (v) the other expensive media like Medicult and Scandinavian medium are used in IVF and embryo culture than for routine sperm preparation.

Method 1

Layering (when there are > 20 million motile sperm/ml) Pipette 2 ml of sperm preparation medium into a 10 ml round-bottomed plastic tube. Gently pipette approximately 1.5 ml of semen underneath the medium (taking care not to disturb the interface formed between the semen and the medium). Tightly cap the tube and allow it to stand at room temperature for up to 2 hours or until a cloudy middle layer forms.

Pipette the resulting top and middle clouded layers into a conical test tube and spin at 200 G for 5 minutes. Remove the supernatant and re-suspend the pellet in 2 ml medium. Re-spin and discard the supernatant. Re-suspend the pellet in 1 ml gamete preparation medium. Count the number of sperms in the sample, gas with 5 percent CO_2 in air, and store at room temperature prior to dilution for lVF.

Alternatively, 2 ml of medium can be layered gently over the semen sample in its container. After 30-45 minutes, an aliquot of this layer is suspended in 1 ml of medium, and processed as above.

Method 2

Direct migration

1. Request the patient to produce semen sample into a clean plastic, sterile, nontoxic container. Allow to liquefy, for 15-30 minutes at room temperature.
   ↓
2. Sperm count 1-Volume, Density, Morphology, Motility, Progression (1-4)
   ↓
3. Very gently layer 5 ml of sperm preparation medium above the semen sample. *Do not mix* If mixing occurs the sample will have to be centrifuged.
   ↓
4. Leave for 15-45 minutes at 37°C in a heated block. Active sperm will swim-up away from the seminal plasma.
   ↓
5. Using a 1 ml syringe, draw off 0.5 ml of sperm preparation medium plus sperm. Note: ensure syringe tip goes no further than halfway into the medium.
   ↓
6. Sperm Count II.
   ↓
7. Adjust contents to 5- 20 million sperm in 1 ml.
   ↓
8. Place sample in test tube rack at room temperature until use.

   NB: Methods (1) and (2) are essentially very similar, though method (1) contains additional washing steps which will result in a "cleaner" sperm sample.

Method 3

Discontinuous 40 and 80 percent Pure Sperm Gradient

To make 80 percent gradient:

- 8 ml of Pure Sperm + 2 ml Sperm preparation medium (or 4 ml Pure Sperm + 1 ml Sperm preparation medium) and 40 percent gradient.
- 4 ml of Pure Sperm + 6 ml Sperm preparation medium (or 2 ml Pure Sperm + 3 ml Sperm preparation medium)
  - Make gradients with 2.0 - 2.5 ml of 80 percent, gently overlaid with 2.0-2.5 ml of 40 percent. Layer up to 2 ml of sample on top of the 40 percent.
  - Spin at 300 G for 20 minutes. Cells, debris and immotile/abnormal sperm accumulate at the interfaces, and the pellet should contain functionally normal sperm (Recovery of a good pellet is influenced by the amount of debris and immotile sperm which impede the travel of the good sperm. A quick 10 seconds first spin of semen or of layered pure sperm and semen to remove debris sometimes helps recovery out of a messy sample).
- Carefully collect the pellet, suspend in a 1 ml Sperm preparation medium, and assess count and motility.

Method 4

Sperm Preparation using *Wash, Spin and Swim up technique*

1. Patient produces sample into plastic-topped sterile semen sample container. Allow to liquefy, 15-30 minutes at room temperature.
   ↓
2. Sperm count 1-volume, density, morphology, motility, progression (1-4)
   ↓
3. Transfer 0.5 ml of semen to a cell culture tube and add 1.5 ml of sperm preparation medium.
   ↓
4. Mix semen with medium. Spin at 200 g for 10 minutes.
   ↓
5. Remove supernatant from pellet and discard. Gently layer a further 1 ml of sperm preparation medium above pellet.
   ↓
6. Allow sperm to swim up for 45 minutes at 37°C in heated block.
   ↓
7. Remove part of upper portion and perform second sperm count.
   ↓
8. Adjust count to 5-20 million sperm/1 ml total. Transfer labelled sample to test tube rack at room temperature.

Method 5

Swim-down technique or layering technique: When the semen sample is oligozoospermic, this technique is used. To 1 ml of culture medium the semen sample is added by layering it gently on top of the culture medium. The sample is left undisturbed for about 1 hour in an incubator or at room temperature (around 30°C). The bottom 0.5 ml is aspirated and the sample is assessed for sperm parameters. Alternatively, culture medium can be layered on the semen sample, and the top 0.5 ml aspirated after incubation.

Sperm preparation techniques are extremely useful in obtaining a motile, sperm rich sample devoid of seminal plasma for use in routine ARTS.

REFERENCES

1. Pandiyan N (Ed): Handbook of Andrology. TR Publications: Chennai, 1999.
2. Jequier AM, Crich JP: Semen Analysis: A Practical Guide. Blackwell Scientific publications: Oxford, 1986.
3. Obstetrics and Gynecology for the Postgraduates: Male Infertility 1:282, N Pandiyan,; Ratnam SS, K Bhasker Rao, Arulkumaran S (Eds): 1999.
4. Lundquest F: Aspects of the biochemistry of human semen. Acta Physiologica Scandinavica 1949; 19(Suppl66):7-105.
5. WHO laboratory Manual for the Examination of Human Semen and Sperm-Cervical Mucus Interaction 3rd edn. Cambridge University Press, 1992
6. WHO Laboratory Manual for the Examination of Human Semen and Sperm-Cervical Mucus Interaction 4th edn. Cambridge University Press, 1999.
7. Amelar RD: Coagulation, liquefaction and viscosity of human semen. J Urol 1962;87:187-90.
8. Marshburn PB, Kutteh WH: The role of antisperm antibodies in infertility. Fertil Steril 61(5):799-811.

MALE INFERTILITY—CURRENT TRENDS IN THE MANAGEMENT OF AZOOSPERMIA AND OLIGOASTHENOTERATOZOOSPERMIA

A Rajasekaran, R Jayaganesh

INTRODUCTION

"For decades, various therapies have been proposed to improve sperm parameters in cases of male factor infertility. Administration of antiestrogens and androgens have been found to be ineffective. No peer-review data are available to demonstrate the benefit of the use of intra-uterine insemination or the correction of varicocele. The conventional treatment for male factor infertility has little value and has been revised and abandoned."

Styptoe and Edwards (1978) of Bourn Hall, Cambridge made history producing the first test tube baby (*In vitro* Fertilization and embryo transfer) resulting in the birth of Louis Brown. Eventhough this epoch making discovery was largely beneficial for tubal factor infertility in the female it could not be effectively utilized in male factor infertility. To be successful at least 500,000 sperms are required for IVF and ET. In severe male factor infertility with very few and/or poorly motile sperms with increased number of sperm abnormalities IVF has not proved to be successful. The Belgium group Palermo and Van Steirteghem (1992) achieved pregnancy utilizing a micro-manipulation technique, intracytoplasmic sperm injection ICSI.

Intracytoplasmic sperm injection (ICSI) has been major break through in the 'reproductive revolution'. The main advantages are that it offers couples the possibility of having a child that is genetically related to both partners, even if the male is suffering from severe subfertility. Until recently the alternatives available for these couples were donor insemination or adoption.

Intracytoplasmic sperm injection (ICSI) is an effective treatment even for cases of extreme oligoasthenoteratozoospermia. It has to be considered as the method of choice and should replace ineffective conventional therapies (Devroey P *et al* 1998). "There no longer seems to be any category of male factor infertility that cannot be treated with ICSI. Even for men with azoospermia caused either by obstruction or by germinal failure, ICSI may be performed successfully. Of all the factors studied, the only factor that seems to matter (as long as spermatozoa are retrieved) is the age of the wife and her ovarian reserve" (Silber 1998). ICSI has changed the practice of andrology enabling men previously thought to be irreversibly infertile the chance to initiate their own biological pregnancy. ICSI is actually the assisted fertilization technique with the highest incidence of pregnancies and "take home babies" (Garcea 1998). The leading European ICSI group in Belgium achieved a transfer rate of 92 per cent after 2820 consecutive treatment cycles, and a pregnancy rate of 34 per cent per transfer (Van Steirteghem *et al*, 1995).

INDICATIONS FOR ICSI IN MALE INFERTILITY

Absolute Indications

1. Patients with immotile cilia syndrome.
2. Cases where nonejaculated samples (Sperms aspirated from the epididymis or testis) are used.
3. Globozoospermia—in acrosome deficient sperms successful pregnancy has been reported with ICSI (Ludin *et al* 1994).
4. Poor fertilization with previous IVF cycles.
5. Frozen-thawed sperms with poor survival.

The main advantage of ICSI is that the outcome is not directly related to either number of sperms, their motility or their morphology.

ABNORMAL SPERM PARAMETERS AND ICSI

Necrozoospermia

Occasionally patients may present with 100 per cent immotile sperms. The infection, e.g. *E. coli* chronic prostatitis or immobilizing antisperm antibodies have been attributed as the possible factors. Absolute necrozoospermia, a condition in which all sperms are dead has to be distinguished from conditions such as axonemel defects ('immotile cilia syndrome'). Nonviability of the sperms rather than immotility affects fertilization.

Oligoasthenoteratozoospermia

The cause of oligoasthenoteratozoospermia (OAT syndrome) is still unknown. As regards teratozoospermia, a high risk of fertilization failure (11/18 patients) after IVF (76% for ICSI against 15% for IVF) has been reported (PAYNE *et al* 1994). Asthenozoospermia is defined as a very low proportion of rapid progressively motile spermatozoa of less than 5 per cent in the fresh sample. In a controlled comparison study between conventional IVF and ICSI, it was concluded that a low rate of rapid progressive sperm motility is associated with a high rate of complete fertilization failures after conventional IVF (Verhe Yen *et al* 1999).

Azoospermia vs Aspermia

Aspermia refers to the absence of ejaculation and azoospermia, the absence of sperms or its precursors in the ejaculate.

Causes of Aspermia

- Anejaculation due to spasm (functional)
- Obstruction to ejaculatory ducts
- Retrograde ejaculation
  For purpose of ICSI, the sperms could be obtained from any of the following sources in case of aspermia
- Nocturnal emissions
- Vibratory/electroejaculatory sample
- Prostatic massage
- Retrograde ejaculation—retrieval of sperms from bladder
- Transrectal aspiration from dilated seminal vesicle/seminal vesicle cyst.

Azoospermia (Obstructive)

- Postinfective causes affecting cauda or body of the epididymis—smallpox/tuberculosis/non-specific infections

- Postsurgical obstruction—hydrocoele/inguinal hernia repair/vasectomy
- Congenital bilateral absence of vas/blind ending vas/spermatocele
- Ejaculatory duct obstructions.

Azoospermia (Nonobstructive)

Defective or incomplete or absent spermatogenesis resulting in absence of sperms or its precursors. The following histopathological conditions could be identified.
- Sertoli cell only syndrome (SCOS)/germ cell aplasia
- Maturation arrest
- Hypospermatogenesis
- Fibrosis and atrophy
- Postmumps orchits
- Cryptorchidism
- Torsion testis
- Chronic epididymoorchitis
- Surgical implantation of testis into thigh (filarial)
- Postchemotherapy.
  1. The clinical parameters are unable to predict which men with nonobstructive azoospermia will have sperms retrieved by TESE.
  2. Patients should not be excluded for TESE based on FSH level, age and prior histopathological pattern or cytology results.

Surgery in Obstructive Azoospermia

- Microsurgical vasovasal anastomosis (VVA)
- Microsurgical vasoepididymal anastomosis—VEA— (side to side/vasotubular)
- TUR of ejaculatory duct orifice
- Alloplastic spermatocele (a discarded procedure).

Microsurgical Vasovasal anastomosis The success depends upon the time interval between vasectomy and VVA, and the site and extent of the segment excised. The microsurgical two-layered mucosa to mucosa anastomosis ensures proper approximation, better continuity and prevents fibrosis.

Micro VVA Results (Goldstein 1998)
Patency sperm appearance more than 80 per cent
Pregnancy (in 2 yrs)— 63 per cent.

Microsurgical vasoepididymal anastomosis (Micro VEA) The cases with chronic epididymitis, tuberculous epididymitis and scarred epididymis are not suitable for surgical correction.

Bilateral congenital absence of vas is excluded from VEA for obvious reasons. There remains only a small group of patients for VEA, *viz* obstructions limited to cauda epididymis sparing the caput and body of the epididymis.

> *Results* (Schelegal and Goldstein, 1993)
> *Patency*—Sperm appearance in ejaculate 70 per cent
> *Pregnancy*—43 per cent.

Vasotubular anastomosis establishes precise approximation between the mucosa of the vas lumen to the opened-out dilated epididymal tubules. Excellent microsurgical expertise is necessary for technical success. In cases where micro-VEA fails, reoperation on the scarred epididymis is often unsuccessful. Following VEA spontaneous closure of communication can also occur. Collection of epididymal fluid and cryo-preservation of sperms at the time of VEA is beneficial for subsequent use for ICSI.

Micro-VEA in the Era of ICSI

Surgery if successful provides sperms for natural conception or Intrauterine insemination (IUI). In our country the cost of VEA is much less than for ICSI. ICSI has the disadvantage of hormonal manipulation and related problems in the female. For VEA, to be successful, proper case selection and excellent microsurgical skill and facilities should be available. If VEA fails retrieval of sperms from epididymis or testis could be made use of for ICSI during subsequent cycles.

VASOGRAPHY: IS IT ALWAYS NECESSARY?

In a classical case of normal sized testes, distended epididymis and presence of vas, the vasography is not necessary. In cases where obstructions are suspected, *viz.* inguinal hernia surgery or after undescended testes surgery the site of obstruction could be assessed by vasography. Blind injection of contrast into the vas may produce intravasation and fibrosis. Using the operating microscope, partial division of the vas and injection of non-ionic contrast and approxi-

mation of cut ends by resuturing is the preferred method.

ICSI IN AZOOSPERMIA

In couples in whom the male is absolutely azoospermic, it is possible to get biological pregnancy using his own sperms. Earlier to the invention of ICSI except for surgical reconstruction in obstructive azoospermia the alternatives available in other cases were only adoption or donor sperm insemination. ICSI has revolutionalised the treatment of male infertility to such an extent that it can be carried out even in cases of failed reconstruction and in cases of non-obstructive azoospermia. The first successful attempts at sperm aspiration combined with ICSI were reported by Silber *et al*, and Tournaye *et al* 1994. ICSI with aspirated epididymal spermatozoa in men with congenital absence of the vas deferens (CAVD) yielded a pregnancy rate of 47 per cent and a delivery rate of 33 percent. Furthermore, there was no difference in pregnancy rate with epididymal spermatozoa retrieved for any cause of obstruction, whether it was failed vasoepididymostomy, CAVD, or simply irreparable obstruction.

Soon after the MESA-ICSI procedure was developed in 1994, it was discovered that testicular spermatozoa could fertilize as efficiently as ejaculated spermatozoa and also result in normal pregnancies. The development of TESE meant that even patients with zero motility of the epididymal spermatozoa or of ejaculated spermatozoa, or even men with no epididymis could still have their own genetic child, so long as there was normal spermatogenesis.

In the majority of patients with testicular failure (caused either by maturation arrest, Sertoli cell only syndrome, cryptorchid testicular atrophy, post-chemotherapy azoospermia, or even Klinefelters syndrome), very tiny number of spermatozoa or spermatids can usually be extracted from extensive biopsies of the testicle and utilized for ICSI (Devroey *et al* 1995, Silber, 1995).

The indications for ICSI with epididymal sperms are listed below:

• Congenital bilateral absence of vas deferens

- Failed vasoepididymostomy
- Failed vasectomy reversal
- Young syndrome
- Obstruction of both ejaculatory ducts
- Anejaculation due to spinal cord injury.

The indications for ICSI with testicular sperm are:

- Impossibility of retrieving motile epididymal spermatozoa
- Hypospermatogenesis
- Partial germ-cell aplasia (Sertoli-cell-only syndrome)
- Incomplete maturation arrest
- Klinefelter syndrome.

SPERM RETRIEVAL METHODS FOR ICSI

Which method is to be preferred:
- From the epididymis
  1. Percutaneous epididymal sperm aspiration (PESA)
  2. Microepididymal sperm aspiration (MESA)
- From the testis
  1. Fine-needle aspiration cytology (TEFNA)
  2. Testicular sperm extraction (TESE)— multiple tiny incisions, open biopsy.

Percutaneous epididymal sperm aspiration (PESA): In case of obstructions to epididymis or vas, local injection of 1 percent lignocaine is given along the side of the vas near the external ring. By stabilizing the epididymis between the index finger, thumb and forefinger a 23-gauge butterfly needle is inserted and connected to 20 ml aspirating syringe. Opalescent fluid will be seen to enter the tubing when the tip of the needle is moved in and out. The fluid is flushed into the culture medium and after processing the sample with density gradient centrifugation or swim up depending on the quality of sperms, they are used for ICSI.

This is a quick and simple method and can easily be preformed on an outpatient basis. In a series of 181 PESA-ICSI cycles epididymal spermatozoa were recovered in 151 cycles (83%). The fertilization rate was 54.7 per cent and ongoing pregnancy rate 34 per cent per ICSI cycle (Meniru 1998). The main criticism of the PESA technique is that blind percutaneous puncture may cause inadvertent damage to the fine epididymal structures and produce uncontrolled bleeding, causing postinterventional fibrosis.

Micro epididymal sperm aspiration (MESA): It requires surgical expertise to identify the dilated epididymal tubule under the operating microscope and for selectively cannulating the tubule; a small "window" opening is adequate to expose the epididymis. If no fluid is found or if no sperms are present in the fluid, small bits of testicular tissue could be obtained by rotating the testis.

This procedure is invasive which requires basic knowledge of epididymal anatomy and of microsurgical techniques. Use of an operating microscope is preferable. The procedure causes minimal fibrosis and less risk of creating obstructions to epididymal tubule. Microsurgical epididymal sperm aspiration (MESA) is the preferred method when performed concomitantly with a vasoepididymostomy. The number of sperms retrieved is high, which facilitates cryopreservation (Devroey et al 1995). In a retrospective analysis on the use of epididymal spermatozoa for ICSI no difference was seen in fertilization clinical pregnancy rate either with fresh or frozen-thawed epididymal spermatozoa (Tournaye et al 1999).

From the Testis

Fine needle aspiration cytology (TEFNA): This procedure would be performed using 21-gauge needle or 19-gauge needle with local anesthesia. In patients with normal spermatogenesis a sperm recovery rate of 96 per cent may be obtained. This is a minimally invasive procedure, which could be used for cytological assessment.

The Testicular Sperm Extraction (TESE)

The use of testicular sperm injection for ICSI was first introduced for obstructive azoospermia in 1992 (Craft et al 1993) and subsequently for nonobstructive azoospermia (Silber et al 1995). Testicular sperm extraction (TESE) combined with ICSI is becoming the first line of treatment in nonobstructive azoospermia. In cases of azoospermia with defective spermiogenesis, open testicular biopsy is found to be more effective than needle biopsy. However, to enhance the diagnostic accuracy multiple sites were necessary for TESE.

Testicular sperm extraction (TESE) and ICSI may be the sole-treatment available in cases of non-obstructive azoospermia. In patients with normal spermatogenesis TESE gives 100 per cent recovery rate (Tourney *et al* 1996a). In patients with 47, XXY Klinefelter syndrome, spermatozoa may be recovered and the first babies born were reported recently. (Tourney *et al* 1996b). In order to minimise tissue damage when taking multiple excisional biopsies, small tissue samples may be taken using a microsurgical approach as proposed by Schlegel (1999). After opening the tunica albuginea, under magnification the more distended seminiferous tubules may be selected for micro-excision. The major advantage of the open approach is the possibility of freezing testicular tissue and of performing ICSI whenever the final histopathology shows spermatozoa. The Cryopreservation of testicular spermatozoa may prevent repeat surgery when pregnancy does not occur after ICSI.

Microdissection Testicular Sperm Extraction (Modified TESE)

To minimise the risks of inflammatory changes and devascularization and for better sperm retrieval, microdissection TESE has been advocated (Schlegel 1999).

Even though time consuming, the subtunical vessels were identified under surgical microscope and avoided. The testicular tissues were observed for morphologically normal tubules, small samples taken from most dilated tubules and observed for the presence of spermatozoa. In a study of 116 azoospermic patients with different etiology, sperm recovery rate of 62/116 (53%) reported (Medhat Amer *et al* 2000).

IVF AND ICSI

In a recent review, the ESHRE task force on ICSI (Tarlatzis and Bili 1998) reported that in 1995 a total of 23,932 ICSI cycles were performed worldwide by 101 centers. The procedure seems to be safe, as the incidence of major and minor congenital malformations in the group of children born after ICSI is similar to those reported for *in vitro* fertilization (IVF) or in the general population.

In contrast to IVF where there is natural selection of sperms and oocytes, ICSI involves an invasive procedure using a sperm chosen on morphological criteria. Hence, doubts were raised on the quality of zygotes and subsequent development with ICSI in contrast to IVF. The concerns raised in ICSI were, the possibility of injection of abnormal sperm which can affect the oocyte, damage to cytoplasma structures and subsequent impairment on embryonic development. For the majority of patients, ICSI can be performed with spermatozoa obtained from the ejaculate.

The risk of failure of fertilization after conventional IVF with normospermia semen has been a frustrating experience. Unexplained lack of fertilization after IVF is observed in about 8 per cent of the cycles. Total failure of fertilization after IVF as well as very low fertilization rates are repetitive phenomena indicating a possible underlying, undiagnosed sperm-oocyte pathology (Calderon *et al* 1995, Roest *et al* 1998). After ICSI, fertilization failures rarely occur (2.8%). A treatment combining IVF and ICSI on sibling oocytes has therefore been advised in order to avoid or reduce the proportion of failed fertilization cycles. For patients with borderline semen ICSI has shown a better performance than conventional IVF in terms of fertilization rate and absence of fertilization failure. (Aboulghar *et al* 1995, 1996; Calderon *et al* 1995).

FACTORS INFLUENCING ICSI RESULTS

ICSI results are influenced by:

Intrinsic changes in oocytes fragmentation of DNA in sperm.

Maternal age and ovarian reserve has no effect on fertilization and cleavage of embryos, but affects embryo implantation, pregnancy and delivery rates (Silber, 1997).

Age

• Under 20s—46 percent live deliveries/cycle
• Under 30-36—34 percent live deliveries/cycle

• Under 37-39—13 percent live deliveries/cycle
• More than 40—4 percent live deliveries/cycle.

Congenital Malformations in Children Born after ICSI

More than 20,000 children have been born worldwide with the use of ICSI (De Mouzon, 1997). The primary concern has been whether this spermatozoa with impaired motility and morphology in the seminal fluid or immature spermatozoa derived from epididymis and testis would result in genetic aberrations and malformations in the children. In a study of 1139 infants the total no. of identified anomalies was 87 (7.6%) of which 40 were minor. The increased rate of congenital malformations was attributed to high rate of multiple works. The only specific malformation noted with ICSI was Hypospadias which may be related to Paternal subfertility (UB Wennerholm *et al* 2000).

"There appears to be some risk of transmitted chromosomal and aberration of *de novo,* mainly sex chromosomal aberrations, transmitting infertility problems to the offspring." The couple may be reassured that until now there seems to be no higher incidence of congenital malformations in the child using epididymal or testicular sperms.

Influence of Antisperm Antibodies on ICSI

Antisperm antibodies have no influence on ICSI outcome. The motile (living) sperm is the single most important criteria for success. In ICSI the natural selection of sperm is not there. We are not able to distinguish between good and poor quality sperm other than by crude assessment of gross morphology and nuclear decondensation.

Effects of male factor in repeated spontaneous abortion (6.5–21%) may be attributed to the following factors. Chromosomal, anatomic, hormonal, immunological, unexplained. The sperm characteristics are likely to influence the quality of conception.

Round Spermatids for ICSI

Wherever there are early round spermatids there will also be elongated mature spermatids with a tail (Silber *et al* 1996). If the round cells are spermatids then a better search would have revealed the presence of mature sperms.

386 oocytes retrieved—140 (2PN) 36 per cent, 98 embryos transferred 2. (2%) implantation and ongoing pregnancies

CONCLUSION

In conclusion, ICSI has revolutionized the management of male infertility during the past decade.

• ICSI may only be used when the male's sperm function is impaired to such an extent that regular IVF is not a genuine option.
• There should be careful selection of spermatozoa to be injected. The immotile sperms and sperms with severe morphological abnormalities should not be used.
• Couples applying for ICSI should be provided with detailed information about the known and theoretical risks of the treatment. Couples should be able to balance the respective pros and cons of ICSI and the available alternatives, particularly DI. Consent should be obtained individually.
    1. In view of the risk of transmitting genetic abnormalities, an extensive family history should be drawn up and adequate counselling should be provided.
    2. Relevant preconception genetic testing, in particular karyotyping, of the males should be a precondition of all ICSI treatments.
    3. The option of prenatal diagnosis should be offered to all women who become pregnant as a result of ICSI.

FURTHER READINGS

1. Aboulghar MA, Mansour RT, Serourgi et al. The role of intracytoplasmic sperm injection and conventional in vitro fertilization for sibling oocytes in cases of unexplained infertility and borderline semen. J Assist Reprod Genet 1986;13:38-42.
2. Aboulghar MA, Mansour RT, Serourgi, Amin YM. The role of intracytoplasmic sperm injection (ICSI) in the treatment of patients with boderline semen. Hum Repro 1995;10:2839.
3. Calderon G, Belili Aran B et al. Intracytoplasmic sperm injection versus conventional in vitro fertilization. First Results Hum Reproduction 1995;10:2835-39.
4. Claudio A, Benadiva MD, John Nulsen MD, Linda Siano MS et al. Intracytoplasmic sperm injection overcomes previous fertilization failure with conventional in vitro fertilization 1998.
5. Craft I, Tsirigotis M, Courtauld E, Farrer-Brown G. Testicular needle aspiration as an alternative to biopsy

for the assessment of spermatozoa. Hum Reprod 1997;12:1484-87.

6. Craft I, Bennetv Nigholson. Fertilising ability of testicular spermatozoa. Lancet 1993;342-864.

7. De Mouzon J, Lancaster P. World collabrative report on in vitro fertilization: Preliminary data for 1995. J Assist Rerprod Genet 1997;14(Supple):251-65.

8. Devroey P, Liu J, Nagy Z et al. Normal fertilization of human occytes after testicular sperm extraction and intracytoplasmic sperm injection. Fertil, Steril 1994;62:639-41.

9. Devroey P, Liu J, Nagy Z et al. Ongoing pregnancies and birth after intracytoplasmic sperm injection with frozen-thawed epididymal spermatozoa. Hum Reprod 1995;12:903-06.

10. Gu Salom, M Romero, J Minguezy et al. Pregnancies after ICSI with cryopreserved testicular spermatozoa. Hum Reprod 1996;11:1309-13.

11. Hasani SAL, Demirel LC et al. Pregnancies allowed after frozen, thawed pronuclear oocytes obtained by intracytoplamic injection with spermatozoa extracted form frozen thawed testicular tissues from non-obstructive azoospermia men. Hum Reprod 1999;14: 2031-35.

12. Iruine DS. Epidemiology and etiology of the male infertility. Hum Reprod 1998;13(Suppl):33-44.

13. Jezer D, Knuth JA, Schulzeu. Successful TESE inspite of high serum FSH and azoospermia-correlation between testicular morphology TESE results. Semen analysis and serum hormone values in 103 infertile men. Hum Reprod 1998;13:1230-34.

14. Kaan Osmanagaglu, Herman Tournaye et al. Cumulative delivery rates after intracytoplasmic sperm injection 5 year follow up of 498 patients. Hum Reprod 14: 2651-55, Fert Steril 1999;72:1041-44.

15. Liv J, Nagy ZP et al. Analysis of 76 total fertilization failure cycles out of 2732 intracytoplasmic sperm injection cycles. Hum Reprod 1995;10:2630-36.

16. Medhat Amer, Ahamed Ateyah et al. Prospective cooperative study between microsurgical and conventional testicular sperm extraction in non obstructive azoospermia: Follow up by serial ultrasound examinations. Hum Reprod 2000;15:653-56.

17. Mineru G, Bortha S, Podisindly B et al. ICSI: with epididymal sperm-percutaneous retrieval. In Ne Frontier, Filicori M (Eds): Proceedings of the Symposium: Treatment of Infertility. Boca Raton: Florida, 1998;22-24:363-74.

18. Oates RD, Mulhall, J Burgessc, et al. Fertilization and pregnancy using intentionally cryopreserved testicular tissue as sperm source for ICSI in 10 litre non-obstructive azoospermia. Hum Reprod 1997;12:734-39.

19. P Devroey P, M Vandervorst, P Nagy, A Van Steirteghem et al. Do we treat the male or his gamete? Hum Reprod 1998;13(S1):178-85.

20. Palermo G, Joris H, Devroey P et al. Pregnancies after intracytoplasmic injection of single spermatozoon into an oocyte. Lancet 1992;340:17-18.

21. Payne D, Fiarerty SP, Jefery R et al. Successful treatment of severe male factor infertility in 100 consecutive cycles using intracytoplasmic sperm injection. Hum Reprod 1994;9:2051-57.

22. Robert Fisher. Treatment of infertility new frontiers. 1998;403-09.

23. Roest J, Van Heusden AM, Zeilmaker GH, Verhoeff A. Treatment policy after poor fertilization in first IVF cycle. J Asst Reproduction Genet 1998;15:18-21.

24. Silber S. Intracytoplasmic sperm injection today: a personal review. Hum Reprod 1998;13(Suppl 1):208-17.

25. Schlegel, Su LM. Physiological consequences of testicular sperm extraction. Hum Reprod 1997;12:1688-92.

26. Schlegel PN, Godlstein M. Microsurgical vasoepididymostomy. Refinements and results. J Uro 1, 1993;1 50:1165-68.

27. Schlegel PN. Testicular sperm extraction. Micro dissection improves sperm yield with minimal tissue excision. Hum Reprod 1999;14:131-35.

28. Silber S, Van Steirteghem AC, Liu J et al. High fertilization and pregnancy rates after intracytoplasmic sperm injection with spermatozoa obtained from testicle biopsy. Hum Reprod 1995;10:148-52.

29. Silber S, Van Steirteghem AC, Liu J et al. Normal pregnancies resulting from testicular sperm extraction and intracytoplasmic sperm injection for azoospermia due to maturation arrest. Fertil Steril 1996;1:110-17.

30. Stanwell-Smith RE, Hendry WF. The progress of Male subfertility—a survey of 1025 men referred to a fertility clinic. Br J Urol 1984;56:422-28.

31. Tarlatzis BC, Bili H. Survey on intracytoplasmic sperm injection report from the ESHRE ICSI task force. Hum Reprod 1998;13(Supp):165-77.

32. Tournaye H, Camus M, Vandervorst M et al. Sperm retrieval for ICSI. Int J Androl 1997b;20,S3,69-73.

33. Tournaye H, Liu J, Nagy Z et al. Correlation between testicular histology and outcome after intracytoplasmic sperm injection using testicular sperm. Hum Reprod 1996a;11:127-32.

34. Tournaye H, Meedad T, Silber S et al. No differences in outcome after intracytoplasmic sperm injection with fresh or frozen-thawed epididymal spermatozoa. Hum Reprod 1999;14:90-96.

35. Tournaye H, Staessen C, Liebaers I et al. Testicular sperm recovery in 47, XXY Klinefelter patients. Hum Reprod 1996b;11:1164-649.

36. UB Wennerholm, Bergh1, L Hamberger 1, K Ludin1, L Nilsson1, M Wikland3 and B Käällén 2. Hum Reprod 2000;15(4):944-48.

37. Van Steirteghem A, Nagy P, Joris H et al. The development of intracytoplasmic injection. Hum Reprod 1996;11(Suppl):59-72.

38. Verheyen G, Tournaye Staessen C, De Vos A et al. Hum Reprod 1999;14:2313-19.

SEXUAL DYSFUNCTION IN MALE INFERTILITY

SS Vasan

INTRODUCTION

In India approximately 15 per cent of couples are unable to initiate a pregnancy without some form of assistance or therapy and in this, the male factor contributing to infertility is around 50 per cent. These patients are said to be "primarily infertile". In approximately 1 percent of these couples there are factors other than seminal abnormalities, which prevent conception. It is imperative that these groups of patients are properly diagnosed and treated to enable them to achieve conception.

The use of standard techniques for evaluating medical problems in general, such as complete history, physical examination, and laboratory tests which are beyond the scope of this chapter, are essential for this purpose. Some of the uncommon problems seen in males leading to infertility are:

- Nonconsummation of marriage
- Ejaculatory disturbances.

Treatment of these problems entails proper understanding of the physiology of erection and ejaculation. The majority of contemporary knowledge on the physiology of erection has been assembled during the past 30 years. It consists of basic biological response and mechanics of pelvic floor muscles and sphincters during erection and ejaculation.

BIOLOGICAL BASIS OF SEXUAL RESPONSE

The stimuli from a receptive female and/or sexual act itself leads to the release of dopamine (DA) in at least three integrative hubs. The nigrostriatal system promotes somatomotor activity, the mesolimbic system subserves numerous types of motivation; and the medial preoptic area (MPOA) focuses the motivation onto specific sexual targets, increases sexual rate and efficiency, and coordi-nates genital reflexes. The previous (but not neces-sarily concurrent) presence of testosterone is permissive for DA release in the MPOA, both during basal conditions and in response to a female. One means by which testosterone may increase DA release is by upregulating nitric oxide synthase, which produces nitric oxide, which in turn increases DA release. Finally, while DA is facilitative to sexual activity, 5-HT (5 hydroxy tryptamine) is generally inhibitory. 5-HT is released in the LHA (lateral hypothalamic area), but not in the MPOA, at the time of ejaculation. Thus, reciprocal changes in DA and 5-HT release in different areas of the brain may promote sexual activity and sexual satiety, respectively. Other factors such as medication, alcohol and other health problems, can modify the biological impact of hormones on libido.

As to mediators in the cavernosal level acetylcholine and nitric oxide (NO) released from the endothelium are involved along with noradrenaline, VIP (vasoactive intestinal polypeptide), CGRP (calcitonin gene-related peptide) and prostaglandins. Nitric oxide and VIP play the most important roles in the phase of erection. Erection takes the following course (simplified): erotogenic stimuli lead to the stimulation of the parasympathetic nerve→ vasodilating substances are released→the sinusoids are filled with blood (tumescence stage)→the venoocclusive mechanism starts to work→thus complete erection occurs. Then the contractions of the musculature of the perineum compress the proximal portions of the corpora cavernosa: this leads to rigid erection. Detume-scence (which occurs as a rule after ejaculation) is due to released noradrenaline (active stage) and the reduced tonus of the smooth muscles of the blood vessels (released endothelin and neuropeptide Y).

PELVIC FLOOR MUSCLES AND SPHINCTERS DURING ERECTION AND EJACULATION

The pelvic floor muscles involved in maintaining an erection consists of puborectalis (PR), levator ani (LA) and external anal (EAS) and urethral sphincters (EUS). The increased PR activity might express the prostatic secretions into the posterior urethra. Levator ani contraction seems to elevate the prostate and partially straightens the prostato-membraneous urethral kink that might occur during erection. The EAS and EUS contractions are believed to abort the urge to defecate or urinate and prevent leak of feces, flatus, or urine during coitus. The rhythmic EUS contraction at ejaculation might act as a "suction ejection pump," sucking the genital fluid into the posterior urethra, while being relaxed and ejecting it into the bulbous urethra upon contraction.

NONCONSUMMATION OF MARRIAGE

The main factor associated with an unconsummated marriage is the intense social pressure to accomplish hasty sexual activity with an unfamiliar woman (some men having had no social contact with their new bride) and in the presence of relatives waiting nearby for evidence of the bride's virginity and confirmation of sexual act. This initial problem will then be further compounded with resultant erectile failure caused by anxiety about sexual performance. In addition to psychological causes and a lack of sexual education, the social circumstances in which partners are obliged to initiate and complete the sexual act are important factors in the etiology of a nonconsummated marriage.

Inability to consummate the marriage is caused by:
• Premature ejaculation in 23 percent
• Erectile dysfunction in 61 percent
• Combination of factors in 16 percent.

Erectile dysfunction in some form or other may contribute to the problem. It is the clinician's obligation to establish the etiology of impotence, namely end organ vascular failure versus neurologic dysfunction versus psychosexual dysfunction, classify the severity of that dysfunction, and select a therapy that is not only acceptable to the patient but also addresses his pathology. The most commonly utilized diagnostic tests for erectile dysfunction are as follows:

Combined injection and stimulation test or Pharmaco testing It consists of intracavernous injection and visual rating of the subsequent erection. It is simple, minimally invasive, and performed without monitoring equipment. Hemodynamic investigations suggest that a positive injection test is associated with normal venoocclusion, but not necessarily with normal arterial function. When the penile response to pharmacotesting is suboptimal or equivocal, diagnostic testing with duplex Doppler assessment should be performed.

Nocturnal penile tumescence (NPT) NPT to measure man's nocturnal erections have been measured by each of the following methods: stamp test, snap gauges, strain gauges, NPTR (Rigiscan, Osborn Medical Systems), and sleep lab NPTR. Normal nocturnal penile tumescence and rigidity (NPTR) depends on both the integrity of the corticospinal efferents to the penis and vascular responsiveness of the penile tissues to those nerve signals. When nocturnal erections are of appropriate duration and strength, the central and peripheral neuroeffectors and intra-corporal regulators of penile hemodynamics are intact. Unfortunately, abnormal NPTR is of little value in determining the etiology or classifying the severity of vascular impotence, the most prevalent kind of end organ failure.

Blood flow studies Insufficient penile blood flow and inefficient corporal veno-occlusion is implicated in up to 30 per cent of patients, and in their evaluation numerous diagnostic tests have been employed to evaluate penile hemodynamics. The more popular ones are color duplex doppler ultrasound, selective internal pudendal pharmacoangiography, and dynamic infusion cavernosometry/cavernosography. Duplex ultrasound, which measures penile blood flow, provides an objective, minimally invasive evaluation of arterial pattern in a suboptimal/equivocal erectile response.

The diagnosis and demonstration of venous leakage requires complete smooth muscle relaxation. Veno-occlusive dysfunction is associated with poorly sustained erections; this pathology has traditionally been evaluated with dynamic infusion cavernosometry and cavernosography. DICC is an invasive test, and is now primarily reserved for patients considering the option of vascular reconstructive procedure.

Neurological assessment The sacral reflex arc of erection consists of somatosensory afferents via the dorsal and pudendal nerves and autonomic efferents via the pelvic and cavernous nerves. These afferents have been measured indirectly by somatosensory evoked potentials (SSEP) and bulbocavernosus reflex (BCR) latency. These at present are used in research situations, as it does not principally aid in patient management.

Penile EMGs (CC-EMG) have been used to measure corpora cavernosal smooth muscle electrical activity and is far from standardized. Computer-assisted interpretations of penile electrical potentials may eventually differentiate afferent nerve pathologies so long inferred in diabetes, spinal cord injury and following radical pelvic surgery.

Erectile dysfunction evaluation is based on clinical judgement and not all these tests may be necessary for evaluation. Proper evaluation of nonconsummation will aid in treatment planning. Various options in management are psychotherapy, sexual education, oral medications (sildenafil citrate), intracavernosal injection agents and specific treatment directed for organic cause. Most cases respond to medications and counseling with surgical option being reserved for resistant organic causes.

EJACULATORY DISTURBANCES

The most widely accepted theory to explain ejaculation consists of two phases (Hermabessiere S, 1999):

- A phase of accumulation of the various constituents of semen inside the prostatic urethra
- A phase of expulsion with opening of the striated sphincter, while the smooth sphincter of the bladder neck remains closed

These events are mediated by the sympathetic nervous system via T_{10}-L_3 level preganglionic fibers. Ejaculation is the forceful expulsion of semen from the posterior urethra through the urethral meatus in an antegrade fashion. This event is secondary to the rhythmic contraction of periurethral and pelvic floor smooth muscles, mediated by parasympathetic ($S_{2,3,4}$) outflow and somatic efferents, and occurs in conjunction with closure of the bladder neck, which is sympathetically stimulated.

Ejaculatory disorders include
- Retrograde ejaculation
- Anejaculation
- Premature ejaculation
- Deficient or retarded ejaculation.

On the basis of the history and simple investigations, the various disorders are relatively easy to differentiate. History taking should include information about the ability to ejaculate, including nocturnal emission and the ability to experience an orgasm.

Premature Ejaculation

Deficiency in ejaculation appears to be caused by sympathetic, motor pudendal or suprasacral lesion. An altered perception of genital sensations due to a lesion in the afferent pudendal pathway appears to be present in premature ejaculation (MetzME, 1997).

It is proposed that there are two basic kinds of premature ejaculation:
- Biogenic and
- Psychogenic

The traditional assumption among sex therapists is that premature ejaculation is almost universally caused by psychological features and is easily treated with sex therapy behavioral techniques. This is questionable as results from systematic investigations have shown that behavioral treatments for premature ejaculation remain beneficial to only a minority of men three years after treatment ends, suggesting that this male dysfunction is difficult to treat effectively with behavioral techniques.

With proper assessment and identification a specific diagnosis of premature ejaculation can be reached and accurate treatment designed to address the particular type of disorder with long-term benefits can be achieved.

Commonly used medications in this disorder are Fluoxetine, Paroxetine and Clomipramine either singly or in combination. Recently there has been emphasis on pelvic floor rehabilitation as a form of treatment for this disorder.

Retrograde Ejaculation

Retrograde ejaculation is an uncommon cause of male infertility. Antegrade ejaculation requires intact anatomy and innervation of the bladder neck. Retrograde ejaculation can be defined as the escape of seminal fluid from the posterior urethra, into the bladder. The etiology may be anatomic, neurogenic, pharmacologic, or idiopathic. Anatomic causes include prostatectomy (open or transurethral) or bladder neck surgeries (Y-V plasty, transurethral incision of the bladder neck). Neurogenic causes include spinal cord injury, retroperitoneal surgery, and diabetes mellitus. Pharmacologic agents implicated in causing retrograde ejaculation include neuroleptics, tricyclic antidepressants, alpha-blockers used in the treatment of prostatism and certain anti-hypertensives. Also congenital and idiopathic causes have been described (Glander HJ, 1998).

It should be suspected in any case of persistent low volume ejaculate (< 1. 5 ml), absent ejaculate or rarely azoospermia. It can easily be differentiated from partial ejaculatory obstruction by transrectal ultrasound.

Investigation which Aid in the Diagnosis

- Demonstration of sperm in the postmasturbation urine
- Analysis of the ejaculate
- Determination of the secretion markers of the adnexa
- Ultrasonographic (abdominal and transrectal) examination of the genital organs.

The patient is instructed to void immediately following ejaculation and the diagnosis of retrograde ejaculation can be confirmed by examination of postejaculate urine (PEU). A sample of the specimen is evaluated microscopically for sperm density and motility. Alternatively, the specimen may be centrifuged and the pellet resuspended in a medium, such as human tubular fluid, and then analyzed for sperm density and motility. Presence of more than 15 sperms/HPF is confirmatory of retrograde ejaculation.

Principles of Management of Retrograde Ejaculation

- Conversion of retrograde into antegrade ejaculation by drug therapy
- Harvesting of sperm from postejaculatory urine
- Surgical treatment.

In the treatment of retrograde ejaculation, an initial trial of medical therapy is warranted. The agents commonly utilized are alpha-adrenergic agonists such as ephedrine, pseudoephedrine, imipramine, and phenylpropanolamine. When pharmacological attempts to restore antegrade ejaculation fail, the spermatozoa should be recovered from postejaculation urine, to be applied in one of the modern techniques of assisted reproduction. The successful recovery of viable spermatozoa from the urine is dependent upon careful regulation of pH and osmolarity of the urine at the time of ejaculation. Careful handling of the retrieved spermatozoa enables isolation of sperm cells with good quality for insemination of ovulated oocytes (*in vivo*) or retrieved oocytes (*in vitro*) and is timed to coincide with the wife's ovulation.

Protocol for Urinary Alkalization

Patient is instructed to use Sodium bicarbonate tablets 2 gm TID and Sudafed 60 mg TID since 3 days prior to anticipated day of ovulation and to monitor his urinary pH with pH strips to assess the efficacy of alkalization.

On the day of sample collection pH and osmolarity of spontaneous urine is measured. The aim is that the pH should reach 7.3 and the osmolarity should be 280 mosmol, if not dissolve 2.0 gm sodium bicarbonate in 200 ml of distilled water and administer to the patient. After 30 min repeat the measurement and if the desired value has not been attained, repeat the procedure by reducing the amount of sodium bicarbonate and measure again in 30 minutes (this is the time the sodium bicarbonate needs to reach the bladder).

It should be remembered that the reducing bicarbonate is dependent on pH level and if the correct pH and osmolarity are reached, the patient is instructed to empty his bladder completely just prior to ejaculation (the closer the better). Then catheterize the bladder, drain it to completion, and administer a small volume of media. The patient then ejaculates and collects this antegrade sample. Then re-catheterize, collect the bladder sample and if needed irrigate the bladder with media to collect the rest of the retrograde specimen prior to sending them all off to the laboratory for processing. It is necessary to use media at room temperature and minimal lubrication while catheterizing to enhance sperm recovery.

Most cases of retrograde ejaculation can be managed either by conversion to antegrade by pharmacological manipulation or sperm recovered from the bladder by urinary alkalization, and surgical treatment is anecdotal in the era of assisted reproduction.

Anejaculation

Anejaculation and ejaculatory dysfunction are the terms used to describe the inability of a man to have an ejaculation. It is a relatively uncommon disorder that can occur as a result of spinal cord injury, retroperitoneal lymph node dissection, or other retroperitoneal surgery, diabetes mellitus, transverse myelitis, or multiple sclerosis. In addition, the etiology may be psychogenic or idiopathic. The nerves that are responsible for carrying the signal for ejaculation exit the spinal cord and course along the aorta in the posterior part of the abdomen. These nerves are most commonly injured after spinal trauma resulting in paraplegia or quadriplegia, major bowel or vascular surgery, or surgery for testicular cancer. In the past men with ejaculatory dysfunction were considered infertile because they could not ejaculate but presently there are treatment options available.

Anejaculation resulting from damage to the afferent or efferent neural pathways (reflex arc) responsible for emission and/or ejaculation can be treated with electroejaculation. In cases where the reflex arc is intact or is partially damaged, vibratory stimulation is useful. Some researchers have tried medical therapy in both these types and were generally unsuccessful.

<u>VIBRATORY STIMULATION</u>

Vibratory stimulation (VS) employs a custom-designed mechanical vibrator (store bought vibrators do not work for many patients) that is applied to the underside of the glans penis and set to vibrate at a designated frequency and wave amplitude. This vibration travels along the sensory nerves to the spinal cord and may induce a reflex ejaculation. This technique only works in patients with an intact ejaculatory reflex arc. The results are dependent on the level of spinal cord injury and are most effective in patients with upper cord lesions. This is an office procedure that requires no anesthesia or sedation to perform. However it is suggested that all patients irrespective of the level of injury in the spinal cord have an initial trial with vibratory therapy as many a times the lesion may be incomplete. When vibratory stimulation is unsuccessful, electroejaculation often works quite well.

After standard bladder preparation (detailed below), a hand-held, electrically-driven vibrator is applied initially to the dorsum of the glans and then to the frenulum and penoscrotal area. The slow movement of the vibrator often identifies a "trigger" point, which is often be reproducible from one cycle to another. The selection of a frequency of 100 Hz and a peak-to-peak amplitude of 2.5 mm may be important for successful ejaculation. Patients who ejaculate using this form of stimulation need to be trained properly in its usage and ejaculatory interval may vary from 10 to 180 min depending on the pathology. People who are likely to respond to vibrators develop penile tumescence and pelvic floor contractions. In the absence of these signs electroejaculation is a better option. Most patients who respond to vibratory stimulation will exhibit antegrade ejaculation, but catheterization must be performed because these patients frequently have incomplete closure of the bladder neck and may also have a significant retrograde component.

Researchers from the University of Miami School of Medicine, Miami, Florida, have hypothesized that presence of bulbocavernous and hip flexion reflexes are useful in predicting response of penile vibratory stimulation. When both reflexes were present, 80 pe rcent of the men ejaculated in response to stimulation compared to only 8 per cent of men in whom neither reflex was present. Poor prognostic indicators are spinal cord injury within the last 6 months, the absence of reflex hip flexion and lesion below T_{12} level.

Electroejaculation

Initially used in veterinary medicine and animal husbandry, electroejaculation produces seminal emission by sinusoidal electrical stimulation of sympathetic efferent fibers and smooth muscle. The best site for inducing seminal emission is in front of the bifurcation of the aorta, between the rectum and obturator nerves, where both preganglionic and postganglionic sympathetic fibers reside. Unfortunately, because electroejaculation does not stimulate the somatically mediated events of ejaculation or coordinate bladder neck closure essential to antegrade emission, pulsatile expulsion of seminal fluid does not occur. Rather, semen either dribbles from the meatus or is deposited retrograde into the bladder (Ohl DA, 1989).

A complete urologic evaluation is required prior to electroejaculation in order to detect and treat any urinary tract infections. Men with spinal cord injuries often have a problem of poor sperm production as well as ejaculatory difficulty. A diagnostic trial of electroejaculation is attempted to obtain and examine the quality of the semen specimen. Good quality samples are frozen for future use as a back-up. A fresh specimen is obtained at the time of the women's ovulation. Unlike vibratory stimulation, electroejaculation is uniformly successful irrespective of the duration and level of the spinal lesion.

Electroejaculation is performed with a device known as an electroejaculator (Figure 15.1). A specially designed electric probe is inserted into the rectum next to the prostate (Figure 15.2). A current generated by the machine is applied to stimulate the nerves and produce contraction of the pelvic muscles resulting in ejaculation. The procedure begins by first catheterizing the patient in supine position and emptying the bladder completely. The use of betadine is to be avoided because of its spermicidal effect. Instead, the urethra is lubricated with glycerin for catheterization. The pH of urine should be assessed to

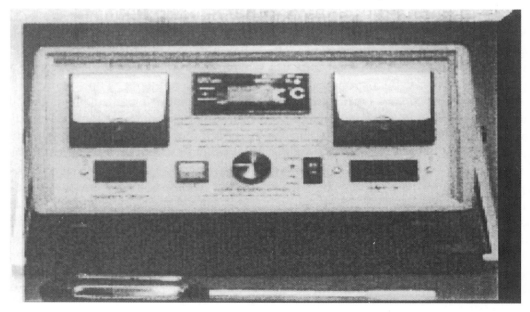

FIGURE 15.1: Electroejaculator

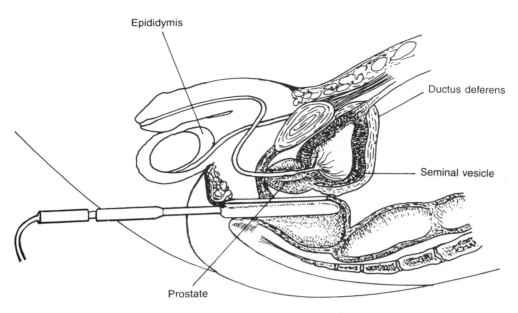

FIGURE 15.2: Electroejaculation probe

ensure its alkalinity (pH > 7.0). Oral sodium bicarbonate may be used if necessary. Because retrograde ejaculation occurs frequently in this procedure, an additional 10 cc of the medium is instilled into the bladder to help preserve any sperm inside the bladder. The catheter is then removed. Although it is possible to perform the procedure in lithotomy position, lateral decubitus position is preferred, as it allows easier access to both the penis and rectum.

Rhythmic delivery of current is performed by manually turning the dial to increase the voltage delivery progressively for a few seconds. After a few initial stimulations, the voltage is reduced to zero. Voltage is then gradually increased until erection/ejaculation has occurred. The voltage at which the first erection/ejaculation occurs is noted and it is then increased to a level 30 to 50 per cent higher, depending on patient's tolerance and the rectal temperature which is constantly monitored and displayed. Ejaculation may be entirely retrograde and in such cases, sweating, piloerection, goose bumps on the thighs, buttocks, and partial erection may be the only signs that the patient is adequately stimulated and ejaculated. The number of stimulations, the current, and the voltage necessary to produce a maximum erection are noted, as this information will be useful for subsequent procedure if needed. The ejaculate is collected directly into a cup containing sperm friendly buffer.

The collected semen specimen is processed in the andrology laboratory and if the specimen is of very good quality, then it can be used for intrauterine insemination (IUI). If there are few sperms or the sperms have low motility then the specimen can be used with *in-vitro* Fertilization/ICSI to establish a pregnancy. Electroejaculation must be performed under general anesthesia in all patients who have abdominal and perirectal sensation. Anesthesia is not required for spinal cord injured men who have high level injuries and are without sensation. Anyone who has a history of autonomic dysreflexia must have blood pressure and heart rate monitored as electroejaculation may cause a significant increase in blood pressure.

Initial results in terms of the ability to obtain motile sperm were variable, but with refinements in the equipment and techniques, sperm can now be obtained in approximately 90 per cent of anejaculatory patients. These patients have excellent sperm densities averaging 180 to 300 million/cc. Despite successes in the induction of ejaculation, sperm motility has continued to be low, limiting fertility in these patients. Mean sperm motilities of 20 per cent have been reported in several series. This poor motility appears to be secondary to intrinsic factors such as elevated scrotal temperature and recurrent genitourinary tract infection rather than to the electroejaculation procedure. The use of assisted reproductive techniques (ARTs), especially ICSI, has become increasingly important in this patient population. Because these patients often have supranormal sperm densities with low motility, semen processing with Percoll gradients may be beneficial in removing non-motile sperm, white blood cells, and debris before insemination.

Research on persistent low motility in these patients suggests that psychogenic anejaculation is associated with increased incidence of anti-sperm autoimmunity explaining poor motility. The majority of antibodies were directed against the sperm heads. Surface antibodies were mainly IgA isotype whereas serum antibodies were IgG isotype. Further research on sperm motility and effects of electrical current on sperm behavior *in-vitro* exhibited a significant two-fold decrease in motility percentage and viability. Superoxide dismutase (SOD) activity decreased significantly in sperm subjected to direct electric current in comparison to the control groups. These studies indicate that *in-vitro* and *in-vivo* electrical stimulation generates reactive oxygen species, which affects superoxide dismutase (SOD) activity, which in part is responsible for decreased sperm motion and viability.

Electroejaculation and vibratory stimulation have enabled many men who suffer from ejaculatory failure to conceive children of their own, but it is imperative to plan for multiple sittings to maximize benefit.

Patient Preparation

Pretreatment : 24 to 48 hour's alkalization with sodium bicarbonate, 2 gm peroral TID
1. Bladder wash + medium optional*
2. May need
   • antibiotics, if there is a history of urinary tract infection

---

* Several proprietary media are available for sperm preservation

• Alpha-agonist (e.g. Sudafed) to prevent retrograde ejaculation
• Nifedipine (sublingual), if there is autonomic dysreflexia

Currently, employing this technique, semen can be obtained in more than 90 per cent of neurologically impaired men. More than 40 per cent of the couples achieve pregnancy with IUI or IVF. Pregnancy rates are slightly better among couples in whom the male partner had spinal cord injury (43%) or idiopathic anejaculation (33%) than in those who had undergone retroperitoneal lymph node dissection (20%) or had diabetes (0%).

Retarded Ejaculation

Retarded ejaculation is the persistent difficulty or inability to ejaculate despite the presence of adequate sexual desire, erection, and stimulation. Ejaculatory episodes are either partial, without pleasure or with pain. The causes of this dysfunction may be organic, i.e., medical illness or drug induced (particularly medications with anti-adrenergic effects), the result of surgical interventions, or secondary to inhibiting psychological factors. With regard to psychological determinants, fear, guilt and resentment have all been implicated.

Medical therapy is helpful in patients with severe psychological factors and behavioral therapy or vibratory therapy helps most patients.

ORGASMIC DISTURBANCES

Primary absolute anorgasmia is the impossibility to have an orgasm and ejaculation during any kind of sexual activity while awake, in men with normal erectile function and nocturnal emission. Though some men are occasionally found to have a neurological basis for the problem (occult spinal dysraphism with tethered cord, MS, etc.) but primarily it is psychogenic with very few cases reported in literature. Primary modality of treatment of this condition is by
• Sexual behavioral therapy—where in majority are refractory to treatment.
• Electroejaculation—may require multiple sittings and usually successful

• Vasal aspiration and ICSI is used in resistant cases

Secondary anorgasmia is mainly associated with psychotropic drugs such as sertraline and gebapentin. Clinicians are increasingly faced with the need to identify, treat, and counsel patients regarding psychotropic drug-induced sexual dysfunction. Antipsychotic and antidepressant drugs have both rational mechanisms to explain their effects on sexual function and established literature documenting these effects. Sexual dysfunction secondary to the use of antidepressants, especially clomipramine or SSRI's is an adverse effect that is often underestimated and according to earlier studies, this can affect approximately 60 percent of the patients. These patients may present with decrease in libido, alterations in the ability to reach orgasm/ ejaculation, erectile dysfunction and anorgasmia. These dysfunctions appear to be related to the increase in serotonin, which occurs anorgasmia. These dysfunctions appear to be related to the increase in serotonin, which occurs with the stimulation of serotonin 5HT receptors. Nefazadone, amantadine, cyproheptadine, sildenafil, serotonin antagonist mianserin are some of the drugs used in secondary anorgasmia but are ineffective. Failing drug therapy, electroejaculation or vibratory stimulation is generally successful.

SUMMARY

Fertility related concerns are significant for the spinal cord injured male because of his young age and loss of ejaculatory function. Fortunately, using electroejaculation and vibratory stimulation, the successful recovery of sperm has become routine. However, because of the poor quality of the sperm obtained, the ARTs of IUI and *in vitro* fertilization have had only modest pregnancy results. The revolutionary technique of intracytoplasmic sperm injection (ICSI), which involves the injection of a single sperm into an oocyte, is particularly applicable for these patients and has been very successful in initiating pregnancies. The potential for improvement in semen recovery and processing is great and must be considered a challenge for the immediate future. Finally, fertility issues in men may be quite complex and clearly needs a multidisciplinary management approach.

FURTHER READINGS

1. Broderick GA. Evidence based assessment of erectile dysfunction. Int J Impot Res 1998;2(Suppl):S64-73, discussion S77-9.
2. Chung PH, Verkauf BS, Mola R et al. Correlation between semen parameters of electroejaculates and achieving pregnancy by intrauterine insemination. Fertil Steril 1997;67(1):129-32.
3. Eid JF.Electroejaculation. AUA Update Series, Volume XI, Lesson 1992;10:73-80.
4. Glander HJ. Disorders of ejaculation. Fortschr Med 1998;116(26):26-28,30-31.
5. Hermabessiere J, Guy L, Boiteux JP. Human ejaculation: physiology, surgical conservation of ejaculation. Prog Urol 1999;9(2):305-09.
6. Hirsch IH, Sedor J, Jeyendran RS et al. The relative distribution of viable sperm in the antegrade and retrograde portions of ejaculates obtained after electrostimulation. Fertil Steril 1992;57(2):399-401.
7. Hora M, Vozeh F. The physiology of erection. Urologicka klinika LF UK a FN, Plzen Cas Lek Cesk 1997;136(12): 363-66.
8. Hull EM, Lorrain DS, Du J et al. Hormone-neurotransmitter interactions in the control of sexual behavior. Behav Brain Res 1999;105(1):105-16.
9. Malossinni G, Ficarra V, Caleffi G. Retrograde Ejaculation. Arch Ital Urol Androl 1999;71(3):185-96.
10. McMahon CG, Touma K. Predictive value of patient history and correlation of nocturnal penile tumescence, colour duplex Doppler ultrasonography and dynamic cavernosometry and cavernosography in the evaluation of erectile dysfunction. Int J Impot Res 1999;11(1): 47-51.
11. Metz ME, Pryor JL, Nesvacil LJ et al. Premature ejaculation: A psychophysiological approach for assessment and management. J Sex Marital Ther 2000;26(4):293-320.
12. Michetti PM, Rossi R, Travaglia S et al. Primary absolute anorgasmy in the male. Report of three clinical cases. Minerva Urol Nefrol 1999;51(1):23-26.
13. Nehra A, Werner MA, Bastuba M et al. Vibratory stimulation and rectal probe electroejaculation as therapy for patients with spinal cord injury: semen parameters and pregnancy rates. J Urol 1996;155(2): 554-59.
14. Ohl DA, Bennett CJ, McCabe M et al. Predictors of success in electroejaculation of spinal cord injured men. J Urol 1989;142:1483-86.

15. Ohl DA, Sonksen J, Menge AC et al. Electroejaculation versus vibratory stimulation in spinal cord injured men: Sperm quality and patient preference. J Urol 1997; 157(6):2147-49.

16. Rajasekaran M, Hellstrom WJ, Sparks RL et al. Sperm-damaging effects of electric current: Possible role of free radicals. Reproductive Toxicology 1994;8(5):427-32.

17. Shafik A. Pelvic floor muscles and sphincters during erection and ejaculation. Arch Androl 1997;39(1):71-78.

18. Sonksen J, Biering-Sorensen F, Kristensen JK. Ejaculation induced by penile vibratory stimulation in men with spinal cord injuries: The importance of the vibratory amplitude. Paraplegia 1994;32(10):651-60.

19. Witt MA, Grantmyre JE. Ejaculatory failure. World J Urol 1993;11(2):89-95.

20. Zaragooshi J. Unconsummated marriage: clarification of aetiology; treatment with intracorporeal injection. BJU Int 2000;86(1):75-79.

ASSISTED REPRODUCTION FOR MALE FACTOR INFERTILITY

Nalini Krishnan

INTRODUCTION

Male infertility is a multifactorial syndrome which covers a wide variety of disorders. Male factor as the sole cause or as a contributory cause for infertility is seen in approximately 40 to 50 percent of infertile couples. In more than 50 percent of infertile men, the cause is unknown, and it could be congenital or acquired.

ETIOLOGY (TABLE 15.1)

TABLE 15.1: Etiological factors in male factor infertility and subfertility

Abnormality	Cause or pathogenesis
Absence of testicular tissue	Anorchism[1] bilateral castration
Impaired sperm production and function	Klinefelter's syndrome[2] or variants AZF-gene deletions (y-deletions)[3] Hypogonadotropic hypogonadism Cryptorchidism[5,6] Testicular cancer Varicocele Age Genitourinary infections Environmental agents • Temperature • (Ir) Radiations • Medications • Occupational exposure • Stimulants • Drugs, alcohol, tobacco abuse • Nutritional deficiency trace elements (Selenizm Zn), vitamins
Impaired sperm transport	Sperm antibodies[8, 9] Epididymal blockage of vas deferens Ejaculatory failure Impotence Vasectomy
Disturbance in sperm-egg inter- actions	Disturbance could be at various levels • Sperm capacitation • Cumulus passage • Sperm egg fusion • Egg activation

MALE HISTORY

Medical History

- Especially genitourinary infections
- Systemic diseases
- Actual medications.

Surgical History

- Especially abdominal and genital surgery.

Social History

- Smoking habits
- Psychological/social impact of the subfertility on the male partners and on his or her relationship
- Prior or actual exposure to toxins and/or high temperature, environmental and/or occupational.

Prior Fertility History

- Infertility, infecundity, pregnancies, children in a previous relationship?

Sexual History

- Use of (sperimicidal) lubricants
- Sexual dysfunctions.

Any Prior Work-up for Infertility

- Assessment of sperm morphology according to WHO or Kruger standards.

CLINICAL EVALUATIONS

Clinical examinations and evaluations cannot be overemphasized. A detailed and meticulous history with particular attention to potential risk factors followed by a careful physical examination encompassing the following:
- General examinations
- State and level of virilizations
- Presence of gynecomastia

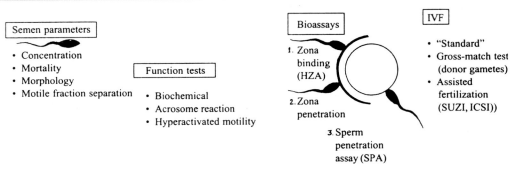

Figure 15.3: The sequential, multi-step diagnostic scheme for male factor patients in assisted reproductions[10]

- Phallic competence
- Testicular size (calibrated orchidometer is recommended)
- Presence of epididymis, vas deferens
- Prostatic status
- Varicocele palpable or made palpable by Valsalva maneuver.

DIAGNOSIS (FIGURE 15.3)

Routine Semen Analysis

Routine semen analysis though still the most important source of informations regarding the fertility status of the male, is more an assessment of the potential for fertility rather than a test for its fertilizing capacity (Table 15.2). Therefore more specialized tests are necessary to determine conclusively the fertilizing capacity of the sperms.

TABLE 15.2: Normal values of semen parameters[11] from WHO 1992	
Parameter	*Normal range*
• Semen volume	2 mL or more
• pH	7.2-8.0
• Sperm concentrations	20 million/mL or more
• Total sperm count	40 million or more
• Motility	50% or more with forward profession
• Morphology	30% or more normal forms
• Vitality	75% or more live
• White blood cells	less than 1 million/mL

Specialized Tests of Sperm Functions

- Sperm antibodies
- Hypo-osmotic sperm tail swelling test (HOS)[12]
- Reactive oxygen species (ROS)
- Hyperactivation of sperm motility

- Acrosin content[13]
- Acroseme reaction[13a]
- Hamster egg sperm penetration assay
- Hemizona binding test.[14]
- Computer-assisted sperm analysis (CASA)[15]
- Cervical mucous penetration.

The Hormonal Profile to Differentiate between Gonadotropin Deficiency and Primary Testicular Dysfunctions

Gonadotropin Deficiency

- Profound fall in testosterone level
- No reciprocal increase in FSH or LH.

Primary Testicular Dysfunctions

- Serum FSH level increased proportion to the amount of spermatogenic tissue lost
- Serum LH increases when testicular dysfunction is severe
- Testosterone level is maintained
- Free unbound testosterone level is decreased (Fig. 15.4).

TREATMENT FOR MALE FACTOR INFERTILITY

The key to successful treatment is in identifying the cause. Unfortunately in male factor infertility for approximately 50 percent of the cases, the cause is unknown. Assisted reproductive techniques (ART) can help bypass the abnormality in many patients without actually correcting the cause.

Medical Treatment

Specific treatment of hormonal abnormalities in men is frequently effective.

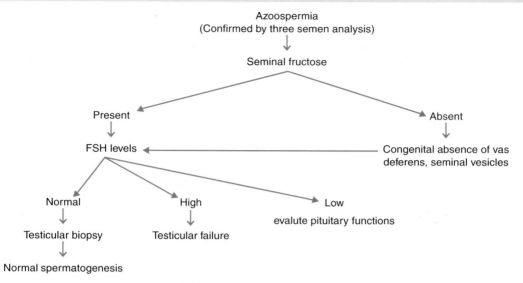

FIGURE 15.4: Approach to azoospermia

No production of GnRH and subsequent lack of pituitary release of LH and FSH resulting in absence of puberty. So initial treatment is with testosterone injections leading to the onset of puberty and development of secondary sexual characteristics.

Intramuscular injections of FSH (as hMCa) and LH (hCG) leads to fertility and sperm production.

Pulsatile GnRH replaces deficient hypothalamic hormones. Abnormally high levels of prolactins (due to pituitary tumor) can also lead to a lack of FSH and LH with a resultant drop in testosterone and sperm production. Bromocriptine administration reverts the hormonal levels to normal and restores sperm productions. Treatment of infections with antibiotics is advocated.

Surgical Interventions

Surgical intervention is necessary when there are obstructions in the reproductive tract. Varicocele is the 'distention of the pampiniform plexus in the scrotum in response to increased venous pressure. It is seen in 35 percent of men with primary infertility and in 81 percent of men with secondary infertility and is associated with reduction in testicular size and abnormalities in spermatogenesis. The treatment is varicocelectomy and it is shown to improve testicular volume and sperm count.

In vas deferens or epididymal obstructions microsurgery with reconstruction of the lumen is advocated.

In vasectomy cases microsurgical recanalization vasovasostomy[16] is beneficial.

The ejaculatomy duct which is formed by the union of the ampulla of the vas deferens and the duct of the seminal vesicle enters the prostatic urethra. Obstruction can develop which may be partial or complete and may be located high or low. Treatment is resection of the constricted/obstructed portion along with a small area of the prostate.

Assisted Reproduction

The term ART (assisted reproductive technology) encompasses numerous fertility enhancing procedures and processes which vary greatly in their costing, degree of invasiveness, laboratory requirements, technique and the level of expertise.

Assisted reproductive technologies provide efficient means to overcome multiple sperm abnormalities and also allow the completion of sperm diagnostic testing (Table 15.3).

Intrauterine Insemination (IUI)

Intrauterine insemination has been reported since the late 1950's,[23-31] and summerized by Allew *et al* in 1985.[32] Among the ARTs, IUI is the least

TABLE 15.3: Comparative study of the various procedures in ART

	IUI	SIFT*	GIFT*18	ZIFT*19	TET*20	IVF	ICSI
Ovarian stimulation	a. Natural cycle b. Stimulated cycle	a. Natural cycle b. Stimulated cycle	Stimulation	Stimulation	Stimulation	Stimulation	Stimulation
*Tubal patency	Necessary	Necessary	Necessary	Necessary	Necessary	Not necessary	Not necessary
Oocyte retrieval	No	No	Yes	Yes	Yes	Yes	Yes
Insemination	Prepared sperm injected directly into the uterine cavity using an insemination catheter	Prepared spermatozoa transferred directly into the fallopian tubes using a very long catheter	both oocytes and spermatozoa transferred into the fallopian tube using a GIFT catheter	In vitro insemination for 18-20 hrs in an incubator -CO_2 till 2PN stage	(in18-20 hrs (in a CO_2 incubator) till 2PN stage	18-20 hrs later cleaned and incubated further for 48-72 hrs	Microinjection of a single morphologically normal looking sperm into a denuded metaphase II oocyte
Transfer of zygote/ embryo	—	—		2PN zygote transferred to the fallopian tube	Day 2 2-8 cell embryos transferred to the fallopian tube using catheter along	Day 3/Day 5 embryos/blastocysts transferred to the uterine cavity using an ET catheter	Day 3/Day 5 embryos/blastocysts transferred to the uterine cavity using an ET catheter
*Semen parameters	> 3 × 10^5 motile sperms 10% or more (grade A hyperactive)	Similar to IUI	5 × 10^4-1 × 10^6 sperms/oocyte	50 × 10^3-1 × 10^6 sperms/oocyte	Similar to ZIFT		Severe oligoasthenospermia theoretically a single sperm is required

*SIFT, GIFT, ZIFT, TET—do not offer increased pregnancy rates and hence are not routinely practised.

ZIFT (Devroey et al, 1989)
TET (Balmaceda et al, 1988)
IVF (Ewards RG et al, 1980)
GIFT (Brinsden, PR et al, 1992)
ICSI (Palermo et al, 1992)

expensive, least invasive, least stressful and least hazardous. With the advent of new sperm preparation techniques higher pregnancy rates have resulted.

Indications for IUI Male Factor

- Ejaculatory abnormalities
- Oligo/oligoasthenospermia
- Antisperm antibodies.

Sperm Processing Techniques

Simple wash[33]
- Ideal for a near normal semen sample with minimal/no dead sperms, leukocytes, cellular and acellular debris.

Swim-up[34]
- Suited for samples which have a higher percentage of motile sperms.

Percoll gradient[35]
- Harvests highly motile morphologically normal sperms and reduces bacterial contamination.

Albumin columns[36]
- Separates progressively motile sperm from non-motile forms and debris. It is also used to separate X and Y bearing sperms.

Glass-wool filtrations[37,38]
- Recovery of motile sperm is high. Modified version retains the functional integrity of the membrane. This technique is good for asthenozoospermic and high viscosity samples.

Sperm migration
- Hyaluronate which is a linear polysaccharide mimicks cervical mucus. Sperms swimming through it have decreased oxidative damage.

Migration sedimentations
- Liquefied semen is layered around the outer of two concentrically arranged tubes which are then filled with medium. Sperms swim through the medium and sediment in the inner tube.

Membrane separation[40] of sperm from semen Antisperm-antibody positive sperm
- Physical separation by a semipermeable fibrous polyester which allows only sperms to pass through, are used.
- Various methods have been suggested:

- Elution of antibodies from the sperm surface by washing and centrifugation.[41]
- Treatment with low pH or high ionic strength media.[41]
- Absorption of ASA with immunobeads.[42]
- Absorption with protein A.[43]
- Absorption of ASA by collection of ejaculate into high serum concentration media.[44]
- Protease digestion of sperm-bound ASA.[45]
- Isolation of immunodepleted sperm using percoll.[46]

Sperm Concentrations and Tuning of Insemination

There is an increase in the pregnancy rate in general when increasing numbers of motile, spermatozoa are inseminated, but there is no obvious advantage of using concentrations of more than 20 million motile sperms. In case of severe male factor pooling of sequential ejaculates may be considered.

The timing of insemination is important and should be performed as close as possible to the time of ovulation.

The ideal timing would be the day after LH rise (15.8 ± 2.6 hrs) after the LH peak or about 30 to 33 hours after LH rise in the urine).

Predictive Parameters and Success in an IUI Program[58]

- Not much difference in success rates between primary and secondary infertility
- Pregnancy rate/cycle drops significantly after the third treatment cycle
- Ovulation induction with hMG yields better results after IUI treatment compared to CC-treated cycles
- Conception rates were similar for idiopathic, female factor only and male factor subfertility
- No individual parameter can predict success
- More than 3×10^5 motile spermatozoa with 10 percent grade A motility after preparations Success rates are similar to cases with normal sperm characteristics.
- Cycle fecundity of IUI in poor responder cancelled IVF cycles was similar to that in planned IUI cycles.

In conclusion there is no single perfect procedure for all types of semen and therefore the choice of the procedure should be customized for a given sample.

In Vitro Fertilization (IVF)

The birth of Louise Brown in July 1978[49] heralded an important milestone in the treatment options for infertile couples. The standard or conventional *in vitro* fertilization (IVF) procedure was originally developed to treat infertility due to tubal factor. But soon couples with other categories of infertility including male factor infertility benefitted.[50,51]

The standard IVF procedure involves controlled ovarian hyperstimulation. The oocytes are retrieved transvaginally with ultrasound guidance and under intravenous sedation. These retrieved oocytes are incubated for a duration which is dependent on the degree of maturity and then inseminated for 18 to 20 hours using prepared sperm samples. After confirmation of fertilization they are further cultured for another 48 hours and the resultant embryo/embryos are transferred back to the uterine cavity.

Diagnostic Sperm Parameters in Relation to IVF

The initial diagnostic test done to assess sperm function is the standard semen analysis.[11] As said earlier in the chapter that it is an assessment of the potential for fertility rather than a test for its fertilizing capacity. But Mahadevan *et al* (1984) reported that of conventional semen analysis parameters, motility was the single best predictor of fertilization rate *in vitro* with failure of fertilization consistently occurring with less than 20 percent motility.[52]

A study in 1993 showed that assessment of motility in a prepared (for IVF) sample can be combined with morphology analysis, prior to processing, to provide excellent IVF predictive ability.[53]

Sperm morphology Most studies using different criteria have found sperm morphologic parameters to be predictive for IVF outcome. Severe teratozoospermia is associated with poor IVF performance, including reduced as well as delayed fertilization, poor embryo quality, and reduced clinical and live born pregnancy rates.[54]

Presence of white blood cells A concentration of more than 10^6/mL is considered to be abnormal and is referred to as leukocytospermia.[11] Seminal leukocytes have been identified as a major source of reactive oxygen species and is associated with decreased fertilization.

Sperm penetration assay (SPA) A normal SPA result is predictive of successful IVF while an abnormal result appears to be of less predictive value, especially in the setting of abnormal semen parameters.[55,56] A number of preparation methods which modify the SPA have been developed that may yield a positive SPA result. These methods which can be applied to improve IVF results are Percoll gradients, TES and TRIS (test)—yolk buffer incubation, follicular fluid, use of a hyperosmolar medium and of a calcium ionophore.

Sperm-zona pellucida binding tests Human zona is selective for binding of morphologically normal sperm. The hemizona assay (HZA) uses the matched halves of a microbisected zona to compare binding capacities of a proven fertile semen specimen and a test specimen.[57]

Acrosomal status and function Breakdown of the acrosome as a final step in capacitation can be induced by the ZP and is necessary for its penetration. In semen samples with poor morphology, the proportion of sperm with normal intact acrosomes following swim-up was correlated with fertilization *in vitro*. Thus demonstrating the importance of acrosomal status in assessing the functional capacity of spermatozoa.

Hypo-osmotic swelling test The hypo-osmotic swelling test (HOS) evaluates the functional integrity of the human sperm membranes. An abnormal HOS test result has substantial predictive value, whereas a normal result is not predictive of IVF success.

Semen processing in relation to IVF Semen processing techniques have been discussed earlier in this chapter.

Insemination using high concentrations of motile sperm and microinsemination techniques.

In cases of abnormal semen analysis fertilization is more likely to occur when higher concentrations of motile sperm are used. Concentrations upto 5×10^6/mL have been used with success.

Microinsemination techniques involve concentrating the prepared sperm specimen in a small volume for oocyte insemination.

Viscous Semen Samples

These samples benefit from collection directly into medium or by the use of proteolytic enzymes during processing.

Factors which Influence the Success of IVF

Women who register for an IVF program are extremely anxious to know their chances of success and as to what is the actual "take-home-baby-rate". The following factors which influence the success of IVF are as follows.

Maternal age: Maternal age plays a very important role in the success rate and outcome of IVF. The pregnancy rate falls as the maternal age increases over 40 years.
- 30-34 yrs—24.4%
- > 40 yrs—14.7%

There is a progressive decrease in the mean number of oocytes retrieved, fertilized oocytes and cleaved embryos with increasing maternal age. There is also a significant increase in the proportion of babies born with chromosomal abnormalities with increasing maternal age.

Etiology of infertility Highest fertilization and cleavage rates are seen among patients with tubal factor and lowest among those with male factor infertility.

Number of embryos transferred There is an increase in the pregnancy rate when more than one embryo is replaced.

Embryo cryopreservation The additional pregnancies from replacement of cryopreserved embryos have effectively increased the success rate of a couple by 10 percent but the stage at which the embryos are cryopreserved are of importance. 2PN zygotes have a better success rate that blastocysts.

Semen parameters Reduced semen quality increases the likelihood of failed fertilization.

Intracytoplasmic Sperm Injection (ICSI)

The development of ICSI[22] has been a major break through in reproductive medicine, offering definite hope to infertile couples especially with severe male factor infertility.

Indications for ICSI (Table 15.4)

- Severe male factor infertility
- Azoospermia (obstructive)
- Repeated fertilization failure with conventional IVF
- *In vitro* matured oocytes
- Cryopreserved oocytes
- High titers of antisperm antibodies
- Only immotile spermatozoa available
- Acrosomeless spermatozoa (round-headed)

TABLE 15.4: The non-existent, relative and absolute indications for ICSI[48]

IVF as first choice	IVF and ICSI in combination	ICSI as first choice
Normal sperm sample	Poor or no fertilization in first cycle Less than 0.8×10^6 spermatozoa after preparation Sperm morphology < 5% normal Antisperm antibodies	Poor or no fertilization in two IVF cycles Epididysmal testicular spermatozoa Globozoospermia Immotile spermatozoa Frozen-thawed spermatozoa with poor survival preimplantation genetic diagnosis

- Fertilization of oocytes prior to PGD (preimplantation genetic diagnosis)
- Immotile cilia syndrome
- Poor post-thaw survival of cryopreserved sperm sample.

Despite the meteoric rise of ICSI and the instant success and acceptance worldwide it should be approached with caution since the long-term effects are largely unknown and unexplored. Indiscriminate use of ICSI should not be undertaken when conventional IVF would serve the purpose very well.

It has to be emphasized that comparisons between ICSI and conventional IVF in terms of success rates are not relevant since they are performed on different categories of infertility. Transferring cases of unexplained infertility and poor fertilization in conventional IVF to ICSI did not enhance their success rate.[47]

In spite of all the debates and controversies surrounding ICSI it has to be acknowledged that ICSI has come to stay. It has been accepted as a miracle cure since what were known as crucial and important parameters (count, motility, morphology and functional capacity) and indicators for the outcome of conventional IVF *no longer mattered* and were successfully by-passed by the technique.

REFERENCES

1. Coulam CB. Testicular regression syndrome. Obstet Gynecol 1979;53:44.
2. Griffin JE, Klilsan JD. Disorders of sexual differentiation. In Klalsh PC, Relak A, Stamey TA (Eds): Campbell's Urology. WB Saunders: Philadelphia, 1992;2.
3. Chandley AC. Chromosome anomalies and Y chromosome microdeletions as causal factors in male infertility. In Devroey P, Tarlatzis BC, Steirteghem AV (Eds): Current Theory and Practice of ICSI. Hum Reprod 1998;13.
4. Handelsman DJ, Swedloff RS. Male gonadal dysfunction. Clin Endocrinol Metab 1985;14:89.
5. Cendran M, Keating MA, Huff DS. Cryptorchidism, orchiopexy and infertility: A critical long-term retrospective analysis part II. J Urol 1989;142:559.
6. Lee P. Fertility in cryptorchidism: Does treatment make a difference? Endocrinol Metab Clin N Am 1993; 22(3):479.
7. Wong WY et al. Male factor subfertility possible causes and the impact of nutritional factors. 2000;7.3(3):435-42.
8. Adeghe JHA: Male subfertility due to sperm antibodies: A clinical review, 1992.
9. Clarke GN. Sperm antibodies and human fertilization. Am J Reprod Immunol Microbiol 1988;19:65.
10. Oehninger S, Acosta AA, Veeck L et al. Recurrent failure of in vitro fertilization: Role of the hemizona assay (HZA) in the sequential diagnosis of specific sperm/oocyte defects. Am J Obstet Gynecol 1991;164:1210-15.
11. World Health organization: WHO Laboratory Manual for the Examination of Human Semen and Semen Cervical Mucus Inter action (2nd ed): Cambridge University Press: Cambridge, 1992.
12. Jayendran RS, Vander ven HH, Zanaveld LJ: The hypoosmotic swelling test: An update. Arch Androl 1992;29(2):105.
13. van der ven HH, Kennedy WP, Kaminski JM et al. Human sperm acrosin as a fertility marker. J Androl 1987;8:20.
13a. Fenichel P, Parinaud J (Eds): Human Sperm Acrosome Reaction John Libbey Eurotext, Colloque INSERM, 1995;236:460.
14. Oehninger S, Franken D, Alexander N et al. Hemizona assay and its impact on the identification and treatment of humans sperm. Andrologia 1992;24(6):307-21.
15. Wang C, Leung A, Tsoi WL et al. Computer-assisted assessment of human sperm morphology: Usefulness in predicting fertilising capacity of human spermatozoa. Fertil Steril 1991;55:989-93.
16. Belker AM, Thomas AJ Jr, Fuchs EF et al. Results of 1469 microsurgical vasectomy reversals by the vasovasostomy study group. J Urol 1991;141:505.
17. Oehninger S. An update as the laboratory assessment of male infertility. Hum Reprod 1995;10(Suppl-1):39-45.
18. Brinsden PR, Asch RH. Gamete intrafallopian transfer. In Brinsden PR, Rainsbury PA (Eds): A Textbook of in vitro Fertilization and Assisted Reproduction. Parthenon Publishing Group: New Jersey 1992;227-36.
19. Devroey P, Staessen C, Camus M et al. Zygote intrafallopian transfer as a successful treatment for unexplained infertility. Fertil Steril 1989;52:246-49.
20. Balinaceda JP, Gastaldi C, Remohi J et al. Tubal embryo transfer as a treatment for infertility due to male factor. Fertil Steril 1988;50:476-79.
21. Edwards RG, Steptoe PC, Purdy JM. Establishing full term human pregnancies using cleaving embryos gram in vitro. Br J Obstet Gynecol 1980;87:737-56.
22. Palermo G, Joris H, Devroey P et al. Pregnancies after intracytoplasmic injection of a single spermatozoon into as oocyte. Lancet 1992;340:17-18.
23. Mastroianni L Jr, Laberge JL, Rock L. Appraisal of the efficacy of artificial inseminations with husband's sperm and evaluations of insemination technique. Fertil Steril 1957;8:260-66.

24. Farris EJ, Murphy DP. The characteristics of the two parts of the partitioned ejaculation and the advantages of its use for intrauterine insemination. Fertil Steril 1960;11:465-69.

25. Cohen MR. Intrauterine insemination. Int J Fertil 1962;7:235-40.

26. Barwin BN. Intrauterine insemination of husband's sperm. J Reprod Fertil 1974;36:101-06.

27. Glass RN, Ericcson RJ. Intrauterine insemination of isolated motile sperm. Fertil Steril 1978;29:535-38.

28. White FM, Glass FH. Intrauterine insemination with husband's serum. Obstet Gynecol 1978;47:119-21.

29. Kremer J. A new technique for intrauterine insemination. Int J Fertil 1979;24:53-56.

30. Dmowski WP, Gaynor L, Lawrence M et al. Artificial insemination homologous with oligospermic semen separated an albumin columns. Fertil Steril 1979;31:58-62.

31. Harris SJ, Milligan MP, Masson GM et al. Improved separation of motile sperm in asthenospermia and its application to artificial insemination homologous. Fertil Steril 1981;36:219-21.

32. Allen NC, Herbert CM III, Maxson WS et al. Intrauterine insemination: A critical review. Fertil Steril 1985;44:569-80.

33. Hanson FM, Rock J. Artificial insemination with husband's sperm. Fertil Steril 1951;2:162-74.

34. Lopata A, Patullo MJ, Chang A et al. A method for collecting motile spermatozoa from human semen. Fertil Steril 1976;27:677-84.

35. Gorus FK, Pipeleeos DG. A rapid method for the fractionation of human spermatozoa according to their progressive motility. Fertil Steril 1981;35:662-65.

36. Ericsson RJ, Langevin CN, Nishino M: Isolation of fractions rich in human Y sperm. Nature 1973;246:421-24.

37. Paulson JD, Polakoski K, Leto S. Further characterization of glass wool column filtration of human semen. Fertil Steril 1979;32:125-26.

38. Jayendran RS, Peraz-Pelaez M, Crabo BG. Concentration of viable spermatozoa for artificial insemination. Fertil Steril 1986;45:132-34.

39. Wikland M, Wik O, Steen Y et al. A self-migration method for preparation of sperm for in vitro fertilization. Hum Reprod 1987;3:191-95.

40. Agarwal A, Manglona A, Loughlin KR. Filtration of spermatozoa through L membrane: A new method. Fertil Steril 1991;56:1162-67.

41. Haas GG Jr, D' Cruz OJ, Denum B. Effect of repeated washing on sperm bound immunoglobulin. G J Androl 1988;9:190-96.

42. Jeulin C, Soumah A, Da Silva et al. In vitro processing of sperm with autoantibodies: Analysis of sperm populations. Hum Reprod 1989;4:44-48.

43. Clarke GN, Hyne RW, Du Plessis Y et al. Sperm antibodies and human in vitro fertilization. Fertil Steril 1988;49:1018-25.

44. Byrd W, Kutteh WH, Carr BR. Treatment of antibody-associated sperm with media containing high serum content: A prospective trial of fertility following intrauterine insemination in men with high sperm antibodies. Am J Reprod Immunol 1994b;31:84-90.

45. Kutteh WH, McAllister D, Byrd KI et al. Antisperm antibodies: Current knowledge and new horizons. Mol Androl 1992;4:183-93.

46. Almagor M, Margalioth EJ, Yaffe H. Density differences between spermatozoa with antisperm autoantibodies and spermatozoa covered with antisperm antibodies from serum. Hum Reprod 1992;7:959-61.

47. Peterson K, Gabrielsen A, Mikkelsen A KI et al. ICSI does not overcome an oocyte defect in previous fertilization failure with conventional IVF and normal spermatozoa. 12th Annual Meeting of ESHRE, Maastricht, 1996;Abstrack No 107.

48. Hamberges L, Lundin K, Sjogren A et al. Indications for intracytoplasmic sperm injection. Hum Reprod 1998;13(Suppl 1):128-33.

49. Steptoc PC, Edwards RG. Birth after the re-implantation of a human embryo (Letter). Lancet 1978;2:366.

50. Mahadevan MM, Trounson AO, Leeton JF. The relationship of tubal blockage, infertility of unknown cause, suspected male infertility, and endometriosis to success of in vitro fertilization and embryo transfer. Fertil Steril 1983;40:755-66.

51. Batten D, Vargyas JM, Sato F et al. Th correlation between in vitro fertilization of human oocytes and semen profile. Fertil Steril 1985;44:835-38.

52. Mahadevan MM, Trounson AO. The influence of seminal characteristics on the success rates of human in vitro fertilization. Fertil Steril 1984;42:400-05.

53. Daucan WW, Gleu MJ, Wang GJ et al. Prediction of in vitro fertilization rates from semen variables. Fertil Steril 1993;59:1233-38.

54. Kniger TF, Menkveld R, Stander FSH et al. Sperm morphologic features as a prognostic factor in in vitro fertilization. Fertil Steril 1986;46:118-23.

55. Margalioth EJ, Navot D, Laufer N. Correlation between the zona-face hamster egg sperm penetration assay and human in vitro fertilization. Fertil Steril 1986;45:665-70.

56. Coetzee K, Kvuger TF, Menkveld R et al. Usefulness of sperm penetration assay in fertility predictions. Arch Androl 1989;23:207-12.

57. Burkman LJ, Coddington CC, Franken DR et al. The hemizona assay (HZA): Development of a diagnostic test for the binding of human spermatozoa to the human hemizona pellucida to predict fertilization potential. Fertil Steril 1988;49:688-97.

58. Ombelet W, Cox A, Janssen M et al. Artificial insemination (AIH) Artificial insemination 2: Using the husband's sperm. In Acosta AA, Kruger TF (Eds): Diagnosis and Therapy of Male Factor in Assisted Reproduction. Parthenon Publishing: Carnforth, UK, 1995;397-410.

Section 4

Female Factor Infertility

• Arati R Rao

16

Uterine and Cervical Factors in Infertility

While the major causes of infertility are anovulation and tubal disease, the less prevalent though still significant causes involve the uterus and the cervix. Together, these factors account for almost 10 percent of all cases of female infertility.

THE ROLE OF THE CERVIX IN REPRODUCTION

The cervix stands as the gatekeeper to the female reproductive tract. For fertilization of the ovum to occur in the Fallopian tube, the cervix must permit the sperms to pass through. This is facilitated by the changes in the mucus secreted by the columnar cells lining the cervix, brought on by the hormonal variations in the menstrual cycle.

The preovulatory mucus is secreted under the influence of high estrogen and low progesterone concentrations seen just before ovulation. This mucus which is thin and acellular, will permit the passage of sperms into the uterus, and henceforth into the uterus and fallopian tubes for fertilization to occur (Figure 16.1).

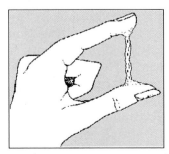

FIGURE 16.1: Preovulatory mucus

Similarly, the postovulatory mucus that is secreted under the influence of high progesterone and low estrogen levels, is thick, viscid and cellular; factors that render it impenetrable to sperms (Figure 16.2).

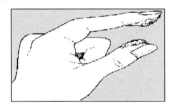

FIGURE 16.2: Postovulatory mucus

TABLE 16.1: Characteristics of cervical mucus	
Preovulatory	*Postovulatory*
Copious	Minimal
Watery	Thick
Acellular	Cellular
Low viscosity	Viscid
Spinnbarkeit and ferning	—
Allows sperm to pass through	Impenetrable to sperm
Associated with opening of the cervical os	Associated with closing of the cervical os

ETIOLOGY OF THE CERVICAL FACTOR

The cervix as the cause of female infertility is seen in less than 5 percent of all women. Factors that reduce the quality or the quantity of sperm, affect sperm viability and ultimately fertility (Table 16.2).

The cervix could become scarred or stenosed from previous surgery resulting in destruction of the cervical glands or obstruction to the sperm.

TABLE 16.2: Etiology of the cervical factor
1. Stenosis
2. Scarring
3. Infection
4. Immunological
5. Malposition
6. Congenital defects

Some of the common surgical procedures resulting in the above conditions include electrocauterization, LEEP, cone biopsy, etc. Occasionally, prenatal exposure to DES (Diethylstilbestrol) can cause stenosis and other cervical abnormalities.[1]

Chronic infection can destroy the endocervical glands, which are responsible for mucous secretion. Also, the accompanying leukocytic infiltration can destroy the sperms.

Antisperm antibodies-both IgG and IgA may be present in the cervical mucus. These will not only cause disordinate movements of the spermatozoa, but will also render them unable to penetrate the mucus.[2]

Even in the absence of humoral antibodies, upto 10 percent of infertile women will have antisperm antibodies in the cervical mucus—hence it is imperative to study the cervical mucus when there is poor sperm survival despite negative serological tests for antisperm antibodies.[3]

Lastly, and probably the commonest cause is the malpositioning of the cervix that is seen with acutely retroverted uteri. Here, the cervix will not be accessible to the pool of semen in the posterior vaginal fornix.

INVESTIGATION OF THE CERVICAL FACTOR

Careful questioning and a detailed history taken at the initial interview could indicate whether the cervix is the cause of infertility in a couple (Table 16.3).

TABLE 16.3: History to be elicited for assessing the cervical factor	
1. Surgery on the cervix	• Cone biopsy
	• Electrocauterization
	• LLETZ
	• Cryosurgery
2. Cervico-vaginal infections–chronic vaginal discharge, pruritis	
3. Prenatal exposure to diethylstilbestrol	

History of chronic vaginal discharge or irregular spotting per vaginum could indicate the presence of a chronic cervicovaginal infection.

Similarly, a history of surgery on the cervix may be associated with stenosis or scarring leading to a deficient mucus production. Prenatal exposure to diethylstilbestrol, although rare must be asked for.

Physical examination should include an adequate visualization of the cervix. This would not only reveal any anatomical defect, but also the presence of infection, and the state of the cervical mucus in synchrony with the phase of the menstrual cycle.

CERVICAL MUCUS SCORING

The cervical mucus is scored on a point system, based on its characteristics which are hormone dependant.

Insler's cervical score is based on the volume, ferning, Spinnbarkeit formation and the diameter of the external os.

Moghissi's cervical score, in addition to the volume, ferning and Spinnbarkeit formation also assesses the viscosity and cellularity

These scoring systems aid the systematic assessment of the cervical factor in an infertile woman.

A higher preovulatory cervical score indicates an adequate estrogen production from the growing follicles, while a lower cervical score is seen in the postovulatory phase under the influence of progesterone

POSTCOITAL TEST

The Sims-Huhner post-coital test is a simple method of identifying a cervical cause of infertility.[4]

Ever since its introduction in the 1900's, the validity of this test has been questioned time and again; with authors claiming both high and low predictive values.[5-7] However, it still forms a part of the basic investigations advised by the American Society of Reproductive Medicine for the initial evaluation of an infertile couple.

The test is a simple office procedure, which provides information on the coital technique and cervical mucus-sperm interaction (Figure 16.3).

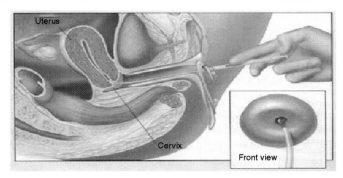

FIGURE 16.3: Postcoital testing

The Timing of the Postcoital Test

This test must be performed in the preovulatory or ovulatory phase of the menstrual cycle when the sperms will survive in the cervical mucus. If done at any other time the results may be grossly misleading.

In the 28-day menstrual cycle, the test should be carried out between D12 and 14. But if the cycles are irregular, the test may have to be repeated every 2 days to get an accurate result.

Some authors suggest regularization of the menstrual cycle by treatment with clomiphene citrate and then performing the test between D12 and 14.[8]

The couple is advised abstinence for a period of 2 to 4 days before the test, and then to report 10 to 12 hr after intercourse.

Though the sperm can be detected in the cervix approximately 90 seconds after intercourse, reporting later has the dual advantage of ascer-

taining whether the sperm can live for extended periods in the cervical mucus (sperm-mucus interaction) and allows for sexual relations in relatively "stress free" circumstances.[9]

The Procedure of the Postcoital Test

With the patient in the lithotomy position, a bivalve speculum, lubricated with warm water is inserted to allow for adequate visualization of the cervix. Vaginal secretions from the ectocervix are gently wiped off. Endocervical mucus is collected using a nasal forceps, tuberculin syringe or a plastic bacteriological loop. The mucus is evaluated for the following factors:

1. Volume of mucus
2. Clarity of mucus
3. Spinnbarkeit formation
4. Degree of cellularity
5. Number of motile sperm per high power field
6. Ferning

Clinical Significance of the Postcoital Test

The results of the postcoital test have been interpreted in many ways by different authors. Given below are some of the methods used for interpretation (Tables 16.4 and 16.5).

From the tables below it is evident that the average predictive value for all tests is approximately 30 percent. Eimers JM *et al*, who concluded their study with the fact that a positive result of the postcoital test was a strong indicator of

TABLE 16.4: Results of the postcoital test		
Results	*Qualification*	*Probability of pregnancy (%)*
No sperm seen	Negative	10
1 to 5 sperms/hpf or > 5 sperms with poor or no motility	Bad	24
< 5 sperms/hpf with medium motility or > 5 sperms/hpf with poor motility	Poor	40
< 5 sperms/hpf with good motility or > 5 sperms/hpf with medium motility	Fair	42
6 to 20 sperms/hpf with good motility	Good	44
> 20 sperms/hpf with excellent motility	Excellent	33
All tests		30

TABLE 16.5: Results of the postcoital test	
Results	*Probability of pregnancy (%)*
Negative	10
Positive with non-progressive motility of sperm	25
Positive with progressive motility of sperm	40
All tests	30

fertility in the subsequent year, described a more optimistic outcome.[10] However, in another study conducted by Glazener *et al*, the prognostic power of the postcoital test was found to be effective only when the infertility was less than 3 years of duration and when definite female factors were not found[10a] (Figures 16.4a and b).

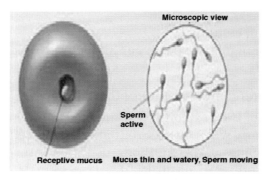

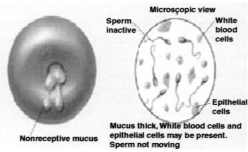

FIGURES 16.4A AND B

Abnormal Postcoital Test

The occurrence of an abnormal or negative post-coital test calls for definitive measures. Some of the factors that should be considered include the following:

1. Inappropriately timed test—this is probably the most common reason for an abnormal postcoital test.
2. Abnormal semen sample.
3. Absent or incomplete penile penetration.
4. Insufficient or inadequate vaginal ejaculation.
5. Cervical factor—Infection, destruction of the lining cells following prior surgical procedures.
6. Medications—antiestrogens especially clomiphene citrate are found to be associated with poor quality and quantity of cervical mucus.

Assessment of antisperm antibodies is indicated when there are no sperms, immotile sperms or those with abnormal or non-progressive motility.

Management of an Abnormal Postcoital Test

The management protocol for an abnormal post-coital test is given in the Flow Chart 16.1.

OTHER TESTS FOR SPERM-MUCUS INTERACTION

A number of tests have been developed to assess sperm-mucus interaction at various levels; though many of these may not be applicable in day-to-day practice. Some of these tests are described here.

Fractional Postcoital Test

Samples of cervical mucus collected from three different levels within the endocervical canal are analyzed. Usually a uniform distribution of sperms throughout the endocervical canal is seen. Some correlation could be identified between the sperm concentrations at different levels, though no association with pregnancy rates could be identified.[11]

Kurzok Miller In Vitro Sperm Penetration Test

Sperm penetration into the cervical mucus is assessed *in vitro*, on a glass slide. Though this test is easy to perform and quite accurate, it fails to reproduce the *in vivo* environment.

A modification of this test uses the sperm penetration meter, which has the added advantage of mimicking the *in vivo* conditions quite accurately.

Kremer's Capillary Tube Mucous Penetration Test

Square glass capillary tubes are used to assess sperm migration, velocity and direction through the cervical mucus.[12,12a]

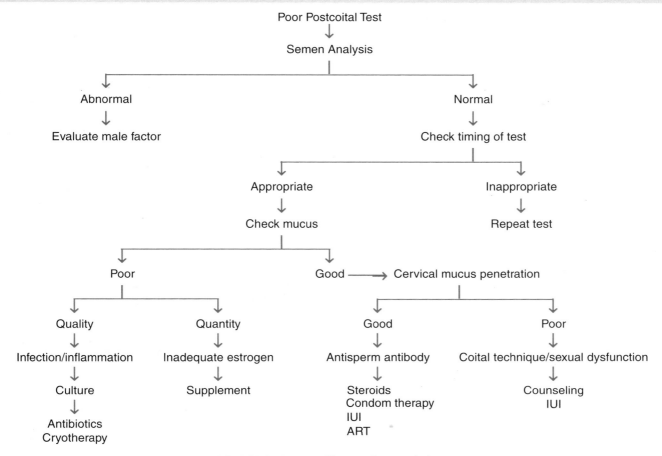

FLOW CHART 16.1: Abnormal postcoital test

TREATMENT OF CERVICAL FACTOR

Any infection is treated with appropriate antibiotics. Oral Doxycycline (100 mg 12th hrly) is usually used for a period of 2 weeks. It must be remembered that both the partners have to be treated simultaneously.

If there is no response, Cryotherapy to eliminate infection in the gland crypts may be necessary.

Oral mucolytics (e.g.-guaifenesin) have no role in improving the quality of the cervical mucus.

Poor mucus due to estrogen deficiency has been treated by estrogen supplementation from D8 to D16 of the cycle. This, however, does not result in significant improvement in the quality of the mucus.

The presence of antisperm antibodies can be treated by condom therapy that ensures no further exposure to sperm or by corticosteroid supplementation, which would act as an immuno-suppressant, by reducing the antibody production, as well as weakening the antigen-antibody association.

Some studies have shown significant reduction in the concentration of antibodies, especially IgG, while others have shown no effect.[13, 14] Pregnancy rates too do not show much difference. Considering these factors, there is no consensus on the use of corticosteroids for treatment of antisperm antibodies.[14a]

Persistently abnormal cervical factor would require intrauterine insemination—a process that completely bypasses the cervix altogether.

Assisted reproductive techniques especially intracytoplasmic sperm injection, has been used with considerable success in the treatment of antisperm antibodies. This is supposed to overcome any possible negative effect of the antibodies, which could affect sperm- zona binding leading to lower fertilization rates.[15] In fact the use of ICSI has resulted in much better fertilization as well as pregnancy rates in these women.[16]

POINTS TO REMEMBER

The cervical factor although rare, is an important cause of infertility in the female.

Though the validity of the Sims Huhner post-coital test is being questioned in current infertility investigation protocols, it does have a definite role in certain situations.

Immunological factors—presence of antisperm antibodies is a common cause of the cervical factor infertility.

Corticosteroids have not proven to be of much benefit for the treatment of antisperm antibodies.

Intrauterine insemination and ART have much better results in terms of fertilization, implantation and pregnancy rates in women with anti-sperm antibodies.

Estrogen supplementation and mucolytics have no role in the treatment of poor quality cervical mucus.

Effect on future fertility potential must always be kept in mind while performing any surgery on the cervix.

CERVICAL CHANGES DURING THE MENSTRUAL CYCLE

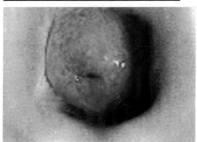

FIGURE 16.5A: The menstrual phase

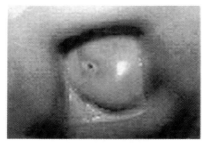

FIGURE 16.5B: The early follicular phase (Cervix is firm, os closed)

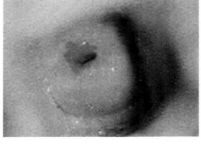

FIGURE 16.5C: The ovulatory phase (Cervix is soft, os open; mucus is thin, watery, acellular)

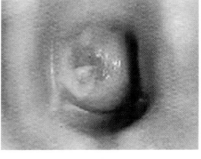

FIGURE 16.5D: The postovulatory phase (Cervix is firm, os closed, mucus is thick, scanty, cellular, viscid)

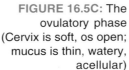

FIGURE 16.5E: The luteal phase (Cervix is firm, os closed, no mucus)

REFERENCES

1. Burke l, Antonioli D et al. Evolution of Diethylstilbestrol associated genital tract lesions. Obstet Gynecol 1981;57:79.
2. Kremer J. The immunology of cervical sterility: Its assessment and management. Contracept Fertil Sex (Paris). 1979;7(2):141-46.
3. Bronson RA et al. Factors affecting the population of the female reproductive tract by spermatozoa. Their diagnosis and treatment. Semin Reprod Endocrinol 1986;4:387.
4. Huhner M: Sterility in the female and treatment. Rebman, New York, 1913.
5. Griffith et al. The validity of the post-coital test. Am J Obstet Gynecol 1990;162:616-20.
6. Eimers JM et al. The validity of the post-coital test for estimating the probability of conceiving. Am J Obstet Gynecom 1994;171(1):65-70.
7. Glastein IZ et al. The reproducibility of the post coital test:A prospective study. Obstet Gynecol 1995;85:396-400.

8. Wilcox AJ et al. Timing of intercourse in relation to ovulation: Effects on probability of conception, survival of the pregnancy and sex of the baby. NJEM 1995;333: 1517.

9. Siebel MM et al. The emotional aspects of infertility. Fertile Steril 1982;37:137.

10. Eimers JM et al. The validity of the post-coital test for estimating the probability of conceiving. Am J Obstet Gynecol 1994;171(1):65-70.

10a. Glazener CM, Ford WC, Hull MG. The prognostic power of the post-coital test for natural conception depends on duration of infertility. Hum Reprod. 2000;15(9): 1953-57.

11. Drake et al. A reassessment of the fractional post-coital test. Am J Obstet Gynecol 1979;133:382.

12. Kremer J. A simple sperm penetration test. Int J Fertil 1965;10:209.

12a. Kroeks MV, Kremer J. The fractional post-coital test performed in a square capillary tube. Acta Eur Fertil. 1975;6(4):371-75.

13. Alexander NJ et al. Pregnancy rates in patients treated for antisperm antibodies with prednisolone. Int J Fertil 1982;28:83-67.

14. Haas GG et al. A double blind placebo controlled study of the use of methylprednisolonein infertile men with sperm associated immunoglobulins. Fertil Steril 1987;47:295-301.

14a. Bals-Pratsch M, Doren M, Karbowski B, Schneider HP, Nieschlag E. Cyclic corticosteroid immunosuppression is unsuccessful in the treatment of sperm antibody-related male infertility: A controlled study. Hum Reprod 1992;7(1):99-104.

15. Lahteenmaki A et al. Treatment of severe male immunological infertility by intracytoplasmic sperm injection.Hum Reprod 1995;10:2824-28.

16. Daitoh T et al. High implantation rate and consequently high pregnancy rate by IVF-ET treatment in women withantisperm antibodies. Fertil Steril 1995;63: 87-91.

THE ROLE OF THE UTERUS
IN REPRODUCTION

The uterus not only serves as a conduit for the transfer of sperm from the vagina/cervix, into the fallopian tube, but also has the very important function of nurturing the embryo and carrying the fetus to term.

Infertility is explained by uterine factors in only a minority of cases; in approximately 5 percent. Uterine pathology such as fibroids, congenital anomalies, polyps, etc. are more often associated with miscarriages than with infertility.[1]

TABLE 16.6: Uterine causes of infertility—anatomical
1. Intrauterine adhesions
2. Leiomyoma
3. Endometrial polyps
4. Adenomyosis
5. Congenital uterine defects
6. Infections-tuberculosis

Intrauterine Adhesions

Intrauterine adhesions responsible for infertility usually follow curettage for a pregnancy related complication (Figure 16.6).

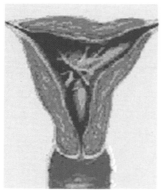

FIGURE 16.6: Diagrammatic representation of intrauterine scar tissue

Scar tissue in the uterine cavity can affect implantation, as well as increase the risk of miscarriage.

Asherman's syndrome is defined by the National Fertility Association, as the presence of scar tissue within the endometrial cavity. It usually follows endometrial curettage after a spontaneous, incomplete or elective abortion. Another more likely cause is curettage for post-partum hemorrhage.

Intrauterine adhesions have been classified (depending on their extent and nature) into mild, moderate and severe (Table 16.8).[2]

TABLE 16.7: Uterine causes of infertility-functional
1. Luteal phase defect
2. Thin-non receptive endometrium
3. Integrin deficiency

TABLE 16.8: Classification of intrauterine adhesions
• Mild—thin, filmy; consisting mostly of endometrial tissue
• Moderate—thick fibromuscular, covered by endometrial tissue
• Severe—dense connective tissue

Another classification proposed by March CM, Israel R *et al* is based on the degree of occlusion of the uterine cavity (Table 16.9).[3]

TABLE 16.9: Classification of intrauterine adhesions	
A —	Less than 1/4th of uterine cavity involved; thin flimsy adhesions;ostia and fundus minimally involved or clear.
B —	1/4th to 3/4th of uterine cavity involved; no agglutination of walls;ostia and upper fundus only partially involved.
C —	More than 3/4th of uterine cavity involved; agglutination of walls or thick bands seen;osta and upper cavity occluded.

Leiomyoma

Leiomyomas are benign tumors of the uterine musculature.

It is rather difficult to assess their effect on fertility, as many women with leiomyomas have no difficulty in conception.[4] Nevertheless, it has been postulated that fibroids could hamper fertility in a number of ways—from mechanical obstruction to alterations in blood flow, which could adversely affect implantation.

Probably the more common types of fibroids that adversely affect reproduction (unless very large) are the submucus and the intra-cavitary types. Sub serous fibroids rarely affect fertility.[5, 6]

TABLE 16.10: Effect of leiomyomas on fertility
Alter uterine contractility–affect sperm transport
Obstruct uterine cavity/tubal ostia–affect sperm transport
Distort uterine cavity–affect sperm transport
affect embryo transport
Alter position of the cervix–compromises exposure to semen
Associated endometrial thinning/infection/altered vascularity–affects implantation embryo growth

Endometrial Polyps

Most small endometrial polyps do not affect reproduction, but the larger polyps can, very much in the same manner as a submucous myoma. Sometimes small polyps may be present at the tubal ostia.

Mucus polyps must be differentiated from hyperplastic endometrium and myomata.In contrast to the myomas, which are fixed, the polyps gently float when the uterine cavity is being distended with fluid.

Adenomyosis

Adenomyosis is the growth of the endometrial lining of the uterus within the uterine myometrium.

Congenital Uterine Anomalies

Anomalies of the Mullerian system are seen in about 2 to 3 percent of all women; and, approximately 25 percent of these will have associated infertility. Though in general, congenital uterine defects in isolation are more often found to be associated with recurrent pregnancy loss than infertility.The most common congenital defect associated with infertility is the septate uterus.

The American Fertility Society (1988) has categorized Mullerian anomalies into the following seven classes.[7]

Class 1—Hypoplasia/Agenesis

This includes entities such as uterine/cervical agenesis or hypoplasia. The most common form is the Mayer-Rokitansky-Küster-Hauser syndrome,

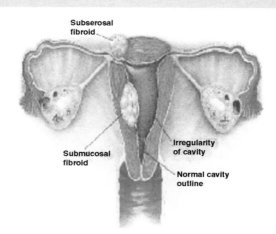

FIGURE 16.7: Diagrammatic representation of the uterine cavity distorted by submucous fibroids

which is combined agenesis of the uterus, cervix, and upper portion of the vagina. Patients have no reproductive potential aside from medical intervention in the form of in vitro fertilization of harvested ova and gestational surrogacy.

Class 2—Unicornuate Uterus

A unicornuate uterus is the result of complete, or almost complete, arrest of development of 1 müllerian duct .If the arrest is incomplete, as in 90 percent of patients, a rudimentary horn with or without functioning endometrium is present. If the rudimentary horn is obstructed, it may come to surgical attention when presenting as an enlarging pelvic mass. If the contralateral healthy horn is almost fully developed, a full-term pregnancy is believed to be possible (Figure 16.8).

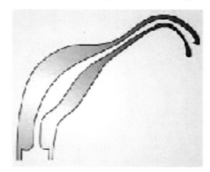

FIGURE 16.8: Unicornuate uterus—Complete development of one and failure of development of the other müllerian duct

Class 3—Uterus Didelphys

This anomaly results from the complete nonfusion of both müllerian ducts .The individual horns are

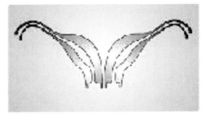

FIGURE 16.9: Uterus didelphys—Complete but separate development of each müllerian duct

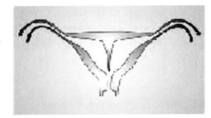

FIGURE 16.11: Septate uterus—The midline septum may be fibrous or muscular and of varying lengths

fully developed and almost normal in size. Two cervices are inevitably present. A longitudinal or transverse vaginal septum may be noted as well. Didelphys uteri have the highest association with transverse vaginal septa but septa also may be observed in other anomalies. Consider metroplasty; however, since each horn is almost a fully developed uterus, patients have been known to carry pregnancies to term.

Class 4—Bicornuate Uterus

A bicornuate uterus results from the partial nonfusion of the müllerian ducts. The central myometrium may extend to the level of the internal cervical os *(Bicornuate Unicollis)* or external cervical os *(Bicornuate Bicollis)*. The latter is distinguished from didelphys uterus because it demonstrates some degree of fusion between the two horns, while in classic didelphys uterus, the two horns and cervices are separated completely. In addition, the horns of the bicornuate uteri are not fully developed; typically, they are smaller than those of didelphys uteri. Some of these women are candidates for metroplasty.

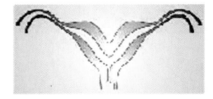

FIGURE 16.10: Bicornuate uterus—Partial fusion of the lower uterine segments. The upper segments remain separated

Class 5—Septate Uterus

A septate uterus results from failure of the resorption of the septum between the two uterine horns. The septum can be partial or complete, in which case it extends to the internal cervical os.

Histologically, the septum may be composed of myometrium or fibrous tissue. The uterine fundus is typically convex but may be flat or slightly concave (< 1 cm fundal cleft). Women with septate uterus have the highest incidence of reproductive complications. Differentiation between a septate and a bicornuate uterus is important because septate uteri are treated using transvaginal hysteroscopic resection of the septum, while if surgery is possible and/or indicated for the bicornuate uterus, an abdominal approach is required to perform metroplasty.

Class 6—Arcuate Uterus

An arcuate uterus has a single uterine cavity with a convex or flat uterine fundus, the endometrial cavity, which demonstrates a small fundal cleft or impression ($\geq$ 1.5 cm). The outer contour of the uterus is convex or flat. This form is often considered a normal variant since it is not significantly associated with the increased risks of pregnancy loss and the other complications found in other subtypes.

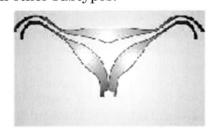

FIGURE 16.12: Arcuate uterus—Mild thickening of the fundal myometrium results in a fundal cavity indentation with a normal outer contour

Class 7—Diethylstilbestrol Related Anomalies

From the 1940s to the 1970s, several women have been treated with diethylstilbestrol (an estrogen

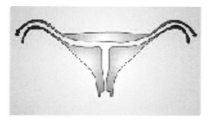

FIGURE 16.13: Diethylstilbestrol exposed uterus—Diethylstilbestrol causes myometrial hypertrophy—resulting in an irregular, small, T Shaped uterine cavity

analog prescribed to prevent miscarriage). The drug was withdrawn once its teratogenic effects on the reproductive tracts of male and female fetuses were understood. The uterine anomaly is seen in the female offspring of upto 15 percent of women exposed to DES during pregnancy. Female fetuses who are affected have a variety of abnormal findings that include uterine hypoplasia and a T-shaped uterine cavity. Patients also may have abnormal transverse ridges, hoods, stenoses of the cervix, and adenosis of the vagina with increased risk of vaginal clear cell carcinoma.

Tuberculosis

One of the commonest symptoms of pelvic tuberculosis is primary infertility. This is most commonly due to Tuberculous salpingitis. It may be seen in 60 to 70 percent of women even though the fallopian tubes may be patent-indicating abnormal tubal/endometrial function.[8]

Ovulatory disorders with tuberculosis may present with absent, excessive or non-cyclical menstruation, largely attributable to ovarian involvement (40% of cases) and uterine (endometrial) tuberculosis (30%).

Local tuberculous lesions may appear on the cervix and vagina.

It has also been suggested that any woman with infertility that cannot be attributed to a specific cause should be investigated for tuberculosis.

The luteal phase defect is characterized by a defect in which the endometrium either is not exposed to enough progesterone or does not respond properly to the progesterone that is produced. As a result the endometrium does not undergo the changes necessary to allow implantation to occur.

However, one must add that many investigators have failed to find any correlation between luteal phase defects and fecundity in infertile women.[9, 10]

The luteal phase defect is covered in detail elsewhere in this manual.

Endometrial receptivity Endometrial receptivity for the implanting embryo has come under intense scrutiny over the last few years, as this is regarded as the rate-limiting step in reproduction. Normal endometrium usually develops to a thickness, as measured by ultrasound, of around eight to ten millimeters.

Integrins Integrins are the proteins that are responsible for intercellular adhesion, and thus play an important role in implantation. Deficiency of the same will obviously have a deleterious effect on implantation.

INVESTIGATION OF THE UTERINE FACTOR

Pertinent history that would indicate the involvement of the uterus should include the following:

1. History of prenatal exposure to Diethylstilbestrol
2. Menstrual history—for example, a woman with significant intrauterine adhesions may complain of oligomenorrhea or amenorrhea.

    Pelvic Tuberculosis can present with a spectrum of menstrual disorders ranging from primary or secondary amenorrhea (14.3%), menorrhagia (19%), metrorrhagia and oligomenorrhea. Dysmenorrhea is very uncommon.
3. Prior surgery on the uterus-including D and C, therapeutic abortions, etc.
4. History suggestive of Tuberculosis/exposure to the infection—Previous H/o peritonitis, appendicectomy with slow healing, pleurisy, prolonged illness in childhood, family H/o tuberculosis and childhood contact.

Physical examination should pay attention to the size, position and mobility of the uterus and the presence of any palpable pelvic pathology.

The importance of assessing the uterine cavity cannot be underestimated in an infertile patient. To lose a pregnancy after assisted reproduction due to a preventable or correctable uterine factor is indeed a tragedy! Methods of assessing the uterine factor are listed below in Tables 16.11 and 16.12.

TABLE 16.11: Methods of assessing the uterine factor
1. Hysterosalpingogram
2. Ultrasound
3. Hydrosonography
4. Doppler study of uterine blood flow
5. Hysteroscopy
6. Magnetic Resonance imaging
7. D and C with endometrial biopsy

Table 16.12: Evaluation of endometrial receptivity
1. Assess luteal phase defect
2. Transvaginal ultrasound
3. Doppler study of uterine blood flow patterns
4. Endometrial biopsy—integrin assay

A Hysterosalpingogram is performed after the cessation of menses and before ovulation; it allows visualization of the intrauterine cavity. This test is particularly helpful in detecting uterine abnormalities such as a bicornuate uterus or septate uterus, scar tissue, polyps, and

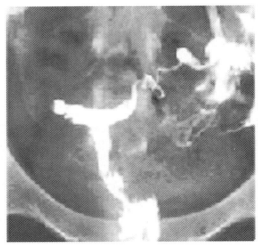

FIGURE 16.16: Diethylstilbestrol exposed hypoplastic T shaped uterus

fibroids as well as establishing the patency of the fallopian tubes. The most important disadvantage of the HSG is that it does not show the external contour of the uterus—a fact that makes it hard to differentiate between septate and bicornuate uteri as well as identify the presence of a non-communicating horn.

Ultrasound has been discussed elsewhere. Transvaginal ultrasound is an easy, rapid and non-invasive method of assessing the endometrium.

While extensive research has been carried out on whether the thickness and reflectivity of the endometrium as assessed by ultrasound can be used to predict implantation, there is yet no consensus on the same. It has been suggested that a hyperechoic endometrium of 6 mm or less in the preovulatory phase is associated with a 100 percent negative predictive value for conception.[11, 12]

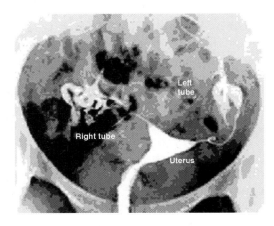

FIGURE 16.14: A normal hysterosalpingogram (Uniform triangular uterine cavity with copious spill from both tubes)

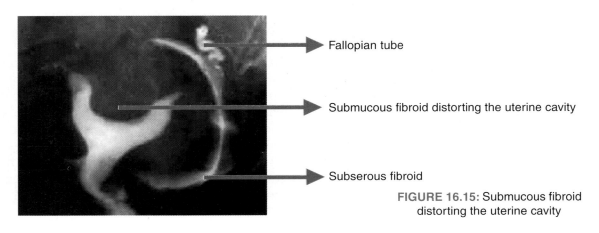

Fallopian tube

Submucous fibroid distorting the uterine cavity

Subserous fibroid

FIGURE 16.15: Submucous fibroid distorting the uterine cavity

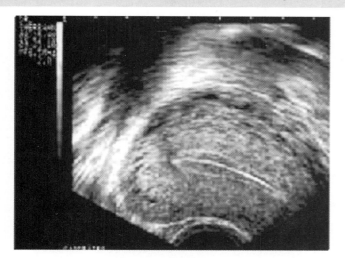

FIGURE 16.17: Ultrasound picture of the characteristic "triple line" endometrium seen in the preovulatory phase

Hydrosonography involves instillation of Saline into the uterine cavity followed by ultrasound. The rationale behind this is that distension of the cavity would allow for visualization of intrauterine pathology such as polyps.

Uterine perfusion assessed by Doppler has also been used to assess endometrial receptivity and predict implantation. Higher uterine flow rates are associated with a positive pregnancy outcome, while a negative outcome was seen with absent diastolic flow.[13, 14]

Some studies have failed to find any association between uterine blood flow and pregnancy rates.[15]

Magnetic resonance imaging is a very useful tool for the diagnosis of uterine anomalies. It provides high-resolution images of the uterine body, fundus, and internal structure, and in addition helps to evaluate the urinary tract for associated anomalies. The disadvantages of this technique are that the image quality is operator dependant, and the prohibitive cost. MRI cannot be performed in patients who have pacemakers, are claustrophobic or are obese.

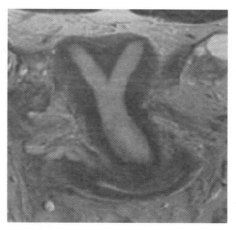

FIGURE 16.19: MRI image of a septate uterus

Of all these methods, the "gold standard" or the ideal technique would be the direct visualization of the uterine cavity by *Diagnostic Hysteroscopy*. Before starting any form of Assisted Reproduction therapy, the uterine cavity must be assessed either by a Diagnostic Hysteroscopy or a Hysterosalpingogram.

While the American Society of Reproductive Medicine includes only the Hysterosalpingogram as the base-line investigation for the uterine factor, diagnostic hysteroscopy is gradually gaining popularity as a first-line investigation.[16]

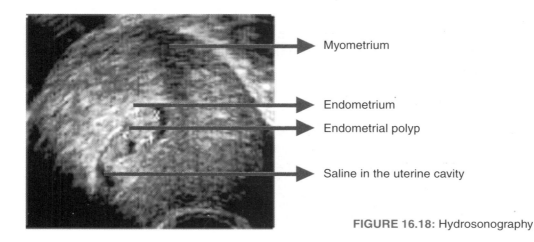

Myometrium

Endometrium

Endometrial polyp

Saline in the uterine cavity

FIGURE 16.18: Hydrosonography

TABLE 16.13: Indications for diagnostic hysteroscopy

1. History of IUCD use
2. History of surgery on the uterus
3. History suggestive of endometritis
4. History suggestive of pelvic inflammatory disease
5. History of tuberculosis
6. Long-standing unexplained infertility
7. Recurrent miscarriages
8. Intrauterine lesion suspected on hysterosalpingogram or ultrasound
9. Failure of implantation in upto 3 IVF cycles

TABLE 16.14: Indications for operative hysteroscopy

1. Intrauterine adhesions
2. Submucous fibroids
3. Endometrial polyps
4. Septate uterus

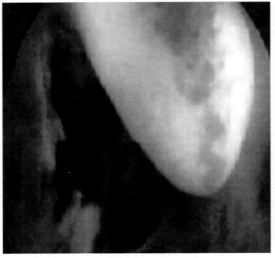

FIGURE 16.21: Endometrial polyp at hysteroscopy

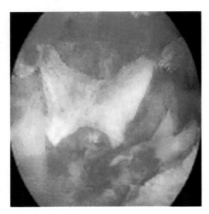

FIGURE 16.20: Hysteroscopic appearance of intrauterine scar tissue (white)

One of the overwhelming advantages of Hysteroscopy is that it not only permits adequate direct visualization of the uterine cavity and diagnosis of intrauterine lesions, but also allows for therapeutic intervention at the same sitting.

Pregnancy rates after such procedures have been found to be very good in both infertility and following recurrent miscarriages.[17]

The diagnosis of pelvic tuberculosis may be confirmed by histopathological examination, direct smear with Ziehl-Neelsen staining, culture and polymerase chain reaction (Table 16.15).

Operative Hysteroscopy, as well as the role of ultrasound, Doppler study of uterine blood flow, Hysterosalpingogram and the role of endometrial biopsy in evaluating the uterine factor in infertility are discussed elsewhere in this manual. Though many methods have been described to assess endometrial receptivity, their usefulness is severely limited by the fact that the positive predictive value of these tests is negligible. Better modalities have to be established to accurately predict a receptive endometrium.

TABLE 16.15: Investigations for tuberculosis

Biopsy of suspect lesions	Ziehl-Neelsen staining
Pre-menstrual endometrial aspiration	Culture in Lowenstein Jenson medium
Collection of first day menstrual discharge	Histopathological examination

Polymerase Chain Reaction–Genus specific 16S rRNA PCR Test.
Species specific IS 6110 PCR Test.
Roche Amplicar MTB PCR Test.
Amplified Mycobacterium Tuberculosis Direct detect test (AMDT)

Other tests (not widely used)–Luciferase and fluorescent techniques
High performance liquid chromatography (HPLC)
DNA probe

Treatment of the Uterine Factor

Ashermans syndrome/intrauterine adhesions are quite effectively treated by hysteroscopic lysis of the scar tissue. This is usually followed by replenishment of the endometrial lining by estrogen supplementation for a period of at least 2 months following surgery.

An IUCD is also inserted to prevent scar tissue from reforming and causing recurrence of adhesions during this time. The same is removed once the medications are discontinued.

An alternative approach would be to perform a second look hysteroscopy, about 6 weeks later and remove any residual adhesions if present. Details of the surgical procedure are described elsewhere in this manual.

Leiomyomata of the uterus can be managed in a variety of ways—both medical and surgical.

There are a number of drugs that can be used to treat fibroids (Table 16.16). With the trend towards non-invasive therapy, these could represent a major treatment option.

TABLE 16.16: Drugs used in the treatment of fibroids
i. Combined oral contraceptive pills
ii. Progesterone-oral/parenteral
iii. GnRH analogs
iv. RU 486
v. Gestrinone

Myomectomy is a procedure used to excise fibroids out of their uterine bed. This can be done either by laparotomy or laparoscopically. Submucous fibroids may be excised using the operative hysteroscope. This is the most common procedure used for the treatment of "infertility associated" fibroids.

Most of the other techniques described briefly below are not very well accepted because of the inadequate information available of their effect on future fertility.

Cryomyolysis uses a probe to freeze the tumor, and cause shrinkage and death of the cells.

Myoma coagulation is a laparoscopic procedure where electric current is applied to the tumor which causes coagulation of its blood supply as well as the smooth muscle cells. This approach is best used either alone or in combination with laparoscopic myomectomy when multiple tumors are encountered. It helps avoid tedious laparoscopic removal of multiple fibroids.

Selective uterine artery embolization has been documented to stop growth and promote shrinkage of fibroids in addition to controlling hemorrhage. Though most studies do not report any deleterious effect on fertility, further studies are necessary to document the same before the safety index of this procedure can be established.

Septate uterus is treated surgically. The intervening septum is removed either by hysteroscopy or laparotomy. Review of literature revealed successful pregnancies in upto 80 percent of women who have undergone metroplasty.

Tuberculosis has to be treated with a complete course of chemotherapy. Genital tuberculosis has the advantage of lower bacteria load, and hence responds well to short course chemotherapy. In general, standard drug treatment should include Rifampicin, INH, Pyrizinamide and Ethambutol for 2 months followed by administration of 2 drugs, i.e. INH and Rifampicin for four more months unless resistance to either agent exist. If the patient is HIV positive-drug treatment should be continued for 9 months.

Some of the common regimes used are listed in Table 16.17.

TABLE 16.17: Chemotherapy regimes for genital tuberculosis		
Regime-I	First 2 months daily INH, Rifampicin and Pyrizinamide	Next 2 months 3 times a week INH and Rifampicin
Regime-II	4 months 3 times a week INH, Rifampicin and Pyrizinamide	May promote multidrug resistance
Regime-III	First 2 months daily INH, Rifampicin, Pyrizinamide and SM or Ethambutol	Next 2 months 3 times a week INH, Rifampicin add SM or Ethambutol if resistance is anticipated

Endometrial biopsy has to be repeated 6 months to 1 year after therapy, to test for cure.

Restoration of fertility depends upon the severity and the extent of the disease process. Some authors have indicated that spontaneous conception is possible within 2 to 9 months of starting anti-tuberculosis therapy.[18] If the fallopian tubes are already blocked, permanent sterility is likely, but if they are open and scarred, there will always be the risk of tubal implantation. Tubal reconstruction is not advised.

Miscarriages are also common with intra-uterine pregnancies in these women.

Probably, the best treatment option for conception would be *in vitro* fertilization and embryo transfer.

Irreparable uterine factors may prevent a woman from conceiving or carrying a pregnancy to term, but does not preclude her from having her own genetic offspring. The use of IVF with a gestational host would allow for embryos from such a woman and her partner to be transferred to the uterus of a gestational host who could carry the pregnancy to term.

REFERENCES

1. Bulletti C et al. Reproductive failure due to spontaneous abortion and recurrent miscarriage. Hum Reprod Update 1996;2:118-36.
2. Valle R F et al. Intrauterine adhesions, Hysteroscopic diagnosis, classification, treatment and reproductive outcome. Am J Obstet Gynecol 1988;158:1459-70.
3. March CM, Israel R et al. Hysteroscopic management of Intra-uterine adhesions. Am J Obstet Gynecol 1978; 653.
4. Buttram V C Jr et al. Uterine leiomyomata: Etiology, symptomatology and management. Fertil Steril 1981;36: 433.
5. Bajekal N et al. Fibroids, fertility and pregnancy wastage. Hum Reprod Update 2000;6(6):614-20.
6. Eldar-Geva T et al. Effect of intramural, subserosal and submucous fibroids on the outcome of assistd reproductive technology treatment. Fertil Steril 1998;70(4): 687-91.
7. The American Fertility Society classifications of adnexal adhesions, distal tubal occlusion, tubal occlusion secondary to tubal ligation, tubal pregnancies, mullerian anomalies and intrauterine adhesions. Fertil Steril 1988;49(6):944-55.
8. Parikh FR et al. Genital tuberculosis—A major pelvic factor causing infertility in Indian women. Fertility and Sterility 1997;67(3):497-500.
9. Wentz AC et al. The impact of luteal phase inadequacy in an infertile population. Am J Obstet Gynecol 1990; 162:937.
10. Driessen F et al. The significance of dating an endometrial biopsy for the prognosis of an infertile couple. Int J Fertil 1980;25:112.
11. Shoham Z et al. Is it possible to run a successful ovulation induction program based solely on ultrasound monitoring? The importance of endometrial measurements. Fertil Steril 1991;56:836.
12. Gonen Y et al. Prediction of implantation by the sonographic appearance of the endometrium during controlled ovarian hyperstimulation for in vitro fertilization. J In Vitro Fertil Embryo Transf 1990; 7:146.
13. Steer CV et al. The use of transvaginal color flow imaging after in vitro fertilization to identify optimal uterine conditions before embryo transfer. Fertil Steril 1991;57:372.
14. Sterzik K et al. Doppler sonographic findings and their correlation with implantation in an IVF program. Fertil Steril 1989;52:825.
15. Bassil S et al. Uterine vascularity during stimulation and its correlation with implantation in IVF. Hum Reprod 1995;10:1497.
16. Golan A et al. Diagnostic Hysteroscopy: Its value in an IVF-ET unit. Fertil. Steril 1992;58:1237-39.
17. Ubalsi F et al. Fertility after hysteroscopic myomectomy. Hum Reprod Update 1996;(1):81-90.
18. John M, Kukkady Z. Genital tuberculosis and infertility. International Journal of Gynecology and Obstetrics 1999;64:193-94.

• Sadhana Desai • Partha G Roy

17

Tubal Factor of Infertility and Assisted Reproduction

INTRODUCTION

Impaired tubal function is one of the important causes of female infertility. It is responsible for 25 percent of female infertility (Sorensen 1980). The degree of tubal obstruction, presence of endosalpingeal destruction and presence of peritubal adhesions are the factors which cause this type of female infertility. For many years the standard treatment of tubal factor of infertility used to be surgery.

However results of tubal surgery using conventional techniques were rather poor. After introduction of microsurgery from 1970 onwards the results have improved. The birth of Louise Brown in 1978 by IVF/ET started a new era in infertility treatment (Edward RG 1987). The assisted reproductive technology was originally meant only for women with tubal factor of infertility, especially women with irreparably blocked tubes, women with history of failed tuboplasty, women with history of bilateral salpingectomy due to either PID or due to previous ectopic pregnancies. With advancements in ART over a period of years, ART technology has now become less invasive and more popular. With more and more ART centers being established all over the world, the treatment for all the causes of tubal infertility has witnessed a shift from microsurgery to IVF/ET.

TUBAL SURGERY VS ART

In the year 1990 operative laparoscopy was introduced to promote fertility in women with tubal disease and tubal microsurgery by laparotomy were partially replaced by laparoscopic microsurgery. Today women with pelvic adhesions, women requiring recanalization of fallopian tubes following tubectomy operations are treated by microsurgery rather than by ART procedures (Oelsner G *et al* 1994).

In patients with flimsy adhesions, cumulative pregnancy rate after 24 months is 68 percent following microscopic adhesiolysis (Diamond E, 1979). This is clearly better than five IVF cycles. Adhesiolysis is, therefore, the preferred treatment in such cases. However, the pregnancy rate sharply falls to 19 percent in the presence of dense adhesions following microscopic adhesiolysis. Therefore, patients with dense adhesions and frozen pelvis are best treated by IVF. In women with proximal tubal obstruction it is found that the term pregnancy rate with tubocornual anastomoses or by tubal catheterization procedures are 45 percent when affected segment of isthmus is < 1 cm. It falls to 22 percent when affected segment of isthmus is > 1 cm. The success rate of microsurgery for distal tubal obstruction strictly depends on pre-existing tubal disease (Donnez *et al* 1986a). Large hydrosalpinx give poor outcome while fimbrial phimoses can be treated successfully by laparoscopic microsurgery. Today, IVF and tubal microsurgery must be considered as complementary rather than competitive procedures.

Tubal Infertility and Factors Affecting the ART Results

In past two decades besides tubal infertility, ART is also indicated for other causes of infertility namely male fertility (ICSI procedure), unexplained infertility and endometriosis. Therefore, it is now possible to compare the pregnancy rates following IVF in women with tubal factor of infertility vs women with other factors of infertility.

Templeton *et al* in 1996 noticed that women with tubal factor of infertility had lower implantation rate than women with unexplained fertility undergoing ART, although the author found no difference in live birth rate in these two groups.

Many factors affect the IVF success rate in tubal infertility including the age of the women, the quality of controlled ovarian stimulation, the quality and number of embryos transferred, endometrial receptivity and most important of all the cause of the tubal damage and presence of hydrosalpinx.

It has been shown by Csemiczky *et al* from Sweden that high tubal damage is associated with low pregnancy rate in women undergoing IVF/ET. This study from Stockholm, Sweden showed that patients with milder tubal damage had considerably higher take-home baby rate per started cycle (48%) than patients with severe tubal damage who had take-home baby rate of 6 percent only. The authors also found lower ovarian response in women with severe tubal damage.This group of women needed more gonadotropin ampoules per cycle and had lower E2 levels prior to ovum pick up.

ROLE OF HYDROSALPINX IN SUCCESS OF IVF

In recent years, there has been great debate regarding whether presence of hydrosalpinx adversely affects the IVF success rate and whether the surgical removal of hydrosalpinx prior to IVF improves the pregnancy rate or not.

A meta-analysis of fifteen published retrospective studies comprising of 5592 patients by E Camus *et al,* 1999 showed negative consequences on pregnancy rate, implantation rate, live birth rate in women with tubal infertility with hydrosalpinx undergoing IVF than women with tubal infertility without hydrosalpinx undergoing IVF.

The main mechanisms by which the presence of a hydrosalpinx may exert a negative effect on IVF outcome are considered to be, flushing the embryos into a damaged fallopian tube at the time of embryo transfer and leakage of hydrosalpinx fluid into the uterine cavity rendering environment toxic to embryo *in vivo* (Mukherjee *et al* 1996) or flushing out the embryo from the uterine site.

It has been suggested that adrenergic denervation and subsequent disturbance of ovum myosalpingeal transport might explain the poor pregnancy rate in cases with hydrosalpinx (Donnez 1986).

The epithelial endometrial alpha v beta 3 integrin levels as a marker of endometrial receptivity were also found to be significantly reduced in concentration in patients with hydrosalpinx as compared to controls (Meyer *et al* 1997).

However, in a prospective randomised multicentric trial of nine Nordic IVF Centres, (Strandell *et al* 1999) which had recruited 204 patients, it was shown that salpingectomy can be recommended for only a subgroup of women in whom bilateral hydrosalpinx is enlarged enough to be visible on ultrasound.In this series the diagnosis of hydrosalpinx was made by prior HSG or diagnostic laparoscopy in women where reconstructive surgery had been rejected.

Hydrosalpinx with a diameter > 3 cm prior to COH has high chances of enlargement during ovarian stimulation and reflux of fluid into the endometrial cavity impairing implantation of the embryo. Instead of salpingectomy, ultrasonographic aspiration of hydrosalpinx at the time of ovum pick up, just prior to ovarian stimulation has been recommended by VanVoorha *et al* 1986, while others recommend proximal tubal interruption. Indiscriminate salpingectomies of women with hydrosalpinx are clearly not the consensus.

The hydrosalpinx that is visible on transvaginal sonography is now proposed as a new clinical entity, (de Wit. *et al* 1998), although diagnostic and pathophysiological features of this sub-group is poorly defined. Several authors describe enlargement of hydrosalpinx during ovarian stimulation (Hill *et al* 1986, Andersen *et al* 1996, Bloechle *et al* 1997, Sharara FI, McClamrock HD. 1997). The mechanism of enlargement of hydrosalpinx during ovarian stimulation is unknown. In experimental conditions, distal occlusion results in a very slow distension of the mechanically increasing hydrosalpinx taking more than 12 weeks. It is speculated that uterine proximal zone contractions play a fundamental role in movements of both uterine and tubal fluid. The wave frequency of junctional zone is higher in IVF cycles than in spontaneous cycles (Fanchin R *et al* 1998) and (IJlanda *et al* 1999).

The altered fluid movements caused by junctional zone contractions during ovarian stimulation in the presence of thin walled hydrosalpinx could be responsible for an adverse effect, viz. by acting as a mechanical barrier to embryo implantation (Mansour *et al* 1991, Edwards 1992). The fluid component itself has no cytotoxicity or adverse effect on normal development of human embryos and their implantation.

The adverse effects of hydrosalpinx in natural cycle IVF where there is no ovarian stimulation and no increased pressure in the hydrosalpinx by the enlarged ovary are also reported by some authors. Zeyneloglu *et al* in meta-analysis of 2 retrospective studies have shown that adverse effect was present in such cycles, while Fahy *et al* in 1995 observed higher success rate during IVF in natural cycles in women with tubal disease as compared to unexplained infertility. A prospective study by Janssens *et al* in 1999 in 50 women with tubal infertility also confirms this finding. It is felt that the time has not yet arrived to recommend indiscriminate preventive salpingectomy for hydrosalpinx.

TUBAL INFERTILITY AND IMPLANTATION RATE

Endometrial damage occurring simultaneously with acute phase of tubal damage may be responsible for alteration in uterine receptivity (Strandell *et al* 1999). Hydrosalpinx also adversely affects implantation in donor oocyte programme (Cohen MA *et al* 1999) with lower implantation rate 7.1 vs 19.3 percent and higher miscarriage rate, 75 vs 14.9 percent and a higher ectopic pregnancy rate. The authors suggest that the intrauterine environment is altered by the same pathogens that cause hydrosalpinx. *Chlamydia trachomatis* infection of endometrium should be considered as a possible cause of decreased implantation in recipients of donated oocytes (Mansour RT *et al* 1991). Chlamydia infection causes tubal infertility and increases the risks of tubal pregnancy. Successful treatment of chlamydia infection improves the pregnancy outcome. Higher proportion of chlamydia infection are asymptomatic and may not be recognized clinically.

However, chlamydia can be identified in endometrial tissue with the use of PCR analysis. Either chlamydia organisms or tissue reaction to infection may be responsible for impaired implantation.

Research is required to see whether a prophylactic course of an appropriate antibiotic before recipient cycle can improve implantation rate in women with tubal factor of infertility (Sharara *et al* 1997).

Tuberculosis is another etiological factor which besides causing tubal infertility affects the endometrium in 50 percent of women (Desai SK *et al* 1997) thus reducing the pregnancy rate. When the disease affects endometrium it may cause intrauterine adhesions or fibrosis of basal layer of endometrium in severe form and then the endometrium does not respond to exogenous estrogen therapy. During periovulatory phase endometrium remains < 8 mm, affecting the success of IVF/ET. The color Doppler study of endometrium in these women also shows high resistance flow in spiral vessels of endometrium. Desai SK *et al* 2000 in their study of assisted reproduction in histopathologically proved cases of genital TB, showed that no pregnancy occurred when ET was less than 8 mm at the time of ovum pick up.

Whenever tuberculosis causes intrauterine adhesions the synechiae are very thick and hysteroscopic synechiolysis is not very successful in these cases. Gurgan T *et al* 1996 reported that total corporeal synechiae due to tuberculosis carry a poor prognosis and synechiae recur in 3 to 4 months. Then surrogacy is the only option in this group of women.

Tubal Infertility and Ovarian Function

Whenever there is tubal infertility due to genital TB, the ovaries also get involved by the disease process in 50 percent of cases, leading to impairment of ovarian function either causing cycle cancellation or poor ovarian response even in the young patients. The authors found this in 42 of the women of histopathologically proved endometrial TB and blocked tubes undergoing IVF. There were three cycle cancellations and 4 young women between the age of 24–29 years were found to be poor responders. Gurgan *et al* also have found poor ovarian response in women undergoing IVF due to tubal factor of infertility due to genital TB as compared to other causes of tubal infertility. Subjects with genital TB had higher basal FSH levels, required more exogenous gonadotropin for controlled ovarian stimulation, reached lower peak E2 levels and yielded fewer oocytes and embryos when compared to women with tubal factors of infertility.

It is advisable to do FSH/LH estimation on day 3 of period or to do clomiphene challenge test in this group of women irrespective of the age prior to IVF-ET.

Whether impaired ovarian function occurs in women with pelvic adhesions is not clear. Oelsner *et al* and Hill *et al* found neither the stage of ovarian disease nor a history of pelvic adhesions or presence of frozen pelvis had any significant impact on efficiency of IVF/ET while Bowman *et al* suggest correlation between pelvic adhesions and ovarian compromise. It is suggested that women with pelvic adhesions due to chronic inflammation have lower fertility and low folliculogenesis on ovarian stimulation due to increased levels of follicular fluid, histamine concentration and due to interference by diffusion of gonadotropin into follicular fluid.

Ectopic Pregnancy and Tubal Infertility

Although IVF/ET is recommended for women who have history of repeated ectopic pregnancies, it has been noticed that occurrence of ectopic pregnancy is not completely prevented by IVF. The incidence of ectopic pregnancy following IVF/ET for tubal factor of infertility is found to be 6 percent while it is negligible following IVF for male factor of infertility. It is the underlying tubal pathology rather than the IVF/ET procedure which pre-disposes to ectopic pregnancy. Hence, the patients with tubal factor infertility undergoing IVF/ET should be counseled regarding occurrences of ectopic pregnancy.

Conventional IVF Vs ICSI for Couples with Tubal Factor of Infertility and Normozoospermia

Whenever a couple with tubal factor of infertility and normal sperm count come for ART conventional IVF is recommended. The ICSI procedure is usually for male factor of infertility.

However, unexpected fertilization failure after IVF in couples with tubal infertility and normal sperm count has been described upto 12.5 percent by Andre Van Stretghem *et al* 1999. Undefined and repetitive sperm oocyte interactive defect may be present in such couples with tubal infertility. Hence it may be worth doing ICSI in some of the sibling oocytes in order to prevent disappointment following fertilization failure.

No large scale well documented outcome of children after ICSI with normozoospermic semen are available. Follow-up study of 1082 karyotypes of ICSI children demonstrated a slightly increased risk of chromosomal anomalies. It is to be seen whether these findings are linked to the technique itself or to the severe andrological infertility of treated patients.

CONCLUSION

ART is the only solution for tubal infertility due to surgically irreparable blocked tubes. However, counseling of patient is required regarding low take-home baby rate in the presence of associated endometrial or ovarian pathology. The couple should also be informed about small risk of getting ectopic pregnancy.

A thorough pre-IVF evaluation including hysteroscopy and basal ovarian function tests are advisable even if the patient is young in women with tubal factor of infertility.

TAKE HOME MESSAGE

1. Check for the cause of tubal factor of infertility. If it is due to pelvic infection then check for chlamydia and tuberculous infection as causal factor as these affects the endometrium and prevent implantation.
2. Presence of bilateral hydrosalpinx on ultrasonography has adverse effect on ART success rate. It requires treatment either in the form of salpingectomy or salpingostomy or USG guided aspiration of Hydrosalpinx prior to ovum pick up in patients undergoing ART.
3. In case of Genital Kochs, in more than 50 percent of the patients endometrium gets affected and thereby may affect implantation. Before taking the patient for IVF, it is necessary to do the following:
   a. Hysteroscopy + D&C for adhesions
   b. Periovular endometrial thickness for fibrosis
4. Absolute contraindication for ART in patients with genital kochs are:
   a. Grade III-IV intrauterine adhesions
   b. Endometrial thickness < 8 mm which does not respond to exogenous estrogen therapy.

BIBLIOGRAPHY

1. Aboulghar MA, Mansour RT, Serour GI, Sattar MA, Awad MM, Amin Y. Transvaginal ultrasonic needle guided aspiration of pelvic inflammatory cystic masses before ovulation induction for in vitro fertilization. Fertil Steril., 1990;53(2):311-14
2. Andersen AN, Lindhard A, Loft A. et al. The infertile patient with hydrosalpinges-IVF with or without salpingectomy? Hum.Reprod 1996;11:2081-84.
3. Bloechle M, Schreiner TH, Lisse K. Case Report: recurrence of hydrosalpinges after transvaginal aspiration of tubal fluid in an IVF cycle and the development of a serometra. Hum. Reprod 1997;12,703-05.
4. Boeckx W. Reconstructive microsurgery of the rabbit oviduct. Thesis at the Catholic University of Leuven, 1982;108.
5. Bowman MC, Cooke ID, Lenton EA. Investigation of impaired ovarian function as a contributing factor to infertility in women with pelvic adhesions. Hum Reprod 1993;8(10):1654-56.
6. Camus E. Human Reproduction, Pregnancy rate after IVF in Cases of tubal infertility with and without hydrosalpinx-a meta-analysis 1999;14,1243.
7. Cohen MA et al. Human Reproduction Hydrosalpinx adversely affects implantation in donor oocyte programme 1999;14(4):1087.
8. Csemiczky G, Landgren BM, Fried G, Wramsby H, High tubal damage grade is associated with low pregnancy rate in women undergoing in-vitro fertilization treatment. Hum Reprod 1996;11(11):2438-40.
9. Dechaud H, Daures JP, Arnal F et al. Does previous salpingectomy improve implantation and pregnancy rates in patients with severe tubal factor infertility who are undergoing in vitro fertilisation? A prospective randomized pilot study. Fertil Steril 1998a;69:1020-25.
10. Diamond E. Lysis of postoperative pelvic adhesions in infertility. Fertil Steril 1979;31:287-95.
11. Desai SK et al. Chapter on Genital Tuberculosis and Infertility-Infertiltiy & TVS-Current concepts, edited by S Desai & G Allahbadia published by Jaypee Brothers. 1995.
12. Desai SK, Roy PG, Hansotia MD-ART in histopathological proved endometrial TB-paper read in XVI FIGO World Congress at Washington DC, 5-8th September, 2000.
13. de Wit W, Gowrising CJ, Kuik DJ et al. Only Hydrosalpinges visible on ultrasound are associated with reduced implantation and pregnancy rates after in vitro fertilization. Hum Reprod 1998;13:1696-1701.
14. Donnez J, Casanas-Roux F. Prognostic factors influencing the pregnancy rate after microsurgical cornual anastomosis. Fertil Steril 1986a;46:1089-92.
15. Donnez J, Caprasse J et al. Loss of adrenergic innervation in induced rabbit hydrosalpinx. Gynecol. Obstet invest 1986;21:213-16.
16. Edwards RG. Why are agonadal and post-amenorrhoeic women so fertile after oocyte donation? Hum Reprod 1992;7:733-34.
17. Edwards RG, Steptoe PC, Purdy JM. Establishing full term human pregnancies using cleaving embryos grown in vitro. Br J Obstet Gynaecol, 1980;87:737-56.

18. Fahy UM, Cahill DJ et al. in vitro fertilization in completely natural cycles. Hum Reprod 1995;10:572-75.

19. Fanchin R, Righini C et al. Uterine contractions at the time of embryo transfer alter pregnancy rate after in vitro fertilization. Hum Reprod 1998;13:1968-74.

20. Gurgan T, Urman B, Yarali H. Results of in vitro fertilization and embryo transfer in women with infertility due to genital tuberculosis. Fertil Steril 1996;65(2):367-70.

21. Hill GA, Herbert CM, Fleischer AC et al. Enlargement of hydrosalpinges during ovarian stimulation protocols for in vitro fertilization and embryo replacement. Fertil Steril 1986;45:883-85.

22. Hochuli E. Surgical treatment of tubal sterility macrosurgery versus microsurgery? Geburtshilfe Frauenheilkd 1979;39:927-31.

23. IJland MM, Hoogland HJ, Dunselman GAJ et al. Endometrial wave direction switch and the outcome of in vitro fertilization. Fertil Steril 1999;71:476-81.

24. Imoedemhe DA, Wafik Ah, Chan RC. In vitro fertilzation in women with "frozen Pelvis": Clinical outcome of treatment. Fertil Steril 1988;49(2):268-71.

25. Janssens RMJ, Lambalk CB et al. Successful IVF in natural cycles after four previously failed attempts in stimulated cycles; a case report. Hum Reprod 1999;1 4:2497-98.

26. Kunz G, Beil D, Deininger H et al. The dynamics of rapid sperm transport through the female genital tract: evidence from vaginal sonography of uterine peristalsis and hysterosalpingography. Hum Reprod 1996;11, 627-32.

27. Leyendecker G, Kunz G, Wildt L et al. Uterine hyperperistalsis and dysperistalsis as dysfunctions of the mechanism of rapid sperm transport in patients with endometriosis and infertility. Hum Reprod 1996;11: 1542-51.

28. Mahadevan MM, Wiseman D, Leader A, Taylor PJ. The effects of ovarian adhesive disease upon follicular development in cycles of controlled stimulation for in vitro fertilization. Fertil Steril 1985;44(4):489-92.

29. Mansour RT, Aboulghar MA, Serour GI, Riad R. Fluid accumulation of the uterine cavity before embryo transfer: a possible hindrance for implantation.J. In vitro Fert Embryo Transf 1991;8:157-59.

30. Meyer WR, Castelbaum AJ et al. Hydrosalpinges adversely affect markers of endometrial receptivity. Hum Reprod 1997;12:1393-98.

31. Mooms Y, Rosenwak Z. Chlamydia trachomatis infection of endometrium should be considered as a possible cause of decreased implantation in recipients of donated oocytes who have history of tubal disease. Fertil.Steril. 1999;71:15-21.

32. Mukherjee T, Copperman AB et al. Hydrosalpinx fluid had embryotoxic efects on murine embryogenesis; a case for prophylactic salpingectomy. Fertil Steril 1996;66: 851-53.

33. Nagata Y, Honjou K sonoda M, Makino I Tamura R, Kawarabayashi T, Peri-ovarian adhesions interfere with the diffusion of gonadotrophin into the follicular fluid. Hum Reprod 1998;13(8):2072-76.

34. Ng EHY, Yeung WS, Ho PC. The presence of hydrosalpinx may not adversely affect implantation and pregnancy rates in in vitro fertilization treatment. J Assist Reprod Genet, 1997;14:508-12.

35. Ng EHY, Ajonuma LC, Lau EYL et al. Adverse effects of hydrosalpinx fluid on sperm motility and survival. Hum Reprod 2000;15:772-77.

36. Oehninger S, Scott R, Muasher SJ, Acosta Aa, Jones HW Jr. Rosenwaks Z. Effects of the severity of tubo-ovarian disease and previous tubal surgery on the results of in vitro fertilization and embryo transfer. Fertil Steril 1989;51(1):126-30.

37. Oelsner G, Sivan E, Goldenberg M et al. Should lysis of adhesions be performed when in-vitro fertilization and embryo transfer are available? Hum Reprod 1994;9: 2339-41.

38. Puttemans PJ, Brosens I, Delattin P et al. Salpingoscopy versus hystersalpingography in hydrosalpinges. Hum Reprod 7;2:535-40.

39. Schlaff WD, Hassiakos DK, Damewood MD et al. Neosalpingostomy for distal tubal obstruction: prognostic factors and impact of surgical technique. Fertil Steril 1990;54:984-90.

40. Sharara FI, Mc Clamrock HD. Endometrial fluid collection in women with hydrosalpinx after human chorionic gonadotrophin administration: a report of two cases and implications for management. Hum Reprod 1997;12:2816-19.

41. Shrivastav P, Gill DS, Jeremy JY, Craft I, Dandona P. Follicular fluid histamine concentrations in infertile women with pelvic adhesions. Acta Obstet Gynecol Scand 1988;67(8):727-29.

42. Sorensen SS. Infertility factors. Their relative importance and share in an unselected material of infertility patients. Acta Obstet Gynecol Scand., 1980; 59:513-20.

43. Spandorfer SD, Liu HC, Neuer A et al. The embryo toxicity of hydrosalpinx fluid is only apparent at high concentrations: an in vitro model that simulates in vivo events. Fertil Steril 1999;71:619-26.

44. Strandell A, Lindhard A, Waldenstrom U et al. Hydrosalpinx and IVF outcome; a prospective randomized multicentre trial in Scandinavia on salpingectomy prior to IVF. Hum Reprod 1999;14:2762-69.

45. Strandell A, Waldenstrom U et al. Hydrosalpinx reduces in vitro fertilization/embryo transfer pregnancy rates. Hum Reprod 1994;9:861-63.

46. Stretghem Andre Van Conventional IVF Vs ICSI in sibling oocytes for couples with tubal infertility and normozoospermic semen. Hum Reprod 1999;14(10): 2474.

47. Templeton A et al. Women with tubal disease have lower implantation rates than women with unexplained infertility. Lancet 1996;88:573-76.

48. Van Voorha. Hum Reprod ultrasonographic aspiration of hydrosalpinx is associated with improved pregnancy, embryos and implantation rate. 1986;13:736-37.

49. Winston RM. Microsurgery of the fallopian tube: from fantasy to reality. Fertil Steril 1980a;34:521-30.

50. Zeyneloglu HB, Arici A, Olive DL. Adverse effects of hydrosalpinx on pregnancy rates after in vitro fertilization-embryo transfer. Fertil Steril 1998;70: 492-99.

• Sulochana Gunasheela • Reeta H Biliangady

18

Evaluation of Fallopian Tube in Infertility

INTRODUCTION

The oviduct that runs from the cornual region of the uterus, ending near the vicinity of the ovary, has gained its name as "fallopian tube" since this was first described in the year 1561 by Gabriele Fallopio.[1] He called it "the seminal duct originating from the cornu uteri and looking like a nerve after a short distance it begins to broaden and coil like a tendril. It shows an extremitas of the nature of skin and color of flesh, the utmost end being very ragged and crushed like the fringe of worn-out clothes. Further, it has a great hole which is held closed by the fimbriae which overlap one another."

Dionis in 1724 pointed out the importance of tubal motility. He even described the accurate etiology of tubal pregnancy, "if the egg is too big or if the diameter of the tube fallopiana is too small, the egg stops and gets no further, but shoots forth and takes root here."

The movement of cilia was first recognized by Purknje and Valentin in 1834 who noticed that small particles moved and rotated on the mucosal surface of rabbit's oviduct. He described, "The forces which led the egg out of the ovary and then through the oviduct, are in part the vibratory movements of the cilia of the epithelium of the infundibulum and in part the independent motion of the latter."

From the beginning of the 20th century extensive diagnostic procedures have been developed for the investigation of tubal pathology.

The introduction of hysterosalpingography and laparoscopic chromopertubation have given extensive information regarding tubal anatomy, physiology and pathology over the last 100 years. With further improvement in instrumentation and development of endoscopic equipment the lumen of the tube has been looked at from the cornual to the fimbrial end. Tubal patency is assessed by X-ray salpingography or intraperitoneal visualization through laparoscopy. Pathological lesions of the mucosa like loss of ciliary movements, bald areas and inflammatory hypertrophy of the muscular segments caused by nonspecific inflammatory lesions like endometriosis may all contribute to dysfunctioning of anatomically patent tubes. Most of these can be identified by direct visualization of the tubal lumen through a falloposcope.

Damage resulting from infection is the most common cause of tubal infertility. In 1950, Westman[1] found that tuberculosis and infections resulting from abortion and childbirth, and those of unknown origin occurred with equal frequency in women with pelvic inflammatory disease. Current studies have shown that the most common cause are sexually transmitted "nonspecific" infections and postabortal and postpartal salpingitis.

INVESTIGATION OF TUBAL PATHOLOGY

A multidisciplinary approach should be adopted as every type of investigation has its merits and demerits. But one must know that at least with the beginning of the new millennium, inconclusive tubal tests like transcervical instillation of air or even CO_2 under pressure through the genital canal should be totally condemned. The information obtained from these kind of tests is too ambiguous when compared to dangers involved like tubal rupture, air embolism spread of tubal infection, etc.

The tubal investigation must start from the simplest and end up in the most sophisticated method, if required, and from the least invasive to the most invasive, keeping in mind the cost efficacy, safety and the practical utility of the information obtained from each procedure. Ultrasound examination of the anatomy of the uterus, tubes and ovaries may give sufficient information in order to rearrange the protocol or supercede one modality of investigation over the other, and thereby chalk out a treatment schedule.

Hysterosalpingography

Hysterosalpingography (HSG) should be the first test for investigation of the fallopian tubes. It provides accurate information about the anatomy of the uterine cavity and proximal fallopian tube like no other simple test can furnish. The details of the uterine cavity can be made out more clearly by HSG than by ultrasound in certain situations like marginal synechiae or total or partial septae in uterus (Figure 18.1). The proximal fallopian tube is difficult to negotiate either by transcervical cannulation or falloposcope. But an HSG can delineate this hairline lumen. HSG is best performed immediately after the menstrual period is over because of the following reasons: (i) there is no fear of committing the blunder of doing an HSG in a gravid uterus—this accident can happen if HSG is done in the postovulatory or premenstrual period, and (ii) the endometrial thickness is at its minimum and the uterine cavity will be outlined clearly. Hypertrophic and polypoid endometrium does produce serrations and irregularities of the uterine lining. This type of endometrium can be blown off from its moorings and cause an obstruction at the cornual ostium

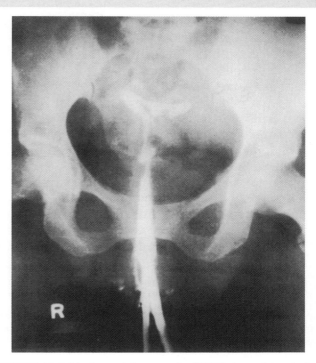

FIGURE 18.1: Hysterosalpingography (HSG) shows intrauterine synechiae with partial visualization of tubes establishing superiority of HSG over laparoscopy

preventing the flow of dye into the intramural segment of the tube. The general rule of getting a pregnancy test done before conducting an HSG on any woman who is having a long-standing period of amenorrhea cannot be overemphasized.

One of the advantages of HSG is that it can be performed in the radiology department without anesthesia. Some authors like Palmar and Decherney[2, 3] and many others have claimed that HSG also has a therapeutic effect.

An assortment of cannulae is available in the market like Shirodkar's screw tip cannula, Rubin's rubberbung cannula, etc. About 5 to 10 cc of water-soluble iodine containing medium is injected through the cannula which is introduced through the cervix and 2 to 3 consecutive films may be taken. The first one shows the uterus and the medial portion of the tube, the second shows the whole length of the tube, and the third one may be taken after injecting a few mL of air. This will further drive the dye out of the tubes into the peritoneal cavity. The authors are against the use of Foley's catheter for the purpose of HSG, as the

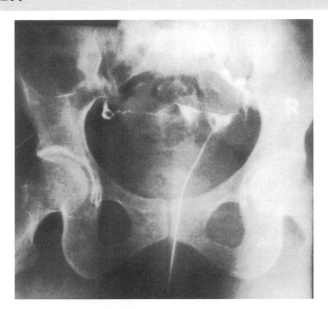

FIGURE 18.2: Bulb of Foley's catheter has obliterated visualization of almost the whole of uterine cavity, however tubes have been delineated

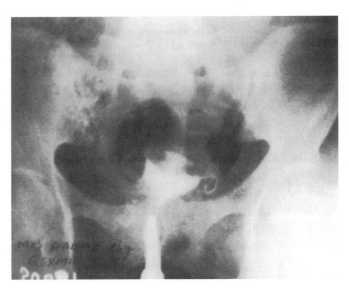

FIGURE 18.3: A case of tubercular pathology of uterus and tubes. Note a hazy margin of the uterus and stiffened tubes ending half-way along their course. Direct infiltration of dye into uterine musculature adds to diagnosis

bulb of the Foley's catheter will occupy the whole of the uterine cavity. This negates the advantages of HSG over laparoscopic assessment of the uterus and tubes (Figure 18.2). The latter modality cannot delineate the uterine cavity unless the procedure of hysteroscopy is also included in it. HSG can delineate synechiae and septae in the uterine cavity (Figure 18.3) and also delineate fistulation and sinus formation through the myometrium. It can show direct infiltration of the dye into the parametrium. The pathology in the uterine cavity is often corroborated by the resistance of flow into the tubal lumen (bilateral cornual block apparent or real) and fistulation of dye along the length of the tubes (suggestive of tubercular pathology also seen in the uterine myometrium Figure 18.3). One must be aware of a false diagnosis of synechiae and tubal block caused by introducing the HSG cannula making a false passage in the myometrium. Figure 18.4 shows a similar situation which was discovered during a hysteroscopic examination done within a few days.

Hysterosalpingography can outline a communicating hydrosalpinx which may or may not be visible during a real-time sonographic examination. A persistent hydrosalpinx with a bipolar block is more likely to be seen during a

sonographic examination than during HSG. Sometimes one can see unilateral or bilateral segmental hydrosalpinges which also show patency. All such cases have to be re-evaluated by laparoscopy (Figures 18.5 to 18.7).

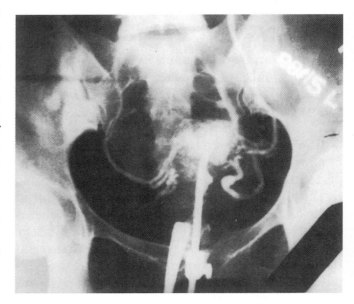

FIGURE 18.4: Note nonvisualization of either uterine outline or tubes. HSG cannula had made a false passage into the myometrium which was identified during hysteroscopy conducted within a few days

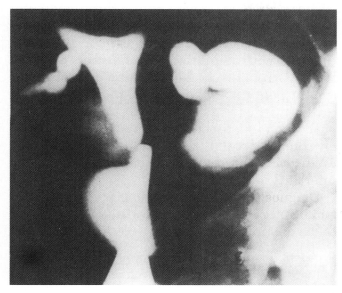

FIGURE 18.5: Hysterosalpingography (HSG) showing a voluminous hydrosalpinx. May require salpingectomy

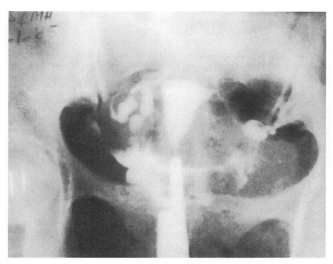

FIGURE 18.6: Picture shows segmented hydrosalpinx on right side without patency. This case requires laparoscopy

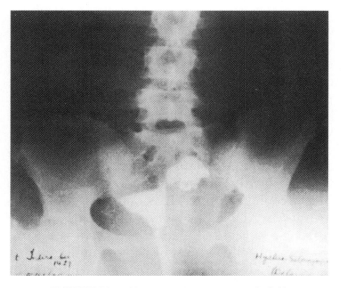

FIGURE 18.7: Hysterosalpingography (HSG) shows well-established hydrosalpinx

Laparoscopic Evaluation of Tubes

Laparoscopic evaluation of tubes has come to become very popular as a part of infertility investigation. The advantage of this procedure is that, many a time a therapeutic procedure can also be conducted at the same sitting when a diagnosis of tubal pathology is made. However, the investigation needs to have special training since it is invasive and requires general anesthesia. Most clinicians would use this as secondary to an X-ray salpingography.

The advantage of laparoscopy is that while HSG is performed in a matter of a few seconds using 5 to 10 ml of radiopaque dye, laparoscopy is performed in a leisurely manner using 100 to 200 ml of fluid (saline or RL) tinted with methylene blue. An assistant dilates the cervical canal beyond the internal os and inserts a cannula similar to that used during HSG. While the fluid is pushed through the uterus by an assistant, the laparoscopist observes the entry of dye into the tubal lumen. The tube not only gets a bluish discoloration but also gets distended from segment to segment and ultimately the fimbriae open and the dye outflow through the fimbria is visualized. Kinks in the tubes can be straightened through accessory instruments which can also milk the dye along the tube.

In cases where a unilateral obstruction is observed, an atraumatic forceps can be applied to the medial end of the patent tube so that the dye is selectively forced through the contralateral tube. This kind of manipulative benefits are not available during an X-ray salpingography.

Laparoscopy also gives the advantage of identifying the nature of pathology that has afflicted the tube. Tubal fistulae in the presence

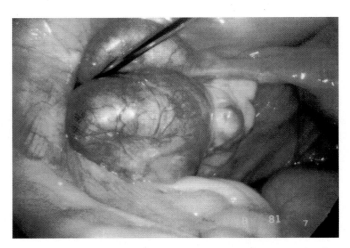

FIGURE 18.8: Laparoscopic view of thin walled communicating hydrosalpinx. See bluish discoloration of the tube caused by methylene blue dye instillation

of intercurrent or burnt-out disease, false passages, juxta fimbrial diverticulae which rupture during instillation of fluid can all be recognized. Distal tubal obstruction may be seen as unilateral or bilateral hydrosalpinges (Figure 18.8). As a rule, tubal pathology is usually bilateral and symmetrical. Since communicating hydrosalpinges periodically empty into the uterine cavity, they may be missed out during an ultrasound examination. In fact, a persistently visible hydrosalpinx recognized by a sonologist, usually shows a state of advanced disease since the block is usually bipolar. The tubal rugae and cilia are permanently lost in such cases. These types of tubes cannot be salvaged by any kind of surgery. On the other hand, they can cause trouble during monitoring of induction of ovulation and oocyte recovery for IVF. Large communicating hydrosalpinges which are periodically pushing inflammatory fluid into the uterine cavity can produce embryo toxicity and nonimplantation during an IVF procedure. The laparoscopist must be able to recognize an unhealthy tube which is beyond salvage and he or she must be in a position to take a decision on removing the tube with a view to enhancing success rate in a subsequent IVF procedure. On the other hand, general peritoneal inflammations can produce agglutination of fimbriae resulting in medium-sized hydrosalpinx. On opening the fimbrial ostium, one

frequently sees the inner lining of the infundibular portion of the tube looking quite healthy. One can proceed to evert the lining of the fimbrial end and finish off with a fimbrioplasty. Severely diseased tubes with multiple fistulae may be excised for the purpose of biopsy. One frequently gets surprised by a histological diagnosis of an unexpected pathology, like tuberculosis, and may proceed to give antitubercular treatment thereby eventually eradicating the systemic disease though not the infertility.

Diagnostic laparoscopy also gives a chance for looking at other causes of infertility like minimal and substantial endometriotic lesions. Endometriomata can be drained at the same time and a subsequent treatment program charted out.

Transcervical Tubal Cannulation

Despite all the advantages mentioned regarding laparoscopic evaluation of tubes, in about 20 per cent of cases when a laparoscopic examination fails to establish tubal patency, one gets the feeling that the tubes are entirely normal and the cause of non-establishment of patency was probably a functional and not due to an organic block. This has been corroborated by several workers.[3-6]

This kind of tubal obstruction caused by tubal spasm can be overcome by the procedure called transcervical tubal cannulation under c-arm fluoroscopic control. This is done by radiologists by injecting a dye through a radiopaque catheter which is inserted transcervically and the tip is wedged into the ostium at the cornual end. The dye injected under pressure can overcome the tubal spasm and delineate the whole length of the tube a procedure called selective salpingography (Figure 18.9). When resistance is encountered at any segment of the tube, a guide wire is passed coaxially and advanced beyond the tip of the catheter. The catheter is pushed along the guide wire, beyond the obstruction and dye is injected. By this method not only functional obstruction can be recognized but organic obstructions can also be treated.

According to our experience in 80 per cent of the patients referred for transcervical

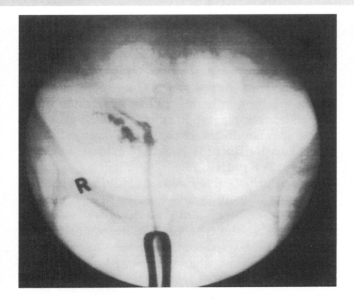

FIGURE 18.9: A case of bilateral tubal pregnancy, left tube has been excised. Right tubal pregnancy treated with methotrexate. Right tubal patency established by selective salpingography

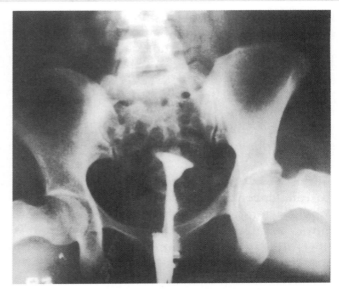

FIGURE 18.10: Bilateral cornual block. Normal uterine cavity with bilateral tubal block. Laparoscopy could not establish patency either. Tubes appeared normal. TTC established bilateral patency

cannulation, both the tubes have been opened up and in another 10 per cent of the cases at least one tube has been opened up. But it must be emphasized that the referred cases were those with tubes appearing entirely normal on laparoscopy (Figure 18.10). It has also been seen that false passages did occur during this procedure especially where proximal tubal endometriosis has been suspected.

Hysteroscopic Tubal Cannulation with Combined Laparoscopic Manipulation

Hysteroscopic tubal cannulation with combined laparoscopic manipulation is an alternate method to transcervical cannulation under fluoroscopy. This can be done where the facility of C-arm fluoroscopic control is not available. But it is a fairly invasive procedure as compared to the above. A special catheter is inserted through the operating channel of the hysteroscope and the cannula is wedged into the cornual end along with a guidewire (Figure 18.11). The wire and the cannula are advanced under the guidance of the laparoscopist. The procedure demands the skill of an expert hysteroscopist and laparoscopist at the same time. Moreover the catheter used is

disposable which can make the procedure expensive. However, Das *et al*[7] have shown that by this procedure they have been able to establish proximal tubal patency and obtained a pregnancy rate of 55 per cent which was superior to the 51 per cent success obtained by resecting and anastomosis of a proximal tubal block.

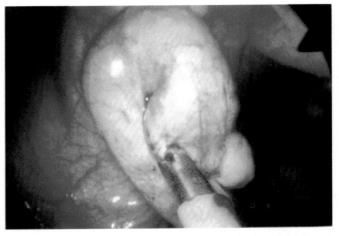

FIGURE 18.11: Laparoscopy instruments being introduced through a puncture made over the fimbrial end of the hydrosalphinx

Fallopian Tube Catheterization under Ultrasound Guidance

Fallopian tube catheterization under ultrasound guidance is a simplified technique to evaluate patency and open up proximally obstructed tubes.[8] The system consists of a catheter guide cannula with a ball-shaped tip and a catheter made of polyester elastomer. The guide is pushed into the uterus under ultrasound guidance without cervical dilatation and gently advanced towards the uterine cornua. Once the tip of the guide is in place, the tubal catheter is inserted through the guide cannula and advanced 5 cm into the tube and an electrolyte solution is instilled. The flow and distribution of fluid in the tube and pelvis is displayed on real-time ultrasound.

Sonosalpingography

Sonosalpingography is a simple and minimally invasive technique that can be done by using the same procedure as an X-ray salpingography. A screw type cannula is inserted beyond the internal os and normal saline is instilled through the cannula into the uterine cavity. The flow of fluid can be followed along the tube and the trickle of fluid can be seen along the lateral end of the tube forming a pool in the pouch of Douglas. However, this method is inferior in resolution when compared to fluoroscopic imaging of the uterus and tubes. But it can be used in situations where a previous X-ray examination has been technically faulty or inconclusive and a laparoscopic examination has been done by a novice without giving proper information about the uterus and tubes. This procedure also has some therapeutic value as the authors have seen some pregnancies occur soon after the procedures.

Falloposcopy and Salpingoscopy for Endoscopic Evaluation of Tubal Lumen

Kevin *et al*[9] first described the transcervical examination of tubal lumen and called it falloposcopy. They used a flexible hysteroscope with an outer diameter of 3.5 to 5.5 mm. Later a falloposcope with a 0.5 mm outer diameter was devised. With this the mucosa of the entire length

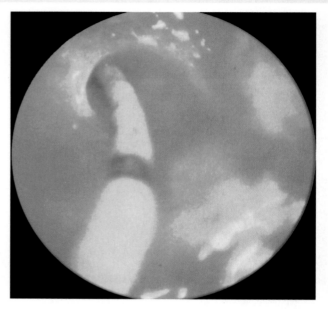

FIGURE 18.12: Tubal ostium being catheterized during hysteroscopy

of the tube could be visualized in 90 per cent of the cases. Falloposcopy helps to differentiate physiological blocks from true anatomic blocks.

Henry Suchet *et al*[10] used a rigid hysteroscope for salpingoscopy in 1985. The instrument was introduced through the fimbrial end of the fallopian tube using normal saline as a distending medium (Figure 18.12). They described the normal well-formed folds of the fallopian tube running parallel to one another in normal tubes and loss of folds, intratubal adhesions in diseased ones (Figure 18.13).

This procedure requires distention of the abdomen and establishment of a primary laparoscopic visualization of pelvic organs. Hysteroscope or falloposcope would be introduced through an accessory portal. The tubal fimbria has to be held by a grasping forceps, while the falloposcope is pushed into the infundibular portion of the tube. The tube is continually distended by normal saline or Ringer lactate instilled through the channel built in the outer sheath of the falloposcope. The flow of fluid is maintained by a pressure head. The procedure, however is cumbersome for an everyday infertility specialist. In addition to the complications of laparoscopy, a novice can possibly cause damage

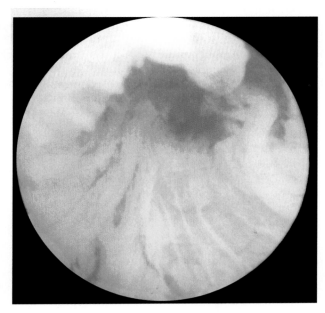

FIGURE 18.13: Falloposcopic view of the normal mucosal folds of the tube

to the fimbria when it is held with the forceps while advancing the falloposcope through the ostium. Maintaining the distention of the tube while the fluid is leaking through the fimbrial ostium is an added burden to the technique. However, experts have shown an excellent demonstration of tubal lumina, both normal and abnormal, by this technique (see Picture Tubal Infertility— Brosen and Gorden).

Gynecoradiological Procedure with Measurement of Tubal Perfusion Pressure (TPP)

Gynecoradiological procedure with measurement of tubal perfusion pressure (TPP) was devised by Karande *et al*[8] of the Center for Human Reproduction, Illinois, Chicago. This procedure consists of a more detailed evaluation of the uterus and tubes as compared to HSG using a digitalized recording system that allows replay and enhancement of the findings in place of the usual spot films of an ordinary HSG. It also involves the assessment of tubal perfusion pressure which is representative of the fallopian tubal resistance using water soluble contrast. The pressure is measured using a pressure transducer which is connected to a computer and is displayed on the monitor screen. While performing a selective salpingography, the TPP of each tube is measured individually. Women with high TPP show low pregnancy rates. Hence, it is a technique which determines not only the patency but also the capability of a tube to achieve pregnancy. In their study, women with endometriosis showed an increased incidence of asymmetrical tubal filling during the initial HSG as compared to controls and they also demonstrated significantly elevated TPP than women without endometriosis. The drawback of this procedure is that it requires the use of expensive gadgetry.

CONCLUSION

In conclusion, it must be understood that all kinds of tubal patency tests have their merits and demerits. Of all the tests described above, laparoscopy still has the place of "gold standard". Selective transcervical tubal cannulation takes a better place than laparoscopy in patients who have an absolutely normal looking pelvis as patency can still be established in 90 per cent of these patients by transcervical cannulation. Thus, this would give a lot of hope to the patients who would otherwise have to proceed to an unnecessary laparotomy or an expensive procedure like IVF. Any other type of evaluation is more of academic interest than what is accessible to a practical infertility therapist.

REFERENCES

1. Westman A. Etiology, diagnosis and surgical treatment of infertility. Acta Obstetrica et Synecologica Scandinavica 1950;30:186.
2. Palmar A. Ethiodol hysterosalpingogrphy for the treatment of infertility. Fertil Steril 1960;11:3112.
3. De Cherny AH. Anything you can do I can do better....... or differently! Fertil Steril 1987;48:374.
4. Sulak et al. Histology of proximal tubal occlusion. Fertil Steril 1987;3:48.
5. Sulak PJ, Letlerie GS, Codington CC et al. Histology of proximal tubal occlusion. Fertil Steril 1987;48:437.
6. Thurmand AS, Novy M, Rosin J. Terbutaline in diagnosis of interstitial fallopian tube obstruction. Invest Radiol 1988;23:209.
7. Das et al. Hysteroscopic cannulation for PTO. Fertil Steril 1995;63:5.
8. Lisse, Sydow. Fallopian tube catheterization and recanalisation under ultrasonic observation— a simplified

technique to evaluate tubal patency and open proximally obstructed tubes. Fertil Steril 1991; 56(2):198.

9. Karande et al. Tubal perfusion pressures and endometriosis. Fertil Steril 1995;64:6.

10. Henry, Suchet J. Endoscopy of the tube. Acta Eur Fertil 1985;16:139.

11. Kevin JF, Williams DB, San Romano GA. Falloscopic classification of treatment of fallopian tube lumen disease. Fertil Steril 1992;57:731.

12. Boxdemer CW. In Hafex ESE, Blandau RJ (Eds): History of the Mammalian Oviduct, University of Chicago Press: 1968;3-26.

13. Cornier E. Ampulloscopic per coclioscopique. J Obstet Gynecol Biol Reprod (Paris) 1985;14:459.

14. De Cherny AH, Kort H et al. Increased pregnancy rate with oil soluble hysterosalpinography. Fertil Steril 1980;33:407.

• Prakash Trivedi • Shyam V Desai
• Nikhil S Jani • Kusum Zaveri • Indira Hinduza

19

Female Infertility Surgery

HYSTEROSCOPIC CANNULATION FOR PROXIMAL TUBAL BLOCK

Prakash Trivedi

INTRODUCTION

Transvaginal cannulation of fallopian tube and Transcervical balloon tuboplasty (Confino, 1986) has attracted a great deal of interest recently. Tubal occlusion is the main cause of infertility in about one-third of all infertile couples. Further 10-20 percent of all tubal blocks are in the proximal part of the fallopian tube. Traditional treatment for proximal tubal occlusion by tubocornual anastomosis is tedious and an invasive surgical procedure without encouraging pregnancy rates. Further, treatment by *in vitro* fertilization and embryo transfer is very costly and with still lower pregnancy rates. Tubal cannulation utilizes transvaginal route and avoids incisional surgery. With recent advances in bioengineering with dedicated catheters and cannulas transvaginal tubal cannulation has been less invasive and more cost effective treatment for Proximal Tubal Obstruction. This can be done by hysteroscopic, fluoroscopic, ultrasonic, tactile and falloposcopic techniques. We will highlight the hysteroscopic methods of tubal cannulation along with our own experience and international data available.

The complex, narrow and tortuous nature of the intramural tube has lead to difficulties in the development of hysteroscopic tubal cannulation techniques. Bio-engineers have custom designed and miniaturized guidewires, cannulas and flexible endoscopes, which have the ability to negotiate the tubal lumen based on *in vivo* observations.

Functional *in vivo* Anatomy of Proximal Tubal Region

The intramural oviductal lumen is a potential space 1.5 to 2.5 cm in length straight or slightly curved. The intramural lumen diameter of 0.2–0.4 mm is due to collapse and contraction of oviductal wall. *In vivo* actually the intramural oviduct is of 0.8–1.2 mm in diameter and can accommodate cannulas, which can stretch the lumen marginally due to healthy elasticity. Apart from diseases directly affecting the promixal tube, this can further be distorted by peritubal adhesions, fibroid of uterus and broad ligament, ovarian pathology and infections. Each ostium is situated at the apex of the uterotubal gutter and can be seen hysteroscopically at the bottom of a saucer-shaped depression as a sharp membranous ring, which measures 0.8–1.2 mm in diameter. Therefore, if one passes a flexible, smooth-walled, J-shaped directional cannula through internal os and directs it towards the left or right, it will follow the uterotubal gutter towards the respective tubal ostium.

A description and illustration of the passage of a wire probe through the intramural segment of the human oviduct using a transvaginal approach was first published by Gardener in 1856. Less flexible cannulas and endoscopes will tend to get stuck in the intramural bulge as it narrows to about 1–1.5 mm beyond ostia. That is why the importance of over the wire or coaxial cannulation systems to keep the lumen coaxially aligned with the tubal lumen, for advancement. Smaller cannulas with diameter of 0.6 mm may negotiate most intramural lumens without coaxial assistance. Greater attention to coaxial alignment is necessary during hysteroscopic cannulation techniques as the distension medium converts the uterine cavity into a three-dimensional structure.

Around 1-1.5 cm from the ostium the intramural portion narrows further, the isthmic portion takes a 40-60° bend as it exits beyond the uterotubal junction. This is the common place where tubal perforations can take place during cannulation in spite of having significant muscular layers. The ampullary portion is cavernous and thin walled wherein overenthusiastic cannulation can also lead to perforation if cannula is advanced too much further.

Tubal obstruction can be due to chronic Salpingitis, Salpingitis Isthmica Nodosa (SIN), Intratubal Endometriosis, amorphous material, e.g. mucus plug or spasm.

Presence of tubal disease lateral to the proximal tubal obstruction will affect success of the procedure adversely.

METHODS OF HYSTEROSCOPIC TUBAL CANNULATION

Different methods of hysteroscopic tubal cannulation have been attempted without rigorous randomized scientific assessment and with simplistic success rates of cannulation with or without subsequent pregnancy rates.

Essentially there are three methods of hysteroscopic tubal cannulation:
  a. Flexible guide wire through a catheter
  b. Falloposcopically guided cannulation
  c. Transcervical balloon cannulation and linear eversion catheters

Flexible Guide Wire through a Tubal Catheter

Here through operative hysteroscopy instrument channel a fine diameter catheter (5 Fr) with J shaped curve at the tip is passed and the 30° forward oblique Hysteroscopic cable is rotated on the side opposite to the tubal ostium planned to be cannulated. The tubal catheter is loaded with a memory and curve going away from the cable. The tubal ostium is centralized and the catheter

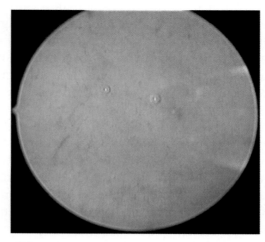

FIGURE 19.1A: Hysteroscopy—left tubal ostia

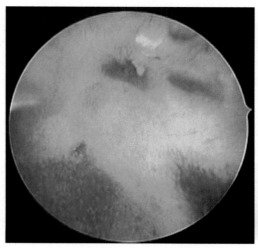

FIGURE 19.1B: Hysteroscopy—right tubal ostia

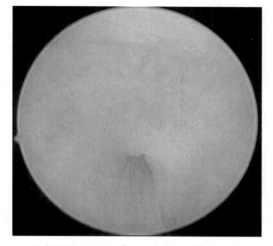

FIGURE 19.2A: Cannulation of left ostia

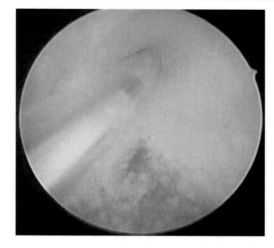

FIGURE 19.2B: Cannulation of right ostia

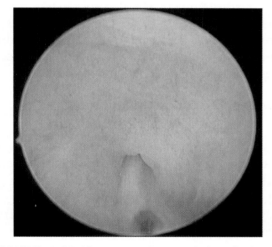

FIGURE 19.3A: Hysteroscopic cannulation of left ortia

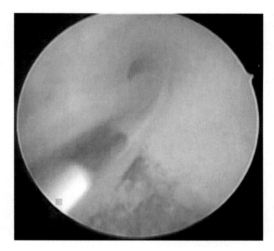

FIGURE 19.3B: Hysteroscopic cannulation of right ortia

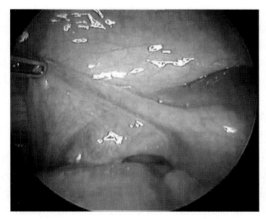

FIGURE 19.4A: Laparoscopic cannulation of left tube

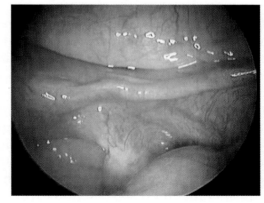

FIGURE 19.4B: Laparoscopic cannulation of right tube

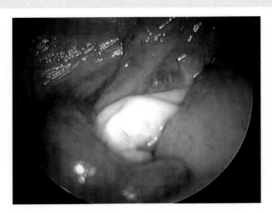

FIGURE 19.5A: Cannulation of left tube

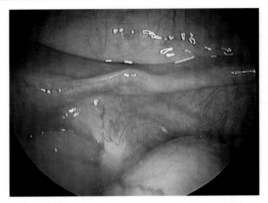

FIGURE 19.5B: Cannulation of right tube

is advanced to wedge into the tubal ostium. Through this catheter a fine flexible guide wire– Terumo is passed and tubal cannulation is done gently by advancing the Terumo wire. Simultaneous laparoscopy notices the path of cannulation of the guide wire preventing tubal perforation by aligning the tubal lumen laparoscopically avoiding acute curvature of the tube.

If the guide wire curls on itself then advancing the outer catheter reduces the effective length of guidewire, thus stiffening for further advancement. If still resistance is felt then there can be bad occlusion of lumen. If the movement of guidewire is smooth then the terumo wire is withdrawn and selective salpingography is done for the cannulated tube. The same procedure is repeated on the opposite side rotating the operating hysteroscope by 180°.

The same principle is further improved by the Novy's curved catheter-cannula, wherein on platinum tip guide wire, there is a tubal catheter, which goes inside the curved cannula. Here for selective tubal patency only the platinum tip wire is removed and dye can be pushed through the catheter. This device is costlier than a combination of tubal catheter with a terumo guide wire, which is very economical.

Letterie and Sakas evaluated histologic findings in 15 patients (27 tubal segments) at Laparotomy after failed tubal cannulation. They found that 93 percent of these patients had severe disease, suggesting that tubal cannulation might distinguish functional obstructions from true occlusion.

Perforation is reported in upto 10 percent attempted procedures. Use of appropriate flexible catheter may decrease the risk of perforation. When perforation occurs, it is left to heal spontaneously. Infection is rare.

Transcervical tubal cannulation should not be performed in presence of known pelvic infection and in cases of known distal tubal disease.

Falloposcopic Guide Cannulation

This system has a flexible optic, which goes through the cannulation system, which further goes through the cervix. The small flexible optics of falloposcopy helps to additionally have a good view of the intratubal coarse adhesions, etc. however technically it is a skillful and difficult procedure. There is continuous irrigation between the falloposcope and the cannula. The falloposcope should not be pushed too much outside the cannula and specially on white out areas to avoid perforation. There is a scoring system depending on adhesions, dilatation, epithelial appearance, endotubal vascularity and degree of patency. Many clinicians strongly feel that falloposcopy still is a research tool with practical limitations.

Linear Eversion Cannula/ Catheter and Balloon Catheters

A novel alternative to direct probing is by linear eversion catheter (LEC) wherein; there is a plastic polymer catheter of 2.8 mm outer diameter with a sliding stainless steel inner body 0.8 mm in diameter. The outer and inner bodies are connected at their tips by a polyethylene membrane or balloon some 20 cm long and 50 μm thick. The inner lumen of the balloon is constructed of a material that is flexible enough to conform the fallopian tube path but retains sufficient radial integrity to maintain an open internal lumen under balloon pressures. The balloon is inverted in on itself and the hydraulic pressure from the proximal end forces its inner lumen to become outer, thereby advances along the tubal lumen. Even the falloposcope can be within the LEC effectively. This system overcomes the difficulties of guide wire techniques to anatomic irregularities and transcervical balloon tuboplasty (TBT) is further advancement in this direction, conceived in analogy to vascular recannalization of coronary arteries first done in 1986. Here there is a double balloon catheter blocking the internal os and proximal balloon to seal the cervical canal. Hysterosalpingography is performed. Then a third balloon catheter is introduced preloaded with a selective salpingography catheter with a guide wire. The balloon is inflated and blocked area is dilated, then contrast material is injected to confirm tubal patency.

The results of TBT are 90 percent unilateral patency, 80 percent bilateral patency, 33 percent pregnancy within 6 months, 5 percent ectopic pregnancy and 70 percent have maintained tubal patency even after 6 months. Hysteroscopically guided TBT seems to be more difficult compared to fluoroscopic TBT.

AUTHOR'S EXPERIENCE

We performed hysteroscopic cannulation along with concurrent laparoscopy in 127 cases between February 1994 to May 2003. Proximal tubal obstruction was confirmed on hysterosalpingo-graphy and laparoscopy. We used different cannulation devices, more often Novy's curved catheter with platinum tip guide wire when cost was not a consideration or used fine terumo guide wire with regular tubal catheter, which was more economical.

At least one tube was cannulated in 75 percent of 127 cases. 40 percent patients have conceived

and no ectopic pregnancy so far. There were 6 tubal perforations, more with platinum tipped wire than terumo wire. In 11 cases cannulation was abandoned as anatomy of the cornua was badly distorted. These results are far satisfactory compared to the period prior to February 1994, when hysteroscopic tubal cannulation was frequently more traumatic rather than a rewarding procedure specially due to poor design in catheters, cannulas and guide wires.

Proximal tubal block due to obstructive intraluminal adhesion, nonobstructive debris were reversible by cannulation and aqua flushing with catheters but severe intraluminal diseases could be traumatic, nonreversible with reduced therapeutic effect.

CONCLUSION

Proximal tubal obstruction is one of the common causes for infertility. Management with Microsurgical Tubocornual Anastomosis or IVF is more invasive or costly with less result.

With the good quality of dedicated tubal cannulation catheters Hysteroscopic or Fluoroscopic tubal cannulation is the procedure of choice, which is minimally invasive, skillful and effective. The complications are not of much significance. This procedure avoided a laparotomy.

We are convinced that hysteroscopic or fluoroscopic tubal cannulation is a safe and effective procedure for treatment of proximal tubal obstruction, better than conventional laparotomy and cheaper than IVF.

BIBLIOGRAPHY

1. Confino E, Triberg, Gleicher N. Transcervical balloon tuboplasty. Fertil Steril 1986;46:963.
2. Daniell IF, Miller W. Hysteroscopic correction of cornual occlusion with resultant term pregnancy. Fertil Steril 1987;48:490.
3. Gardener AK. The causes and creative treatment of sterility with a preliminary statement of the physiology of generation. New York: De WH and Davenport, 1856.
4. Kerin J, Daykhovsky L, Grundfest W, Surrey E. Falloposcopy: A microendoscopic transvaginal technique for diagnosing and treating endotubal disease

incorporating guide wire cannulation and direct balloon tuboplasty. J Reprod Med 1990;35:606.

5. Letterie GS, Sakas EL. Histology of proximal tubal obstruction in cases of unsuccessful tubal canalization. Fertil Steril 1991;56:831-35.

6. Lisse K, Sydow P. Fallopian tube catheterization and recanualization under ultrasonic observation a simplified technique to evaluate tubal patency and open proximally obstructed tubes. Fertil Steril 1991;52:198.

7. Novy MJ, Thurmond AJ, Patton P, Uchida BT, Rosch J. Diagnosis of cornual obstruction by Transcervical follopian tube cannulation. Fertil Steril 1988;50:434.

8. Stern JJ, Peters AJ, Coulam CB. Transcervical tuboplasty under ultrasonographic guidance: A pilot study. Fertil Steril 1991;56:359.

9. Sulak RT, Letterie GS, Coddington CC, Haystip CC, Woodward JF, Klein JA. Histology of proximal tubal obstruction. Fertil Steril 1987;43:437.

LAPAROSCOPIC TUBAL MICROSURGERY

Prakash Trivedi

INTRODUCTION

Microsurgical techniques have become the gold standard for tubal surgery in the last two decades with its excellent results as revealed by Gomel 1995, Winston 1977.

Laparoscopic microsurgery is a technique that synergies the potential of classical microsurgery and laparoscopy. With further evolution of technology this tool is poised for as yet undiscovered applications. This can overcome deficiencies inherent to both laparoscopy and laparotomy. Laparoscopy avoids the inherent disadvantages of laparotomy, i.e. predisposition to desiccation of tissues, long incisions, need for retraction, pelvic and bowel packing with its adhesiogenic potential. Also limited depth of field and small field of vision with the operating microscope is a limitation. Avoiding this along with the already inherent advantages laparoscopic surgery has of magnification, meticulous hemostasis, precise suture placement, lavage, maximal patient comfort with minimal access are well known.

PRINCIPLES OF MICROSURGERY

Here we have two major concepts:
  a. Microsurgical Technique
  b. Microsuturing

Microsurgical technique through laparoscope or open surgery involves delicate surgical style with fine atraumatic instrumentation, magnification, accurate dissection and reconstruction, meticulous hemostasis, minimal energy and intermittent irrigation to avoid desiccation of tissues. The pathological area is removed with little damage to adjacent normal tissue, encouraging better healing and less adhesion.

Microsuturing involves use of 6-0 to 10-0 microsutures, small needle with nonabsorbable sutures with reduced foreign body reaction to achieve better results.

Traditional microsurgery with laparotomy predisposes tissue desiccation, retraction, packing, which is all adhesiogenic. Further the Operating Microscope has only vertically downward vision with limited depth and small field of view specially for one or two persons only. Thus macroscopic mobilization to elevate adnexa becomes mandatory.

Operative laparoscopy doesn't have inherent disadvantage of laparotomy alongwith wide view, better depth and same vision for all the members of the team. As handling of tissue is in closed environment adhesion formation is also reduced. These new approach synergies advantages of two modalities into one. Laparoscopic Tubal Microsurgery is useful for tubotubal anastomosis for reversal of sterilization, cornual anastomosis and cuff salpingostomy for hydrosalpinges. Also salpingo ovariolysis of varying degree and correction of endometriosis or fibroids can be done simultaneously by operative laparoscopy. Preliminary evaluation by Hysterosalpingography and Laparoscopy is beneficial for planning surgical approach and define prognostic outcome.

Equipment and Instruments for Laparoscopic Microsurgery

Magnification at 25-40 times is essential to identify healthy mucosa and muscularis before anastomosis can be performed. For microsuturing, magnification at 10-15 times is adequate.

The telescope has a magnification factor of 3-5 times and this is increased to 7 times when the telescope is brought very close to tissue. The use of an endoscopic camera with a television monitor (20 inches) provides a 'multiplier' effect, which further magnifies the image. Recent cameras with a zoom factor further enlarge the image.

Magnification requires a corresponding high resolution to be usable, and this is provided by the three-chip cameras available today, which are capable of 800 lines of horizontal resolution, and this is complemented by monitors capable of 800 lines of resolution. The three-chip camera is also indispensable for accurate color resolution. An 8-0 suture, which is 45 μm in diameter, is easily seen using such a video system.

To further enhance contrast, some companies have built in digital enhancement in their cameras or as an add-on unit. This enhances small vessels and edge detail, thus improving discrimination. An extremely sensitive autoiris built into the camera provides rapid control of illumination, avoiding the dreaded 'white-out' when the telescope is brought close to tissue. This is particularly important in microsuturing as the telescope has to be frequently panned in and out during the case.

Microinstruments

- Sandblasted tips reduce glare when the telescope is brought close to it, thus allowing the suture and magnified tissue to be visible without distraction.
- The terminal serration of the jaw is specially designed to be able to pick tissue atraumatically, leaving no petechia or abrasion. Jaw apposition occurs precisely over its whole length so that 8-0 suture may be grasped anywhere without slippage. This greatly aids intracorporeal suturing as there is no need to grasp the suture at a designated portion of the jaw.
- The serrations and edges of the jaw have been treated so that 8-0 nylon or Prolene is not crushed or cut during normal use for suturing.
- The handle design has been chosen as having least friction and maximal transmission of finger movement to the instrument tip, another prerequisite for precision microsurgery. The handle angle to the shaft of 130° complements the set-up described above and allows the elbows to be at rest and adducted to the body during microsurgery.

Slightly more rigid needle is necessary for laparoscopic microsuturing than for classical microsurgery. Furthermore, it is often easier to insert the needle directly into tissue without the use of a counterpressing grasper. To achieve this the needle needs low force penetration characteristics and superior rigidity. Suitable examples include the BV 175-6 needle swaged to 7-0 and 8-0 polypropylene or a BV 130-5 needle swaged to 8-0 polypropylene.

Plain polyglactin is the most difficult to see laparoscopically and becomes limp when wet. Monofilament sutures tend not to fray and allow easier intracorporeal suturing.
- Trocars—reusable 3 mm trocars are available with the Ultramicro Series or 5 mm trocars with 3 mm reducers may be used.
- Suction irrigation—3 mm suction irrigators are available and provide a more suitable jet for microsurgery than the 5 mm counterparts.

Stents are not used as it can be traumatic to cannulate the distal fallopian tube, and hysteroscopic cannulation creates a distraction to the rhythm of surgery and the possibility of contamination.

Uterine manipulators having a terminal opening tend to be lodged in the endometrium and cause intravasation of dye and a false diagnosis of a proximal block therefore side holes are better.

Energy—a 150 um microneedle tip unipolar electrode is used for incision and dissection, powered from a low voltage generator. Power settings of 15-20 W for cutting and 15 W for fulguration are adequate. When the mesenteric vasculature is inadvertently cut causing more vigorous bleeding, a microbipolar electrode of 1 mm diameter is used.

PREQUISITES OF SURGEON

Experience of Classical Microsurgery Necessary

Laparoscopic Skills

Advanced suturing skills with 4-0 to 6-0 sutures are also necessary before embarking on 7-0 and 8-0 microsuturing. Intracorporeal knotting is indispensable as extracorporeal techniques for 7-0 and 8-0 sutures are impractical and crude can cause 'cutting through' or disruption of tissue.

The art of laparoscopic microsuturing is highly skills based. The Ultramicro instrumentation prevents frustration from broken sutures and facilitates the correct technique of intracorporeal microsuturing.

After a significant number of surgeries we have come to the conclusion that 6-0 PDS W9091T with 8 ml 3/8, round bodied needle is the most suitable suture material for laparoscopic tubal recanalization.

SURGICALTECHNIQUE

Patient is under general anesthesia and modified lithotomy position. We find ipsilateral ports convenient for dissection as well as suturing in laparoscopic tubal recanalization. Dilute methylene blue is injected with a Rumi's cannula which allows manipulation of the uterus and also inject methylene blue whenever necessary.

Operative laparoscopy is done with four punctures, one 10 mm optics with three-chip camera at umbilicus. Two 3 or 5 mm trocar on left and right side lateral to inferior epigastric vessels one inch above the imaginary Pfannenstiel's line. The fourth puncture is in the level of umbilicus on left side exactly above the left lower port. These two ports of the left side permits ipsilateral laparoscopic suturing with 3 mm or 5 mm microsuturing instruments. Dilute vasopressin (1:30) is injected in the serosal aspect of the tube on both proximal and distal segments to improve dissection and have better hemostasis. Serosal aspect is incised with scissors or Micro needle monopolar electrode at very low wattage. The serosa incision is taken to dissect it by 5 mm or more from the muscularis. This allows proper suturing of muscularis without inversion as serosa is shaved off for some distance (5-10 m). The muscularis is incised with 5 mm Guillotine or occasionally straight scissors avoiding the mesosalpingeal vessel. With straight or curved injector patency of both signals are checked.

Most important suture is 7-0 or 8-0 at 6 O'clock muscularis to muscularis with knots remaining out of the lumen. Mesosalpinx is approximated with 6-0 prolene. Then 12 O'clock suture is placed and kept untied. Then 9 O'clock and 3 O'clock sutures are placed with same material. Mesosalpingeal window is closed with 6-0 nylon or prolene. Seromuscularis is approximated with 7-0 or 8-0 prolene and chromo pertubation is done to check patency and thorough lavage is given.

Types of Anastomosis

Isthmo-Isthmic Anastomosis

Isthmo-Isthmic anastomosis is comfortable as both the lumen are similar in size with thick muscularis.

Ampullary–Ampullary Anastomosis

The awkwardness in these cases is due to the thin muscularis and the tendency for prolapse or extrusion of the mucosal folds. The angled probe can be used to delineate the muscularis as well as push the redundant mucosa back into the lumen after tying the muscularis sutures.

Tubal-Cornual Anastomosis

A linear slit at 12 O'clock is made in the cornual muscularis using the microneedle electrode after synthetic vasopressin injection. This allows some mobility of the interstitial tube so that it can be aligned to the needle and needle holder to effect suturing.

Hydrosalpinges

Here a cruciate incision is made with focussed beam of CO_2 Laser with metal backstop or with microelectrode with low watts current. The cuff is made and sutured with 5-0 material, however with CO_2 Laser a swiftlase is used to give flowering or everting effect. Results with Cuff Salpingostomy done laparoscopically is improved over laparotomy due to less adhesion, however overall pregnancy rate are low.

Fimbrioplasty

Fimbrial or prefimbrial narrowing is seen with normal looking remaining tube. A Maryland forceps or Babcock type of Grasper is introduced inside the lumen and Grasper is opened in two directions at 90° gently. This give excellent results in terms of tubal patency and pregnancy rate.

AUTHOR'S EXPERIENCE

We performed Laparoscopic tubal recanalization or reanastomosis in 32 cases till May 2003 for those who had undergone previous tubal ligation. Indication of reanastomosis in all cases was for reversal of sterilization. In majority of cases the indication was loss of one live male issue by accidental causes or remarriage. The patients belonged to the age group of 26-40 years. 50 percent of cases had previous cesarean section. In 40 percent of cases only one tube was available for recanalization due to longer segment loss or absent tube.

Type of anastomosis performed were isthmo-isthmic in 14 percent of cases, isthmo-ampullary in 72 percent of cases, ampullo-ampullary in 14 percent of cases. No tubocornual anastomosis was done. Proximal tubal length was < 2 cm in 30 percent of cases and > 2 cm in 70 percent of cases.

RESULTS

Out of 32 cases of laparoscopic tubal recanalization, we had 80 percent unilateral and 60 percent bilateral tubal patency rate as judged by postoperative HSG with a 40 percent pregnancy rate in a follow up period of less than 2 years. There was one ectopic pregnancy. However, in 50 percent of our cases there was history of previous LSCS and in 40 percent of cases only one tube was available for recanalization. Apart from advanced age, fibroids, etc. added to affect the results in terms of pregnancy rate.

There were no major complications. In the group of fimbrioplasty or fimbrial dilatation (38 cases) there was 54 percent pregnancy rate. However results with cuff salpingostomy Hydrosalpinges (24 cases) was only 11 percent pregnancy rate.

DISCUSSION

Laparoscopic microsurgery will introduce a new dimension to Tubal surgery. It is important to realize that learning curve is considerable and technically demanding. Proficiency and experience in laparoscopic suturing is an essential prerequisite for this procedure.

Various workers have reported pregnancy rates to the tune of 50-71 percent (Prado 1993, Silva 1991, Putman 1990, Koh 1996, Reich 1993 *et al*). These results are comparable to the open microsurgery, which is known to be the gold standard for this procedure. Our results of 40 percent could be attributed to other factors in case selection like average age of patients, other factors of infertility and non-availability of both tubes for anastomosis in 40 percent cases. Further evaluation is therefore, needed before we come to a final conclusion. Surgical time of first seven cases was a mean of 180 minutes and later it reduced to 120–130 minutes. The patients were discharged in 80 percent cases on the next day.

Open microsurgery has proved its worth. What is striking is that laparoscopic microsurgery is likely to give comparable results because here we are extremely close to all principles of microsurgery including magnification, meticulous hemostasis, less tissue handling and desiccation, precise placement of fine sutures and perfect apposition. The additional advantages are avoidance of bowel packing and retraction, faster patient recovery and sutureless closure of abdomen. If at all there is any limitation it is only related to technical feasibility and slightly more operating time. This can be overcome by experience and attainment of high laparoscopic suturing skills aided by technical advancements. We found that three chip camera along with instruments of Koh's ultra micro series not only helped in better tissue identification, but also at every step of suturing we could feel the difference since microsutures were used with micro instruments instead of very large regular laparoscopy instruments. There was improved ease of suturing due to better transmission of hand movements and comfortable hand position due to shorter length of needle holder. Assistant appreciated very good anatomy. Unlike open microsurgery, in laparoscopic tubal reanastomosis, the entire team, i.e. surgeon and all assistants have the same magnified view, which makes surgery more comfortable.

Various other modalities of tubal anastomosis have been tried by laparoscopic surgeons like fibrin glue by Sedbom 1989 and Laser welding by Baggish 1981, Choe 1984, etc.

Validation of laparoscopic microsurgery as a discipline requires that the results of reversals of sterilization performed with this technique are equal or better than those with the open microsurgical technique. Koh reports cumulative pregnancy rates of 35.5 percent at three months, 54.8 percent at six months, 67.7 percent at nine months, and 71 percent at 12 months with an ectopic pregnancy rate of 5 percent (Koh and Janik, 1996). The surgical duration in the first ten cases fell from a mean of 5.9 hours in the first five to 3.1 hours in the later five cases. Current operating times range from 60-120 minutes for midtubal anastomosis, and up to 240 minutes for difficult cornual cases. The patients are discharged the same day (75%) or the next morning within 23 hours (25%).

It has been possible to perform ureteric microdissection and anastomosis, vascular repair, intramural myomectomy repair, and bowel repair using the techniques described above. Intra-uterine fetal surgery and pediatric surgery will also find applications, as will vascular and coronary surgery in time.

Laparoscopic microsurgery will introduce a new dimension to reproductive surgery and overtime will replace laparotomy for microsurgery. It is important to realize, however, that the learning curve is considerable and the technique may not be attainable by all despite their best efforts. The reproductive surgeon of tomorrow will be an expert in microendoscopy and laparoscopic microsurgery with sufficient numbers of cases to maintain and develop his expertise.

BIBLIOGRAPHY

1. Baggish MS, Chong AP. CO_2 laser microsurgery of the uterine tube. Obstet Gynecol 1981;58:111.
2. Gomel V. From microsurgery to laparoscopic surgery; A progress. Fertil Steril 1995;63:464-68.
3. Koh CH, Janik GM. Laparoscopic microsurgical tubal anastomosis. In Adamson GD, Martin DC (Eds): Endoscopic Management of Gynecologic Disease Philadelphia: Lippincott, Raven 1996a;119.
4. Prado J, Venegas J. Application of microsurgical principles to the reversal of tubal sterilization. Revista Chilena de Obtetricia y Ginecologica 1993;58(4): 298-303.
5. Putman J, Holder A, Olive D. Pregnancy rates following tubal anastomosis. Pomeroy partial salpingectomy versus electrocautery. Journal of Gynecologic Surgery 1990;6(3).
6. Reich H, Mc Glynn F, Parente C, Sekel L, Leire M. Laparoscopic tubal anastomosis. Journal of American Association of Gynaecologic Laparoscopists 1993;1: 16-19.
7. Sedbom E, Delajahircres JB, Boudovis O. Tubal desterilization through exclusive laparoscopy. Hum Reprod 1989;4:158.
8. Silva PD, Schapes AM, Meisch JK. Outpatient microsurgical reversal of tubal sterilization by a combined approach of laparoscopy and minilap. Fertil Steril 1991;55:696.
9. Winston RML. Microsurgical tubocornual anastomosis for reversal of sterilization. Lancet 1977;1:284.

HYSTEROSCOPIC SURGERY IN INFERTILITY

Shyam V Desai, Nikhil S Jani

INTRODUCTION

Infertility is seldom, if ever a physically debilitating disease. It may, however, severely affect the couple's psychological harmony, sexual life and social function. The incidence calculated by health services is approximately 16.7 percent and forms a common complaint in any gynecological clinic. It is small wonder that as we approach the second millennium, infertility diagnosis and treatment stand out as one of the most rapidly evolving areas in medicine. With recombinant FSH, micromanipulation and egg donation, rapid strides being taken in assisted reproduction, the limits of the reproductive lifespan are blurred. Endoscopic surgery is not far behind and we have several advances in technology over the years such as in fiberoptics, camera technology and documentation that have revolutionized the procedure with benefits to the surgeon and to the patients.

Operative intervention is possible following a diagnostic hysteroscopy under the same anesthesia. Many operative procedures can be carried out through the hysteroscope and these include metroplasties, adhesiolysis, myomectomy and tubal cannulation, so many intrauterine pathologies diagnosed can be treated simultaneously under one anesthesia.

Anesthesia

General anesthesia is preferred for hysteroscopic surgery and most other endoscopic surgery as well. This has been proven to be the safest anesthesia and is most comfortable for the patient who is likely to be in the lithotomy position for an hour or more. However minor surgical procedures such as a polypectomy can be carried out under local anesthesia such as a paracervical block.

Distension Media

The *distention medium* depends on the modality used to carry out the operative procedure. If instruments such as the hysteroscopic scissors are used, any standard irrigating fluid such as normal saline, Lactated Riner's solution or 5 percent or 10 percent glucose in water may be appropriate. When the electrosurgical resectoscope is used, 1.5 percent glycine or Sorbitol are preferred. Liquid media have the advantage of being cleared from time to time by aspiration or by flushing.

Instruments

The instruments used vary depending upon the choice of the surgeon. However the preference is often for rigid instruments rather than semirigid or flexible ones as the latter are fragile and often do not perform the job adequately.

The resectoscope with its attachments, *viz.* Collin's knife and loop is commonly used and helps to perform most hysteroscopic surgeries competently. However, in certain situations the hysteroscopic scissors is often preferred, as the resection of a septum or the division of adhesions can be carried out without the use of electric current, which may be of importance to prevent a decrease in the vascularity of the endometrium.

OPERATIVE HYSTEROSCOPY

Intrauterine Adhesions

Adhesions of the Asherman's syndrome are a recognizable cause of infertility. Adhesions such as these may occur following a traumatic curettage especially in the puerperium or a therapeutic abortion or even a myomectomy.[1]

The adhesions can be classified depending upon the basis of their extent and nature as follows:
• Mild—flimsy and composed of endometrial tissue
• Moderate—composed of fibromuscular tissue and covered with endometrium

- Severe—composed of fibromuscular tissue only and partially or totally occluding the uterine cavity.

March and Israel classified adhesions depending upon the extent of the obliteration of the uterine cavity as seen on hysteroscopy.[2]

Class	Findings
A Minimal	• Less than one fourth of uterine cavity involved, thin or flimsy adhesions. Ostial areas and upper fundus minimally involved or clear.
B Moderate	• One-fourth or three-fourth of uterine cavity involved, no agglutination of walls. Ostial areas and upper fundus only partially occluded.
C Severe	• More than three-fourth of uterine cavity involved, agglutination of walls or thick bands, ostial areas and upper cavity occluded

Hysteroscopic surgery permits the lysis of adhesions after classifying the extent of the problem. It is a safe and complete treatment option which gives a favorable outcome in most cases and should be offered to patients with this pathology. Adhesions which are flimsy can be separated easily with manipulation of the diagnostic hysteroscope but dense adhesions require to be divided with a semirigid or rigid scissors or with the resectoscope using Collin's knife and a cutting current. If scissors are used, the distending medium could be saline or glycine, however if the resectoscope/ Collin's knife is used, the distending medium is 1.5 percent glycine which does not conduct the monopolar current. Adhesions in the cervical canal are divided first before tackling the adhesions in the body of the uterus and the fundal region. It should be remembered that perforation of the uterus occurs easily especially when the adhesions are located at the cornual regions. It is of importance that all adhesions should be lysed under vision to avoid this. In 90 percent of patients it is possible to restore normal anatomy at the first sitting. However, some patients with extensive disease may require repeat procedures to complete the adhesiolysis. In one study 192 patients who had hysteroscopic adhesiolysis 71 (41.4%) became pregnant, 29 (36.7%) had a spontaneous abortion,

2 had premature deliveries, and 45 had a term pregnancy. Eight patients required manual removal of the placenta or postpartum curettage. Placenta accreta can also complicate the delivery and 2 patients in this series required an obstetric hysterectomy. Magos has reported hysteroscopic management of Asherman's syndrome to be the "Gold Standard".[3] Another study of 105 cases found a significant increase in the viable pregnancy rate from 14.7 to 97.4 percent. [4]

Leiomyomata Uteri

The correlation between fibroids and infertility is unclear though submucous fibroids do predispose to habitual abortions and infertility.[5] Hysteroscopic myomectomy should be considered for any patient with a symptomatic submucous myoma. The major symptom that patients with submucous fibroids present with is menorrhagia and the diagnosis is usually confirmed by a transvaginal ultrasonography (TVS). A thorough preoperative assessment with an HSG is mandatory to determine the size and attachment of the myoma,[5] in some cases an MRI and TVS may be required.

Submucous fibroid as seen on hysteroscopy are pale, smooth, firm and rounded and may be pedunculated or sessile. Fibroids bulge into the cavity and the endometrium can be seen to be thinned out over them with prominent vessels.

Neuwirth and Amin described the first hysteroscopic myomectomy in 1976".[6]

The resectoscope and the cutting loop are used for piecemeal resection of the submucus leiomyoma. With 1.5 percent glycine as the distending medium the resectoscope is introduced into the cavity and the anatomical landmarks are identified. The location and size of the leiomyoma is noted. If the myoma is pedunculated, it is better to resect most of the myoma before cutting the stalk. If the stalk is cut early, the myoma will spin around with the irrigating fluid making its removal difficult. Resection is carried out with the resectoscope and cutting loop with a 50 watt current. As the chips of myometrium accumulate within the cavity, vision may be obscured and a periodic curettage of the cavity is necessary for clear access to the lesion.

This is continued until the normal configuration of the uterine cavity is achieved. However, it may not be possible to remove partially intramural myomas completely at one sitting especially if less than half of the tumor presents submucosally.

Single lesion less than 5 cm in diameter which protrudes for 75 percent of its volume into the uterine cavity can be resected in a one-step procedure. Lesions more than 5 cm and which protrude between 50 to 75 percent within the cavity and those that are smaller than 2.5 cm and which protrude less than 50 percent into the cavity can be managed with GnRH suppression followed by a single step procedure.[7]

Resection of the fibroid is carried out with the resectoscope but may also be carried out with an electrosurgical snare. This procedure obviates the need for opening the uterine cavity as was done in the past and is one of the major surgical advances for the treatment of fibroids.

The GnRH analogs also allow for improvement of the hemoglobin in anemic patients. The analogs should be administered for 2 to 3 months before the procedure. Larger or multiple lesions may require two or more sittings.

Pregnancy rates of upto 66 percent have been reported after hysteroscopic myomectomy by use of the Nd:YAG laser for myomectomy.[7-9] Fernandez et al have reported improvement in symptoms in 62 percent patients. However, 27 percent pregnancy rate, and 10 percent delivered at term.[10]

Polyps

Large polyps are uncommon but it is reasonable to postulate that they may hinder implantation. A polyp situated close to the cornual region may hinder conception. Grasping it with a grasper is usually sufficient to excise it, though at times cauterization of the base and extraction may be required. Resection of a polyp is easier than resection of a fibroid and at times transecting its base and removing the compressible mass through the cervix with a grasping forceps may be easy. Liberis has reported 86 percent success rate in hysteroscopic polyp removal.[11]

Uterine Anomalies

The appearance of an intrauterine septum on hysteroscopic examination is characteristic. The uterine cornuae are obviously separated by a central fibrous band. It is unlikely that anomalies of the reproductive tract which occur in 1 of every 700 women are a cause of infertility, but they have been implicated in the etiology of habitual abortion. The septate uterus leads to a diminished uterine capacity, reduced vascularity within the septum leading to first and second trimester wastage. Golan et al found septa in 23 percent of women with a missed abortion.[12] Edstrom first introduced hysteroscopic septum resection in 1974.[12]

Resection of the septum may be carried out using hysteroscopic scissors or the Collins knife and resectoscope with a 30 watt cutting current. The use of the Nd:YAG laser has also been reported by Baggish et al.[14] A laparoscopic evaluation to differentiate between a bicornuate uterus and a septum is advisable, though a preoperative MRI can give the same information. The procedure of septum cutting is a remarkably bloodless procedure and the entire operation takes about 10 to 15 minutes with good distention and vision. The distending medium used is 1.5 percent glycine when an electrocautery is used. When hysteroscopic scissors are employed, Hyskon, normal saline, or sorbitol can be used.

The division of the septum results in the fibromuscular tissue retracting into the uterine wall and the uterine cavity assumes a capacious appearance. The hysteroscope should not be inserted too far beyond the internal os and the surgeon should attempt to maintain both cornual areas in view. A difficult anomaly to treat is the broad-based septum as it is difficult to keep both the ostia under vision, besides the chances of uterine perforation are more in these cases.

Septal tissue is relatively avascular, however, as the fundal region is approached the vascularity increases. Incision should be stopped short of the myometrium and a useful marker to indicate the proximity of the myometrium is the appearance of blood vessels in the hitherto avascular operative site. A panoramic view of the uterine cavity should be obtained from time to time to ensure proper orientation.

Some workers prefer to use GnRH-analogs prior to surgery so that the endometrium thins out, mucous debris is less and the vascularity of the uterus diminishes, however most surgeons prefer to carry out the procedure in the early proliferative phase. It is important to maintain traction on the cervix throughout the surgery so that the long axis of the uterus is parallel to the sacrum. This reduces the chances of uterine perforation.

Israel and March after carrying out hysteroscopic septectomy in 91 patients found a significant improvement in the pregnancy outcome.[15]

DeCherney treated 72 patients with a septum hysteroscopically, 58 percent of these had a successful pregnancy outcome.[16] The patients with habitual abortions will certainly benefit from this procedure when no other causative factor is found. As compared to the Tomkins or Jones metroplasty this procedure is simpler and definitely less invasive. Birinigi L *et al* have reported 36 deliveries in their series of 66 cases of Meteroplasty with normal delivery in 28 cases.[17] It can be performed on an outpatient basis, without an abdominal or uterine scar and minimal postoperative morbidity. The use of estrogens has been advocated ~ by some workers while others have inserted an intrauterine contraceptive device (lUCD) postoperatively. The ability to intervene surgically with the hysteroscope has several advantages for the infertile patient and the gynecologist. An operation that is carried out without incisions followed by a rapid recovery and minimal discomfort is accepted more easily than one which is accompanied by pain and discomfort. In addition, the absence of wound infection, reduced operating time and absence of scarring of the uterus are substantial benefits to the patient who is likely to conceive in the future.

REFERENCES

1. March CM, Israel R, March AD. Hysteroscopic management of intrauterine adhesions. Am J Obstet Gynecol 1978;653.
2. Sugimoto O. Diagnostic and therapeutic hysteroscopy for traumatic intrauterine adhesions. Am J Obstet Gynecol 1966;96:1027.
3. Magos A. Reprod Biomed Online. Hysteroscopic treatment of Asherman's syndrome. 2002;4(Suppl 3): 46-51.
4. Valle RF, Sciarra JJ. Intrauterine adhesions-hysteroscopic diagnosis classification, treatment and reproductive outcome. Am J Obstet Gynecol 1988;58: 1459-70.
5. Buttram JC Jr, Reiter RC. Uterine leiomyomata-etiology, symptomatology, and management. Fertil Steril 1981;36:433-45.
6. Neuwirth RS, Amin HK. Excision of submucous fibroids with hysteroscopic control. Am J Obstet Gynecol 1976;126:95-99.
7. Coddington CC, Collins RL, Shawker TH et al. Long acting gonadotropin releasing hormone analogue used to treat uteri. Fertil Steril 1986;45:624.
8. Donnez J et al. Nd: Y AG laser and enlarged submucous fibroids. Fertil Steril 1990;54:999.
9. Donnez J, Nicolle M: Hysteroscopic surgery. Cllrr Opin Obstet Gynecol 1992;4:439.
10. Fernandez H, Sefrioui O, Virelizier C et al. Hysteroscopic resection of submucosal myomas in patients with infertility. Hum Reprod 2001;16(7):1489-92.
11. Liberis V, Dafopoulos K, Tsikouras P. Removal of endometrial polyps by use of grasping forceps and curettage after diagnostic hysteroscopy. Clin Exp Obstet Gynecol. 2003;30(1):29-31.
12. Edstrom K: Intrauterine surgical procedures during hysteroscopy. Endoscopy 1974;6:175-84.
13. March CM. Hysteroscopic resection of submucus myomas. Contempt Obstet Gynaecol 1990;35:59-66.
14. Baggish MS, Baltoyannis P. New techniques for laser ablation of the endometrium in high risk patients. Am J Obstet Gynecol.
15. Israel R, March CM. Hysteroscopic incision of the septate uterus. Am J Obstet Gynecol.
16. DeChemey AH, Russell JB, Giaebe RA et al. Resectoscopic management of Mutterian fusion defects. Fertil Steril 1986;45:726.
17. Birinyi L, Gyenes O, Major T. Orv Hetil. Debreceni Egyetem Orvos-es Egeszsegtudomanyi Centrum, Altalanos Orvostudomanyi Kar 2003;144(20): 979-83.

ROLE OF MICROSURGERY IN INFERTILITY MANAGEMENT

Kusum Zaveri, Indira Hinduza

INTRODUCTION

Microsurgery is less than 100 years old. No instrument of microsurgery and no microsurgeon can be found in the history of Egyptian or Greek medicine. Kurt Swolin[1] was the first to introduce microsurgical concepts into infertility surgery. He developed a microsurgical technique for salpingostomy in 1967 for hydrosalpinx repair. In comparision to many other surgical specialities, the introduction of microsurgery into gynecology occurred relatively late. Gomel[2] and Winston[3] were the first to employ microsurgery to perform tubocornual anastomosis for pathologic cornual occlusion and reversal of sterilization, and tubotubal anastomosis, for repair of pathologic occlusion and to restore fertility in previously sterilized patients. Microsurgery was introduced into gynecology to improve the outcome of infertility surgery, as the results yielded by conventional surgery were disappointing. Adhesion formation after peritoneal surgery is a major cause of infertility especially after appendicectomy and gynecologic surgery. Microsurgery acts as a prophylactic measure for prevention of infertility due to such adhesions, and also enhances results of infertility surgery when surgical causes exist.

What is Microsurgery?

Microsurgery may be broadly defined as surgery performed with the use of an operating microscope, specialized instruments and fine sutures which allows accurate tissue dissection, precise placement of sutures, minimized tissue trauma and restoring anatomical and physiological function of an organ as close to normal as possible. Surgery under magnification is one of the aspects integrated with philosophy of tissue care design to minimize trauma in microsurgery.

The principles of microsurgery are:

1. *Atraumatic technique* It includes gentle and delicate handling of tissue by avoiding sharp instruments and toothed forceps and also the use of glass or teflon rods for retraction. While packing the intestines, the intestines as well as the uterus is handled in such a way that tissue abrasion does not take place.

2. *Avoidance of foreign body in peritoneal cavity* Foreign material like glove powder is prevented from entering the peritoneal cavity by washing hands with ringer lactate.

3. *Irrigation* Drying of serosal surface due to exposure to atmosphere and operating light is avoided by continuous irrigation with ringer lactate containing heparin.

4. *Haemostasis* Bleeding points are exposed by a jet of irrigating solution and not by swabbing. Bleeding is stopped with bipolar cautery or microelectrode using unipolar current. Meticulous hemostasis is achieved with minimum charring, heating and damage to normal tissue.

5. *Complete excision of pathological tissue* Complete excision of pathological tissue is essential to ensure functional results. Excision of tissue is viewed under operating microscope until healthy tissue is encountered.

6. *Magnification* Magnification permits the appreciation of both normal and pathologic morphological details and facilitates proper excision of pathological tissue. With the use of magnification, bleeding points are visible and can be cauterized individually which leads to least tissue destruction and preservation of blood supply helps to prevent fibrosis for the proper functioning of the tube and prevention of adhesions.

7. *Pelvic lavage* The pelvis should be lavaged with the irrigating solution in order to wash out debris and tiny blood clots at the end of surgery.

Tubal Surgery

Proximal Tubal Occlusion (PTO)

Approximately 25 to 30 percent of involuntary infertility can be attributed to diseases of the fallopian tubes.[4] Occlusion at the cornual region account for 20 percent of operations performed for tubal disease.[5] Diagnosis of PTO is done by conventional techniques like hysterosalpingography (HSG) and laparoscopy. In the seventies, selective salpingography added new dimensions to it.

A variety of pathological conditions have been reported for proximal tubal occlusion including chronic inflammation, salpingitis isthmica nodosa, endometriosis and obliterative fibrosis. Treatment for proximal tubal block traditionally has evolved microsurgical resection and anastomosis achieving pregnancy rates between 54 to 69 percent.[2, 3] A more recent approach to cornual occlusion involves the transcervical cannulation using either fluoroscopic, hysteroscopic or tactile guidance. Pregnancy rates of 34 percent [6,7] have led to suggest that tubal cannulation can be offered as the first choice in the management of PTO. Unsuitable cases for tubal cannulation require tubocornual anastomosis, which is preferred over tubal implantation. Both these techniques require microsurgical approach. Cornual opening being very small, magnification is very important in tubocornual anastomosis. To prevent adhesions, microsurgical principles have to be observed in tubocornual anastomosis and tubal implantation.

In 1977, there was a transition from macrosurgical implantation to microsurgical anastomosis. Gomel[2] and Winston[3] described microsurgical technique for tubal anastomosis in women with PTO. They reported postoperative term pregnancy rates (PR) of 37 to 56 percent respectively. The proposed advantages of the microsurgical tubocornual anastomosis over implantation are as follows:

1. Function of the uterotubal junction will be preserved;
2. Less disruption of the cornual blood supply;
3. No weakening of the uterine musculature, with a presumably low risk of dehiscence in subsequent pregnancies[8, 9]
4. No need for lower segment cesarean section (LSCS) to deliver patients.

Macrosurgical Implantation Results

Grant[10] reported in 73 patients PR of 25 percent and an ectopic PR of 4.1 percent. Diamond[11] presented the results of two macrosurgical implantation techniques, one with reamer and prosthesis and the other fundus splitting technique. Total ongoing PRs were 42 percent and 16 percent respectively and the ectopic PR was 16 percent.

Microsurgical Tubocornual Anastomosis Results

Winston[3,12] and Gomel[2,13] reported term PRs after microsurgical anastomosis of 38 percent and 56 percent respectively. Diamond[11] compared his microsurgery and macrosurgery results in patients with tubal disease where PR was 56 percent and 16 percent respectively.

Selective salpingography and transcervical cannulation under fluoroscopic, hysteroscopic or tactile sensation guidance are effective at establishing patency in appropriately selected patients and are less invasive and less expensive than surgical alternatives.

Tubal implantation has a lower success rate and is indicated only in cases of complete obliteration of intramural fallopian tube. Even in tubal implantation all the principles of microsurgery must be observed otherwise adhesions will further reduce the success rate.

Midtubal Block

Midtubal block due to pathological condition is not very common. Etiology of pathological block is tuberculous salpingitis, endometriosis, salpingitis isthmica nodosa, tubal pregnancy and congenital structural abnormalities. Genital tuberculosis is one of the common etiological factors for midtubal block among the pathological conditions in India. Reversal of sterilization patients forms a bulk of midtubal block.

Tubal sterilization is currently a most popular form of birth control methods in India. However some women eventually regret their decision due to change in personal, social or economical status and request reversal of tubal sterilization. Exact figures for reversal in India are not known. Siegler et al[14] reported 1 percent of women undergoing surgical sterilization seek reversal of the procedure. Accidental death of a child, change in marital status and change in economical status are the most common reasons in India. Garcia[15] reported the first microsurgical re-anastomosis of the fallopian tube; since that time the pregnancy success rates have improved two fold with microsurgical techniques when compared with traditional tubal reversal. The over all success in terms of intrauterine pregnancies after reversal of sterilization using microsurgery ranges from 60-80 percent[2,3,16,17] and with clips best results up to 95 percent[18,19] are achieved. Type of anastomosis, length of tube, condition of fimbria, interval between sterilization and reversal play a role in success rate of pathological mid tubal block and reversal of sterilization.

Microsurgical end to end anastomosis is done, by excising the blocked portion and achieving hemostasis on the cut surface by bipolar cautery. The tissue must be trimmed until healthy mucosa and muscle can be seen. Complete excision of the pathologic segment is essential to ensure a functional result. The tissue is excised under the operative microscope till normal looking tissue is encountered. The sign of healthy tissue are: Presence of four to five mucosal folds with fine linear blood vessels, regular circular inner muscle coat without white fibrous or gritty tissue in it, absence of extravasation of dye in tubal lymphatics and no diverticuli.

In tubal anastomosis every effort is made to align the two segments of the tube properly so that tubal transport will not be disrupted. Anastomosis is done in two layers. After excluding the mucosa, inner and outer layers are sutured by 8/0 absorbable or non-absorbable synthetic suture material under magnification.

During the last few years, laparoscopic reversal was tried with glue, one stitch or two stitch techniques but success rate was disappointing. Koh[20] published the first true microsurgical laparoscopic technique for tubal anastomosis with new microsurgical instrumentation. Pregnancy rate was 71 percent and ectopic pregnancy rate was 3.2 percent with one year follow-up. Till date ~100 successful pregnancies worldwide are recorded. The largest published series [21] shows a pregnancy rate of 75.5 percent by laparoscopic reversal, which compares favorably with the oldest series of microsurgery by Dubuisson et al.[17]

The many different means available to carry out this anastomosis show that there is as yet no one best method of laparoscopically guided sterilization reversal. Some authors[22] propose a combined technique of laparoscopy and minilaparotomy but nothing is comparable to conventional microsurgery by laparotomy. Handling long instruments, suturing the tissue, visualization of tubal lumen and tying intracorporeal knots are the difficulties with laparoscopic reversal, but the most important would be the magnification, which cannot be achieved as much as with an operative microscope for perfect anastomosis. Microsurgery by laparotomy with end to end anastomosis has best results and remains a method of choice for midtubal block, pathological or reversal of sterilization.

In case of discrepancy in lumen it is preferable to carry out the anastomosis by microsurgery than laparoscopically. Yoon et al have reported 87.1 percent pregnancy rate after bilateral tubal anastomosis using laparoscopic techniques. They further mentioned that laparoscopic reversal is a procedure of choice for surgeons who have extensive experience with both tubal anastomosis by laparotomy and advanced laparoscopic techniques.[23]

At present the results of laparoscopy except by those of Yoon cannot match those of laparotomy and microsurgical tubal anastomosis still remains the standard surgical method.

Distal Tubal Occlusion

Distal Tubal Occlusion (DTO) is diagnosed by HSG and laparoscopy. Salpingoscopy and falloposcopy have added prognostic value and help to make a decision between surgery and assisted reproduction techniques (ART). Damage to fallopian tubes with subsequent tubal occlusion continues to be a very common cause of infertility. Distal occlusion may be a result of acute pelvic infection, intra-abdominal or appendicular infection, pelvic surgery and endometriosis. The goals of surgical treatment are to repair the obstruction either by exposing the remaining fimbriae or creating neosalpingostomy and restoring the normal tubo-ovarian relationship with free mobility of the adnexae. The crude pregnancy rate ranged from 20 to 35 percent, with 10 to 50 percent[24-27] of these pregnancies being tubal ectopics in conventional surgery. Many studies using microsurgical techniques have been published showing crude pregnancy rates between 30 to 40 percent after neosalpingostomy with 10 to 30 percent[24, 28-30] of these being tubal ectopics. Results of microsurgery and macrosurgery do not show significant difference in terms of pregnancy rate.

Pregnancy outcome after reconstruction tubal surgery, for terminal block is thought to be related to the extent of pelvic adhesions and of tubal disease. Based on various parameters several classifications have been proposed to access the extent of tubal disease in order to predict pregnancy outcome.[31-35] However, none of the devised classifications included a direct evaluation of the status of ampullary mucosa among the parameters, although status of this endosalpinx could be the most important prognostic factor in terms of reproductive outcome.

Transfimbrial salpingoscopy, represents a valuable adjunct to the evaluation of the distal tube. The ability to directly visualize intraluminal adhesions and mucosal abnormalities provides valuable information not otherwise obtained employing more traditional diagnostic techniques.

Prognostic value of salpingoscopy was compared with American Fertility Society (AFS) scoring system for adnexal adhesions and DTO[36] in patients with tubal infertility undergoing reconstructive tubal surgery. There was a significant correlation between salpingoscopic grade I-II v/s grade III-V and the achievement

of a term pregnancy for both the salpingo-ovariolysis and the salpingo-neostomy group of patients. There was no significant correlation between the AFS scores and the achievement of a term pregnancy for both groups of patients.

In a prospective study by De Bruyne[37] the prognostic value of salpingoscopy was evaluated in patients undergoing salpingo-ovariolysis or salpingo-neostomy by microsurgical laparotomy for post-pelvic inflammatory disease (PID). There was significant difference when cumulative intrauterine pregnancy rates for salpingoscopic classes I-II v/s III-V were compared both in salpingo-ovariolysis and salpingo-neostomy groups.

A recent prospective study[38] demonstrated that the combination of HSG and laparoscopy is less accurate for diagnosis of tubal infertility than the endoscopic inspection of the tubal mucosa. Several studies on hydrosalpinx have shown that when salpingoscopy can exclude the presence of mucosal adhesions > 50 percent intrauterine and <5 percent tubal pregnancy rate can be predicted following reconstructive surgery.[39-42] However, tubal endoscopy has not yet gained widespread clinical acceptance.[43]

Marconi and Quintana[44] reported that during falloposcope scoring, it is possible to access the tubal epithelium. The frequency of mucosal flattening and vascular alterations is not different between pregnant and non-pregnant patients, whereas the presence of intraluminal adhesions and nuclear staining with methylene blue was not conducive to the occurrence of subsequent pregnancies.

During diagnostic laparoscopy, treatment can be attempted at the same sitting and conditions like terminal tubal block can be corrected. Laparoscopy and microsurgery has shown equally good results and hence terminal block is corrected by laparoscopy. Recent reports suggest that surgical correction of the hydrosalpinx may improve the outcome of IVF-embryo transfer. Further studies are needed to verify if this subgroup of patients could benefit from salpingostomy.[45-47]

Based on salpingoscopy results, selection for tuboplasty can be more meaningful. Patients with normal tubal mucosa should undergo salpingoovariolysis and salpingo-neostomy, whereas those with abnormal tubal mucosa of class III-V should not undergo salpingo-neostomy but should be referred for ART.

Ectopic Pregnancy

Early diagnosis of ectopic pregnancy by repeated measurement of serum human chorionic gonadotropin, ultrasonographic and laparoscopic examinations have permitted conservative surgical treatment of unruptured tubal pregnancy.[48,49] The value of conservative management of ectopic tubal pregnancy has been well established.[50-52] When conservation or laparoscopic treatment is contra-indicated microsurgical laparotomy approach is chosen. Linear salpingostomy is performed on the anti-mesosalpinx with either electrodiathermy or laser beam. Through this 10-15 mm incision, the products of conception are gently removed. Hemostasis is achieved. All blood clots are removed and thorough peritoneal wash with ringer lactate and heparin is given.

Ovarian Surgery

Sequelae of ovarian surgery can be an important factor in infertility. In endometriosis the removal of an ovarian endometrioma can result in extensive tubo-ovarian adhesion formation. Nevertheless, conservative infertility surgery appears to be more successful than medical treatment. However, wedge resection of the ovaries in Stein-Leventhal syndrome has been superseded by medical treatment because of the sequelae to surgery. Similarly, removal of a benign ovarian tumor or cyst in patients desiring fertility can result in serious fertility problems due to adhesions. Progress in surgical techniques particularly gynecologic microsurgery can be applied in ovarian surgery to minimize surgical trauma and retain maximal function of the delicate tubo-ovarian structures.

Myoma

Fibroids are the commonest solid tumor. At least 30 percent of all women are estimated to have leiomyomas during their life time and 80 percent of them are asymptomatic. Myomectomy is a controversial procedure for infertile women. In the absence of additional factors impeding conception, some investigators have suggested conservative surgery,[53,54] whereas others favor expectant management.[55,56] These uncertainties arise because of the pathogenetic mechanisms through which fibroids cause infertility are still hypothetical and controlled data on the efficacy of intervention are lacking. Data on the outcome of IVF-ET in matched women with and without myomas could clarify the issue indirectly, but the published results are not consistent.[57]

Myomectomy often causes adhesion formation and posterior or fundal incisions are associated with more adhesions than anterior. Adnexal adhesion may impair fertility. Similarly utericuloplasty is a rare indication for treatment of infertility. Like myomectomy utericuloplasty also has an incision on the surface of the uterus which may lead to adhesions and produce infertility. Microsurgery is commonly associated with surgery done under magnification. During any surgery done on the uterus magnification is not as important as the principles of microsurgery, which are required to reduce adhesion formation. No adjuvant treatment has been demonstrated to be effective in preventing adhesion formation to uterine incision sites. Recently barrier material such as polytetrafluoroethylene (PTFE) barrier has been used and found to be effective in reducing adhesions.[58]

Laparoscopic myomectomy has been reported to be an effective technique that is associated with a low rate of patient morbidity.[59,60] Because myomectomy is often performed to preserve the uterus for future pregnancy, maintaining the integrity of uterine wall is of utmost importance. However three case reports of spontaneous uterine rupture during pregnancy after laparoscopic myomectomy have raised questions concerning the safety of this technique for women who desire future pregnancy.[60, 61]

One of the concerns regarding laparoscopic myomectomy has been adequate reconstruction and healing of the uterine defect with subsequent ability for the uterus to withstand the strain associated with pregnancy and labor.

At laparotomy, closure of the excision site is usually accomplished by a multilayer suture; whereas, in operative laparoscopy, suturing can be cumbersome and tedious and restoration of the uterine wall integrity to an equivalent manner may be difficult. Furthermore, extensive use of thermal energy to achieve hemostasis laparoscopically may also compromise uterine tissue. The procedure of laparoscopic myomectomy is rather new and may not be efficacious for patients who desire future pregnancy. Gomel[62] suggested a combination of laparoscopy and minilaparotomy for large myomas and it will have benefit of adequate uterine repair and easy removal of specimen.

Abdominal myomectomy is a mainstay of conservative reproductive surgery.[63-66] The results in surgical series adds further evidence in favor of a potential treatment benefit of the procedure in terms of an increased pregnancy rate in infertile women and a decreased abortion rate in women with a history of miscarriages.[67]

Endometriosis

The incidence of endometriosis is 2 to 7 percent in women in the reproductive age group. It is significantly higher varying from 20 to 25 percent in infertile subjects. Laparoscopy remains the most important modality in diagnosis of endometriosis, and ultrasound is for chocolate cyst. Although originally proposed for tubal disease, microsurgical principles in a broader sense can also be applied in situations characterized by severe and extensive anatomical alterations like those caused by advanced endometriosis. In these difficult situations the use of an operating microscope or magnifying loops may not always be practical, but apart from this, microsurgery may substantially improve the chance of reconstructing a functional genital apparatus.

Ovarian endometriomas do not respond well to medical treatment with danazol or luteinizing hormone releasing hormone agonists.[68] Therefore surgical treatment remains the main treatment modality. Simple drainage of endometriomas by laparoscopy or by transvaginal approach has been shown to be inadequate because of the high incidence of recurrence.[69]

Laparoscopy is now the treatment of choice for physical elimination of minimal and mild endometriotic lesions and for excision of endometriomas not associated with particularly dense extensive adhesions. The controversies arise in cases with the really severe forms.

Although the advantages of endoscopic surgery are obvious in terms of limited morbidity, hospitalization and possibly costs, the doubt still persists that treatment of the more severe forms of pelvic endometriosis at laparoscopy may not be optimal compared with laparotomy[70] using microsurgical techniques. The cleavage planes are better identified at microsurgical laparotomy due to perception of the depth of the field and direct palpation of the tissues.

The field of vision is restricted, laparoscopic instrumentation can not be defined as atraumatic, tissue handling may not be as delicate and precise as at laparotomy, suturing can be difficult and the direct manual tactile sense, which is invaluable in very difficult cases is limited. Severe endometriosis requires a high level of surgical expertise to be both efficacious and safe and provides a realistic test of surgical skills.[71]

Adjuvants to Microsurgery

Peritoneal adhesions that develop as a normal consequence of wound healing continue to be a significant cause of postoperative complications 80-90 percent of pelvic adhesions are attributable to preceding surgery. Five to twenty percent arise from inflammatory causes. Postoperative adhesions can lead to bowel obstruction, chronic pelvic pain, and infertility. A great deal of effort has been dedicated to various surgeons to reduce postoperative adhesions by developing a variety of surgical techniques and use of several agents. Innumerable adhesion preventing agents have been used throughout the history of surgery.[3] However, at least 50 percent of patients still develop significant adhesions.[72]

SurgicalTechnique

- To adhere to strict microsurgical technique of maintaining atraumatic tissue handling and meticulous hemostasis, avoiding abrasions and serosal drying and by choosing the least reactive suture material one can minimize subsequent adhesion formations. Use of crystalloid solution as an irrigation solution may reduce serosal trauma.
- Use of lasers along with other microsurgical principles, performing adjunctive surgical procedures like uterine or adnexal suspension may help to reduce postoperative adhesion formation.

Still other researchers advocate use of laparoscopic surgery over open surgical methods.

An early second look laparoscopy with adhesiolysis has also been recommended.

But as recent studies have demonstrated that microsurgical techniques alone will not prevent adhesion formation hence researchers attempted to reduce adhesion formation by identifying drugs and biocompatible material as adhesion barriers.

Pharmacologic Agents

a. Reduction of the inflammatory reaction, fibrinous exudation and fibroblastic proliferation (Drugs like glucocorticoids, NSAIDs, progestins, promethazine, colchicine have all been used but they have a low efficacy with higher rate of adverse reactions).

b. Inhibition of fibrin deposition and coagulation, use of heparin during peritoneal irrigation may reduce adhesions but higher efficacy may not be achieved in all patients.

c. Enhancement of fibrinolysis Use of plasminogen activators, apoproteins and fibrinolytic enzymes like pepsin, trypsin, chymotrypsin, streptokinase and hyaluronidase have all been tried but are not yet proven to be efficacious in preventing postoperative adhesion formation.

Barrier Agents

They cause separation of serosal surfaces. Earlier Dextran was used intraoperatively to separate serosal surfaces but the side effects were considerable: Nowadays the commonly used agents are:

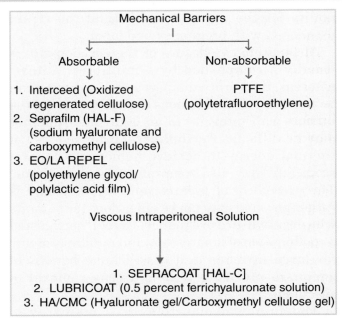

Out of the above only interceed (TC7) and PTFE are commercially available. A 66-80 percent reduction in postoperative adhesions formation was demonstrated by their use. Recently lazaroids (non-steroidal–PNU 83836E) and steroidal (PNU 4006F) have been tried as fibrinolytic agents.

Miscellaneous Procedures

i. Postoperative hydrotubation has been used with little or varied success outcome

ii. Peritoneal grafts or omentectomy

iii. Splints: like Mulligan hood, Roland's spiral have been used with low success rates

iv. Prevention of contamination by prophylactic use of antibiotics is recommended by most researchers.

ABANDONED ADJUVANTS

There have been agents in the past which have shown no effect at all or an actual increase in adhesion formation as compared to that in controls (In animal studies and clinical experience).

These include fish bladder, carp peritoneum, ox peritoneum, shark peritoneum, amniotic membrane, silk or rubber sheets, olive oil, mineral oil, camphorated oil, liquid paraffin, gelatins, lanolin, sodium ricinolate, albumin, oxidized cellulose, agar, callodion, chyle, epinephrine solution and amniotic fluid. They have long since been abandoned.

Till date no single agent/treatment has been proven uniformly effective in prevention of adhesion formation. Surgical techniques that limit tissue ischemia as well as the use of mechanical barriers provide clinical benefits to the patients of today.

CONCLUSION

The development of microsurgery, operative laparoscopy and assisted reproductive technology in the last 30 years, have improved the outlook for infertile couples. Microsurgery and ART must be considered complementary rather than competitive procedures. Intelligent patient selection is the key in making the best therapeutic choice. Tubocornual anastomosis for proximal block, reversal of sterilization, myomectomy, utericuloplasty, advance stage endometriosis and hemodynamically unstable patients of ectopic pregnancy, microsurgery is the treatment of choice. Microsurgery has added advantage over ART that it gives a chance to patients to restore natural fertility and get opportunity to have more than one pregnancy. Operative laparoscopy is preferred for salpingo-ovariolysis, fimbrioplasty, salpingostomy and tubal pregnancy. Like microsurgery, in operative laparoscopy most of the microsurgical principles are followed except small incision. Thus laparoscopic surgery is also a type of microsurgery.

Poor candidates for microsurgery due to inadequate tubal length, extensive cornual scarring, distal fimbrectomy, inoperable tubes like tuberculous salpingitis, distal tubal block with extensive endosalpingeal damage and bipolar block are treated with ART.

REFERENCES

1. Swolin K. Fifty fertility operations: Literature and methods. Acta Obstet Gynaecol Scand 1967;46:234.
2. Gomel V. Tubal reanastomosis by microsurgery. Fertil Steril 1977;28:59-65.
3. Winston RM. Microsurgical tubocornual anastomosis for reversal of sterilization. Lancet 1977;1:284-85.
4. Musich J, Behrman S. Surgical management of tubal obstruction at the uterotubal junction. Fertil Steril 1983;40:423-40.
5. Kistner RW, Patten GW. Surgery of the oviduct. In Atlas of Infertility Surgery. Boston: Little Brown, 1975;95.
6. Confino E, Friberg J, Gleicher N. Priliminary experience with transcervical balloon tuboplasty. Am J Obstet Gynecol, 1988;159:370-75.
7. Novy MJ, Thurmond AS, Patton P, Unchide BT, Rosch J. Diagnostics of cornual obstruction by transcervical fallopian tube cannulation. Fertil Steril 1988;50:434-40.
8. Green-Armytage V. Tubo-uterine implantation. J Obstet Gynaec Br Emp 1957;64:47-49.
9. Woolam GL, Pratt JH, Wilson RB. Uterine rupture following tubal implantation. Report of 2 cases. Obstet Gynecol 1967;29:415-19.
10. Grant A. Infertility surgery of the oviduct. Fertil Steril 1971;22:496-503.
11. Diamond E. A comparison of gross and microsurgical techniques for the repair of cornual occlusion in infertility: A retrospective study, 1968-1978. Fertil Steril 1979;32:370-76.
12. Winston RM. Microsurgery of the fallopian tube: from fantasy to reality. Fertil Steril 1980;34:521-30.
13. Gomel V. An odyssey through the oviduct. Fertil Steril 1983;39:144-56.
14. Siegler AM, Hulka J, Peretz A. Reversibility of female sterilization. Fertil Steril 1985;43:499-510.
15. Garcia CR. Oviductal anastomosis procedures. In Richard RM, Prager DJ (Eds): Human Sterilization. Springfield IL: Thomos Charles C. 1972;116.
16. Swolin K. Spontanheilung nach querresektion der tuba fallopii. Acte Obstet Gynecol Scand 1967;46:219-22.
17. Dubuisson JB, Chapron C, Nos C, Morice P, Aubriot FX, Gamier P. Sterilization reversal: fertility results. Hum Reprod 1995;10:1145-51.
18. Donnez J. La trompe de fellope. Histophysiologic normale et pathologique. These Universite Catholique de Louvain 1984.
19. Owen E. Reversal of female sterilization. Review of 252 microsurgical salpingoplastics. Med J Aust 1984;141:276-79.
20. Koh CH. Microsurgical laparoscopic tubal resection and anastomosis: techniques and results. References en gynecologic obstetrique. (Review), Congres Vichy, IFS, 1995;102-04.
21. Yoon TK, Sung HR, Cha SH, Lee CN, Cha KY. Fertility outcome after laparoscopic microsurgical tubal anastomosis. Fertil Steril 1997;67:18-22.
22. Gomel V. From microsurgery, to laparoscopic surgery: A progress. Fertil Steril 1995;63:464-468.
23. Yoon TK, Sung HR, Kang HG, Cha SH, Lee CN, Cha KY. Laparoscopic tubal anastomosis: Fertility outcome in 202 cases. Fertil Steril 1999;72:1121-26.
24. Luber K, Beeson CC, Kennedy JF, Villaneuva B, Young PE. Results of microsurgical treatment of infertility and early tubal second-look laparoscopy in the post-pelvic inflammatory disease patient: Implications for in vitro fertilization. Am J Obstet Gynecol 1986;154:1264.

25. Lavy G, Diamond MP, DeCherney AH. Ectopic pregnancy: Its relationship to tubal reconstructive surgery. Fertil Steril 1987;47:543.

26. Bateman BG, Nunley WC Jr, Kitchin JD III. Surgical management of distal tubal obstruction are we making progress? Fertil Steril 1987;48:523.

27. Williams KM, Gritlin WT. Distal tuboplasty: Is it appropriate? South Med J 1988;81:872.

28. Kitchin JDIII, Nunley WC Jr, Bateman BG. Surgical management of distal tubal occlusion. Am J Obstet Gynecol 1986;155:524.

29. Marana R, Quagliarrello J. Distal tubal occlusion: Microsurgery versus in vitro fertilization a review. Int J Fertil 1988;33:107.

30. Jacobs LA, Thie J, Patton PE, Williams TJ. Primary microsurgery for postinflammatory tubal infertility. Fertil Steril 1988;50:855.

31. Rock JA, Katayama KR, Martin EJ, Woodruff JD, Jones HWJ. Factors influencing the success of salpingostomy techniques for distal fimbrial obstruction. Obstet Gynecol 1978;52:591-96.

32. Hulka JF. Adnexal adhesion: A prognostic staging and classification system based on a five-year survey of fertility surgery results at Chapel Hill, North Carolina. Am J Obstet Gynecol 1982;144:141-48.

33. Boer-Meisel ME te Velde EL, Habbema JDF, Kardaun JWPF. Predicting the pregnancy outcome in patients treated for hydrosalpinx: a prospective study. Fertil Steril 1986;45:23-29.

34. Mage G, Pouly JL, de Jolimere JB et al. A preoperative classification to predict the intrauterine and ectopic pregnancy rate after distal tubal microsurgery. Fertil Steril 1986;46:807-10.

35. American Fertility Society: The American Fertility Society classifications of adnexal adhesions, distal tubal occlusion, tubal occlusion secondary to tubal ligation, tubal pregnancies, Mullerian anomalies and intra-uterine adhesions. Fertil Steril 1988;49:944-55.

36. Marana R, Muzii L, Rizzi M, dell'Acqua S, Mancuso S. Prognostic role of laparoscopic salpingoscopy of the only remaining tube after contralateral ectopic pregnancy. Fertil Steril 1995;63:303-06.

37. DeBruyne F, Hucke J, Willers R. The prognostic value of salpingoscopy. Hum Reprod 1997;12:266-71.

38. Dechaud H, Daures JP, Hedon B. Prospective evaluation of falloscopy. Hum Reprod 1998;13:1815-18.

39. Puttemans P, Brosens I, Delattin P, et al. Salpingoscopy versus hysterosalpingography in hydrosalpinges. Hum Reprod 1987;2:535-40.

40. De Bruyne F, Puttttemans P, Boeckx W, Brosens I. The clinical value of salpingoscopy in tubal fertility. Fertil Steril 1989;51:339-40.

41. Marana R, Muzii L, Rizzi M, et al. Prognostic role of laparoscopic salpingoscopy of the only remaining tube after contralateral ectopic pregnancy. Fertil Steril 1995;63:303-06.

42. Puttemans PJ, De Bruyne F, Heylen SM. A decade of salpingoscopy. Eur J Obstet Gynecol Reprod Biol 1998;81:197-206.

43. Surrey ES. Microendoscopy of the human fallopian tube. J Am Asso Gynecol Laparosc 1999;6:383-89.

44. Marconi G, Quintana R. Methylene blue dyeing of cellular nuclei during salpingoscopy, a new in vivo method to evaluate vitality of tubal epithelium. Hum Reprod 1998;13:3414-17.

45. Anderson AN, Lindhard A, Loft A et al. The infertile patient with hydrosalpinges-IVF with or without salpingectomy? Hum Reprod 1996;11:2081-84.

46. Puttemans PJ, Brosens IA. Salpingetomy improves in-vitro fertilization outcome in patients with a hydro-salpinx: blind victimization of the Fallopian tube? Hum Reprod 1996;11:2079-81.

47. Aboulghar MA, Mansour RL, Serour GI. Controversies in the modern management of hydrosalpinx. Hum Reprod Update 1998;4:882-90.

48. Kadar N, Caldwell BV, Romero R. A method of screening for ectopic pregnancy and its indications. Obstet Gynaecol 1981a;58:162-65.

49. Kadar N, DeVore G, Romero R. Discriminatory hCG zone: Its use in the sonographic evaluation for ectopic pregnancy. Obstet Gynaecol 1981b;58:156-60.

50. Bukovsky I, Langer R, Herman A, Caspi E. Conservative surgery for tubal pregnancy. Obstet Gynecol 1979;53:709.

51. DeCherney AH, Maheux R, Naftolin F. Salpingostomy for ectopic pregnancy in the sole patent oviduct: Reproductive outcome. Fertil Steril 1982;37:619.

52. Valle JA, Lifchez AS. Reproductive outcome following conservative surgery for tubal pregnancy in women with a single fallopian tube. Fertil Steril 1983;39:316-19.

53. Buttram VC, Snabes MC. Indications for myomectomy. Semin Reprod Endocrinol 1992;20:378-90.

54. Verkauf BS. Myomectomy as a fertility-promoting procedure. Infertility and Reproductive Medicines Clinics of North America 1996;7:79-89.

55. Paulson RJ. Value of myomectomy in the treatment of infertility (letter). Fertil Steril 1993;59:1332.

56. Peacock LM, Rock JA. Indications for and technique of myomectomy. Infertility and Reproductive Medicines Clinics of North America 1996;7:109-27.

57. Ramzy AM, Sattar M, Amin Y, Mansour RT, Serour GI, Aboulghar MA. Uterine myomata and outcome of assisted reproduction. Hum Reprod 1998;13:198-202.

58. The Myomectomy Adhesion Multicenter Study Group. An expanded polytetrafluoroethylene barrier (Gore-Tex* Surgical Membrane) reduces post-myomectomy adhesion formation. Fertil Steril 1995;63:491-93.

59. Nezhat C, Nezhat F, Silfen SL et al. Laparoscopic myomectomy. Int J Fertil 1991;36:275-80.

60. Dubuisson JB, Chapron C, Chavet X et al. Fertility after laparoscopic myomectomy of large intramural myomas: Preliminary results. Hum Reprod 1996;11: 518-22.

61. Stringer NH, Strassner HT. Pregnancy in fine patients after laparoscopic myomectomy with the harmonic scalpel. J Gynaecol Surg 1996;12:129-33.

62. Nezhat CH, Nezhat F, Roemisch M, Seidman DS, Tazuke SI, Nezhat CR. Pregnancy following laparoscopic myomectomy: Preliminary results. Hum Reprod 1999;14:1219-21.

63. Garcia CR, Tureck RW. Submucosal leiomyomas and infertility. Fertil Steril, 1984;42:16-19.

64. Tulandi T, Murray C, Guralnick M. Addition formation and reproductive outcome after myomectomy and second-look laparoscopy. Obstet Gynecol 1993;82:213-15.

65. Acien P, Quereda F. Abdominal myomectomy: Results of a simple operative technique. Fertil Steril 1996;65:41-51.

66. Dubuisson JB, Lecuru F, Foulot H, Mandelbrot L, Aubriot FX, Mouly M. Myomectomy by laparoscopy: A preliminary report of 43 cases. Fertil Steril 1991;56:827-30.

67. Vercellini P, Maddalene S, De Giorgi O, Pesole A, Ferrari L, Crosignani PG. Determinants of reproductive outcome after abdominal myomectomy for infertility. Fertil Steril 1999;72:109-14.

68. Rana M, Thomas S, Rotman C, Dmowski WP. Decrease in the size of ovarian endometriomas during ovarian suppression in stage 4 endometriosis. Role of preoperative medical treatment. J Reprod Med 1996;41:384-92.

69. Zanetta G, Lissoni A, Dalla Valle C, Trio D, Pittelli M, Rangoni G. Ultrasound-guided aspiration of endometriomas: Possible applications and limitations. Fertili Steril 1995;64:709-13.

70. Candiani GB, Vercellini P, Fedele L, Bianchi S, Vendola N, Candiani M. Conservative surgical treatment for severe endometriosis in infertile women: Are we making progress? Obstet Gynecol Surv 1991;46:490-98.

71. Peel KR. The implications of the changing nature of gynaecological surgical practice on training. Br J Obstet Gynaecol, 1995;102:177-78.

72. Tevfik Yoldermir, Sermet Sagol, Saban Adakan, Kemal Oztekin, Serdar Ozsener, Nedim Karadadas. Comparison of the reduction of postoperative adhesions by two barriers, one solution, and two pharmacologic agents in the rat uterine model. Fertil Steril 2002; 78:335.

• Rakesh Sinha • Neelam Sood

20

Endometriosis and Infertility

A SURGICAL MANAGEMENT

Rakesh Sinha

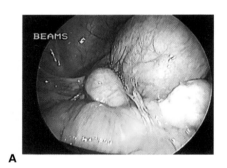 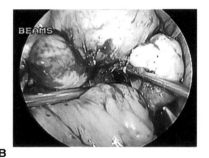 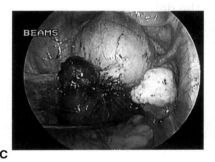

A **B** **C**

FIGURES 20.1A TO C: BEAMS—(A) Severe posterior bowel adhesions, (B) Adhesiolysis, and (C) Final view

Few clinical conditions in gynecological practice have been as enigmatic and challenging as endometriosis.

The challenge of endometriosis stems from the fact that even after decades of study of its etiology and pathogenesis, it still remains a "disease of theories".

With improved networks of diagnosis, most of stage I of the revised American fertility society classification not recognized in the past are now recognized and treated. Among the noninvasive methods ultrasound is particularly helpful in ovarian pathology.

Laparoscopy has opened new doors to treatment of endometriosis particularly in cases of endometriosis with infertility.

DIAGNOSIS OF ENDOMETRIOSIS: LAPAROSCOPIC APPEARANCES

Knowledge of the anatomic distribution of endometriosis is essential to focus on these areas during laparoscopy.

The areas most commonly involved with endometriosis include:[1]

1. Anterior and posterior cul de sac
2. Ovaries
3. Posterior broad ligaments
4. The uterosacral ligaments.

Endometriosis involves the left side of bilateral pelvic structures more frequently than the right. The area of pelvic adhesions roughly correlates under the localization of endometriosis.

On diagnostic laparoscopy systematic evaluation of the pelvic structures, should be undertaken to avoid missing lesions, with specific attention to the posterior cul de sac and broad ligament. Ovaries appearing larger than normal size should alert the surgeon to the possibility of an endometrioma. These are rarely larger than 10 cm and develop over several months as a result of intracystic hemorrhage. During the diagnostic portion of the laparoscopic procedure, care should be taken to look for endometriosis in unusual places such as in the canal of Nuck, pelvic brim, Allen-Masters windows (Allen and Master et al, 1995), serosal surface of the small bowel, liver diaphragm and fallopian tube. The peritoneal defects commonly known as Allen-Master defects or windows are frequently associated with endometriosis at their base. As these defects can cause pelvic pain or serve as an area for collection of reflux menstrual blood, it is necessary to open the defects even if endometriosis cannot be seen.

Histologically, endometriosis is comprised of both endometrial glands and stroma but visually it is described as "Red Raspberries, Purple Raspberries, blue berries, blebs and peritoneal pockets" (Sampson 1921, 1924, 1927).

White opacified and red flame like lesions are most common (81%), rest vary from glandular lesions, yellow brown peritoneal patches (17%), circular peritoneal defects (45%) and rarely cribriform peritoneum (9%).[2]

The puckered black brown lesions, "powder burn" lesions are comprised of stroma, glands, fibromuscular scarring and intraluminal debris.[3]

Clinical Features

The cardinal symptoms of endometriosis are:
• Dysmenorrhea
• Pelvic pain
• Infertility
• Dyspareunia
• Menstrual irregularity
• Co-menstrual rectal pain and
• Rectal bleeding if the colon is involved.[4]

Dysmenorrhea

In young patients, cyclic pelvic pain and dysmenorrhea are common with endometriosis. Pain occurs on an increasing number of days, and dyspareunia becomes an increasing problem with aging.

Severe dysmenorrhea is highly predictive of endometriosis, whereas mild and moderate dysmenorrheas are not.

Focal Pelvic Tenderness

Focal tenderness correlates with deep fibrotic endometriosis or other fibrotic pathology; however, 96 percent of lesions with or without tenderness can be fibrotic. There has been significant correlation with depth and volume. Excision is necessary for deep and large lesions. Cul-de-sac nodularity has been more frequent in infertile women with endometriosis. Patients with vaginal endometriosis have an increased risk of deep dyspareunia.

Infertility

Endometriosis is often associated with infertility, the tubes with endometriosis, except in isthmal endometriosis which produces isthmica nodosa, are patent. Other factors contributing to reduced fertility are dyspareunia, ovulatory defects, impaired oocyte transfer, impaired fertilization and impaired implantation.

MEDICAL MANAGEMENT OF ENDOMETRIOSIS

The medical treatment options for women suspected of endometriosis are based on suppression of ovarian function or exclude estrogen activity. This offers the best chance for clinical remission of endometriosis with direct regressive effects on the implants or activation of an auto-antibody reaction by medical therapy further contributory to atrophy. Follow-up studies have shown that endometriosis seems to be a chronic disease with a high rate of recurrence of symptoms after medical treatment. Morphological examination suggests that only permanent deprivation of estrogens can definitively cure the disease.[5]

Although endometriotic lesions have been shown to possess both estradiol and progesterone receptors, the responsiveness of individual endometriotic implants seems to be determined by the relative stromal and glandular components.[6] The Medical Management of Endometriosis in detail is discussed on page 238.

Progestins

The use of progestogens in the treatment of women with endometriosis was based originally on the suggestion that endometriosis regressed during pregnancy. Long-term exposure of endometriotic lesions to the effects of progesterone results in decidualisation and apparent atrophy. Also they reduce the frequency and increase the amplitude of the pulsatile GnRH release, which results in a reduction in FSH and LH secretion and low levels of ovarian steroids.

The most commonly used progesterone is medroxyprogesterone acetate in dose of 10-30 mg orally for more than 6 months. Other forms of progesterone can also be used in different dosages.

Disadvantages of progesterone are break through bleeding and prolonged interval before resumption of ovulatory menses after discontinuance. In today's management they are used mainly for pain relief or other symptoms for long term.

Danazol

Danazol is an impeded androgen derived from ethisterone, it reduces pituitary gonadotrophin secretion and thus reduce ovarian steroidogenesis. It has been shown to be effective in cases of mild and moderate endometriosis, while inducing marked weight gain and occasional androgenic side effects. Danazol is shown to improve symptoms in 66-100 percent with reduction of lesion by 80-90 percent. However, the recurrence rate within 4 years about 40-50 percent.

GnRH Analogues

GnRH agonists reduce or suppress FSH and LH secretion, this is therapeutic principle of the antigonadotrophic action of all GnRH agonists such as buserelin, goserelin, leuprorelin and others. Inhibition of follicular maturation for 6-12 months by inducing a reversible hormonal hypophysectomy prevents dystopic bleeding and will eventually, if regimen is effective, restore fertility by the involution of endometriotic lesion in the ovary and/or the oviduct. Relief of pain and formation of scars, fibrosis, atrophy of endometriotic lesions is observed post-therapy with GnRH agonists in 80 percent of patients.[7]

Peritoneal endometriosis and superficial ovarian implants react well to ovarian suppression, deep infiltrating endometriotic nodules in the bladder, rectum or the rectovaginal septum do not cause symptoms during therapy, they are not significantly reduced in size and early recurrences are characteristic. Ovarian endometriomas larger than 3 cm in diameter reduce in volume, but regrow rapidly and surgical treatment is necessary.[8]

Since endometriosis is a chronic disease which continuously threatens the female during their reproductive life, the efficacy of a therapy is based on recurrence rates. On comparison between Danazol and GnRH treatment follow-up of 5-6 years, 75 percents patients in both cases required repeat medical or surgical intervention.[9]

Repeated GnRH therapy is limited by the side effects of bone loss, though add-back therapy with Norethisterone, Hormone replacement therapy, Tibolone showed good results in endometriosis, they did not completely inhibit demineralization of bone.[10-12]

Ru 486 (Mifeprestone)

The antiprogestrone mifepristone(RU486) has been evaluated by Kettel *et al* (1996) in management of endometriosis, it showed regression of pelvic pain and cramps and 55 percent regression of endometriosis.

Management Strategies in Treatment of Endometriosis

The group of patients with endometriosis not desiring fertility can be tackled as, follows stage I and II-Diagnostic laparoscopy with thermocoagulation, adhesiolysis and resection of implants and residual fibrosis. Thereafter follow-up is directed to look for recurrence and when indicated additional hormonal treatment initiated. In stage III and IV a 3-6 month course of Danazol/GnRH should follow endoscopic surgery.

Patients above 45 years with evident recurrence are subject to definitive surgery, Total Laparoscopic Hysterectomy with Bilateral Salpingo-Oophorectomy being the method of choice.

Infertility patients with incidental finding of endometriosis should be managed with thermocoagulation followed by 6-12 month induction of ovulation. In case of stage II-III or recurrent endometriosis medical management with surgical excision will give the best benefit. Even in case of incomplete resection the chances for pregnancy are best in the first 6-12 month following surgery.

Surgical Treatment of Endometriosis

Surgery is usually the treatment of choice for endometriosis associated infertility, particularly when moderate or severe endometriosis causes anatomic distortion of the pelvis, because it allows the opportunity to restore normal anatomy.

In women who have pain, surgical treatment of all stages of endometriosis may be beneficial. Conservative surgery to remove the disease and restore normal anatomy and definitive surgery (hysterectomy and salpingo-oophorectomy) are options that can be effective in relieving endometriosis-associated pain. Surgery is also effective for removing endometriotic masses. Although endometriosis is not considered a life-threatening disease, it is a life-altering disease that requires timely diagnosis and treatment to minimize the clinical sequelae.

The surgical treatment of endometriosis is accomplished by laparotomy or laparoscopy. Improvements in equipment and operative techniques generally have made laparoscopy the preferred surgical approach. Laparotomy, however, may be more appropriate for removal of large endometriomas, enterostomy, extensive enterolysis, bowel resection, or other situations deemed too complex for the laparoscopy.[15]

The advantages of operative laparoscopy include less tissue trauma and exposure to foreign bodies, improved visualization, possibly less adhesion formation, and lower complication rates.[16] Moreover, laparoscopic incisions are smaller and less painful, allowing for return to daily activities and work within 2-7 days as opposed to 4-6 weeks for laparotomy.[9, 10]

Despite the advantages of operative laparoscopy, the successful application of this surgical approach is dependent on the laparoscopic skills of the surgeon. A good result after laparotomy is generally preferable to less satisfactory results after operative laparoscopy. The surgical treatment of endometriosis may be accomplished by electrosurgical desiccation, laser ablation, or sharp resection.

Surgical Principles

The techniques used during surgery are designed to facilitate the removal of all endometrial implants in an atraumatic, hemostatic fashion in the least amount of time. These goals are especially important in patients with reproductive dysfunction because meticulous surgical techniques that maintain serosal integrity may reduce the risk of de novo adhesion formation. Serosal integrity may, but has not been conclusively proven, be preserved by copious irrigation with physiologic fluids such as Ringer's lactate, which reduces tissue desiccation and maintains clean surgical fields. The success of the operation will be related to how well these goals are achieved. Close adherence to surgical principles (Table 20.1) will increase the likelihood of successful outcome.

TABLE 20.1: Surgical principles in the treatment of endometriosis[17]
• Knowledge of disease and treatment modalities
• Experienced surgeon
• Adequate facilities, personnel and equipment
• Appropriate patient selection
• Careful pelvic evaluation
• Maximum exposure
• Use of magnification
• Minimum tissue trauma
• Excellent hemostasis
• Removal of all diseased tissue
• Confirmation of tissue pathology

Evaluation of outcome of surgical management of endometriosis in various cases is reaffirming the status of surgery in endometriosis.

In general, a pregnancy rate of approximate 65 percent can be expected within 1-2 years after surgery for endometriosis. In a meta-analysis comparing surgery with endometriosis-associated infertility, surgery was superior to non-surgical approaches in improving the crude pregnancy rates.[18] In patients with minimal or mild endometriosis, laparoscopic treatment has been used frequently because treatment can be accomplished easily during diagnostic laparoscopy. The ablation or removal of endometriosis implants, however, potentially can increase the risk for postsurgical adhesion formation. The average rate from several studies evaluating the surgical approach was approximately 58 percent compared with an average pregnancy rate after expectant management of approximately 45 percent.[19] The available evidence supports the surgical approach compared with the nonsurgical approach for invasive, adhesive and/or endometriosis disease.[18] Intuitively, surgical treatment that can potentially correct anatomic defects should result in better outcomes than expectant management or medical treatment, which does not restore normal anatomy. The combined data reveal that medical treatment after surgery is not better than laparoscopy alone) without any postoperative medical R̩.

In the absence of supporting evidence for the postoperative use of medications, the cost, the side effects, and delay in attempting conception argue against a role for medical treatment after surgery. The role for preoperative medical therapy is inconclusive because of the lack of sufficient data for evaluation. In light of the evidence supporting the equivalent, if not better, outcome of laparoscopy compared with laparotomy and in the presence of appropriate equipment and skill, the laparoscopic approach is preferable in most cases of endometriosis-associated infertility.

Because of the ineffectiveness of medical therapy, surgery has been the approach for treating endometriomas. In two retrospective studies, pregnancy rates after laparoscopic treatment of endometriomas in infertility patients were 50 percent (26 of 52) and 52 percent (12 of 23).[20]

Surgical treatment for endometriosis-associated pelvic pain has been poorly studied but appears to be useful. Uncontrolled trials have reported success in relieving pain in 70-100 percent of patients.

In one study, complete relief of pain one year after surgery was reported in 82 percent of patients.[21] Patients with higher stage disease had more pain relief after surgery than did patients with mild disease. The approach of wide excision and drainage has been recommended as an alternative to wedge excision because of less adhesion formation and a recurrence rate (23%) similar to cyst stripping and ablation. In other studies, stripping and ablation, perhaps the most widely used techniques, has been associated with even lower endometrioma recurrence rates(< 5%).

Endometriosis-associated pain may be effectively reduced by definite surgery with hysterectomy and salpingo-oophorectomy. This approach would be considered in patients for whom medical and/or conservative surgical treatment has failed and who can accept loss of fertility.

It is our observation at our center that, adhesiolysis resulted in an improvement in pelvic pain symptoms in approximately 85 percent of patients. Despite the uncertainly of the relationship between adhesions and pain, lysis of adhesions appears reasonable in the presence of endometriosis-associated pain, especially when the location of adhesion and pain correlate.

Presacral neurectomy involves interrupting the sympathetic innervation to the uterus at the level of the superior hypogastric plexus, this technique has variable effects on endometriosis associated pain, specially dysmenorrhea

Laparoscopic uterosacral nerve ablation (LUNA) is another procedure used to reduce pain in endometriosis, pain relief occurred mainly in patients with dysmenorrhea. A success rate of both has been reported as 50-83 percent for short-term relief.

METHODS OF SURGICAL MANAGEMENT

In most cases, operative laparoscopic procedures are aimed at destruction of the endometriotic lesions. This can be achieved by a number of techniques such as excision, electrocoagulation and vaporization.

Sharp Excision

It involves the dissection of endometriotic implants and nodules from surrounding normal tissue. This may be accomplished with laparoscopic scissors and monopolar cautery. The advantage is collection of material for histopathology, disadvantages are the associated bleeding and injury to adjacent structures.

Monopolar Electroexcision of Endometriosis

The concept behind electrocoagulation or desiccation of endometriotic implants is the destruction of tissue by the application of thermal energy. The advantages of the technique are that the lesion may be destroyed without the risk of hemorrhage. The disadvantages include the risk of unrecognized injury to surrounding and adjacent structures, the lack of surgical specimen for histological evaluation and the possibility of incomplete destruction of entire endometriotic lesion.

The monopolar electrocautery uses 90 W of non-modulated current or 50 W of modulated current. Non-modulated current is more useful for peritoneal incisions.

Laparoscopic electroexcision of endometriosis consists of 80 percent blunt dissection to prepare the surgical field and 20 percent electrosurgery to severe abnormal tissue from healthy tissue. In cases of deep peritoneal lesions with fibrosis or where retroperitoneal invasion is suspected, the adjacent peritoneum is dissected and retroperitoneal blunt dissection done to reach the center of the lesion, thus ensuring complete electrocoagulation.

Uterosacral involvement with invasive endometriosis warrants resection of the ligament taking care of the course of ureters by locating the position with visible peristalsis.

Small areas of superficial ovarian endometriosis can be excised by cutting the cortex around the lesion, however, this results in removal of more normal ovarian tissue than with laser vaporization or electrocoagulation.

Vaporization of Endometriosis

Vaporization with Laser energy offers several advantages over bipolar diathermy, endocoagulation of endometriotic implants or ultrasonic energy, namely control of 'star-burst' effect, ability to gauge the depth of the endometriotic implant.

The various lasers available for medical use today offer distinct advantage for vaporization of lesions. The carbon dioxide, KTP (potassium-titanyl-phosphate), Nd:YAG (neodymium:yttrium-argonyl-garnet), argon, and ho:YAG (holmiumYAG) lasers have distinct property differences that allow them to be useful for tissue vaporization under different conditions.

Usually small implants can be excised, vaporized or coagulated; deeper lesions should be vaporized or excised to level of healthy tissue.

For excision, the lesion is outlined by cutting through the peritoneum and into the loose connective tissue with the laser. The underlying loose connective tissue and fat are injected below the peritoneum with irrigating solution to dissect through these layers. This technique is called 'hydrodissection', (or aquadissection) (Nezhat and Nezhat, 1989). Dissection with an irrigating solution is used in vascular areas to avoid inadvertently cutting across large vessels and is used in the broad ligament to push the ureters away from the peritoneum. The fluid acts as a backstop to the CO_2 laser, preventing injury to the tissue beneath the peritoneal lesion. Once tissue has been excised it is removed through the laparoscope.

Advantages

Advantages of excisional method are:
- Creates less smoke
- Leaves less carbon than vaporization
- Provides tissue for diagnosis
- Likely to remove all deep lesions

Disadvantages

- Removes unnecessary peritoneum
- Technically can be more difficult
- Slightly more time consuming

Bladder lesions can be excised in much the same way, re-peritonalization occurs over the resected lesion. However, one must prevent adhesion formation by use of biodegradable cellulose mesh (Interceed). If adhesions are allowed to form, irritative bladder symptoms may follow.

A superficial bowel lesion involving the serosal surface only can be easily removed with a superpulse laser beam of 5-10 w moved rapidly across the colon. As long as the muscularis is not entered, there is no need to close the defect.

The precision and accuracy of the laser beam and especially the "what you see is what you get" effects of CO_2 makes it ideal for surgically treating peritoneal endometriosis.

Ovarian Endometriosis

The first case of ovarian endometrial cysts was described by Ressel in 1899 in a premenopausal women who underwent surgery for a cystic adenocarcinoma of the left ovary in whom the right ovary was enveloped in adhesions of the posterior face of the broad ligament.

The evidence that the perforating hemorrhagic cyst was of endometrial origin was based on the observations that the lining of the cyst was similar to endometrial tissue and that in two patients who underwent surgery at the time of the menstrual period, the histologic changes in the ovarian 'endometrial' tissue corresponded to the phase of the menstrual cycle. Both structural and functional features, therefore, indicated the endometrial origin of these cysts. It is, therefore, not surprising that the endometrioma has been described as a pseudouterine cavity.

The escape of chocolate fluid while freeing the ovary from adhesions and the identification of endometrial implants with the full characteristics of superficial endometrium at the site of perforation led Sampson (1921) to believe that perforation of these cysts was a frequent phenomenon, leading to spilling, adhesions and spread of peritoneal endometriosis.

The endometrioma has typical features, which make the visual diagnosis very reliable, these features include:
• Size not more than 12 cm in diameter.
• Adhesions to the pelvic sidewall and/or the broad ligament.
• 'Powder burns' and minute red or blue spots with adjacent puckering on the surface of the ovary.
• Tarry, thick chocolate-colored fluid content.

Large ovarian endometriomas are characteristically adherent to the posterior side of the uterus or broad ligament or the lateral pelvic wall.

Ovarian endometriomas are often associated with luteal cysts which are multilocular and can pose a diagnostic and surgical problem. Ultrasonography and MRI are diagnostic tools to detect the presence of endometriomas; these are especially useful to detect malignancy. Ovarian cystoscopy has recently been proposed as a useful diagnostic technique for pre-operative identification of endometriotic implants and for the selection of site for biopsy of large ovarian endometriomas.[22]

After careful inspection of the pelvis and in the absence of signs suggesting malignancy, the cyst is first punctured and an aspiration sample is obtained. The cyst is subsequently flushed abundantly with sterile saline at body temperature until the fluid becomes clear using a suction irrigator. The small endoscope is introduced through a suprapubic/lateral port into the cyst and a saline infusion is allowed to run freely to distend the cyst. The 30° angle of the endoscope allows nearly complete visualization of the inside wall of the cyst. The typical features of the large endometriotic cyst are presence of old or recent hemorrhage with puckering and network of implants and vessels.

The complete evaluation and treatment of endometriomas include full adhesiolysis of the ovary and identification of the invagination site, wide opening of the invagination site and resection of the fibrotic ring, destruction of the superficial endometriotic lesions on the ovary and POD.

In contrast to the other ovarian cysts the walls of the small endometrioma do not usually collapse after opening the cyst and in the absence of fibrosis have the pearl-white appearance of ovarian cortex. Removal of the walls can be difficult but with persistence they can be removed completely by segments. Adhesiolysis often results in opening of the cyst and spilling of the chocolate content. Removal of a large cyst from the underlying ovarian stroma is relatively easy except at the site where the capsule is adherent (Nezhat et al., 1992). At this site the adhesions are often very dense and in the absence of a plane of cleavage, removal can be difficult.

Representative biopsies of the cyst are useful in ruling out malignancy and for confirmation of diagnosis. Closing by apposition of the walls and suturing of the cortex is not indicated because the ovarian stroma is not exposed and the ovarian cortex preserved. Theoretically closure of the wall can cause burying of follicles leading to formation of functional cysts. It has often been observed in patients who undergo follicular monitoring post-surgery to have a cyst in the ovary, these are pseudocysts, 2-3 months interval allows spontaneous resorption of these cysts and are not a cause of worry.

The use of gonadotropin releasing hormone (GnRH) agonist can be beneficial postsurgery.

Reduced postoperative adhesion formation is achieved by avoiding any unnecessary surgical procedure such as incision of normal cortex or excision of functional structures.

Lasers are preferable as only minimal of irreversible tissue damage is done from the edge of crater; if lasers are not available then electro-surgical techniques can be used.

At the end of the procedures, copious irrigation and an underwater inspection is performed to ensure hemostasis. Any evidence of bleeding not tackled by laser can be stopped with electro diathermy. H.Reich (1989) recommends leaving one liter of warm heparinised Ringer's lactate solution to prevent subsequent adhesion formation, which usually occurs during the initial stages of the healing process. The idea of this acquaflotation is to prevent surfaces adhering during this phase.

Complications of Surgery of Ovarian Endometrioma

Incomplete adhesiolysis and exposure can result in incomplete surgery, which leads to a higher rate of recurrences.

At the other end of the spectrum is excessive surgery which can result in removing diseased cyst along which normal follicles and functional cysts.

Some of the specific complications of Surgery for endometriomas include:
• Severe bleeding from the hilus of the ovary
• Trauma to the ureters during dissection
• Postoperative adhesion leading to encapsulation of the ovary resulting in pain and cyst formation

• Disturbance of the tubo-ovarian relation by adhesions
• Repeat excision of endometrioma causing ovarian resistance and premature menopause.

It is always to be kept in mind that the first surgery in a young woman for endometrioma determines the ultimate outcome of her reproductive life.

Laparoscopic Treatment of Advanced Endometriosis

Superficial endometriosis can be destroyed by coagulation while infiltrating lesions require dissection, vaporization or excision.[9] Although the depth is related to the size for infiltrating lesions, endometriosis is flattened against the cyst wall in large ovarian endometriomas and does not infiltrate more than 1.5 mm. Thus, exploration, examination and coagulation of the inner lining of very large endometrioma are capable of destroying the endometriosis that lines these.

Although the surgical approach to advanced endometriosis is important, this cannot be used unless lesions are recognized.

Ovarian Endometriomas

Smaller ovarian endometriomas can be biopsied and then the base coagulated or vaporised. Endometriomas that are larger than 2 cm require more extensive surgical strategy. Treatment can consist of drainage, biopsy and coagulation or stripping.[10]

Once the cyst has been drained and lavaged, endometriomas generally have a red or red and brownish appearance on a white fibrotic background. A more uniform brownish appearance is present when these are residual hemorrhagic corpus lutea.

Deep Infiltration

Although coagulation is effective on lesions less than 2 mm depth, deep lesions with infiltration require either vaporization or excision. Stage I and II endometriosis in the cul-de-sac usually do not cause distortion and can be completely resected. In stage III and IV there is distortion of the cul-de sac with the rectum pulled towards the cervix. Careful adhesiolysis and identification is required to excise them.

Bladder and Ureteral Involvement

The majority of lesions overlying the ureter and bladder are in the peritoneum and loose connective tissue and are not adherent to the urinary structures. In cases of previous cesarean sections chances of endometriosis infiltrating through the scar and affecting the bladder can cause bladder endometriosis. These lesions infiltrate the serosal and mucosal layers often, but rarely infiltrating mucosa. At our center we resected endometriotic lesion involving posterior surface of the bladder by transurethral resection using resectoscope with total laparoscopic hysterectomy. The patient has recovered well with complete healing of the bladder lesion.

Rectosigmoid Infiltration

Infiltration of the rectosigmoid is suggested by a palpable mass on per-rectal examination bleeding at the time of menstruation, pain on defecation. As long as the lesions can be delineated by visualization and by mechanical palpation, they can be resected laparoscopically. During surgery use of separate intrauterine, intravaginal and rectal manipulators may be necessary.

CONCLUSION

The laparoscopic treatment of endometriosis is not limited by the stage or size of the disease.

Surgical treatment has been shown to be efficacious for elimination of pain and even infertility. Review of papers suggest that surgical treatment is mainly cytoreductive and requires medical treatment for invisible lesions or lesions not resectable. Each individual case must be evaluated separately and the treatment tailor made to the patient. Surgical management should be undertaken with good skills, surgical principles and with knowledge of the various complications possible especially in case of advanced endometriosis.

REFERENCES

1. Jenkins S, Olive DL, Haney AF. Endometriosis: pathogenetic implications of the anatomic distribution. Obstetrics and Gynaecology 1986;155:1154-59.
2. John A. Roche & Sujatha Reddy. Diagnosis of Endometriosis; Endoscopic Surgery for Gynaecologists: WB Saunder Company Ltd: 1999;353-54.
3. Stripling MC, Martin DC, Chatmen DL, Vander Zwaag R, Poston WM. Subtle Appearance of pelvic endometriosis, Fertility and Sterility 1988;49:427-31.
4. Wild RA, Wilson EA. Clinical presentation and diagnosis. In:Wilson EA (Ed.): Endometriosis. New York, NY: Alan R, Inc 1987.
5. Schweppe KW, Dmowski WP, Wynn RM. Ultra structural changes in endometriotic tissue during Danazol treatment. Fertil-Steril 1981;36:20-26.
6. Schweppe KW. Klinik and Morphologic der endometriose. Schatrauer, Stuttgart 1984.
7. Schweppe KW, Cirkel U. Gn RH analogues in the treatment of endometriosis: effectivity and side effects 4th Annual Meeting ESHRE, Barcelona. 1988.
8. Waller KG, Shaw RW. Gonadotropin-releasing hormone analogue for the treatment of endometriosis: long term follow-up. Fertil-Steril 1993;59:511-575.
9. Wadsworth. Reports of the 4th Interational Congress of GnRH Analogues in Gynaecology. In Lunenfeld (Ed): In press. 1996.
10. Surray ES, Faurnet N et al. Effects of sodium etidronate in combination with low dose norethisterone in patients administered a long acting GnRH agonist,a preliminary report.J.Endocrinol Metab 1993;81:581-86.
11. Cedars ML Lu JKH, Meldum OR. Treatment of endometriosis with a long acting GnRh agoinst + Medroxy-progesterone acetate. Obstet Gynaecol 1990;75:641-45.
12. Moghissi K. Report of the 4th Int. Cong of GnRh-Analogues in Gynaecology. Lunenfeld (Ed): in press 1996.
13. Adamson GD. Lap treatment of endometriosis. In: Adamson GD, Martin DC (Eds.): Endoscopic Management of Gynaecologic disease. Philadelphia: Lippincott–Raven, 1996;147-87.
14. Marcoux S, Maheux R, Berube S et al. Lap Surgery in infertile women with minimal or mild endometriosis. N Engl J med 1997;337:217-22.
15. Luciano AA, Mauzi D. Treatment options for endometriosis surgical therapies: Infertile reproduction med Clin N Am.1992;3:657-82.
16. Operative Lap study Group Post operative adhesion development following operative Lap: evaluation at early second-look procedure:Fertil Steril 1991;55: 700-04.
17. Adamson GD. Lap Treatment of endometriosis In: Adamson GD, Martin DC.eds Endoscopic Management of Gynaec disease. Philadelphia: Lippincott Raven, 1996;147-87.
18. ChapronC, Vercillini P, Barakat H, Vieira M, Dubuisson JB: Management of ovarian Endometriomas; Hum Reprod Update.2002;8(6):591-97.
19. Wardle PG, Mc Laughlin EA, Mc Dermott A et al. Endometriosis and ovulatory disorder: Reduced fertilization in vitro compared with tubal and unexplained infertility; Lancet 1985;2:236-39.

20. Adamson GD, Hurd SI, Pasta DI, Rodriguez BD. Lap endometriosis treatment: Is it better? Fertil Steril 1993; 59(1):35-44.

21. Martin DC, O'Conner DT. Surgical Management of endometriosis-associated pain: Obstet Gynaecol Clinic North Am 2003;30(1):151-62.

22. Brosens IA, Puttemans PJ, Deprest J. The endoscopic localization of endometrial implants in the ovarian chocolate cyst, Fertility and Sterility 1994;61:1034-38.

MEDICAL MANAGEMENT

Neelam Sood

INTRODUCTION

Medical therapy for endometriosis and its associated symptoms including dysmenorrhea, dyspareunia, pelvic pain and lower backache or chronic pelvic is highly successful. The two most common symptoms that have been presented by patients in the clinic are painful periods, chronic pelvic pain and infertility. Infertility is diagnosed as a cause of endometriosis only when a young female presents in the clinic with the history of dyspareunia and chronic pelvic pain. Medical treatment for endometriosis in cases of infertility remains highly controversial. Unit now, no studies have evidence that medical treatment has shown any improvement in infertility associated with endometriosis.

There are various ways endometriosis can be treated but at the same time there is a great controversy regarding the treatment for this mysterious gynecological condition. Three main strategies to be kept in mind while treating the patients of endometriosis are:
• To concentrate in relief of symptoms—therapeutic
• Suppressing the disease—hormonal
• Removing or destroying the ectopic endometrial tissue—surgical.

DIAGNOSTIC APPROACH

• What symptoms do it cause?
• How do I know if I have endometriosis? Self-diagnosis.
　Woman during their reproductive age present with symptoms like
　• Painful period—dysmenorrhea
　• Infertility—dyspareunia (painful sexual intercourse)
　• Abnormal bleeding.

INVESTIGATIONS

Since endometriosis is easy to diagnose, therefore it need not require much of the investigations,

but the following could be the right parameters to guide the physician to plan the treatment according to the severity of the disease.

Serum CA-125

The exact diagnosis of endometriosis is only made by laparoscopy. When patients approach with clear suggestive symptoms of endometriosis—one must think of CA-125. CA-125 is cell surface antigen which is found on the derivatives of the celomic epithelium which includes endometrium too. An increased value of CA-125 is found in patients with severe degree of endometriosis. Some studies have documented, a mean concentration correlate with the degree of endometriosis, somehow are never found with high levels of CA-125. It is advisable to do serum CA-125 in all the cases presenting with endometriosis. CA-125 is quite useful in follow-up cases and is a right parameter to guide the physician to decide the plan of action in these patients. Patients showing improvement or recurrence or deterioration of endometriosis can be checked with repeat serum CA-125.

Antiendometrial Antibody

Antibodies to endometrial tissue have been detected by various immunoassay techniques. Currently these assays are limited to research laboratories only and are difficult to perform. Kennedy *et al* compared the study in 35 women in case of proven endometriosis by laparoscopy. Later these cases were either treated with danazol or nafarelin: blood samples were drawn after and before the therapy. Antibodies to endometrial time were found low in cases after the treatment. Furthermore a significant suppression of antiendometrial antibodies was found in the group treated with GnRH-agonist only.

Placental Protein 14 (PP14)

PP14, varies a lot during the menstrual cycle and due to this reason it may limit the diagnostic utility of this assay. The correlation of PP14 with the respective stage of endometriosis (milder to severe) is found, but in milder cases disease overlaps significantly with values in normal controls.

CA-125 remains the only diagnostic test in severe degree of endometriosis.

TREATMENT OPTIONS

Symptomatic

Since endometriosis is an absolute benign condition, before starting any treatment a general non-specific measures must be considered. A complete thorough infertility evaluation is mandatory in all the women with endometriosis. The use of mild analgesics and oral contraceptives for few months must be tried. The treatment remains cheap and avoids the side effects of medication. The only precaution physician has to bear in mind if patients fail to conceive with therapeutic measures when to interfere so that disease should not progress. There are few studies, which have reported women conceiving in cases of untreated endometriosis. No doubt, the period for these women remained between 1 and 4 years, seems to be unduly prolonged period. The women with mild endometriosis, on an average conceived 7 percent whereas severe cases of endometriosis had 3 percent of monthly fecundity rates. If after several months patients are unable to conceive one must think of other line of treatment. Symptomatic treatment mainly depends on the intensity of endometriosis and secondly the age of the patient when it is discovered? In teenage, when endometriosis is discovered, aim of the treatment has to be based on idea of preserving fertility for future.

Hormonal Suppression

In young patients it is important to control the disease as soon as possible and therefore treatment such as mild analgesics, oral contraceptive pill is safe to start as initial therapy. When ovulation is suppressed, it reduces dysmenorrhea (periodic pain) and dyspareunia (painful intercourse) and breakthrough bleeding as well. The prolonged use of oral contraceptive is used to relieve pain in cases of milder form of endometriosis. Oral contraceptives as combination therapy, i.e. estrogen and progesterone, induces a state of pseudopregnancy change, and this regimen initially stimulates endometrium followed by atrophy of ectopic endometriotic implant. Apparently this treatment acts by manipulation of steroid hormones leading to prevention of stimulation and resolution of endometriotic spots and the whole process takes few months.

Treatment with nonsteroidal antiinflammatory drugs (NSAIDs) could be appreciable in number of woman showing remarkable improvement.

Progestogens

There are several synthetic progestational drugs in the treatment of endometriosis. The most commonly used are: Provera (MPA—medroxyprogesterone acetate), lynestrenol, norethynodrel (NET—trade name primolut N) NET and MPA are the hormonal drugs most commonly used. The maintenance dose is small and very effective in treating endometriosis. In some studies oral MPA was found as effective as danazol. MPA is commonly used and is chosen as first drug of choice for medical treatment of endometriosis. The ectopic endometrial implants would first decidualize and later followed by atrophy. The dosage of MPA varies from 30 mg/day in divided doses for 6 months. The doses of medroxyprogesterone acetate could be a high as 100 mg per day for 3 to 6 months. MPA is also available in injectable form as Depo-Provera 100 mg and has been found effective in treating endometriosis. It is given intramuscular each month. A reasonable approach to have a maintenance dose for a period of six months is important if the patient is comfortable with the chosen drugs. Some patients may present with breakthrough vaginal bleeding, which is the most common side effect. Depression is another significant side effect and unfortunately certain patient might need to stop the drug.

Danazol

In 1970, danazol was introduced in the market for the treatment of endometriosis. In its initial years action of danazol was not clearly understood whether to effective in cases of infertility or pain caused by endometriosis. Danazol is an isoxazole derivative of 17-alpha ethinyltestosterone. Danazol works in several ways at once. The main action of danazol is to stop the production of estrogens and progesterone in the ovaries. Danazol decreases midcycle follicle-stimulating hormone (FSH) and luteinizing hormone (LH) surge, by inducing a state of hypogonadism. There is a remarkable reduction in serum estradiol levels and progesterone with danazol therapy.

Chemically danazol is a combination of 17-alpha-ethinyltestosterone and 2-hydroxymethyl ethisterone, so a mild androgenic activity is exhibited as well. Danazol binds to the androgen receptors thus effecting the endometrial implants directly. Apparently danazol induces a hypoestrogenic, hyperandrogenic state which regresses the proliferation of the ectopic endometerial growth.

Recommended dose Danazol is an expensive drug and is normally prescribed as 600 to 800 mg daily in divided doses. The treatment is given for 4 to 6 months. It is very well absorbed by the gastro-intestinal tract. After an oral dose of 400 mg peak serum levels are obtained in 2 hours, serum levels are undeductable after 8 hours. However, low doses of danazol are not recommended since, chances of pregnancy might occur as ovulation is not suppressed with lower doses. If breakthrough bleeding takes place, the dose has to be increased.

Danazol relieves pain of endometriosis and prevents the growth of ectopic implants. Danazol shows its best effect in the treatment of peritoneal lesions. Danazol is highly effective in treating dysmenorrhea, intermenstrual pain and dyspareunia. Danazol is less effective in cases of ovarian endometriomas. Endometriomas of 3 cm needs surgical treatment, although regression has been seen in larger endometriomas sometimes. Recurrence rate of chocolate cysts are highly common, danazol is not a cure for endometriosis neither has any effect on the regression of adhesions.

Side effects Thin women tolerate danazol better than obese women. Weight gain because of water retention, muscle cramps, fatigue, decreased breast size, hot flushes, hirsutism, changes in mood. About 5 percent of patients develop drug rash, resembling allergic reaction. Although these reactions are reversible but in few cases some of the side effects leave permanent changes. Since danazol has its androgenic properties, enlargement of clitoris occurs in only 1 percent of patients. Women experience an increase in facial hair. The treatment must be stopped at this stage otherwise an increase in size could be permanent.

The ladies who are professional singers should not be advised for danazol therapy, since it does show some change in voice. Serum lipid profile to be checked routinely in patients on long-term therapy.

Gonadotropin-releasing Hormone (GnRH) Agonist

Gonadotropin-releasing hormone agonist has been introduced widely as a treatment of endometriosis very recently. GnRH-agonist is used on the basis of downregulating the GnRH receptors of pituitary creating a state of hypogonadism or pseudomenopause by medical oophorectomy, therefore hypogonadal and hypoestrogenic state is obtained, eventually causing atrophy of the endometriotic implants. The effect of GnRH has been studied in animal models by artificially inducing endometriosis. In clinical trials, the effect of GnRH has remained satisfactorily showing significant reduction of endometriotic implants while reducing the intensity of pain caused by endometriosis after a prolonged use of GnRH.

GnRH-agonists are available in the form of nasal sprays and subcutaneous injections. Nasal spray is administered 200 or 400 mg twice daily. Daily subcutaneous injections are also available by the name of leuprolide. Leuprolide acetate is available in the form of depot as a dose of 3.75 mg monthly. The therapy is given for six months. There are various side effects with GnRH therapy.

Side effects The most severe effect over a term longer than six months is a change in bone mineral density. Headache, loss of libido, hot flushes, breast tenderness, insomnia and depression. The loss of bone can be prevented by giving a small dose of estrogen and progestogen at the same time—a maneuver called—add back. It is justifiable to give small doses as levels of estradiol in the abdomen are dramatically very low, the minimal amount of estrogen does not stimulate the endometriosis (Robert Jansen, MD, overcoming infertility) the bone loss is temporarily and is recovered in 6 to 12 months after the therapy ends.

GnRH-agonist have been shown as effective as danazol is reduction of ectopic endometriotic implants. In summary GnRH-agonist like other drugs provides suppression rather than cure of the disease.

Management of an Infertile Women

Endometriosis and in vitro Fertilization

Assisted reproductive techniques (ARTs) in the management of infertility associated with endometriosis have a great role. In mild cases of endometriosis, intrauterine insemination (IUI) with controlled ovarian hyperstimulation is advised, if tubes are patent. Functional integrity of the tubes remain quite controversial and the question remains unanswered. The anatomical distortion of the tubes because of the endometriosis is quite common. The adnexal adhesions and the endometriomas reducing ovum recovery rate in monkeys have been seen in one of the studies. Ninety brown book in mild to moderate cases, *in vitro* fertilization (IVF) gamete intrafallopian transfer (GIFT) is highly recommendable. In severe cases of endometriosis, though pregnancy outcome is poor yet IVF is the only answer. In such cases the quality of embryos is compromised. In such cases follicular monitoring, poor response from ovaries, very few functional oocytes from ovaries, decreased fertilization rates and poor embryo quality have been noted. There is a poor implantation rate and high abortion rate in such cases.

Inone *et al* compared the studies in cases of endometriosis from stage I to stage IV, the treatment of IVF/ET—reported success rates approximately 30 percent. (94 brown book).

Other schools have reported in such cases, pregnancy rates with IVF/ET in women are comparable to those in women with tubal infertility or establish the relation of endometriosis on pregnancy outcome, overall the success rates is poor in such cases.

The prolong use of GnRH therapy is highly recommendable before ovarian stimulation has been studied. In severe cases of endometriosis, GnRH used for over a period of six months have resulted into an increased number of oocytes retrieved during egg pick-up, good cleavage rate with good embroys grading and pregnancies. Long-term GnRH therapy may reduce, rate of early abortion in patients with minimal and mild cases of endometriosis. Yet sufficient data is not available to establish the effects of long-term use of GnRH in endometriosis.

CONCLUSION

Endometriosis is a common gynecological disorder representing from mild to severe form during reproductive age of a women. Mainly they present with the symptoms of pelvic pain, dysmenorrhea and married women present with the complaints of dyspareunia along with infertility.

Infertility and endometriosis have long been associated with poor understanding as when and where endometriosis impairs infertility. The management of endometriosis especially in cases of infertility remains a challenge for those physician who have long association with these patients. The outcome of infertility due to endometriotic implants has yet to be understood. It is clear that anatomical distortion of pelvic organs could be the reason for infertility in advanced cases for endometriosis, but confusion starts when patients suffering with mild degree of endometriosis present with infertility. The disease remains progressive in some cases despite all the active treatment. Suppression of ectopic endometriotic implants with prolong use of drugs for six months and later followed by stimulation of ovaries with HMG/FSH therapies does help such patients with good pregnancy rates.

Unfortunately in long-standing cases of infertility, neither hormonal suppression nor surgical destruction of endometrial implants has helped to improve fertility. Treatment in such women with endometriosis has to be focused in regard with artificial reproductive technology (ART). Even moderate to severe cases of endometriosis get a chance to conceive in ART. Endometriosis often will need several treatment modalities, currently available are medical or surgical, or combination of both can be used to treat such patients. Somehow combination of both has been proved to be highly satisfactory.

FURTHER READING

1. Adhension study Group. Reduction of postoperative pelvic adhesion with intraperinial dextran 70—a prospective randomized clinical trial. Fertil Steril 1983;40:612-19.
2. Andrews MC, Ansrews WC, Strauss AF. Effect of progestin-induced pseudopregnancy on endometriosis: Clinical and microscopic studies. Am J Obstet Gynecol 1959;78:776.
3. Andrews WC, Larsen GD. Endometriosis, treatment with hormonal pseudopregnancy and/or operation. Am J Obstet Gynecol 1974;118:643.
4. Dlugi AM, Miller JD, Knittle J. Lupron depot (luoprolide acetate for depot suppression) in the treatment of endometriosis: A randomized, placebo-controlled, double blind study. Fertil Steril 1990;54:419.
5. Dmowski WP. Endocrine properties and clinical application of danazol. Fertil Steril 1979;31:237.
6. Dmowski WP, Radwanska E, Binoz Z, et al. Ovarian susspension induxec with buserelin or danazol in the management of endometriosis. Fertil Steril 1989;51:395.
7. Franssen AMHW, Kauer FM, Chadhav DR et al. Endometriosis treatment with gonadotrophin-releasing hormone agonist buserelin. Fertil Steril 1989;51:401.
8. Gilson BS, Gilson J, Bernger M et al. The sickness impact profile: development of an outcome measure of health. Am J Public Health 1975;65:1304.
9. Hammond CB, Rock JA, Parker RT. Conservative treatment of endometriosis dometriosis with conservative surgery. Obstet Gynecol 1978;131:416.
10. Henzl MR, Corson SL, Moghissi K et al. Administrative of nasal naferalin as compared with oral danazol of endometriosis. In Dlugi AM, Rufo SD, Amico JF Seibel MM. A comparison of the effects of buserelin versus danazol of plasma lipoproteins during treatment of pelvic endometriosis. Fertil Steril 1988;49:913.
11. Hill GA. Clinical experience in the treatment of endometriosis with GnRH agonist. Obstet Gynecol Surv 1989;44:305.
12. Hsiu J, Given F, Kemp G. Tumor implantation after diagnostic laparoscopic biopsy of serous ovarian tumors of low malignant potential. Obstet Gynecol 1986;68:90S-93S.
13. Hull ME, Moghissi KS, Magyar DF et al. Comparison of different treatment modalities of endometriosis in infertile women. Fertil Steril 1987;47:40.
14. Jarrwtt JC. Laparoscopy—direct trocar insertion without pneumoperitoneum. Obstet Gynaecol 1990;75:725-27.
15. Jelly RY. Multicentre open comparison of buserelin and danazol in the treatment of endometriosis. Br J Clin Pract 1987;41:61.
16. Kistner RW. Management of endometriosis in the infertile patients. Fertil Steril 1975;26:1151.
17. Kistner RW. The use of newer progestins in the treatment of endometriosis. Am J Obstet Gynecol 1958;75:264.
18. Lemay A, Dodin S, Dewailly KS. Long-term use of low dose LHRH analogue combined with monthly medroxyprogesteron administration. Horm Res 1989;32:141.
19. Mann DR, Collins DC, Smith MM et al. Treatment of endometriosis in monkeys. Effectiveness of gonadotrophin releasing hormone agonist compared to treatment with a progestational steroid. J Clin Endocrinol Metab 1986; 63:1277.
20. Martin DC, Hubert GD, Vandez Zwaag R et al. Laparoscopic appearances of peritoneal endometriosis. Fertil Steril 1989;51:67.
21. Mcarthur JW, Ulfeter H. The effect of pregnancy upon endometriosis. Obstet Gynecol Surv 1965;20:709.
22. Overton CE, Lindsay PC, Johal B et al. A randomized, double-blind, placebo-controlled study of luteral phase dydrogesterone (Duphaston) in women with minimal to mid endometriosis. Fertil Steril 1994;62:701.
23. Pittaway DE, Fayez JA. Serum CA-125 antigen levels increase during menses. Am J Obstet Gynecol 1987; 156:75.
24. Rock JA. Endometriosis and pelvic pain. Fertil Steril 1993;69:950.
25. Sakura Y et al. Histological studies on the therapeutic effects of sustained release microsphere of a potent LNRH agonist (luprorelin acetate) in an experimental endometriosis model in rate. Endocrinol Jpn 1990;37:719.
26. Scheken RS, Malinak LR. Reoperation after initial treatment of endometriosis with conservative surgery. Am J Obstet Gynecol 1978;131:416.
27. Schirock E, Monroe SE, Henzl M et al. Treatment of endometriosis with a potent agonist of gonadotropin-releading hormone (naferelin) Fertil Steril 1985;44: 583.
28. Steingold KA, Cedars M, Lu JKH et al. Treatment of endometriosis with long acting gonadotropin-releasing hormone agonist. Obstet Gynecol 1987;69:403.
29. Telimas S et al. Placebo-controlled comparison of danazol and high dose medroxyprogesterone acetate in the treatment of endometriosis. Gynecol Endocrinol 1987;1:13.
30. Thomas EJ, Cooke ID. Impact of gestrinone on the course of asymptomatic endometriosis. BMJ 1987;294: 272.
31. Ulfedler H: The treatment of endometriosis. Med Sci 1966;8:503.

• PG Paul

21

Ectopic Pregnancy

Ectopic pregnancy is no longer a life-threatening emergency, yet it is a leading cause of first trimester maternal death.[1] Early diagnosis and recent developments in the treatment help us to take a more conservative approach to its management. It occurs in approximately 2 percent of all pregnancies and there has seen a six-fold increase in the prevalence of ectopic pregnancy in the last 30 years.[1]

Causes and Risk Factors

More than 97 percent of ectopic pregnancies are located within the fallopian tube, with the remainder in the interstitial part of tube, abdomen, cervix, or ovaries.[2] Most ectopic pregnancies develop from a delay in ovum transport caused by an abnormality of the fallopian tube. A much smaller percentage of ectopic pregnancies are caused by an abnormality of the fertilized egg or its hormonal environment.

Multiple risk factors for ectopic pregnancy have been identified in two meta-analyses.[3,4] More than 50 percent of women with ectopic pregnancies, however, give no history of any of these factors.[3] Factors associated with a high risk for ectopic pregnancy include fallopian tube surgery, tubal sterilization, previous ectopic pregnancy, diethylstilbestrol exposure *in utero*, intrauterine device (IUD) use, and documented tubal damage. Although tubal sterilization decreases the rate of pregnancy overall, at least one-third that do occur are ectopic. The risk for ectopic pregnancy in IUD users is not increased compared with the general population of women of child-bearing age, but if pregnancy does occur, it is significantly more likely to be ectopic.[5] Factors associated with a moderately increased risk include technology-assisted pregnancies, previous genital infections, and multiple sexual partners. Prior abdominal or pelvic surgery, cigarette smoking, vaginal douching, and early age at first intercourse may also be associated with a slight increase in risk. Likewise, prior elective abortions and previous cesarean deliveries have not been shown to be associated with an increased risk.[6]

Clinical Presentation

The symptoms of ectopic pregnancy are often non-specific, and as many as 50 percent of women with ectopic pregnancies are misdiagnosed on their initial visit.[7] Abdominal pain with amenorrhea is the most common presenting complaint,[8] and clinicians should have a high index of suspicion for ectopic pregnancy in every woman of reproductive age who presents with these symptoms. Vaginal bleeding is present in only 40 to 50 percent of patients and may often be mistaken for a normal menstrual period.[6]

Clinical signs are also non-specific. Abdominal tenderness occurs in approximately 75 percent of women with ectopic pregnancies and may or may not be accompanied by rebound tenderness. Cervical motion tenderness is present in approximately two thirds of patients, and adnexal mass is palpable in only approximately 50 percent. Hemodynamic compromise, manifested by orthostatic hypotension, and shock is seen at initial presentation in approximately 20 percent of patients.[8] Today, with modern diagnostic techniques, more than 80 percent can be diagnosed before rupture, thereby greatly reducing the morbidity and mortality rates.

Diagnosis

Because the presenting signs and symptoms of ectopic pregnancy are neither sensitive nor specific, a high index of suspicion is necessary to make the diagnosis. A pregnancy test for beta-hCG should be included in the early evaluation of any woman of reproductive age that presents with abdominal pain and irregular vaginal bleeding or amenorrhea. Urinary assays for beta-hCG have become so sensitive and specific that they are nearly always positive by the time an ectopic pregnancy becomes symptomatic. None of our patients whose pregnancy test was negative had a live ectopic pregnancy. A dead ectopic pregnancy with a negative pregnancy test can be left alone without treatment.

When a positive pregnancy test has been established, it is important to differentiate an ectopic pregnancy from an intrauterine pregnancy. A combination of sonography evaluation, hormonal testing, and other diagnostic procedures is helpful in distinguishing among these entities.

Sonography

The use of sonography has revolutionized the diagnosis of ectopic pregnancy. Transvaginal sonography is capable of reliably detecting IUP when beta-hCG levels range from 1000 to 2000 mIU/mL (approximately 5 weeks' gestation and within 1 week of missed menses).[11]

If an intrauterine pregnancy can be demonstrated, ectopic pregnancy can be virtually excluded, as heterotopic pregnancy is rare in spontaneous conception. But it is important to examine the adnexal region for an abnormality. There are three sonographic features of tubal pregnancy. First is the demonstration of a live embryo within a gestational sac in the adnexa. It typically appears as an intact, well defined tubal ring in which the yolk sacs and/or the embryonic pole with or without cardiac action are seen within a completely sonolucent sac. An ectopic embryo/fetus is seen in 20 percent of cases.[12]

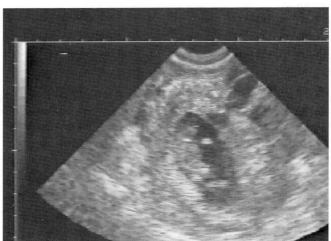

FIGURE 21.1: Transvaginal ultrasound depicting a well-defined tubal ring with a live fetus

The second sonographic feature is that of a poorly defined tubal ring, possibly containing echogenic structures. Typically, pouch of Douglas contains fluid. These features are consistent with a tubal pregnancy, which is aborting.

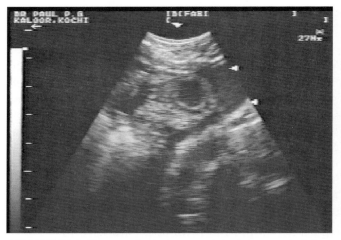

FIGURE 21.2: Transvaginal ultrasound depicting a tubal ring without fetal pole. POD contains fluid and/or blood

The third picture is the presence of varying amounts of fluid in POD representing rupture of the tubal pregnancy. In one study, echogenic fluid alone was seen in 15 percent of patients with ectopic pregnancy.[13] A pseudosac may be present, which can be distinguished sonographically from IUP. A true gestational sac will be eccentrically placed in the endometrial cavity. The use of transvaginal color Doppler sonography can detect the increased blood flow in the tubal artery caused by the implanted trophoblast and allow a rapid diagnosis.

Hormonal Testing

In patients with normal intrauterine pregnancies, the beta-hCG doubling time ranges from 1.5 days in early pregnancy to 3.5 days at 7 weeks' gestation. Ectopic pregnancies and abnormal intrauterine pregnancies have impaired hCG production with prolonged doubling times. The clinical utility of serial beta-hCG measurement is limited because of the inherent delay in determining the pattern of increase or decrease of the hormone. It is also not possible to distinguish an ectopic pregnancy from an abnormal IUP. Finally, approximately 17 percent of patients with ectopic pregnancies have normal beta-hCG doubling times, whereas 15 percent of patients with normal intrauterine pregnancies have serial increase rates of less than 66 percent.[10] When the beta-hCG is below 1500 IU/L and TVS doesn't reveal an ectopic pregnancy, repeat TVS and beta-hCG examination is indicated twice weekly.

Progesterone is produced by the corpus luteum when stimulated by a viable pregnancy. Its level is, therefore, significantly decreased in patients with extrauterine gestations and nonviable intrauterine pregnancies compared with that of patients with normal intrauterine pregnancies. A serum progesterone level of more than 25 ng/mL rules out an ectopic pregnancy with nearly 98 percent sensitivity and strongly favors a viable IUP. Conversely, a progesterone level of less than 5 ng/mL is not compatible with a normal gestation and identifies a nonviable pregnancy with nearly 100 percent sensitivity.[2] Progesterone values between 5 and 25 ng/mL are less sensitive and specific and require additional confirmatory testing to establish a diagnosis. We have not found serum progesterone level estimation useful in our practice.

Uterine Curettage and Culdocentesis

The use of uterine curettage and culdocentesis are obsolete with the availability of transvaginal sonography.

MANAGEMENT

Until recently, surgery was the only feasible option for the management of most patients with ectopic pregnancies. A laparotomy or laparoscopy was needed to visualize the fallopian tube, followed by either a salpingectomy or salpingostomy to remove the ectopic pregnancy. In the past decade, however, medical therapy with methotrexate has gained broad acceptance as an additional first-line treatment option in many patients with ectopic pregnancies.

Surgical Treatment

Surgery remains the treatment of choice for majority of patients with ectopic pregnancy. Laparoscopic approach is usually preferred because of its lower cost, less blood loss, decreased analgesia requirements, and shorter postoperative

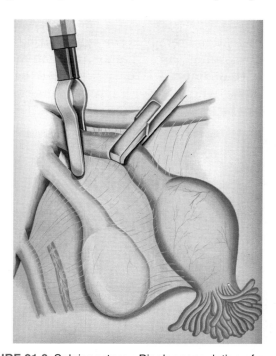

FIGURE 21.3: Salpingectomy: Bipolar coagulation of proximal end of tube after holding it with a grasper introduced through the ipsilateral port

recovery time. Three prospective, randomised trials involving a total of 231 patients have shown definitely that laparoscopic surgery is superior to laparotomy.[14] Laparotomy is indicated in patients who are hemodynamically unstable.

Salpingectomy is the best option in cases of uncontrollable hemorrhage, significant anatomic distortion, recurrent ectopic pregnancy in the same tube, or when future fertility is not desired.[8]

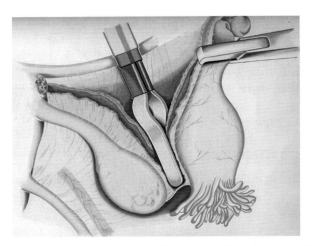

FIGURE 21.4: Salpingectomy: The mesosalpinx is coagulated and then divided in small steps till salpingectomy is completed

Salpingostomy removes the ectopic pregnancy while preserving the fallopian tube. It may be offered to women with unruptured ectopic pregnancies who wish to improve their chances for future fertility.

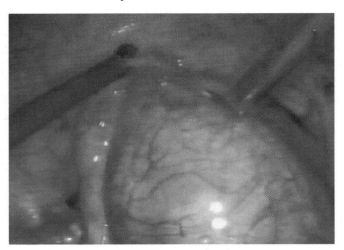

FIGURE 21.5: Laparoscopic salpingostomy for ampullary ectopic

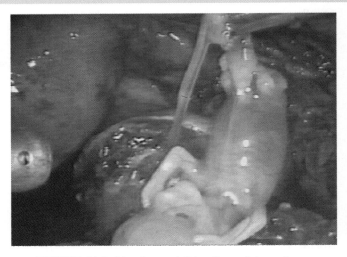

FIGURE 21.6: Live fetus visible after salpingostomy

The risk for persistent ectopic pregnancy (i.e., the persistence of viable ectopic tissue postoperatively) is significantly increased with salpingostomy compared with salpingectomy, so salpingostomy should be reserved for situations in which future fertility is desired and in which fertility is most likely to be improved by sparing the tube. If a patient has only one remaining tube and is interested in future fertility, salpingostomy is the best option. Under these circumstances, the patient should be counseled that, although preserving the remaining fallopian tube offers her some hope for a future pregnancy, the subsequent rate of IUP is low and the risk for a future ectopic pregnancy is high.[15]

Persistent ectopic pregnancy occurs in approximately 8 percent of patients who are treated with salpingostomy.[14] Factors that increase the likelihood of persistent tissue include small ectopic pregnancies (< 2 cm in diameter), early therapy (< 42 days from the last menstrual period), and a high beta-hCG level preoperatively (> 3000 IU/L).[16] A single dose of methotrexate is sometimes used prophylactically in these higher-risk patients when salpingostomy has been performed.[17] We perform urine pregnancy test one week after surgery and if positive, beta hCG level is estimated. If raised, test is repeated after one week to see whether it is regressing. Single dose of prophylactic methotrexate is given if the beta hCG level is not regressing.

Medical Treatment

Methotrexate is a folic-acid antagonist that interferes with DNA synthesis and cell multiplication. It has been used for many years as a chemotherapeutic agent for inhibiting highly proliferative tumor cells and the rapidly growing trophoblastic cells in patients with ectopic pregnancies. Leucovorin rescue is a medication regimen that is given to rescue cells under treatment with methotrexate.

Candidates for medical management with methotrexate must be hemodynamically stable and have no active bleeding or evidence of hemoperitoneum. They should also have gestational sacs of less than 3.5 cm in diameter, a quantitative beta-hCG level of less than 10,000 mIU/mL, and no fetal cardiac motion on transvaginal sonography. Absolute contraindications to treatment with methotrexate include breast-feeding, immunodeficiency, liver disease, blood dyscrasias, active pulmonary disease, peptic ulcer disease, renal dysfunction, or known sensitivity to methotrexate.

Two common regimens have been described: (1) single-dose approach and (2) multi-dose approach. Before initiating either regimen, a complete blood count, liver and renal function tests should be done.

The single-dose approach involves a one-time intramuscular dose of 50 mg/m^2. This regimen has a slightly lower success rate (87%) but has the advantage of being much simpler to administer.[8] The levels of beta-hCG may initially increase after treatment with a single dose of methotrexate,[18] so the first quantitative beta-hCG should not be checked until post-treatment day 4. The level is then rechecked on day 7 and should demonstrate a decrease of at least 15 percent. If it does not decrease, the patient is given another injection.[19] The beta-hCG should then be checked weekly and additional injections given if the weekly beta-hCG values do not decrease appropriately.

Side effects of systemic methotrexate include nausea, diarrhea, oral irritation, and transient transaminase elevations. The individualized, multidose regimen has a side effect rate of 5 percent, and the single dose regimen 1 percent.[18]

High-dose methotrexate can cause bone-marrow suppression, hepatotoxicity, pulmonary fibrosis, and reversible alopecia, but these side effects are unlikely with the lower doses used for ectopic pregnancy.

Most patients have a transient increase in abdominal pain after treatment with methotrexate. Whether this is caused by trophoblastic degeneration and subsequent peritoneal irritation or is a side effect of the methotrexate is not clear. Because it is found in as many as 60 percent of patients, distinguishing patients with this pain from patients with increased abdominal pain from a ruptured tubal pregnancy (which can occur in approximately 5 percent of medically treated patients with ectopic pregnancies) is sometimes difficult.[10] Physicians may counsel these patients about the likelihood of increased abdominal pain after treatment and suggest using a nonsteroidal anti-inflammatory drug for pain management. If increased abdominal pain persists, the patient is evaluated and a hemoglobin level is obtained. If the hemoglobin level is stable, and TVS doesn't show increased fluid in POD, the patient can be managed noninvasively and observed. Otherwise, the possibility of a ruptured ectopic pregnancy should be considered.

In multidose regimen, methotrexate at a dose of 1 mg/kg is administered as sodium salt intramuscularly, followed by leucovorin in a dose of 0.1 mg/kg as calcium salt intramuscularly 24 hours later. Alternate daily doses of methotrexate and leucovorin is continued until serum hCG declines by 15 percent. Upto 4 doses can be given.

In an attempt to increase the success rates of systemic methotrexate treatment, investigators have examined the effects of adding mifeprostone to the treatment protocol. As a single agent, it has not been found to be an effective therapy for ectopic pregnancy. When added to a regimen of methotrexate, however, it resulted in a higher success rate and less need for a second injection or laparotomy. One non-randomised trial involving 30 patients found a decrease in treatment failures from 26 to 3 percent when patients treated with the combination therapy were compared with patients previously treated with methotrexate alone.[21]

Approximately 33-40 percent of patients diagnosed with ectopic pregnancy are eligible for medical treatment.[22] Many studies have demonstrated that methotrexate can be administered by intratubal injection or intramuscularly with similar results. Similarly successful treatment rates are nearly identical among the two protocols,[20] as are rates of subsequent fertility [22] and requirements for postoperative follow-up. The single dose protocol should be reserved for subjects with low or declining hCG values. Multidose protocol is used mainly in the treatment of extratubular ectopic pregnancy.

Expectant Management

Expectant management has poor efficacy and unproven benefit in subsequent reproductive outcome; therefore, its use should be limited to situations in which the EP is suspected but cannot be excluded by transvaginal US. Other conditions for use of expectant management occur when surgery and methotrexate carry higher risk, such as in presence of heterotopic pregnancy or ovarian hyperstimulation syndrome.[14]

Reproductive Outcome

A meta-analysis of 9 studies involving 2,635 patients compared the reproductive outcome of salpingostomy versus salpingectomy.[14] This included 528 patients in the conservative group and 1246 patients in radical group desiring fertility. The rate of subsequent intrauterine pregnancy was 53 percent in conservative group and 49.3 percent in the salpingectomy group. The recurrent EP rates were 14.8 and 9.9 percent, respectively. Another metanalysis reported reproductive outcome after conservative surgery in women with solitary patent tube. Among the 176 women attempting to conceive, there were 54.5 percent IUPs and 20.5 percent recurrent ectopic.[14]

Many other factors influence the subsequent fertility rate, than the type of surgical approach alone. A history of infertility was found to be associated with a decreased fertility rate.[23] Others have found that the status of the contralateral tube at the time of surgery is related directly to the subsequent fertility, regardless of the surgical modality used.[24] Silva *et al*[25] found prior tubal damage to be associated significantly with decreased pregnancy rate: 79 percent pregnancy rate in group without prior damage versus 42 percent in the group with prior tubal damage.

Majority of spontaneous pregnancies after surgical treatment of ectopic pregnancy occur in the first 18 months.[22]

SUMMARY

Ectopic pregnancy is a common clinical condition with high risks for morbidity and mortality. Although its prevalence seems to be increasing, the ability to diagnose and manage this problem continues to improve. Physicians should identify and screen high-risk patients early in their pregnancies and should have a high index of suspicion for ectopic pregnancy in women who present with abdominal pain, amenorrhea, or vaginal bleeding. The diagnosis is commonly made through a combination of hormonal testing and transvaginal sonography. Management options include the traditional surgical salpingectomy or salpingostomy, as well as nonsurgical management with methotrexate in selected patients.

REFERENCES

1. Centers for Disease Control. Ectopic pregnancy-United States, 1990-1992. MMWR Morb Mortal Wkly Rep 1995;44:46-48.
2. Gabbe S, Niebyl J, Simpson J (Eds): Obstetrics: Normal and Problem Pregnancies, 3rd edn. New York, Churchill Livingstone, 1996.
3. Ankum W, Mol B, Van der Veen F, et al. Risk factors for ectopic pregnancy: A meta-analysis. Fertil Steril 1996;65:1093-99.
4. Lonky N, Sauer M. Ectopic pregnancy with shock and undetectable beta-human chorionic gonadotropin. J Reprod Med 1987;32:315-18.
5. Pisarka M, Carson S, Buster J. Ectopic pregnancy. Lancet 1998;351:115-20.
6. Fylstra, D. Tubal pregnancy: A review of current diagnosis and treatment. Obstet Gynecol Surv 1998;53:320-28.
7. Brennan D. Ectopic pregnancy-part I: Clinical and laboratory diagnosis. Acad Emerg Med 1995;2:1081-89.
8. Nieuwkerk P, Hajenius P, Van der Veen F et al. Systemic methotrexate therapy versus laparoscopic

salpingostomy in tubal pregnancy: Part II. Patient preferences for systemic methotrexate. Fertil Steril 1998;70:3.

9. National Center for Health Statistics, US Department of Health and Human Services, Public Health Services, Centers for Disease Control and Prevention: Advanced report of final mortality statistics 1994;43(Suppl).

10. Healy J: Ectopic pregnancy. Linacre Q 1996;63:95-96.

11. Saraj AJ, Wilcox JG, Najmabadi S et al. Resolution of hormonal markers of ectopic gestation: A randomised trial comparing single-dose intramuscular methotrexate with salpingostomy. Obstet Gynecol 1998;92:96.

12. DeCrespigny LC. Demonstration of ectopic pregnancy by transvaginal ultrasound. Br J Obstet Gynecol 1988;95:1253-56.

13. Nyberg DA, Hughes MP, Mack L, Wang KW. Extra-uterine findings of ectopic pregnancy at transvaginal ultrasound: Importance of echogenic fluid. Radiology 1991;178:823-26.

14. Mylene Yao, Togas Tulandi. Current status of surgical and nonsurgical management of ectopic pregnancy. Fertil Steril 1997;67:421-33.

15. Gomel V. For tubal pregnancy, surgical treatment is usually best. Clin Obstet Gynecol 1995;38:353-61.

16. Rulin M. Is salpingostomy the surgical treatment of choice for unruptured tubal pregnancy? Obstet Gynecol 1995;86:6.

17. Graczykowski J, Mishell D. Methotrexate prophylaxis for persistent ectopic pregnancy after conservative treatment by salpingostomy. Obstet Gynecol 1997; 89:118-22.

18. Seifer D: Persistent ectopic pregnancy: An argument for heightened vigilance and patient compliance. Fertil Steril 1997;68:402-04.

19. Kurt Barnhart, Melissa Esposito & Christos coutifaris. An update on the medical treatment of ectopic pregnancy. Obstet & Gynecol Clinics 2000;27:3.

20. Robin F, Lecuru F, Bernard J et al. Use of hystero-salpingosonography for early diagnosis of ectopic pregnancy. Eur J Obstet Gynecol Reprod Biol 1998;79: 217-18.

21. Gazvani MR, Baruah DN, Alfirevic Z et al. Mifepristone in combination with methotrexate for the medical treatment of tubal pregnancy: A randomized controlled trial. Hum Reprod 1998;13:7.

22. Stovall T, Ling F. Single-dose methotrexate: An expanded clinical trial. Am J Obstet Gynecol 1993; 168:6.

23. Dubuisson JB, Aubriot FX, Foulot H, Bruel D, de Joliniere JVB, Mandelbrot L. Reproductive outcome after laparoscopic salpingectomy for tubal pregnancy Fertil Steril 1990;53:1004-07.

24. Pouly JL, Chapron C, Manhes H, Canis M, Wattiez A, Bruhat MA:. Multifactorial analysis of fertility after conservative laparoscopic treatment of ectopic pregnancy in a series of 223 patients. Fertil Steril 1991;56:453-60.

25. Silva PD, Schaper AM, Rooney B. Reproductive outcome after143 laparoscopic procedures for ectopic pregnancy. Obstet Gynecol 1993;81:710-15.

• Mala Arora

22

Role of Fibroids in Infertility

Fibroids, also known as myoma, fibromyoma or leiomyoma are the commonest benign tumors of the female genital tract. They most often occur in the uterus but may also be found in the broad ligament, cervix, ovary and rarely the labia majora. They are found in nearly one in three women in the reproductive age group. They vary in size, shape and position, and may undergo a variety of degenerations. They are more commonly seen in the infertile population, although pregnancy with fibroids in situ is also a common event.

PREVALENCE

The prevalence of fibroids varies from study to study. The prevalence will differ, depending upon the sensitivity of methods used to diagnose uterine fibroids and the population studied. In 100 consecutive hysterectomy specimens assessed histologically 52 percent were shown to have fibroids on routine histopathology, while the incidence rose to 77 percent in the same specimens when the sections were cut at 2 mm intervals.[1]

Ultrasound based studies also show a prevalence of 50 percent in the reproductive age group.[2] However not all of them are symptomatic. In another study Buttram reported that 25 percent of the women have clinically apparent fibroids.[3]

This puts forth a very important point, that, though the prevalence of fibroids is over 50 percent only half of these women will be symptomatic in their lifetime. In this era of frequent ultrasound examinations and medico legal litigations, we are perhaps performing many unnecessary surgeries for the mere presence of fibroids, which is to the detriment of the patients.

The prevalence among Africans is higher than their Caucasian counterparts.[2]

ETIOLOGY

The precise understanding of the triggering factors for development of myomas is important for its prevention. However, these factors are poorly understood at present. The following risk factors have been identified by large epidemiological studies.

Age

Data from the large nurse's health study involving 116,678 nurses, between the age of 25-42 years, showed that the prevalence of fibroids increases as the women's age increases before menopause.[4] In simpler words the prevalence is highest in the fifth decade of life.

Postmenopausal women have a 70-90 percent reduced risk due to shrinkage of fibroids post menopausally.[5] This supports the role of ovarian steroids in the genesis of fibroids.

Race

African and American women had a two to three fold greater incidence from their white, Hispanic or Asian counterparts, at all ages.[4] Incidentally the African women also have a greater propensity to develop collagen rich keloids. This altered collagen production may be the basis of both the keloids and fibroids in Africans.

Menstrual History

Early menarche and late menopause are both associated with a two-fold higher risk of developing fibroids.[6] This may be due to prolonged exposure to ovarian steroids, which have been implicated in its etiology.

Child Bearing

Delivering a child appears to reduce the risk for uterine fibroids by 20-50 percent.[7] Moreover this reduced risk increases with increasing number of live-born children.[8] There exists an almost linear relationship between the number of children and the reduced risk of developing fibroids,[9] i.e. as the number of children increases, the risk of developing fibroids decreases.

The age at which a woman has her first child is not a risk factor for fibroids. However, the risk increases as the interval from her last child increases, independent from the number of live births.

A history of miscarriages or induced abortions does not appear to increase the risk of fibroids.[10] However, a history of infertility has been reported in several studies.[7, 8] Determining the true cause and effect relationship between infertility and uterine fibroids is difficult. It has been shown that submucosal fibroids are the cause of infertility but the presence of other fibroids may also be the effect of infertility. As stated by some, just as fibroadenosis develops in breasts that have been denied their function, so also fibroids develop in the uterus that has been denied its function of child bearing.

Oral Contraceptive Pills (OCP)

The use of OC pills has been shown by some to reduce the risk of fibroids,[5] whereas others have found no association,[11] and still others have found an increased risk of developing fibroids.[12]

Interpretation of literature between OC pills and fibroids is difficult because of two reasons.
1. The earlier higher dose pills have now given way to low dose pills and this may alter the association.
2. The OC pills are often prescribed for treatment of menorrhagia that may be an early symptom of fibroids. Hence the increased association.

Medroxyprogesterone Acetate (MPA)

A study from Thailand has shown a reduced incidence of fibroids in association with the use of MPA.[13] The reduction in risk was more pronounced if the women were using MPA for 5 or more years for contraception. Further studies on this subject are warranted.

Body Mass Index

Obesity has been associated with uterine fibroids. The heavier women are at two to three fold greater risk than the leaner women.[5, 14] Marshall has also concluded that there is an increased risk with weight gain in the reproductive age group, but increased weight at age 18 was not associated with increased risk of fibroids. The explanation for this is as follows:
1. Obesity is often associated with anovulation and increased tonic levels of estrogen unopposed with progesterone
2. Peripheral aromatisation of androgens will lead to higher circulating estrogen levels.
3. Reduced levels of sex hormone binding globulin are seen in obese women, which will lead to a higher level of unbound biologically active estrogen.

Some studies have failed to document this positive association[6,10,15] This is difficult to explain. Some have suggested that obesity makes clinical detection of fibroids more difficult and this may account for the negative association.

Physical Activity

One study has demonstrated that participation in college athletics has been associated with a reduced lifetime prevalence of fibroids.[16]

DIET

One study has reported a two fold increased risk for fibroids in women who consumed a large amount of red meat and a 50 percent reduction in women reporting a high consumption of green vegetables.[17]

Family History

Familial clustering of fibroids has been described as early as 1938.[18] A positive history of uterine fibroids in the mother proves to be the strongest risk factor for development of fibroids. Women whose mothers had a diagnosis of fibroids had a 2.9 times greater risk for uterine fibroids than women whose mothers were known not to have fibroids. Women with a positive history of fibroids tended to be younger when their fibroids were first diagnosed (38 versus 42.5 years), but had the same number of fibroids (4.5 versus 4.0) and the same mean diameter of the largest fibroid (5.3 versus 5.5 cm) on pathological examination of the uterus.[9]

Cigarette Smoking

Most epidemiological studies found that cigarette smokers are at 20-50 percent reduced risk of developing fibroids.[5,14,19] It was earlier thought that this may be the result of a leaner body mass in smokers. However, in all studies the association was independent of BMI. Smoking is known to affect estrogen production and metabolism and leads to earlier menopause, hence the reduced risk of fibroids.

Infectious Agents

An increased incidence of non-uterine leiomyosarcomas has been observed in association with immuno-compromised individuals that are infected with the Epstein-Barr virus.[20] The same has not been substantiated for uterine leiomyomas.

Pelvic Inflammatory Disease (PID)

Women with fibroids reported a higher number of PID episodes than women without fibroids. Whether this is a cause or effect relationship is still not clear. Chlamydia infection was associated with a 3.2 fold increased risk of developing fibroids.[9]

Medical Conditions

Both untreated diabetes and hypertension are associated with an increased risk of fibroids even after adjustment for race and BMI.[21] The risk associated with hypertension appeared to be strongest for women in whom the condition has been diagnosed before the age of 35 or for at least 5 years in the past. Common alterations in smooth muscle may underly both hypertension and fibroids.

In summary, fibroids increase with increasing age and decline after menopause. They also shrink after GnRH agonist administration emphasizing the importance of ovarian hormones in promoting or maintaining the growth of fibroids. The increased prevalence in daughters whose mothers had fibroids suggests a genetic basis. In my personal opinion the genetic predisposition to fibroids requires environmental triggers by way of increased circulation of ovarian hormones especially estrogens and/or alterations in smooth muscle.

GENETICS OF UTERINE FIBROIDS

Pathological evaluation of myoma has revealed that myomas are usually monoclonal tumors, i.e they develop from a single cell line. Initially a study using polymorphic isozymes of X linked glucose 6 phosphate dehydrogenase (G6PD) showed that either A or the B isozyme, but not both were obtained from seven women who were heterozygous for this enzyme.[22] This is the expected result if each tumor is clonal.[9] Furthermore A and B type fibroids were found within the same individual, verifying the independent origin of these neoplasms.

Although most fibroids are chromosomally normal, approximately 40 percent of fibroids have consistent nonrandom chromosomal abnormalities that can be divided into seven main cytogenetic groups
1. Translocation between chromosome 12 and 14
2. Rearrangement of the short arm of chromosome 6
3. Partial deletions in the long arm of chromosome 7

4. Partial deletion in the long arm of chromosome 3
5. Rearrangements in the long arm of chromosome 10
6. Trisomy 12
7. Rearrangement of the X chromosome.

This cytogenetic diversity, together with the variable clinical presentation of fibroids needs further investigations between tumor genotype and clinical phenotype.[23] In one study 12 percent of submucosal fibroids had chromosomal abnormalities as compared to 35 percent of intramural and 29 percent of subserosal.[24]

Besides cytogenetic abnormalities, changes in High Mobility Group (HMG) proteins are noticed in fibroids. These proteins are DNA binding proteins that serve as chromatin architectural factors and regulate gene transcription. They are thought to play a role in cell differentiation and proliferation. Three aberrant splicing variants have been identified in uterine leiomyomas.[25]

Although the causative gene mutation has not been identified yet, researchers believe that a single or multiple gene mutation in the myometrial cell, allows a normal myometrial cell to develop into a myoma. Using microarray analysis, which allows researchers to study many genes at the same time, 12,000 genes were studied both in the normal myometrium and the fibroid tissue of the same patient. They found that 67 genes were upregulated in the myoma and these genes were involved in mitosis, while 78 genes were down regulated in myomas, which were primarily concerned with contractility. This explains why myoma cells multiply faster than normal myometrium and also lose the power of contractility. Furthermore, these gene defects appeared to be inherited from the paternal complement of chromosomes.

Although not translated to useful genetic tests for patients yet, the search for susceptibility genes is on. The center for uterine fibroids at the Brigham and Women's Hospital at Boston is trying to identify genes that predispose women to developing fibroids (www.fibroids.net). Ultimately this could lead to non-invasive treatment options for fibroids such as gene therapy.

CYTOKINES AND GROWTH FACTORS

The genetic predisposition to fibroids is well established. However, the growth promoting factors in susceptible individuals are high circulating levels of ovarian steroids. These steroids are thought to mediate their action via cytokines and growth promoting factors. The following growth factors have been implicated in growth of myomas.[26]

1. Epidermal growth factor
2. Transforming growth factor 3
3. Heparin binding growth factors
4. Insulin like growth factors

Hence drug delivery systems that target these growth factors may slow down the growth of fibroids. One such glycoprotein is interferon, which is currently under investigation for treatment of myomas.

ANATOMIC CLASSIFICATION

According to their position, fibroids are broadly classified into the following categories:

1. Subserous or pedunculated
2. Intramural. These may be further divided into combined intramural-subserous
   - Purely intramural
   - Combined intramural-submucous
3. Submucous
4. Intracavitary or polypoidal
5. Extrauterine for example broad ligament, cervical, vaginal or vulval myoma.

DIAGNOSTIC MODALITIES

Ultrasound imaging with a high frequency transvaginal probe is the most popular non-invasive method employed for the diagnosis of fibroids. In fact, most asymptomatic fibroids are picked up by this investigation. They appear as circumscribed hypoechoic areas in the myometrium, in the case of intramural fibroids, or adjacent to it, in subserous fibroids.

In order to delineate a submucosal fibroid or the submucosal component of an intramural fibroid, installation of 5-10 cc of normal saline into the uterine cavity via a size 8 French Foley's catheter is helpful. This is the technique of sonohysterography, and with the help of a trans-vaginal probe will delineate the distortion of the uterine cavity more effectively than simple scanning. The presence of submucosal component of an intramural fibroid is best delineated by this procedure.

While majority of the uterine leiomyomas require no further imaging, non-uterine leio-myomas may require *Magnetic resonance imaging (MRI)* to confirm the exact location and nature of the tumor.

Hysteroscopy and laparoscopy is required to delineate the size and location of fibroids, the tubal patency and the distortion of the uterine cavity.

There are currently no tumor markers available but in the recent future genetic studies may be available for screening of genetically susceptible women.

SYMPTOMS

Many myomas are asymptomatic and are diagnosed on a routine ultrasound scan. Those that are symptomatic present with

- *Menstrual disturbances*, most often menorrhagia, intermenstrual bleeding and/or dysmenorrhea. In postmenopausal women it may lead to post-menopausal bleeding

- *Pressure symptoms*, on the urinary bladder causing frequency, on the ureter causing hydro-nephrosis, on the rectum causing tenesmus and on the pelvic veins causing venous edema

- *Infertility* (to be discussed later)

- *Recurrent pregnancy loss* Several mechanisms have been postulated.
    1. Submucosal fibroids distort the uterine cavity.
    2. The embryo may implant at a poorly decidualised endometrium.
    3. Fibroids may act as intrauterine contra-ceptive devices and cause subacute endo-metritis.
    4. Increased uterine irritability and contr-actility secondary to rapid fibroid growth may expel the blastocyst prior to proper implantation.

    5. Mechanical compression of conceptus by large fibroids.

- *Pregnancy related complications* These include the following
    1. Preterm labor
    2. Premature rupture of membranes
    3. Placental abruption
    4. Preeclampsia
    5. Malpresentation,
    6. Dysfunctional and/or obstructed labor
    7. Postpartum hemorrhage
    8. Retained placenta
    9. Puerperal infection.

- *Fetal complications*
    1. Decreased Apgar score
    2. Intrauterine growth retardation
    3. Fetal anomalies like limb reduction defects, congenital torticollis.

MYOMAS AND INFERTILITY

Whether uterine myomas cause infertility is still a subject of controversy. Several mechanisms have been proposed for the cause of infertility with fibroids. These are
1. Submucous myomas may act as intrauterine devices and produce subacute endometritis leading to failure of implantation
2. Intramural myomas occurring in the region of the tubal ostia may cause tubal blockage.
3. Compression and dilatation of adjacent vasculature may cause abnormal endometrial maturation which may be inhospitable for embryo maturation.[3]
4. Large intramural, submucous or the combined variety of myomas may cause atrophic or ulcerated endometrium which is hostile to nidation
5. Distortion of the endometrial cavity may increase the travel distance for the sperm.[27]
6. Prostaglandins present in the seminal plasma are believed to increase rhythmic myometrial contractility possibly facilitating sperm transport. Myomas in some way interfere with this mechanism and may decrease fertilization rates.[28]

From the above, it is obvious to the reader, that myomas may depress fertility due to a host of factors. It is the size and location of the myoma that will govern whether fertility is depressed or not. Each embryo that enters the uterine cavity post fertilization will meet a different fate. If it tries to implant close to the myoma, it will be doomed. However, if it implants at a site away from the myoma, it may be able to successfully implant and grow. That is why many myomas are coincidentally present with a pregnancy proving that all these factors may be overcome in some cycles where conception does occur. Hence, the decision to operate on fibroids to enhance fertility is not a simple one.

There is universal consensus that hysteroscopic removal of a submucosal leiomyoma will enhance fertility. The same does not hold true for many intramural and most subserosal myomas that do not cause distortion of the uterine cavity.

Myomas and In Vitro Fertilization

In recent years, Assisted Reproductive Technologies (ART) including in vitro fertilization (IVF) are being employed in women with myomas. IVF offers a unique opportunity to study the effect of uterine fibroids on nidation alone as all other infertility factors including tubal and male factors have been successfully bypassed. Unfortunately no prospective randomized study has evaluated the effect of fibroids and myomectomy on implantation. There are, however, a host of retrospective studies in patients with uterine fibroids with age matched control groups for comparison Farhi et al[29] evaluated by physical examination patients whose uterine size was smaller than 12 weeks , who were scheduled for IVF. Patients with myomas and uterine size over 12 weeks were scheduled for myomectomy prior to IVF and not included in the study. In 46 women that underwent 141 cycles of IVF, 28 patients had a normal endometrial cavity (86 cycles) and 18 patients (55 cycles) had abnormal cavity based on hysteroscopic examination. The overall pregnancy rates were similar in women with myomas (22.1%) and those without (25.1%) Miscarriage rates were also similar. Women whose endometrial cavities were distorted had a significantly lower pregnancy rate of 2.8 percent versus 8.9 percent in patients with normal uterine cavities and 9.7 percent in controls.

Ramzy[30] evaluated 51 patients with fibroids who underwent IVF. Twelve patients with submucous or intramural fibroids larger than 7 cm that encroached on the endometrial cavity were advised to undergo myomectomy prior to IVF. The remaining 39 patients were compared with a control group of 367 women with normal uterine cavities. The pregnancy rates were 38.5 percent in the myoma group as compared to 33.5 percent in the control group. These rates were not significantly different from each other nor were the incidences of miscarriage and other obstetric complications.

On the contrary, Stovall[31] performed a prospective study of 91 ART cycles in women with myomas that did not distort the uterine cavity and were under 6 cm in size. The control group consisted of the next IVF patient of the same age group. He concluded that the pregnancy rate of 37.4 percent in the myoma group was significantly lower than 52.7 percent in the control group. There was no difference in the miscarriage rate between the two groups.

Another study reported similar results[32] but they separated their study group into those with intramural myomas and those with subserosal myomas. Pregnancy rates were 30.1 percent in controls, 34.1 percent in patients with subserosal myomas and 16.4 percent in patients with intramural myomas. The pregnancy rates were significantly lower in the intramural group.

Myomectomy and Infertility

Buttram and Reiter reviewed 1699 cases of myomectomy and determined that 27 percent of these women also had infertility.[3] When all other causes were ruled out, myomas were found to play a role in only 2.4 percent of the cases.[33] Hence it was concluded that, although myomas may be coincidentally present in 25 percent of the cases of infertility, myomectomy would directly benefit only 2.4 percent of these women, where all other infertility factors have been ruled out. The rest will conceive following treatment of an identifiable cause without resorting to myomectomy.

The above concept is important to understand. Most gynecologists feel that operating on fibroids would enhance fertility in all patients with fibroids. On the contrary, myomectomy leads to peritubal adhesions and distortion of the tubo ovarian relationship as well as the uterine cavity in a large number of patients that will actually reduce further fertility potential leaving IVF as the only treatment option postmyomectomy. Hence, the decision to perform myomectomy or not in an infertile patient with fibroids is a crucial one. It must be taken only after all other identifiable factors have been treated, by an infertility specialist, and, pregnancy has not ensued.

TREATMENT OPTIONS

Treatment options may be broadly classified into surgical and medical.

Surgical

In women who have completed child bearing, hysterectomy is the procedure of choice for all symptomatic patients. The role of myomectomy in such patients is limited because of the risk of growth of new myomas with time.

Myomectomy

In women with infertility myomectomy is the procedure of choice Pregnancy rates post myomectomy appear to be variable. A meta-analysis of women with long term-unexplained infertility and myomas demonstrated a conception rate of 59.5 percent after myomectomy and the majority of these conceptions occurred within 1 year of surgery.[33,34] In a retrospective analysis of 51 women with no uterine cavity distortion observed a significantly higher pregnancy rate of 76 percent after myomectomy versus 40 percent before myomectomy.

The approach to myomectomy may be *abdominal or laparoscopic.*

Abdominal Myomectomy

Myomectomy was classically performed via Laparotomy. Since myomectomy is performed as a reproductive procedure. The microsurgical principles inherent to all reproductive pelvic surgeries must be applied, namely atraumatic tissue handling, strict attention to hemostasis, continuous moistening of the pelvic tissues and meticulous approximation of dissected tissue planes. Use of gonadotropin releasing hormone agonist prior to surgery, shrinks the fibroid thereby making it less vascular and also giving better approximation of uterine scar. Two randomized studies have confirmed that injection of Pitressin intraoperatively in the surrounding myometrium helps in reducing blood loss.[35, 36] The uterine incision should preferably be longitudinal as close to the midline as possible as this area is relatively avascular. A correct plane of cleavage should be reached in the pseudocapsule of the myoma. Shelling of the myoma should be by gentle traction and countertraction. The defect in the myometrium should be sutured with interrupted sutures of 2-0 or 3-0 Vicryl. Should the endometrial cavity be breached, it should be repaired with 5.0 Vicryl everting the endometrial edges towards the cavity. Inclusion of endometrial edges in the myometrium may cause foci of adenomyosis.

Laparoscopic myomectomy was described two decades ago.[37-40] However it requires a high degree of training and skill from the operator. Mastering the technique of laparoscopic suturing and intra-abdominal morcellation are crucial.[41] The operation is time consuming.[42] The strength of the uterine scar may be compromised as reported by ten case reports.[43-46]

Laparoscopic Assisted Myomectomy (LAM) has been developed by Nezhat in 1994.[47] The procedure is performed laparoscopically, but the myoma bed is exteriorized by extending the suprapubic port to a minilaparotomy, and adequately suturing the uterus in layers using 4.0 to 2.0 Vicryl.

Prevention of postoperative adhesions is a concern whether the abdominal or laparoscopic route is used. Besides good microsurgical techniques, the use of barrier methods has been shown to be of some use. Removal of more than 5 myomas leads to significantly lower pregnancy rates due to subsequent formation of adhesions. Tulandi[48] performed second look laparoscopy after initial myomectomy and observed a greater degree of adhesion formation after posterior wall myomectomy (93.7%) than with anterior wall myomectomy (55.5%). These adhesions may be prevented by the use of Interceed (Johnson and Johnson, New Brunswick, New Jersey USA)[49] or Gore Tex (WL Gore and associates Inc, Flagstaff AZ USA).[50]

Hysteroscopic Resection

In women with intracavitory defects due to intramural fibroids hysteroscopic resection is superior to laparoscopic myomectomy. This results in less blood loss and postoperative pain, reduced hospitalization and recovery time, lower risk of postoperative pelvic adhesions. The complications reported are uterine perforation, hemorrhage, infection and excessive hypotonic fluid absorption.[51] Uterine rupture during pregnancy has also been reported after hysteroscopic myomectomy.[52] In large myomas it may be worthwhile to perform the procedure in two sittings to minimize the risk of perforation. The recent introduction of a bipolar electrode versapoint (Johnson and Johnson, Somerville NJ) can be used with normal saline as the distension medium, which decreases the complications associated with hypotonic fluid absorption.[53, 54]

Uterine Artery Embolization (UAE)

Percutaneous uterine arterial embolization was first employed to treat leiomyoma in 1995.[55] Later a number of papers have been published.[56-63] Initially it was employed only for poor surgical risk patients, but due to the encouraging response in control of menorrhagia, it may now be employed as primary therapy It is currently not recommended for patients that desire child bearing, because its effect on endometrial maturation and ovarian function is as yet unknown.[65] Most cases reported, underwent UAE after completing child bearing, hence data is limited. However, so far a dozen pregnancies have been reported following the procedure[66] and several have delivered at term. There have been no case reports of uterine rupture unlike following myolysis or laparoscopic myomectomy.

Myolysis

Laparoscopic myolysis is a procedure designed to shrink uterine myomas by coagulating their blood supply. It was first performed in 1980 with the help of Nd:Yag laser.[67] Although other modalities like Diathermy and cryomyolysis was also proposed, the experience with these is limited. Although effective shrinkage of myomas was achieved after laparoscopic myolysis, several cases of uterine rupture in the third trimester have been reported.[68-70] Hence this technique is currently not advisable for women desiring fertility.

Percutaneous Laser Ablation

Thermal ablation of uterine fibroids, using percutaneously placed laser fibers under real time magnetic resonance (MR) guidance, has been performed in a few women.[71] Six weeks later four of these women proceeded with their planned hysterectomy. Circumscribed areas of necrosis were seen in the myomas with minimal damage to surrounding tissue. The remaining women that did not undergo their hysterectomy reported symptomatic improvement. Further patients are continuing to be treated.

High Intensity Focused Ultrasound (HIFU)

High intensity focused ultrasound beams are being employed to treat several human diseases including breast fibroadenomas and benign prostatic hypertrophy. Vaezy and colleagues[72] have tested its use in a nude mouse model. There was tumor regression in half the mice and the other half required retreatment. Pilot studies are currently underway in women with uterine fibroids.

MEDICAL THERAPY

Gonadotropin Releasing Hormone Agonists (GnRHa)

This is a decapeptide that is secreted by the neurons of the hypothalamus in a pulsatile manner. Administration of this compound causes an initial flare up in the level of anterior pituitary hormones FSH and LH followed by their down regulation. This causes a drop in the level of circulating estrogens and progesterone levels. Depot preparations are in the market that will have sustained effect for one month. In 1983, Filicouri was the first to report the use of GnRHa in a patient with leiomyoma..[73] His therapy led to a reduction in the fibroid volume by 77 percent over a course of 90 days. This also led to a rise in hemoglobin concentration from 7.4 gms/dl to 12.8 gms/dl. Since then, the use of GnRHa has gained popularity primarily for pretreatment of patients prior to surgery. This not only builds up the hemoglobin level but also reduces the size of the uterine scar by shrinking the fibroid.

GnRHa successfully reduces myoma size and decreases overall uterine volume. Most studies demonstrate a reduction in myoma volume of 45-60 percent with peak reduction occurring 2-3 months after treatment is initiated,[74, 75] pregnancy rates of 50 percent were obtained in the group pretreated with GnRha before myomectomy versus 8.3 percent in the group treated with GnRHa alone. Kuhlmann[76] also observed a high rate (41%) of spontaneous pregnancy within 6 months of myomectomy in those pretreated with GnRHa. Use of GnRHa may be particularly advantageous in anemic patients, reducing the possibility of blood transfusion during surgery. After the cessation of treatment the uterus rapidly returns to the pretreatment volume within weeks. This rapid regrowth makes this option ineffective for long-term use. The risk of osteoporosis with prolonged hypoestrogenic states is also well documented. It is reasonable to administer them alone to a perimenopausal patient with the hope that natural menopause will begin during treatment thus reducing the probability of myoma regrowth. Its use in the infertile patient is also lucrative. However, no studies are available on the pregnancy rates following its use alone in the infertile population.

Gonadotropin Releasing Hormone and Add Back Therapy

In order to minimize the hypoestrogenic effect of GnRHa, and permit extension of treatment, add back therapy with ovarian steroids has been tried. Friedman[77] reported that adding 20 mg of medroxy proegesterone acetate to leuprolide inhibited the reduction in uterine volume that is obtained when leuprolide is administered with a placebo Most add back regimes have utilized GnRHa first to achieve shrinkage and then added back a low dose of hormone replacement in a continuous or sequential manner, as is used in postmenopausal hormone replacement therapy. Addition of high dose oral contraceptive pills is not recommended.

Tibolone

In a study of postmenopausal women with menorrhagia that were using Tibolone for HRT, it was noticed that these women were more likely to achieve amenorrhea that those on conventional HRT.[78] Subsequently it was tested in premenopausal women that were receiving GnRHa for treatment of leiomyoma.[79] In this trial GnRHa plus tibolone was compared with GnRHa plus placebo. There was no inhibition of uterine shrinkage with tibolone and patients had preservation of bone density as well as symptomatic improvement. There has been no trial assessing the efficacy of tibolone in premenopausal women.

Gonadotropic Releasing Hormone Antagonists

Pilot studies with both daily and depot preparations of Cetrorelix[80-82] showed shrinkage of leiomyoma within 2-4 weeks of treatment equivalent to that seen with GnRH agonist. Studies comparing agonist with antagonists are awaited.

Danazol

In a clinical study 20 women with leiomyoma were treated with 400 mg of danazol for 4 months. Significant volume reduction of leiomyoma was observed that was maintained even 6 months after stopping the treatment.[83] The same authors used 100 mg of danazol for 6 months after GnRH agonist therapy and reported a decrease in rebound seen after discontinuation of therapy.[84]

Mifepristone

Mifepristone, in a dose of 50 mg/day for 3 months, has been administered to normally cycling premenopausal women with symptomatic leiomyoma. The reduction in myoma volume was 49 percent at the end of this period.[85, 86] The clinical benefit was equivalent to that seen with GnRHa with the added advantage of normal circulating levels of estradiol and preservation of bone mass. To date there are no long-term studies reported on this subject.

Selective Estrogen Receptor Modulators (SERMs) Tamoxifen and Raloxifen

In animal studies (rat model) both tamoxifen and raloxifen showed reduction in incidence of uterine tumors by 40-60 percent. (87 Walker CL). No human studies on this compound have been reported so far Theoretically, however, being anti estrogenic they may possess the capability of shrinking myomas.

Growth Factor Directed Treatment

It has been observed that women with acromegaly have a high incidence of leiomyomas. Hence, Lanreotide, a long acting somatostatin analogue that has been used to treat acromegaly, has been tried in seven patients with leiomyoma for 3 months. Shrinkage in myoma volume by 42 percent was observed.[88] Reduction in growth hormone and IGF-1 levels was observed while estrogen levels were maintained.

Interferon

Interferons have clinically been used in a variety of vascular tumors. In leiomyomas too, they might reduce the angiogenic factor, and thus reduce leiomyoma related bleeding. A case report of a woman who was treated with interferon alpha for hepatitis C was shown to have significant shrinkage of a coexistent leiomyoma after 7 months of therapy.[89]

Aromatase Synthetase Inhibitors

Aromatase synthetase inhibitors are potent inhibitors of systemic estrogens, and have been successfully used in the treatment of metastatic breast cancer. They are also being employed for ovulation induction in low doses Theoretically they hold promise in shrinking myomas but need to be clinically tried for this indication. Their oral bioavailability will make them attractive options.[90]

Cytotoxic Gene Therapy for Fibroids

Gene therapy is the treatment modality of the future. It is best defined as the transfer of essential or therapeutic DNA sequences to a patients cell to evoke a clinical benefit. DNA sequence may be transferred to somatic cells via viral vectors or non-viral vectors. Cytotoxic gene therapy seeks to destroy abnormal cells by direct toxic effects. This kind of "Suicidal gene therapy" has been used to treat malignant tumors and is FDA approved for treatment of tumors of the brain and ovary. However, it holds promise for benign proliferative diseases like fibroids. A recent laboratory study has demonstrated the effectiveness of cytotoxic gene therapy on leiomyocytes and leiomyoma cells derived from Eker rats.[91] However in vivo therapy is yet to be tried.

RECURRENCE

Recurrence of myoma is a cause for concern in the infertile woman. Postmedical therapy, most myomas will regrow to their original size within 6 months of cessation of therapy. Postmyomectomy the recurrence rate has been reported as 8.7 percent for women followed up as long as 12 years.[92] Other studies quote a recurrence rate of 30 percent postabdominal myomectomy[93] and 47 percent posthysteroscopic myomectomy.[94] The reoperation rate was 7.5 percent. There is a positive correlation between recurrence rate and the number of myomas removed at the time of surgery.[3]

Decision Making in Fibroids with Infertility

The following table outlines the symptoms supporting surgical intervention in various types of myomas (Table 22.1).

TABLE 22.1: Symptoms supporting surgery

Type of Myoma	Bleeding	Pain	Infertility	Size/ Pressure symptoms
Intracavitary	+	+	+	–
Submucosal	+	±	+	–
Intramural	±	±	±	–
Subserosal	–	±	–	±
Pedunculated	–	±	–	±

The following Flow Chart 22.1 outlines the management strategies.

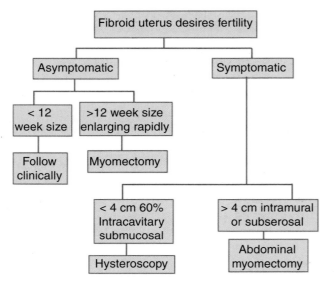

FLOW CHART 22.2: Management guidelines for myoma

CONCLUSION

- The causes of myoma development are poorly understood.
- Its association with infertility is observed but the cause and effect relationship requires further elucidation.
- Treatment of asymptomatic patients with myomas observed on ultrasound scan is controversial.
- In patients with infertility and myoma it is important to rule out all other causes of infertility prior to proceeding with surgical removal, for fear of developing peritubal adhesions.
- Current data suggests surgical treatment is beneficial for patients with uterine cavity distortion.

- Patients who do not have significant uterine cavity distortion and also have no other known causes of infertility, extensive counseling is required explaining the risks and benefits of myomectomy.
- Noninvasive options of uterine artery embolization and high intensity focused ultrasound need further research
- Options for medical treatment are widening with the availability of newer drug molecules.

REFERENCES

1. Cramer SF, Patel A. The frequency of uterine leiomyomas Am J Clin Pathol 1990;94:435-38.
2. Baird DD, Schectman JM, Dixon D, et al African Americans at higher risk than whites for uterine fibroids: Ultrasound evidence [abstract]. Am J Epidemiol 1998;147:S90.
3. Buttram Jr VC, Reiter RX Uterine Lieomyomata: Etiology, symptomatology, and management. Fertil Steril 1981;36:433-45.
4. Marshall LM, Spiegelmau D, Barbieri RL, Goldman MB, et al. Variation in the incidence of uterine lieomyoma among premenopausal women by age and race. Obstet Gynaecol 1997;90:967-73.
5. Ross RK, Pike M, Vessey MP et al Risk factors for uterine fibroids Reduced risk associated with oral contraceptives. BMJ 1986;293:359-62.
6. Samadi AR, Lee NC, Flanders WD et al. Risk factors for self-reported uterine fibroids: a case-control study. Am J Public Health 1996;86:858-62.
7. Marshall LM, Spiegelman D, Barbieri RL, Goldman MB, et al. A prospective study of reproductive factors and oral contraceptive use in relation to the risk for uterine leiomyomata. Fertil Steril 1998;70:432-39.
8. Parazzini F, Negri E, La Vecchia C, et al. Reproductive factors and risk for uterine fibroids. Epidemiology 1996;7:440-42.
9. Van Voorhis BJ, Romitti PA, Jones MP. Family history as a risk factor for development of uterine fibroids: results of a pilot study. J Reprod Med (in Press).
10. Chen CR, BuckGM, Courey NG, et al. Risk factors for uterine fibroids among women under going tubal sterilization. Am J Epidemiol 2001;153:20-26.
11. Parazzini F, Negri E, La Vecchia C, et al. Oral Contraceptive use and risk for uterine fibroids. Obstet Gynaecol 1992;79:430-33.
12. Ramcharan S, Pelligrin FA, Ray R, et al. The Walnut Creek Contraceptive Drug Study: A prospective study of the side effects of oral contraceptives. Bethesda, MD: NIH Publ. No.81-564. Center Popul Res Monogr 1981;3:69-74.
13. Lumbiganon P, Rugpao S, Phandhu-fung S, et al. Protective effect of depot-medroxyprogesterone acetate on

surgically treated uterine leiomyomas: A multicentre case-control study. Br J Obstet Gynaecol 1995;103: 909-14.

14. Marshall LM, Spiegelman D, Manson JE, Barbieri RL, Goldman MB, et al. Risk for uterine lieomyomata among premenopausal women in relation to body size and cigarette smoking. Epidemiology 1998;9:511-17.

15. Parazzini F, Negri E, La Vecchia C, Fedele L, et al Epidemiologic characteristics of women with uterine fibroids: A case-control study. Obstet Gynaecol 1988;72: 853-57.

16. Wyshak G, Frisch RE, Albright NL, Albright TE, Schiff I. Lower prevalence of benign diseases of the breast and benign tumours of the reproductive system among former college athletes compared to non-atheletes. Br. J Cancer 1986;54:841-45.

17. ChiafTarino F, Parazzini F, La Vecchia C, Chatenoud L, et al. Diet and uterine myomas. Obstet Gynaecol 1999;94:395-98.

18. Winkler VDH, Hoffmann W. Regarding the question of inheritance of uterine myoma. Dtsch Med Wochenschr 1938;68:235-57.

19. Parazzini F, Negri E, La Vecchia C, Villa A, et al. Uterine myomas and smoking: Results from an Italian study. J Reprod Med 1996;41:316-20.

20. McClain KL, Leach CT, Jenson HB, et al. Association of Epstien-Barr virus with lieomyoscarcomas in children with AIDS. N.Engl J Med 1995;332:12-18.

21. Faerstein E, Szklo M, Rosenshein N. Risk factors for uterine leiomyoma: A practice-based case-control study.I!: Atherogenic risk factors and potential sources of uterine irritation. Am J Epidemiol 2001;153:11-19.

22. Townsend DE, Sparkes RS, Baluda MC, et al. Unicellular histogenesis of uterine leiomyomas as determined by electrophoresis of glucose-6-phosphate dehydrogenase. Am J Obstet Gynaecol 1970;107: 1168-74.

23. Hu J, Surti U. Subgroups of uterine leiomyomas based on cytogenetic analysis. Hum Pathol 1991;22:1009-16.

24. Brosens I, Deprest J, Dal Cin P, et al. Clinical significance of cytogenetic abnormalities in uterine myomas. Fertil Steril 1998;69:232-35.

25. Kurose K, Mine N, lida A, Nagai H, et al. Three aberrant splicing variants of the HMG1C gene transcribed in uterine leiomyomas. Genes Chromosomes Cancer 2001;30:212-17.

26. Acri A, Sozen 1. Transforming growth factor-beta 3 is expressed at high levels in leiomyoma where it stimulates fibronectin expression and cell proliferation. Fertil Sterif 2000;73:1006-11.

27. Hunt SE, Wallach EE. Uterine factors in infertility: An Overview. Clin Obstet Gynaecol 1974;17:44-64.

28. Coutinho EM, Maia HS. The contractile response of the human uterus, fallopian tubes and ovary to prostaglandins in vivo. Fertil Steril 1971;22:539-43.

29. Farhi J, Ashkenazi J, Feldberg D et al. Effect of uterine leiomyomata on the result of in vitro fertilisation treatment. Hum Reprod 1995;10:2576-78.

30. Ramzy AM, Sartar M, Amin Y, et al. Uterine myomata and outcome of assisted reproduction. Hum Reprod 1998;13:198-202.

31. Stovall DW, Parrish SB, Van Voorhis BJ, et al. Uterine lieomyomas reduce the efficacy of assisted reproduction cycles: Results of a matched follow-up study. Hum Reprod 1998;13:192-97.

32. Elder-Geva T, Meagher S, Healy DL, et al. Effect of intramural, subserosal and submucosal uterine fibroids on the outcome of assisted reproductive technology treatment. Fertil Steril 1998;70:687-91.

33. Verkauf BS. Myomectomy for fertility enhancement and preservation Fertil Steril 1992;58:1-15.

34. Li TC, Mortimer R, Cooke ID. Myomectomy. A retrospective study to examine reproductive performance before and after surgery. Hum Reprod 1999;14: 1735-40.

35. Dillon TF. Control of blood loss during gynaecologic surgery. Obstet Gynaecol 1961;19:428-35.

36. Fredrick J, Fletcher H, Simeon D, et al. Intramyometrial vasopressin as a haemostatic agent during myomectomy. Br J Obstet Gynaecol 1994;101:435-37.

37. Darai E, Dechaud H, Benifla JL, et al. Fertility after laparoscopic myomectomy: Preliminary results. Hum Reprod 1997;12:1931-34.

38. Dubuisson JB, Chapron C, Verspyek E, et al. Laparoscopic myomectomy: 102 cases Contracept Fertil Sex 1993;21:920-22.

39. Hasson HM, Rotman C, Rana N, et al. Laparoscopic myomectomy. Obstet Gynaecol 1992;80:884-88.

40. Nezhat C, Nezhat F, Silfen SL, et al Laparoscopic myomectomy. Int J fertil 1991;36:275-80.

41. Tulandi T, al-Took S. Endoscopic myomectomy: laparoscopy and hysteroscopy. Obstet Gynaecoi Clin Norht Am 1999;26:135-48.

42. Shushan A. Mohamed H, Magos AL, et al. How long does laparoscopic surgery really take? Lessons learned from 1000 operative laparoscopies. Hum Reprod 1999;14:39-43.

43. Dubuisson JB, Chapron C, Verspyek E, et al. Pregnancy outcome and deleveries following laparoscopic myomectomy. Hum Reprod 2000;15:869-73.

44. Foucher F, Leveque J, Le Bouar G, et al. Uterine rupture during pregnancy following myomectomy via coelioscopy. Eur J Obstet Gynaecoi Reprod Biol 2000;92:279-81.

45. Friedmann W, Maier RF, Luttkus A, Schafer AP, et al. Uterine rupture after laparoscopic myomectomy. Acta Obstet Gynaecoi Scand 1996;75:683-84.

46. Hockstein S. Spontaneous uterine rupture in the early third trimester after laparoscopically assisted myomectomy. J Reprod Med 2000;45:139-41.

47. Nezhat C, Nezhat F, Bess O, et al. Laparoscopically assisted myomectomy: A report of a new technique in 57 cases. Int J Fertil 1994;39:39-44.

48. Tulandi T, Murray C, Guralnick M. Adhesion formation and reproductive outcome after myomectomy and

second-look laparoscopy. Obstet Gynaecoi 1970;107: 1168-74.

49. Nordic Adhesion Prevention Study Group. The efficacy of Interceed (TC7) for the prevention of reformation of postoperative adhesions on ovaries, fallopian tubes and fimbriae in microsurgical operations for fertility: A multicenter study. Fertil Steril 1995;63:709-14.

50. The Myomectomy Adhesion Multicenter Study Group. An expanded polytetrafluoroethylene barrier (Gore-Tex Surgical Membrane) reduces post-myomectomy adhesion formation. Fertil Steril 1995;63:491-93.

51. Ubaldi F, Tournaye H, Camus M, et al. Fertility after hysteroscopic myomectomy. Hum Reprod Upd 1995;1: 81-90.

52. Abbas A, Irvine LM Uterine rupture during labor after hysteroscopic myomectomy. Gynecol Endoscop 1997;6: 245-46.

53. Fernandez H, Gervaise A, de Tayrac R. Operative hysteroscopy for infertility using normal saline solution and a coaxial bipolar electrode, a pilot study. Hum Reprod 2000;2:CD000475.

54. Kung RC, Vilos GA, Thomas B, et al. A new bipolar system for performing operative hysteroscopy in normal saline. J Am Assoc Gynaecoi Laparosc 1999;6:331-36.

55. Ravina JH, Herbreteau D, Ciraru-Vinneron N, et al. Arterial embolization to treat uterine myomata. Lancet 1995;346:671-72.

56. Goodwin SC, Vedantham S, McLucas B, et al. Preliminary experience with uterine artery embolization for uterine fibroids. J Vase Interv Radiol 1997;8: 517-26.

57. Worthington -Kirsch RL, Popky GL, Hutchins Jr FL. Uterine arterial embolization for the management of lieomyomas: Quality-of-life assessment and clinical response. Radiology 1998;208:625-29.

58. Goodwin SC, Walker WJ. Uterine artery embolization for the treatment of uterine fibroids. Curr Opin Obstet Gynaecoi 1998;10:315-20.

59. Bradley EA, Reidy JF, Forman RG, et al. Trans-catheter uterine artery embolization to treat large uterine fibroids. Br J Obstet Gynaecoi 1998;105:235-40.

60. Burn P, McCall J, Chinn R, et al. Embolization of uterine fibroids Br J Radiol 1999;72:159-61.

61. Hutchins Jr FL, Worthington-Kirsch R, Berkowitz RP. Selective uterine artery embolization as primary treatment for symptomatic leiomyomata uteri. J Am Assoc Gynaecol Laparosc 1999;6:279-84.

62. Spies JB, Warren EH, Mathias SD, et al. Uterine fibroid embolization: Measurement of health-related quality of life before and after therapy. J Vase Interv Radiol 1999;10:1293-1303.

63. Pelage JP, Le Dref O, Soyer P, et al. Fibroid related menorrhagia: Treatment with super selective embolization of the uterine arteries and midterm follow up Radiology 2000;215:428-31.

64. Bradley SH, Stackhouse DJ, et al. Uterine artery embolization for symptomatic uterine myomas. Fertil Steril 2000;74:855-69.

65. Spices JB, Ascher SA, Roth AR, Kim J, et al. Uterine artery embolization for symptomatic uterine myomas. Fertil Steril 2000;74:855-69.

66. Ravina JH, Vigneron NC, Aymard A, et al. Pregnancy after embolization of uterine myoma: report of 12 cases. Fertil Steril 2000;74:855-69.

67. Donnez J, Squifflet J, Polet R, et al. Laparoscopic myolysis. Hum Reprod Upd 2000;6:609-13.

68. Nkemayim DC, Hammadeh ME, Hippach M, et al. Uterine rupture in pregnancy subsequent to previous laparoscopic electromyolysis: case report and review of the literature. Arch Gynaecol Obstet 2000;264(3): 154-56.

69. Vilos GA, Daly LJ, Tse BM. Pregnancy outcome after laparoscopic electromyolysis. J Am Assoc Gynaecol Laparosc 1998;5:289-92.

70. Arcangeli S, Pasquarette MM. Gravid uterine rupture after myolysis. Obstet Gynaecol 1997;89:857.

71. Law P, Gedroyc WM, Regan L. Magnetic resonance guided percutaneous laser ablation of uterine fibroids. Lancet 1999;354:2049-50.

72. Vaezy S, Fujimoto VY, Walker C, et al. Treatment of uterine fibroid tumours in a nude mouse model using high-intensity focused ultrasound. Am J Obstet Gynaecol 2000;183:6-11.

73. Filicori M, Hall DA, Loughlin JS, et al. A conservative approach to the management of uterine leiomyoma: Pituitary desensitization by a luteinizing hormone-releasing hormone analogue. Am J Obstet Gynaecol 1983;147(6):726-27.

74. Ambramovici H, Dimfeld M, et al. Pregnancies following treatment by GnRH-a (decapeptyl) and myomectomy in infertile women with uterine lieomyomata. Int J Fertil 1994;39:150-55.

75. Cirkel U, Ochs H, Roehl A, et al. Estrogen and progesterone receptor content of enucleated uterine myomata after luteinizing hormone releasing hormone. Acta Obstet Gynaecol Scand 1994;73:328-32.

76. Kulhman M, Gartner E-M, et al. Uterine lieomyomata and sterility, therapy with gonadotropin releasing hormone agonists and leiomyomectomy Gynaecol Endocrinol 1997;11:169-74.

77. Friedman AJ, Barbieri RL, Doubilet PM, et al. A randomized, double blind trial of a gonadotropin releasing-hormone agonist (leuprolide) with or without medroxyprogesterone acetate in the treatment of leiomyomata uteri. Fertil Steril. 1988;49(3):404-09.

78. De Aloysio D, Altieri P, Penacchioni P, et al. Bleeding patterns in recent postmenopausal outpatients with uterine myomas: Comparison between two regimens of HRT Maturitas. 1998;29(3):261-64.

79. Palomba S, Affinito P, Tommaselii GA, et al. A clinical trial of the effects of tibolone administered with gonadotropin-releasing hormone analogues for the treatment of uterine leiomyomata. Fertil Steril 1998;70(1):111-18.

80. Kettel LM, Murphy AA, Morales AJ, et al. Rapid regression of uterine liemyomas in response to daily

administration of gonadotropin-releasing hormone antagonist. Fertil Steril 1993;60(4):642-46.

81. Gonzale-Bareena D, Alvarez RB, Ochoa EP, et al. Treatment of uterine leiomyomas with luteinizing hormone-releasing hormone antagonist Cetrorelix. Hum Reprod 1997;12(9):2028-35.

82. Felberbaum RE, Germer U, Ludwig M, et al. Treatment of uterine fibroids with a slow release formulation of the gonadotropin releasing hormone antagonist Cetrorelix. Hum Reprod 1998;13(6):1660-68.

83. De Leo V, la Marca a, Morgante G. Short-term treatment of uterine fibromyoma with danazol. Gynaecol Obstet Invest 1999;47(4):258-62.

84. De Leo V, Morgante G, Lanzetta D, et al. Danazol administration after gonadotropin releasing hormone analogue reduces rebound of uterine myomas. Hum Reprod. 1997;12(2):357-60.

85. Murphy AA, Kettel LM, Morales AJ, et al. Regression of uterine leiomyomata in response to the anti-progesterone RU 486. J Clin Endocrinol Metab. 1993;76(2):513-17.

86. Murphy AA, Kettel LM, Morales AJ, et al. Regression of uterine lieomyomata to the anti-progesterone RU 486. Fertil Steril 1995;64(1):187-90.

87. Walker CL, Burroughs KD, Davis B et al. Preclinical evidence for therapeutic efficacy of selective estrogen receptor modulators for uterine leiomyoma. J Soc Gynaecol Investig. 2000;7(4):249-56.

88. De Leo V, Morgante G, la Marca a, et al Administration of somatostatin analogue reduces uterine and myoma volume in women with uterine lieomyomata. Fertil Steril 2001;75:632-33.

89. Minakuchi K, Kawamura N, et al. Remarkable and persistent shrinkage of uterine leiomyoma associated with interferon alfa treatment for hepatitis, [letter] Lancet 1999;353:2127-28.

90. Dowsett M, Jones A, Johnston SR, Jacobs S, Trunet P, Smith IE. In vivo measurement of aromatase inhibition by letrozole (CGS 2026) in postmenopausal women with breast cancer. Clin Cancer Res 1995;1;1511-15.

91. Christman GM, McCarthy JD. Gene Therapy and uterine leiomyomas. Clinical Obstetrics and Gynaecology 2001;44(2):425-35.

92. Acien P, Quereda F. Abdominal myomectomy: Results of a simple operative technique. Fertil Steril 1996;65:41-51.

93. Gehlbach DL, Sousa RC, et al. Abdominal myomectomy in the treatment of infertility. Int J Gynaecol Obstet 1993;40:45-50.

94. Vercellini P, Zaina B, Yaylayan L, et al. Hysteroscopic myomectomy: long term effects on menstrual pattern and fertility. Obstet Gynaecol 1999;94:341-47.

• **Mandakini Parihar**
• **Rohan Potdar** • **Sumedha Modi**

23

Enigma of Implantation

INTRODUCTION

Implantation is the most crucial stage in the establishment of pregnancy. In humans, it has been estimated that between 30-70 percent of concepts are lost before or at the time of implantation without women being aware of having been pregnant. Despite improving methods in the *in vitro* fertilization program (IVF), the "take home baby rate" does not still exceed 50 percent. Consequently, it is important to increase the success rate in the IVF program. Therefore, increased knowledge of the implantation process is needed. Our knowledge of what happens during the first week of human life *in vivo* is limited to a handful of observations. *Implantation is the single most important step in management of infertility and is also the most poorly understood part of reproduction.* Failure at this step greatly limits the success of *in vitro* fertilization (IVF) treatments. Implantation is particularly difficult to study, for it requires a blastocyst to interact with a receptive endometrium. According to assumptions based on this and other clinical data, ovulation and fertilization occur in the oviduct on day 14 of an ideal cycle. After fertilization, the zygote floats in the fallopian tube, undergoing mitotic divisions, to enter the uterine cavity at the morula stage, on day 18. On day 19 a blastocyst is formed, which sheds the zona pellucida and on day 20 starts to implant in the endometrium. Meanwhile, the endometrium, under the control of steroid hormones, differen-

tiates and reaches the state of receptivity. The onset of mammalian implantation can be seen as a successful meeting of two separate processes: embryo development and endometrial differentiation. A synchrony between these functions is important, thus defining a bifactorial, transient period when implantation can start, called the *implantation window*.[1, 2]

The aim of this chapter is to understand the physiology of implantation and try and identify the factors responsible for implantation to succeed.

Definition

Implantation is defined as the process by which an embryo attaches to the uterine wall and first penetrates the epithelium and then circulatory system of mother to form the placenta.[1-5]

Time of Implantation

Implantation begins 2-3 days after the fertilized egg enters the uterus on 18-19 day of cycle, i.e. 5-7 days of fertilization.

Preparation for Implantation

Throughout menstrual cycle changes take place that prepare endometrium for implantation. Hormone dependent changes in cell proliferation and cell differentiation occurs in all compartments of endometrium, i.e. glandular epithelium, luminal epithelium and stroma. For successful implantation embryo endometrial interactions must be initiated when embryo and endometrium have reached precise stage of development; embryo must be at blastocyst stage and there should be short lived receptive endometrium.[3-8]

Physiology of Implantation

The three stages in the process of implantation are:

1. Apposition
2. Adhesion
3. Invasion

Apposition

This can be defined as progressively increasing intimacy of contact between trophoblast and uterine epithelium. It occurs by

i. Decrease in uterine fluid volume.
ii. Edema of endometrium
iii. Enlargement of embryo

Apposition depends upon cytokines which lead to progressive interdigitation of microvilli and increasingly intimate association between membranes of blastocyst and endometrium. There is obliteration of uterine lumen with progressively closer apposition of apical end of endometrial cells and trophoblastic cells. The microvilli become shorter, more blunted and irregular and there is *appearance of large bulbous cytoplasmic projections (pinopodes).*[6-10]

Adhesion

Endometrium and embryo now express extracellular matrix component which helps to mediate adhesion through adhesion molecules, e.g. Integrins and selectin. *Integrins* are transmembrane cell receptors for fibronectin and laminin.

Expression of integrin stimulated by insulin like growth factor (IGF) and lack of integrin expression is a cause of infertility.[6-10]

Invasion

Three types of interaction occur between implanting trophoblast and uterine epithelium.

i. Trophoblastic cells invade between uterine epithelial cells on their path to basement membrane.

ii. Epithelial cells lift off the basement membranes, an action that allows trophoblast to insinuate itself underneath epithelium.
iii. Fusion of trophoblast with uterine epithelial cells.

Early embryo secretes a variety of enzymes, i.e. collagenase, plasminogen activator and these are important for digesting intercellular matrix which holds epithelial cells together. Once the intracellular matrix has been lysed this would allow space for implantation and embryo will move through epithelial cells. Then uterine spiral arterioles are invaded by cytotrophoblast and maternal endometrium replaced by cytotrophoblast. Vascular invasion by trophoblast cells need different kinds of molecules especially the selectin factor.[8-10]

Pinopodes are ultra-structural marker of implantation window. Pinopodes are surface epithelial microvilli that exhibit cystic changes. Pinopodes appears when progesterone level is high in luteal phase of menstrual cycle, i.e. day 20-22 in normal cycle, day 18-22 in stimulated cycle. *The life span of pinopodes is 48 hours.* The suggested function of pinopodes is to extract uterine fluid volume which will decrease the uterine fluid volume and facilitate more intimate contact between blastocyst and uterine epithelium. Because of the obvious importance of the endometrial factor, the formation of pinopodes has been studied with the aim of developing a specific marker for uterine receptivity in clinical practice.[10, 11]

Embryonic and Endometrial Synchronization–"Receptive Endometrium"

Endometrium is receptive to blastocyst implantation only during short period in the luteal phase known as *"Implantation Window"*. For successful implantation, embryo-endometrial interactions must be initiated when the embryo and endometrium have reached precise stages of development. This means that the embryo must be at the blastocyst stage of development, and hormone-dependent changes resulting in the development of a short lived receptive endometrium must have occurred. It would be expected that ultimately there would be a time after which transferred embryos would fail to implant because the receptive phase had ended. However, for obvious ethical reasons, it is not possible to conduct these types of experiments in humans.

Animal studies have demonstrated that, depending on the culture conditions, the rate of embryonic development *in vitro* may be retarded or sped up, relative to that which occurs *in vivo*. An additional complication in treatment of infertile patients is the supra-physiological concentrations of ovarian steroid hormones which are the result of ovarian stimulation, which may accelerate endometrial development, thereby increasing the likelihood of asynchrony.[11-13]

Control of Endometrial Receptivity

In animals, the development of endometrial receptivity is regulated by ovarian hormones. In all animals, progesterone during the post-ovulatory period is essential for implantation. Using the artificially induced decidual cell reaction, it has been known since the classical work of Yochim and De Feo (1963) that the amount of estrogen given with progesterone prior to uterine stimulation is crucial. Estrogen in low doses acts synergistically with progesterone to induce endometrial sensitization/receptivity; at high doses, estrogen is inhibitory.[1-3]

TABLE 23.1: Local factors affecting endometrial receptivity[14-21]
Factors (autocrine/paracrine) which mediate implantation and decidualization
• Prostaglandins • Leukotrienes • Integrins • Platelet Activating Factor • Cytokines • Heparin Binding Epidermal Growth Factor (HB-EGF) • Colony Stimulating Factor (CSF) • Leukemia Inhibiting Factor (LIF) • Interleukins (IL) • Glutaredoxin (Grx) • Thioredoxin (Trx) • Variety of Growth Factors

HB-EGF: It is member of endometrial growth factors and important in implantation as:

1. It promote human blastocyst growth and differentiation.

2. It promotes adhesion of blastocyst to uterine wall.

It is present both inside the luminal epithelium and on the surface of pinopodes.

Glutaredoxine (Grx) Levels of Grx and Trx are increased with the presence of pinopodes, suggesting that they play an important role during implantation. It also possibly acts by protecting epithelial cell from apoptotic action of trophoblast cell.

The Surface Morphology of the Human Endometrium

The endometrial epithelium consists of two types of cells that are easily distinguishable by scanning electron microscopy (SEM): the secretory and the ciliated cells. The morphology of ciliated cells does not change much during the cycle. In contrast, the secretory cells bear microvilli (MV) and undergo hormone-dependent changes. The temporal changes of cell surface ultra-structure in the human endometrium have been investigated by SEM throughout the menstrual cycle. In these studies, up to four sequential endometrial biopsy specimens were taken from the same individuals at 48 hours intervals from natural cycles, controlled ovarian hyperstimulation (COH) cycles for IVF, and hormone-controlled (HC) cycles with administration of estradiol and progesterone. Participating patients were either fertile volunteers or patients enrolled in IVF or egg donation cycles, and ethical approval has always been obtained in the various studies which have helped towards solving the enigma of implantation.[21-28]

Natural Cycles

In the *proliferative phase* the cells vary greatly in size and their shapes are either elongated or polygonal. The microvilli (MV) are sparse, the intercellular clefts barely visible and cell bulging is minimal. During the *secretory phase* the morphological changes are distinct and allow dating of the tissue in a 24 to 48 hour interval. This picture is assuming an ideal 28-day cycle as reference. *Day 15-16*, an increase in MV, density and length and the cells begins to bulge, mainly at the central part of their surface. *Day 17*, bulging increases, involving the entire cell apex, and the microvilli reach their maximum development, being long thick, and upright. *Day 18*, the MV start to diminish in size and their tips may appear swollen. *Day 19*, there is a pronounced and generalized cell bulging with a further decrease in MV. Smooth and slender membrane projections begin to form, arising from the entire cell apex (*developing pinopodes*). *Day 20* the MV are virtually absent, and now the membranes protrude and fold maximally (*fully developed pinopodes*). Fully developed pinopodes assume many shapes resembling flowers or mushrooms. *Day 21*, bulging decreases and small tips of MV reappear on the membrane, which are now wrinkled, and the cell size starts to increase (*regressing pinopodes*). *Day 22*, the pinopodes have virtually disappeared, and the MV have become more numerous. *Day 23* is characterized by a further increase in the size of cells, which by *day 24* begin to appear dome shaped and covered with short, stubby MV. By *day 26*, the cell membranes appear degenerate and devoid of MV.[21-28]

Controlled Ovarian Hyperstimulation Cycles

The effects of COH endometrial surface ultra-structure have been examined in oocyte donors undergoing IVF cycles. The stimulation protocol was the long luteal agonist cycle with gonadotropins for stimulations. From each donor, two to four endometrial biopsy specimens were taken at 48 hours intervals between days 14 and 24 of the stimulated cycle (oocyte aspiration designated day 14). The results showed that endometrial morphology is similar to that seen in natural cycles. Again, fully developed pinopodes were detected in only one sample from each donor, indicating a short life span. The cycle day on which pinopodes formed varied between women within a range of 5 days, from days 18 to 22. In the majority of cases, pinopodes formation was significantly accelerated by 1 to 2 days in comparison with natural cycles. This accelerated pinopode formation strongly correlated with preovulatory progesterone rise. The controlled

ovarian hyperstimulation protocols utilized in IVF-ET programs result in concentrations of estrogen and progesterone in the circulation which are substantially higher than normal. Whether these supra-physiological concentrations of steroids, particularly those of estrogen, adversely affect implantation is controversial. Develioglu[25] compared implantation rates in a donor oocyte program with those from a standard IVF program where the recipients in the donor oocyte program had not undergone controlled ovarian hyperstimulation. Implantation rates were higher in the donor oocyte program, suggesting that controlled ovarian stimulation results in an inhibitory hormonal milieu. However, based on a review of the literature, it has recently been concluded that oocyte donation studies have shown that both normal and supra-physiological concentrations of estrogen can allow implantation. However, these results can be interpreted as indicating that *some embryos* are able to implant despite supra-physiological concentrations of estrogens which may have produced a less than perfectly receptive endometrium. *The important question is whether more embryos would be able to implant if estradiol concentrations were in the physiological range in the peri-implantation period?*[21-28]

Hormone Controlled Cycles

The hormone protocol included pituitary down-regulation with a GnRH-a in normal cycling patients. The proliferative phase was induced by a fixed or incremental dose of oral estrogen for 1 to 3 weeks. Then vaginal or intramuscular progesterone was added. The day of progesterone start was designated day 15 (P1). Two or more biopsy specimens were taken from each patient, between days P6 and P10. The surface endometrial morphology was found to be similar to that of normal or COH cycles. The cycle day on which pinopodes formed varied between women within a range of 3 days, from P6 to P8, in most regimens. However, in cycling patients not receiving GnRH-a, these inter-patient variations extended from P6 to P10.

In one study, the correlation between pinopodes and pregnancy was investigated in 17 mock hormonal cycles preceding transfer of donated embryos. Pinopodes were scored according to their number in three grades, abundant, moderate, or few, depending on the percentage of the endometrial surface occupied by pinopodes (> 50%, 20-50%, and < 20%, respectively). Following an identical transfer cycle, all five patients with abundant pinopodes became pregnant, three out of seven with moderate pinopodes became pregnant, and none of the five patients with sparse or no pinopodes became pregnant. In another study, the clinical utility of pinopodes for prediction of the implantation window on an individual basis was explored. Candidate embryo recipients go through a mock Hormone Controlled cycle with biopsy on cycle days 20 and 22 (P6 and P8) for examination by SEM. A transfer cycle follows in which synchronization with the embryo is arranged so that the predicted most receptive day coincides with embryonic age day 6.[26-34]

Importance of Pinopodes in Implantation

The results of these studies suggest that pinopodes are accurate markers of the implanation window. Pinopodes last for less than 2 days in all cases, and the timing of their formation depends both on the hormone treatment applied and on the patient's individual response. On an average, they form on days 20-21 in natural, days 19-20 in COH, and days 21-22 in HC cycles. Such short duration and discrete timing of the window of receptivity could significantly affect the outcome of assisted reproduction treatments. In natural cycles, we may assume that there is an inherent synchrony between the maturing uterus and the developing embryo, ensuring that both will meet at the right stage. In IVF cycles, embryonic development is probably delayed because of the *in vitro* conditions while the uterus may be advanced, resulting in an early closure of the implantation window. Consequently, it would be highly desirable if the window of receptivity in IVF cycles could be postponed for a couple of days. This has been successfully induced in the rat following postovulatory antiprogestin administration, and a similar treatment has been proposed for humans. Indeed, a pilot study showed

that administration of a low dose of mifepristone on days 14 and 15 caused delayed pinopode formation. It is interesting that the number of pinopodes varied between patient, some showing plenty and others only sparse pinopodes, with a strong correlation between pinopode number and implantation success after embryo transfer in a subsequent cycle. These data argue positively for the relevance of pinopodes to implantation and also that menstrual cycles in the same individual are similar. Some women show very few or no pinopodes despite regular ovulation and menstruation. Such cases are usually associated with abnormalities in epithelial morphology, including the presence of large hyperplastic cells or dense microvilli arranged in tufts. It is possible that abnormal endometrial maturation might be a cause of infertility. Thus, examination of endometrial biopsy specimens by SEM for pinopodes may be a useful test in infertility work-up. The most important finding is that the time during which pinopodes develop is predictable and related to the LH surge and serum progesterone levels. The other major finding was that disappearance of progesterone receptor B coincides with development of pinopodes.[26-34]

The cellular and molecular function of pinopodes in humans remains unknown. A suggested function of the pinopodes is to extract uterine fluid.[12, 14] The volume of uterine fluid is significantly decreased at the time of implantation. A decrease in uterine fluid would facilitate more intimate contact between the blastocyst and the uterine epithelium. The smooth surface of the pinopodes and the accompanying loosening of epithelial cell-to-cell contacts may facilitate trophoblast adhesion and/or penetration to the stroma. In an *in vitro* mode, using endometrial epithelial cells growing on stromal cells, human blastocysts adhered only on areas bearing pinopodes. The size of pinopodes in SEM is around 5 mm, arising from the entire cell apex. Considering the shrinkage of the tissue because of dehydration in SEM preparation, their native size may be round 8 mm. With this size, pinopodes are visible in conventional histology as bulbous protrusions of the cell apices. However, the ability of histology to assess pinopodes is limited by the low resolution of light microscopy and by the fact that histology is performed on tissue sections, where only a small area of the surface can be examined. Thus, it appears that SEM is indispensible for detecting and scoring endometrial pinopodes. Examination of endometrial biopsy specimens for pinopodes is a potential test in infertility evaluation both for the optimization of embryo transfer and for supporting other studies on human implantation, which remains the "last frontier" in infertility treatment.[26-34]

Pinopode development closely followed progesterone concentrations: Developing pinopodes were seen during increasing progesterone concentrations and regressing pinopodes were found with decreasing progesterone concentrations. The drastic decrease in progesterone receptor B expression seems to be important. Estrogen receptor expression decreased in the glandular epithelium during the luteal phase, when the serum progesterone concentration was high and the pinopodes started to appear. Estrogen receptor-B has been suggested to modulate estrogen receptor-A-mediated gene transcription in the uterus and to down-regulate progesterone receptor in the luminal epithelium.[4, 25]

In conclusion, serum progesterone concentrations and down-regulation of glandular progesterone receptor B expression are concurrent with development of pinopodes in the endometrium at the time of implantation. It may therefore be possible to predict the implantation window in natural cycles by using the LH surge and thereby increase the success rate of embryo transfer using frozen embryos.[26-34]

Hormones, Genes, and The Implantation of The Fertilized Egg

How the fertilized egg imbeds itself in the uterus is mostly a biological mystery, but in the last year knowledge about the action of genes during implantation has taken a giant leap forward. The initiation of complex interactions between the fertilized egg and the endometrium is determined by a timely interplay of the ovarian hormones estrogen and progesterone. These hormones enter cells and bind to receptor molecules; the resulting molecular complexes regulate gene activity. The proteins created, or expressed, by these genes make the endometrium receptive to the implantation of the fertilized egg. Not all of the newly identified genes will be important for implantation. Once these genes are identified, it may make our understanding of this complex phenomenon easier.[33, 34]

SUMMARY

Blastocyst implantation involves a complex series of events occurring over time. It requires synchronized development of the conceptus and a receptive uterus, attachment of the conceptus to the uterus, transformation of the endometrium to decidua, and finally formation of the definitive placenta. It is arguably the most critical stage in the establishment of pregnancy. In humans, it has been estimated that between 30 and 70 percent of conceptuses are lost before or at the time of implantation, without women being aware that they are pregnant. Endometrium is prepared for implantation by complex activity of cytokines, growth factors and sex hormones. The human endometrium is only receptive for receiving a blastocyst for a short time, during the so called *"implantation window"*, which occurs approximately 7 days after ovulation. The pinopodes on the endometrial surface have been suggested as markers for endometrial receptivity. The pinopodes appear when the progesterone level is high in the luteal phase of the menstrual cycle. It is of importance that the endometrium mature in synchrony with the embryo for a successful implantation. In human *in vitro* fertilization and embryo transfer programs, the low implantation rate after embryo transfer is an important problem. Whether this low rate is a consequence of an inherently low implantation rate in humans, or of an altered physiological state is presently unknown. Based on studies in experimental animals, there are reasons for suspecting that the low implantation rates may be a consequence of an altered physiological state.

REFERENCES

1. Croxatto HB, Diaz S, Fuentealba BA, Croxatto HD, Carrilo D, Fabres C. Studies on the duration of egg transport in the human oviduct: I the time interval between ovulation and egg recovery from the uterus in normal women. Fertil Steril 1972;23:447-58.
2. Psychoyos A. Endocrine control of egg implantation. In: Greep RO, Astwood EB (Eds.): Handbook of Physiology, Vol. II. Endocrinology, Baltimore Williams and Wilkins 1973;187-215.
3. Psychoyos A. Hormonal control of uterine receptivity for nidation. J Reprod Fertil 1976;25(Suppl):17-28.
4. Develioglu OH, Hsiu JG, Nikas G, Toner JP, Oehniger S, Jones HW Jr. Endometrial estrogen and progesterone receptor and pinopode expression in stimulated cycles in oocyte donation. Fertil Steril 1999;71:1040-47.
5. Nikas G, Garcia-Velasco J, Pellicer A, Simon C. Assessment of uterine receptivity and timing of embryo transfer using the detection of pinopodes. Hum Reprod 1997; 12(Suppl):1-69.
6. Develioglu OH, Nikas G, Hsiu JG, Toner JP, Oehninger S, Jones HW Jr. Assessment of endometrial pinopodes by light microscopy. Fertil Steril 2000;74:763-70.
7. Psychoyos A, Nikas G. Uterine pinopodes as markers of uterine receptivity. Assist Reprod Rev 1994;4:26-32.
8. Martel D. Surface changes of the luminal uterine epithelium during the human menstrual cycle, a scanning microscopic study. In: Brux J. Gantrey JP (Eds). The Endometrium: Hormonal Implants. New York: Plenum, 1981:15-29.
9. Nikas G. Cell-surface morphological events relevant to human implantation. Hum Reprod 1999;14(Suppl 2); 37-44.
10. Nikas G, Makrigiannakis A, Hovatta O, Jones HW Jr. Surface morphology of the human endometrium: basic and clinical aspects. Ann N Y Acad Sci 2000;900: 316-24.
11. Nikas G, Develioglu OH, Toner JP, Jones HW Jr. Endometrial pinopodes indicate a shift in the window of receptivity in IVF cycles. Hum Reprod 1999;14: 787-92.
12. Nikas G. Pinopodes as markers of endometrial receptivity in clinical practice. Hum Reprod 1999; 14(Suppl 2):99-106.
13. Weihua Z, Saji S, Makinen S, Chens G, Jensen EV, Warner M, Gustafsson Ja. Estrogen receptor (ER) beta, a modulator of ER alpha in the uterus. Proc Natl Acad Sci USA 2000;97:5936-41.
14. Kennedy TG. Involvement of local indicators in blastocyst implantation. In: Endocrinology of Embryo-Endometrial Interactions SR Glasser, J Mulholland, A Psychoyos (Eds.): Plenum Press, New York, 1994; 183-94
15. Lessey BA, Castelbaum AJ, Sawin SW, Sun J; Integrins as markers of uterine receptivity in women with primary unexplained infertility. Fertil Steril 1995; 63:535-42.
16. Stavreus-Evers A, Aghajanova L, Brismar H, Eriksson H, Landgren B-M, Hovatta O. Co-existence of heparin-binding epidermal growth factor-like growth factor (HB-EGF) and pinopodes in human endometrium at the time of implantation. Molecular Human Reproduction 2002;8(8);765-69.
17. Aghajanova L, Stavreus-Evers A, Nikas Y, Hovatta O, Landgren BM. Co-expression of pinopodes and leukemia inhibitory factor, as well as its receptor, in human endometrium. Fertility and Sterility 2003:79;808-14.
18. Stavreus-Evers A, Masironi B, Landgren B-M, Holmgren A, Eriksson H and Sahlin L. Immunohisto-chemical localization of glutaredoxin and thioredoxin in human endometrium: A possible association with pinopodes. Molecular Human Reproduction 2002;8(6), 546-51.
19. Damsky CH, Ubrach C, Lim K-H, Fitzgerald ML, Mc Master MT Janalpour M, Zhou ur M, Zhou, Logan SK Fisher SJ. Integrin regulate normal trophoblast invasion. Development 1994;120:3657.
20. Diamond Ms, Springer TA. The dynamic regulation of integrin adhesiveness. Curr Bio 1994;4:506.
21. Cooke ID. Failure of implantation and its relevance to subfertility. J Reprod Fertil Suppl 1988;36:155-59.
22. Paulson RJ, Sauer MV, Francis MM, Macaso T, Lobo RA. Factors affecting pregnancy success of human in vitro fertilization in unstimulated cycles. Hum Reprod 1994;9:1571-75.
23. Martel D, Malet C, Gautray JP, Psychoyos A. Surface changes of the luminal epithelium during the human menstrual cycle: A scanning electron microscopic study. In: The Endometrium: Hormonal Impacts. J de Brux, R Mortel, JP Gautray (Eds): Plenum Press, New York: 1981;15-29.
24. Acosta AA, Elberger L, Borghi M, Calamera JC, Chemes H. Doncel GF, et al. Endometrial dating and deter-mination of the window of implantation in healthy fertile women. Fertil Steril 2000;73:788-98.
25. Develioglu OH, Hsiu JG, Nikas G, Toner JP, Oehringer S, Jones HW Jr. Endometrial estrogen and progesterone receptor and pinopode expression in stimulated cycles of oocyte donors. Fertil Steril 1999;71:1040-47.
26. Kolb BA, Najamadi S, Paulsen RJ. Ultra-structural characteristics of the luteal phase endometrium in patients undergoing controlled ovarian hyperstimu-lation. Fertil Steril 1997;67:625-30.
27. Balasch J, Creus M, Fabregues F, Carmona F, Casamitjana R, Penarrubia J, Rivera F, Vanrell JA. Hormonal profiles in successful and unsuccessful implantation in EVF-ET after combined GnRH agonist/ gonadotropin for superovulation and hCG luteal support. Gynecol Endocrinol 1995;9:51-58.
28. Stavreus-Evers A, Nikas G, Eriksson H, Sahlin L. and Landgren B-M. The formation of pinopodes in human endometrium is associated with the concentrations of

progesterone and progesterone receptors. Fertility and Sterility 2001;76:782-91.

29. Bentin-Ley U, Sicgren A, Nilsson L, hamberger L, Larsen JF, Horn T. Presence of uterine pinopodes at the embryo endometrial interface during human implantation in vitro. Hum Reprod 1999;14:515-20.

30. Nikas G, Develioglu OH, Toner JP, Jones Jr HW. Endometrial pinopodes indicate a shift in the window of receptivity in IVF cycles. Hum Reprod 1999;14:787-92.

31. Bentin-Ley U, Sjogren S, Nilsson L, Hamberger L, Larssen JF, Horn T. Presence of uterine pinopodes at the embryo-endometrial interface during human implantation in vitro. Hum Reprod 1999;14:515-20.

32. Paulson RJ, Saucer MV, Lobo RA. Embryo implantation after human in vitro fertilization: Importance of endometrial receptivity. Fertil Steril 1990;53:870-74.

33. Burrows TD, King A, Loke YW. Trophoblast migration during human placental implantation. Hum Reprod Update 1997;2:307.

34. Landgren B-M, Johannisson E, Stavreus-Evers A, HambergerL. And Eriksson H. A new method to study the process of implantation of a human blastocyst in vitro. Fertility and Sterility 1996;65:1067-70.

Section **5**

Ovulation Induction

• RK Bhathena • Duru Shah

24

Superovulation Strategies in Assisted Conception

One in six or seven couples seeks medical advice for difficulty in conceiving. Some of these couples need treatment by *in vitro* fertilization (IVF) which is now widely used to treat many categories of infertility. With increasing recognition that many previously recommended treatments are inadequately effective, the importance of IVF as a treatment option has become obvious, and in many countries the number of IVF treatment cycles have increased many fold times over the last decade.

The aim of any regimen for stimulation of multiple follicles for assisted conception should be to obtain as many follicles as possible from which good quality eggs can be recovered, without having complications like significant ovarian hyper-stimulation. Although Louise Brown was born to a natural cycle,[1] it was soon realized that the conception rate could be significantly improved if more than one embryo was replaced in the uterus.[2] It has been established that the pregnancy rate is influenced by the number of embryos transferred. However, with higher pregnancy rates, the incidence of multiple pregnancies and of early pregnancy losses increases significantly. Most centers therefore restrict the number of embryos transferred to two or three.[3, 4]

Gonadotrophins comprise one of the corner-stones of infertility management, and have been used extensively and effectively over the last three decades. This chapter reviews the progress made in the strategies employed for induction of ovulation with the use of gonadotrophins, with or without gonadotrophin analogues.

Gonadotrophin Preparations

There are three generations of gonadotrophin preparations-a first generation derived from human urine, a second generation of purified urinary gonadotrophins, and a third generation of recombinant preparations.

Human menopausal gonadotrophins (hMG) (menotrophin), prepared from human postmeno-pausal urine, contain both follicle stimulating hormone (FSH) and luteinizing hormone (LH). The commonly available first generation formulation is *Pergonal* (Serono). The first generation preparations have a protein content consisting of only 2 percent FSH, and 98 percent uncontrolled extraneous urinary proteins. Batch-to-batch variability is a potential disadvantage. The woman needs to visit a doctor or a nurse for intramuscular injections.

The second generation products (urofolli-trophin), made by purification of natural human menopausal gonadotrophins, provide more than 95 percent purified FSH, with virtually no LH activity. The commonly available second generation product is *Metrodin High Purity* (Serono).

Batch-to-batch consistency is a potential advantage. The purity allows subcutaneous injections, which may be self-administered, to make the fertility treatment more convenient.

The production of human gonadotrophin preparations depends on the collection of huge amounts of postmenopausal urine. The use of urine sources would imply limited product consistency with varying amounts of LH and human chorionic gonadotrophin (hCG).[5] There would also be a theoretical risk of contamination with urinary products.[6-8]

In the last few years, through the application of recombinant DNA technology, it has been possible to produce human FSH *in vitro* without the need for extraction from human fluids. Recombinant human FSH (follitrophin) (rhFSH) is produced using a hamster ovary cell line, into which genes transcribing human FSH are introduced. Follitrophins are virtually pure FSH and do not contain any LH. As a result of its high purity (> 99%), rhFSH is suitable for both intramuscular and subcutaneous administration. Two rhFSH preparations-follitrophin α- *Gonal-F* (Serono) and follitrophin β- *Puregon (Recagon)* (Organon) are available. Recombinant FSH has been found to be cost-effective.[9]

Following the development of recombinant FSH, recombinant human LH-lutropin α- *Luveris* (Serono) has been produced with superior purity and greater specific activity than hMG which contains only about 2 percent LH. The purity allows subcutaneous injections. Recombinant human LH (rhLH) is useful to treat women with LH deficiency.

Recombinant hCG (choriogonadotrophin alfa) (rhCG) *Ovidrel* (Serono) has superior purity and consistency than urinary hCG. The subcutaneous injection may be self-administered.

Women with Hypogonadotrophic Hypogonadism (WHO Group I Anovulation)

In women with the uncommon WHO group I anovulation (hypothalamic-pituitary failure), the central failure leads to abnormally low serum gonadotrophin secretion and ovarian estrogen production. There is now convincing evidence that in these women, although exogenous preparations containing only FSH are effective in stimulating follicular development, LH needs to be co-administered to obtain adequate follicular steroidogenesis as demonstrated by appropriate estradiol secretion, endometrial growth and luteal phase progesterone secretion.[10, 11]

The traditional standard step-up regimen with gonadotrophins entails initiating the therapy with 75 IU hMG, and increasing the dose, if there is a need, by 75 IU every 4-5 days.[12] When women with anovulatory infertility associated with severe depletion of gonadotrophins are treated with hMG, ovulation is generally achieved in about 90 percent of the cycles, and the pregnancy rate is over 25 percent per cycle.[13]

There is recent evidence that, in WHO group I women, a combination of 150 IU per day of rhFSH and 75 IU per day of rhLH is generally sufficient to obtain optimal follicular development.[14] An alternative option, in these women, would be to use an individualized dose of rhFSH together with 75 IU per day of rhLH.

Women with the Polycystic Ovary Syndrome (PCOS) (Hypothalamic-pituitary Dysfunction) (WHO Group II Anovulation)

A fundamental principle of the management of anovulation in women with PCOS is to initially optimise the woman's health before commencement of therapy, and subsequently offer treatment for regular induction of unifollicular ovulation, with a view to minimize the risk of ovarian hyperstimulation and multiple pregnancy. Obese women should be encouraged to lose weight.

With loss of weight, the endocrine profile is improved.[12] In obese women with hyperinsulinemia, metformin is effective in reducing serum insulin and testosterone levels.[12]

A majority of women with the PCOS ovulate when given antiestrogens, and clomiphene citrate remains the initial modality of treatment. Approximately two thirds of the women conceive over six cycles of treatment.[15] The cumulative conception rate tends to rise for up to 12 cycles.[15] In the United Kingdom, at time present, clomiphene is licensed for use for six months because of a possible link between its long-term (more than 12 months') use and development of ovarian cancer.[16] Since the cumulative conception rates tend to rise up to 12 cycles of therapy, if treatment needs to be continued beyond six months, the woman should be counseled about the possible risks, and may be allowed to continue with the therapy for a few more months.

In women where there is resistance to clomiphene treatment, laparoscopic ovarian electrocautery or gonadotrophin therapy are equally effective therapeutic options.

Laparoscopic ovarian diathermy results in normalization of serum androgens, and persistence of ovulation for several years in a majority of the treated subjects.[17]

Gonadotrophin therapy is indicated for women with the PCOS who have failed to ovulate with clomiphene citrate or have a response to clomiphene that may reduce their chance of conception for instance, persistent hypersecretion of LH.

A proportion of women with the PCOS have relatively high levels of LH which impair normal follicular development. Raised levels of LH in the follicular phase are associated with premature luteinization of the follicle and a relatively high incidence of miscarriage.[13]

While some workers have conducted pharmacokinetic studies that indicate that serum LH levels decrease more significantly after exogenous FSH than after hMG administration, others argue that purified FSH preparations seem to confer no therapeutic advantage over hMG as the LH content in hMG is insignificant in comparison with the endogenous LH secretion.[12,18-20]

Serum LH concentrations usually fall progressively in response to the normal ovarian-pituitary feedback as, after the commencement of the treatment, the dominant follicle grows.[12,13] The fall coincides with the stimulation of follicular development and may be due to suppression of endogenous LH by estradiol.[13] However, some women with the PCOS continue to oversecrete LH in the presence of follicular growth.[12]

In a meta-analysis carried out on FSH versus hMG treatment of eight studies on women undergoing IVF, treatment with FSH resulted in approximately 50 percent higher pregnancy rates.[21] There have been comments in literature about the drawbacks in making conclusions from meta-analyses from studies where the numbers involved are small.[22]

Treatment with gonadotrophins should be commenced within the first 3-5 days of a natural cycle or induced menstrual bleeding, after establishing a thin endometrium (less than 6 mm) and absence of ovarian cysts with transvaginal pelvic ultrasonography. Women with the PCOS have a high level of sensitivity to gonadotrophins. To prevent the risks of overstimulation and multiple pregnancy, in these women low-dose regimens have replaced the traditional standard step-up regimens. A few recent studies suggest that rhFSH may be more efficacious than purified urinary FSH in that a smaller total dose is required in fewer treatment days.[23,24] A low-dose regimen may be commenced with 50-75 IU rhFSH. An adequate response would be indicated by an increase in the growth of one or two follicles and/or a moderate rise in serum estradiol level. If there is an inadequate response or no response, the dose is stepped up by only 37.5-50 IU after 7-10 days. Ovulation is triggered with a single dose of injection hCG-*Profasi* (Serono), *Pregnyl* (Organon), 5000-10,000 IU intramuscularly, or rhCG-*Ovidrel* (Serono), 250-500 mcg subcutaneously when the dominant follicle is equal to or more than 18 mm in diameter and the endometrial thickness is more than 10 mm.[25,26] Injection hCG may not be administered if there are more than 3 follicles equal to or larger than 17 mm in diameter, and/or there are more than 4 or 5 follicles equal to or larger than 14 mm in diameter. Women who develop a large cohort of intermediate follicles (13-15 mm) and have high serum estradiol concentrations appear to be at the greatest risk of developing severe hyperstimulation.[27, 28] In contrast, women who have several large follicles (17 mm size or more) are at a greater risk of multiple pregnancy.[28] In overstimulated cycles, injection hCG is withheld, and the woman counseled. The couple is advised to refrain from sexual intercourse for a few days.

Pituitary Downregulation

When hMG is used alone (or with clomiphene citrate) without downregulation of the pituitary, there is a negative effect on the cycle outcome as a result of the occurrence of LH surges.[29] The LH surge in hMG stimulated cycles may be attenuated and difficult to detect. Clinical management of premature elevation of LH or of an endogenous

LH surge is difficult, and the cycle may need to be cancelled. For these reasons, currently few cycles are performed with hMG alone.[30]

There is evidence that lowering of high endogenous LH levels has a beneficial influence on the conception rate both in women with PCOS and in women undergoing ovulation induction for IVF.[31,32] There is also evidence that hypersecretion of endogenous LH is associated with increased early pregnancy loss.[31, 32]

GnRH Agonist Analogues

Prolonged administration of GnRH agonists is effective in suppressing gonadotrophin secretion from the gonadotrophs of the anterior pituitary by desensitization of these cells. GnRH agonist therapy leads to an initial release of FSH and LH (the flare up effect), followed by decreased responsiveness, and ultimately inhibition of gonadotrophin secretion.

GnRH agonistic analogues are small polypeptide molecules that need to be administered parenterally because they would otherwise be susceptible to gastrointestinal proteolysis. The subcutaneous route is most commonly used. After subcutaneous injection, the agonist is rapidly absorbed and blood concentrations remain elevated for several hours. Buserelin, leuprolide, histrelin and triptorelin are effective when administered subcutaneously as a single daily dose.

The intranasal route (nasal spray) is also being widely used as a convenient alternative to parenteral administration. Buserelin and nafarelin are available as nasal preparations. The intranasal route has some disadvantages. There is marked interindividual variation in absorption. It is estimated that only about 5 percent of the intranasal buserelin dose administered is absorbed in the systemic circulation.[33] Nasal doses need to be administered two to four times daily to maintain effective concentration of the drug.[33]

Depot preparations are particularly useful where long-term pituitary desensitization is needed, as in women with endometriosis or fibroids, but these preparations are also being used in women undergoing controlled ovarian stimulation. Leuprolide and triptorelin are administered once-a-month intramuscularly.

Several different superovulation regimens have been employed to administer GnRH agonists-ultrashort, short and long. The ultrashort and short protocols are based on the initial stimulatory effects of the agonist on the pituitary, leading to gonadotrophin secretion to promote follicular development, before pituitary desensitization occurs. In the short protocol, the GnRH agonist is continued until the administration of injection hCG, whereas in the ultrashort protocol, the agonist is administered for only three days. The short regimens have the advantage of a shorter duration of stimulation, with the use of fewer ampoules of gonadotrophins and low costs.[34]

The long protocols are intended to achieve pituitary downregulation with suppression of endogenous gonadotrophins before stimulation with exogenous FSH. In the long protocol, the GnRH agonist is started either in the midluteal phase (day 21 or 22) of the preceding menstrual cycle or in the early follicular phase (day 1) of the treatment cycle. The agonist therapy is generally continued up to about two weeks, during which time ovarian suppression is confirmed by a plasma estradiol of less than 150-200 pmol/l and/or an endometrial thickness of less than 5 mm on ultrasound scan. Exogenous gonadotrophins and the GnRH agonist are administered together until the day of administration of injection hCG. When the midluteal phase and early follicular phase long protocols are compared as regards treatment time and effectiveness, the results in the literature are contradictory.[34-36] On comparing the long and short protocols, the long protocols tend to result in significantly increased conception rates and live births after IVF.[35]

Although GnRH agonists are useful in controlling the inappropriate endogenous LH surge and improve overall success rates, with the long protocol there is a need for a prolonged period of drug injections and for higher doses and longer duration of gonadotrophin treatment for ovarian stimulation.

GnRH Antagonists

Together with the development of GnRH agonists, other analogues have also been synthesized that get bound to the GnRH receptors in the pituitary but which do not induce the release of gonadotrophins. GnRH antagonists bind competitively to the the receptors and prevent the endogenous GnRH from exerting its stimulatory effects on the pituitary cells. With no intrinsic activity of these compounds, the initial flare up seen with the agonists is avoided, and there is rapid and effective suppression of the endogenous gonadotrophins. The mode of action depends on the equilibrium between the endogenous GnRH and the antagonist utilized. As a result, the effect of the antagonist is dose-dependent.[37, 38]

Two compounds cetrorelix *Cetrotide* (Serono) and ganirelix *Orgalutran* (Organon) are available. Two protocols have been developed for the use of a GnRH antagonist.

In the multiple-dose protocol, controlled ovarian stimulation is commenced in the early follicular phase with exogenous gonadotrophins. The premature LH surge is abolished by the daily subcutaneous administration of 0.25 mg cetrorelix from day 5 or 6 onwards of controlled ovarian stimulation up to the induction of ovulation.[39, 40]

In the single-dose protocol, a single dose of 3 mg cetrorelix is administered around day 6 or 7 of the FSH treatment, when the serum oestradiol level is around 550-750 pmol/l and the follicular size greater than 14 mm.[41, 42]

Both the protocols appear to be effective and safe.[39]

The introduction of GnRH antagonists is a significant contribution towards making infertility treatment more convenient by a reduction in the dose and duration of gonadotrophin therapy for controlled ovarian stimulation.

REFERENCES

1. Steptoe PC, Edwards RG. Birth after reimplantation of a human embryo. Lancet 1978;ii:366.
2. Fishel SB, Edwards RG, Purday JM et al. Implantation, abortion and birth after in vitro fertilization using the natural menstrual cycle in follicular stimulation with clomiphene citrate and human menopausal gonadotrophin. J in vitro Fertil Embryo Transfer 1985;2:123-31.
3. Dawson KJ, Rutherford AJ, Margara RA, Winston RML. Reducing triplet pregnancies following in vitro fertilisation. Lancet 1991;337:1543-44.
4. Baird DT, Pearson SJ. Factors determining response to controlled ovarian stimulation for in vitro fertilisation. In: Templeton A, Cooke I, Shaughn O'Brien PM (Eds.): Evidence-based Fertility Treatment. London: RCOG Press, 1998;274-82.
5. Harlin J, Kahn SA, Diczfalusy E. Molecular composition of luteinizing hormone and follicle stimulating hormone in commercial gonadotrophin preparations. Fertil Steril 1986;46:1055-60.
6. Matorras R, Rodriguez-Escudero FJ. Bye-bye urinary gonadotrophins ? The use of urinary gonadotrophins should be discouraged. Hum Reprod 2002;17:1675.
7. Crosignani PG. Bye-bye urinary gonadotrophins ? Risk of infection is not the main problem. Hum Reprod 2002;17:1676.
8. Balen A. Bye-bye urinary gonadotrophins ? Is there a risk of prion disease after the administration of urinary-derived gonadotrophins? Hum Reprod 2002;17:1676-80.
9. Balasch J, Barri PN. Reflections on the cost-effectiveness of recombinant FSH in assisted reproduction. The clinician's perspective. J Assist Reprod Genet 2001;18:45-55.
10. Hugues JN. The use of recombinant human FSH in ovulation induction. In: Shoham Z, Howles CM, Jacobs JS (Eds): Female Infertility Therapy-Current Practice. London: Martin Dunitz, 1999;115-24.
11. Shoham Z, Loumaye E, Piazzi A. A dose finding study to determine the effective dose of recombinant human luteinizing hormone to support FSH-induced follicular development in hypogonadotropic hypogonadal (HH) women. 51st Annual Meeting of the American Society for Reproductive Medicine, Seattle, Washington DC, 1995;abstract 0-142.
12. Balen A. Polycystic ovary syndrome: mode of treatment. In: Shoham Z, Howles CM, Jacobs JS (Eds.): Female Infertility Therapy-Current Practice. London: Martin Dunitz, 1999;45-67.
13. Baird DT, Howles CM. Induction of ovulation with gonadotrophins: hMG versus purified FSH. In: Filicori M, Flamigni C (Eds): Ovulation Induction: Basic Science and Clinical Advances. Shannon: Elsevier Science, 1994;135-43.
14. The European Recombinant Human LH Study Group. Recombinant human luteinizing hormone (LH) to support recombinant human follicle stimulating hormone (FSH) induced follicular development in LH and FSH deficient anovulatory women: a dose finding study. J Clin Endocrinol Metab 1998;83:1507-14.
15. Kousta E, White DM, Franks S. Modern use of clomiphene citrate in induction of ovulation. Hum Reprod Update 1997;3:359-65.
16. Nugent D, Salha O, Balen AH, Rutherford AJ. Ovarian neoplasia and subfertility treatments. Br J Obstet Gynaecol 1998;105:584-91.
17. Amer SAKS, Banu Z, Li TC, Cooke ID. Long-term follow-up of patients with polycystic ovary syndrome after

laparoscopic ovarian drilling: endocrine and ultrasonographic outcomes. Hum Reprod 2002;17:2851-57.

18. Anderson RE, Cragun JM, Chary RJ et al. A pharmacodynamic comparison of human urinary FSH and hMG in normal women and polycystic ovary syndrome. Fertil Steril 1989;52:216-20.

19. Sagle MA, Hamilton-Farley D, Kiddy D, Franks S. A comparative, randomised study of low-dose human menopausal gonadotrophins and FSH in women with polycystic ovary syndrome. Fertil Steril 1991;55:56-60.

20. Fulghesu AM, Lanzone A, Gida C et al. Ovulation induction with hMG versus FSH after pituitary suppression by GnRH agonist in polycystic ovary disease. A cross over study. J Reprod Med 1992;37: 834-40.

21. Daya S. Follicle stimulating hormone versus hMG for in vitro fertilization: results of a meta-analysis. Horm Res 1995;43:224-29.

22. Gardosi J. Systematic reviews: insufficient evidence on which to base medicine. Br J Obstet Gynaecol 1998; 105:1-4.

23. Coelingh Bennink HJT, Fauser BCJM, Out HJ. Recombinant FSH (Puregon) is more efficient than urinary FSH (Metrodin) in women with clomiphene citrate-resistant, normagonadotropic chronic anovulation: a prospective, multicentre, assessor-blind, randomized, clinical trial. Fertil Steril 1998;69:19-25.

24. Out HJ, Mannaerts BMJL, Driessen SGAJ, Coelingh Bennink HJT. A prospective, randomized, assessor-blind, multicentre study comparing recombinant and urinary FSH (Puregon versus Metrodin) in in vitro fertilization. Hum Reprod 1995;10:2534-40.

25. The European Recombinant Human Chorionic Gonadotrophin Study Group. Induction of final follicular maturation and early luteinization in women undergoing ovulation induction for assisted reproduction treatment-recombinant hCG versus urinary hCG. Hum Reprod 2000;15:1446-51.

26. Chang P, Kenley S, Glasheen T et al. The third recombinant gonadotrophin: results of a large US trial of r-hCG in ART. Fertil Steril 2001;76:67-74.

27. Brinsden PR, Wada I, Tan SL, Balen A, Jacobs HS. Diagnosis, prevention and management of ovarian hyperstimulation syndrome. Br J Obstet Gynaecol 1995;102:767-72.

28. Bhathena RK. The pathophysiology, prevention and management of the ovarian hyperstimulation syndrome. J Obstet Gynaecol 1998;18: 405-07.

29. Devroey P, Naaktgeboren N, Traey E et al. Hormonal evaluation of failed ovarian stimulation in an in vitro fertilization programme. IV World Conference on in vitro Fertilization Melbourne, Australia 1985; abstract 6.

30. Devroey P. Different treatment protocols for different indications. In: Shoham Z, Howles CM, Jacobs JS, (Eds): Female Infertility Therapy-Current Practice. London: Martin Dunitz, 1999;215-20.

31. Homburg R. Detrimental effects of LH hypersecretion. In: Shoham Z, Howles CM, Jacobs JS (Eds.) Female Infertility Therapy-Current Practice. London: Martin Dunitz, 1999;85-91.

32. Homburg R, Levy T, Berkovitz D, et al. Gonadotrophin-releasing hormone agonist reduces the miscarriage rate for pregnancies achieved in women with polycystic ovary syndrome. Fertil Steril 1993;59:527-31.

33. Weissman A, Shoham Z. GnRH and its agonistic analogues: basic knowledge. In: Shoham Z, Howles CM, Jacobs JS (Eds): Female Infertility Therapy-Current Practice. London: Martin Dunitz, 1999;157-66.

34. Balasch J, Howles CM. GnRH agonist protocols: which one to use ? In: Shoham Z, Howles CM, Jacobs JS (Eds): Female Infertility Therapy-Current Practice. London: Martin Duntiz, 1999;189-201.

35. Daya S. Optimal protocol for gonadotrophin releasing hormone agonist use in ovarian stimulation. In: Gomel V, Cheung PCK (Eds): In Vitro Fertilization and Assisted Reproduction. Bologna: Monduzzi Editore, 1997;405-15.

36. Ron-El R, Herman A, Golan A, van der Ven H, Caspi E, Diedrich K. The comparison of early follicular and midluteal administration of long-acting gonadotrophin-releasing hormone agonist. Fertil Steril 1990;54: 233-37.

37. Reissmann T, Felberbaum R, Diedrich K, Engel J, Comaru-Schally AM, Schally AV. Development and applications of luteinizing hormone-releasing hormone antagonists in the treatment of infertility: an overview. Hum Reprod 1995;10:1974-81.

38. Felberbaum RE, Reissmann T, Kupker W et al. Preserved pituitary response under ovarian stimulation with hMG and GnRH-antagonists (Cetrorelix) in women with tubal infertility. Eur J Obstet Gynaecol Reprod Biol 1995;61:151-55.

39. Felberbaum R, Diedrich K. The use of GnRH antagonists in IVF. In: Shoham Z, Howles CM, Jacobs JS (Eds.): Female Infertility Therapy-Current Practice. London: Martin Duntiz, 1999:203-12.

40. Albano C, Smitz J, Camus M, Riethmuller-Winzen H, Van Steirteghem A, Devroey P. Comparison of different doses of gonadotrophin-releasing hormone antagonist Cetrorelix during controlled ovarian hyperstimulation. Fertil Steril 1997;67:917-22.

41. Olivennes F, Bouchard P, Frydman R. The use of a new GnRH-antagonist (Cetrorelix) with a single dose protocol in IVF. J Assisted Reprod Genet 1997;14S:15.

42. Olivennes F, Belaisch-Allart J, Emperaire JC et al. Prospective, randomized, controlled study of in vitro fertilization-embryo transfer with a single dose of a luteinizing hormone-releasing hormone (LH-RH) antagonist (cetrorelix) or a depot formula of an LH-RH agonist (triptorelin). Fertil Steril 2000;73:314-20.

• **Biraj Kalyan**

25

Monitoring of Ovulation Induction

INTRODUCTION

The birth of Louise Brown in 1978 opened up a whole new era of assisted reproductive technologies (ARTs) and offered the hope of parenthood to couples who earlier had none. A key requirement of most of these (ARTs) is multiple follicular development with the availability of many mature oocytes to improve the chances of conception. This has been termed as "controlled" ovarian hyperstimulation or superovulation. Pregnancy rates have been shown to correlate well with the number of embryos transferred, which in turn depend on the number and quality of oocytes obtained. Therefore, obtaining a large number of mature oocytes capable of undergoing fertilization and producing a larger number of good quality embryos is an important strategy in any ART program. A number of drugs and stimulation protocols are available and used for this, a discussion of which is beyond the scope of this chapter. The methods of monitoring or "controlling" the various superovulation regimes, have been discussed in this chapter.

NEED FOR MONITORING OF OVULATION INDUCTION

The retrieval of adequately mature oocytes depends on many factors. With the increasing use of superovulation regimes, close monitoring of ovarian response is necessary for several reasons:

• The development of normal preovulatory follicles by the hyperstimulation regimes so as to yield good quality oocytes of appropriate maturity

• Ovarian response may vary from patient to patient and from one cycle to another

• The use of appropriate dose of ovulation inducing drugs. Response to treatment is assessed during the period of ovarian stimulation to confirm its adequacy. Suboptimal responses call for alteration of the drug treatment protocol or cancellation of treatment cycle

• To help decide the timing of hCG administration and the timing of procedures such as oocyte retrieval or insemination

• To prevent complications such as ovarian hyperstimulation syndrome (OHSS), to minimize its severity and to treat when established. One of the most active areas of precise ovulation monitoring is in the use of controlled ovarian stimulation for the *in-vitro* fertilization (IVF) procedure. The use of estradiol, progesterone, LH and ultrasound as a combined approach for timing of hCG administration prior to oocyte recovery has become standard. Another area necessitating precise monitoring of ovulation is in the timing of intrauterine insemination (IUI) using washed spermatozoa. Because the spermatozoa are being placed directly in the uterine cavity, there is no reservoir effect that occurs when they are deposited in the vagina and picked up by the cervical mucus column. As the spermatozoa must be placed within the uterine cavity at the time that ovulation is occurring, the ability to predict the precise time of ovulation becomes important.

Monitoring Based on Indication and Stimulation Protocol Used

Monitoring of ovulation induction will vary according to the drugs used and the treatment planned. If the procedure planned is an IUI the aim of the ovulation induction is the development of not more than three to four follicles to reduce the risk of high order multiple pregnancies. If however, the treatment planned is IVF, then the ovulation induction is relatively more aggressive, as the surplus embryos can be frozen and replaced in subsequent cycles, thus reducing the cost of subsequent attempts at IVF. Similarly use of gonadotropins requires much more intensive monitoring than use of clomiphene citrate as the risks of ovarian hyperstimulation are greater with gonadotropin use.

TRADITIONAL METHODS

For many years, simple noninvasive methods have been used to predict ovulation. One of the most simple and inexpensive methods has been the use of the thermal shift or the BBT (basal body temperature) changes that occur during the menstrual cycle. The shift in BBT occurs secondary to hormonal changes occurring at the time of ovulation. It is thought that this shift in BBT occurs secondary to the production of progesterone in the dominant follicle immediately before, during the subsequent release of the mature oocyte. The advantage of this method is that it is inexpensive and noninvasive. The main disadvantage is that it can be used only as a retrospective parameter. There is no reproducible change in temperature that will indicate that ovulation is imminent in the next 12, 24, 36 hours. Reliability and reproducibility are lacking when compared to more direct methods such as ultrasound visualization of follicle rupture. Therefore its use to precisely time procedures that must occur around ovulation is limited. Another method is the vaginal squamous epithelial changes which have been utilized for many years to monitor the time of ovulation. As the estradiol

levels rise, more and more cells become superficial and the proportion of basal and intermediate cells decreases. Today this method is no longer used.

Approximately 15 to 20 years ago, monitoring of cervical mucus changes in response to the preovulatory estrogen rise was quantitated and utilized as a predictor of ovulation in ovulation induction regimes. These changes (Spinnbarkeit and cellularity) were organized into a simple scoring system popularized by Insler. However, its ability to document the precise time to ovulation is limited. The cervical mucus begins to change rapidly when the estradiol levels begin to rise. After a moderate rise in estradiol however, there are no further significant changes in the mucus. In addition, the response of the cervical glands varies considerably among individuals. Cervical assessment can therefore alert the physician to an estrogen change, but cannot be relied on for precise timing to avoid excessive stimulation.

CURRENT METHODS

Today, monitoring of patient response is carried out by a combination of ultrasound scanning of the ovaries and uterine endometrium and assay of the serum concentrations of LH, FSH, progesterone and estrogen. It is believed that ultrasonographic findings reflect growth, whereas serum E2 levels primarily detects the functional activity of the follicles. These tests are carried out at different intervals both before and during superovulation. Not all parameters are checked at every monitoring episode and various units have their own particular protocols for such tests. Generally, patients are checked before commencing superovulation to exclude any pathology that contraindicates the proposed treatment, or requires its modification. Assessment at that period also aims to confirm that the patient's physiology is what it should be at that part of the ovarian cycle. Response to treatment is assessed during the period of ovarian stimulation to confirm its adequacy. Suboptimal responses call for alteration of the drug treatment protocol or cancellation of the treatment of cycle. It also used to decide when to schedule hCG administration and oocyte retrieval or insemination and prevent and treat complications such as the hyperstimulation syndrome.

Hormonal Monitoring of Ovulation Induction

Because of the intricate relationship between the hypothalamus, pituitary and ovarian hormones, a more direct method of ovulation monitoring is the use of protein and steroid hormone assays on a daily basis. Endocrine assessment of patients and hormone monitoring are an integral part of any ART program. A well-equipped endocrine laboratory with very reliable assays is a must for this.

Follicle-stimulating hormone levels are monitored in the serum following exogenous gonadotropin administration, to establish the individual threshold above which ovarian response can be observed. Tonically high levels of LH in the late follicular phase have an adverse effect on fertilization and embryo viability and are therefore suggestive of a poor prognosis.

Estrogen concentration in the serum is used to monitor ovarian activity. Although a linear response is observed between estrogen levels and growth of the dominant follicle under normal conditions, development of multiple follicles during gonadotropin induction can cause discrepancies between parameters. The total serum E2 is a function of the state of maturity of all follicles present at a given time. Elevated estrogen levels during gonadotropin induction can be caused by multiple medium-sized follicles or a single dominant follicle. The use of estrogen measurements is necessary to choose the correct moment for administering the ovulatory dose of hCG in order to prevent hyperstimulation. Different programs follow different protocols for hormonal monitoring. With experience, daily estrogen measurements can be avoided although sometimes it may be necessary. Most ART programs today use the GnRH-a long protocol for downregulation followed by gonadotropin administration for ovarian stimulation. Downregulation usually occurs after about 7 to 14 days of GnRH-a when estradiol levels fall to less than 50 pg/mL. At this stage, ovarian stimulation with gonadotropins can be started. Day 7 estradiol level is estimated and depending on this the dosage of gonadotropin is individualized for the duration of the cycle. Gonadotropin dose is adjusted every 3 days so that estradiol levels increase by 50 percent per day.[1] Early follicular phase serum E2 levels may also be predictive of cycle prognosis. Low-serum estradiol concentration after the first few days of stimulation have been seen to be associated with poor outcome and higher cancellation rates.[2-4] E2 levels in the late follicular phase may also be predictive of IVF outcome with higher pregnancy rates seen in cycles with a higher E2/oocyte ratio.[5] The poor outcome seen in cycles with low E2 could be due to the direct effect of E2 on oocyte function and an inadequately estrogenic intrafollicular milieu. An estradiol window of 1000 to 1500 pg/mL is optimum.[6] The risk of hyperstimulation is significant with estradiol levels of more than 3000/pg/mL although there are discrepancies in different studies regarding the predictive value for OHSS using the same criteria.[7-9] There is still a debate on the impact of high E2 levels on the day of hCG administration on implantation/pregnancy rates in patients undergoing IVF.[10,11] The rate of estradiol increase is the same in spontaneous and induced cycles and does not differ in cycles which result in multiple gestation.[12] The level which is reached at the time of hCG administration is more critical than the slope of increase. hCG is usually administered when estradiol levels reach 200 to 300 pg/mL per large follicle. It is difficult to predict based on E2 levels alone, the appropriate timing of hCG administration or whether single or multiple pregnancies would result. The best pregnancy rates are obtained in patients given hCG shortly before the E2 peak.[13]

Serum LH and progesterone levels are monitored to detect the spontaneous premature LH surge and premature luteinization. Since most units now use GnRH in the long protocol, the likelihood of a premature LH surge is negligible. Periovulatory serum progesterone levels are used as a predictor of outcome, and elevated levels in the late follicular phase are suggestive of a diminished chance of conception although there is no consensus on this.[14-17]

In the normal cycle, there is an orderly sequence of events involved in follicular growth and maturation. This is maintained through a delicate balance of gonadotropins, steroids and non-steroidal intraovarian compounds, culminating in the preovulatory gonadotropin surge.[18] In assisted reproduction programs, ovulation is mostly intercepted after hCG administration. The administration of hCG is timed based on arbitrary parameters in an attempt to simulate the events of a normal cycle. In stimulated cycles, because the intricate balance is disturbed, it is likely that hCG is given either before or after the optimal time. There is synchrony of follicular development[19] or anomalies of follicular growth and maturation. Among the cohort of oocytes retrieved, there are likely to be viable, immature and postmature oocytes. The challenge lies in devising a monitoring method that can identify follicles of different quality within a cohort, or better still a stimulation protocol that produces viable oocytes and a synchrony between follicles in the developing cohort.

The main disadvantages of endocrine monitoring are the need for daily blood sampling, with a fairly sophisticated laboratory system capable of running rapid assays, expense and inconvenience.

Ultrasound Monitoring

A frequently used method for prediction of ovulation has come about in the recent past—real-time ultrasound scanning of ovarian follicle development. In 1979 Hackeloer[20, 21] demonstrated a direct correlation between increasing follicular size and estradiol concentration in spontaneously ovulating women. Since then several studies have demonstrated the correlation of follicle growth and hormone concentrations in both stimulated and unstimulated cycles.[22,23] Real-time ovarian ultrasound provides a direct visualization of the developing follicle as well as the disappearance of the follicle at the time of oocyte release. It is a quick and easy method to directly view ovarian follicle development, is non-invasive, requires a short time and has no known harmful effects to the oocyte or reproductive tract.

It has been clearly established now that the vaginal route is superior to the abdominal route for monitoring ovarian function, because of the smaller distance from the probe to the ovary, high resolution of the probes, the absence of a full bladder distorting pelvic organs, improved convenience and patient compliance. The transvaginal scanning technique has been validated under normal, anovulatory and gonadotropin stimulated conditions. Serial ultrasound can be used to monitor follicular growth and determine when ovulation occurs.

Follicular Dynamics

Although a small cohort of follicles will increase in size during the follicular phase, most of these small follicles will not increase in size beyond 10 mm. Follicular diameter of 10 mm acts as a threshold in the further fate of the ovarian follicles.[24] Beyond this size, the growth of the dominant follicle will continue, whereas the non-dominant follicles will undergo atresia. Selection of the dominant follicles is thought to occur by cycle days 5 to 7 but is not sonographically apparent until cycles days 8 to 12. Follicles destined to ovulate will increase linearly in size at the rate of 1 to 2 mm/day reaching a diameter of 18 to 24 mm before ovulation. Sometimes the follicle may enlarge upto 3 to 4 cm and still ovulate. The amount of estrogen produced by the dominant follicle increases as it grows, and there is a linear correlation between follicular diameter and E2 levels. There is also significant correlation between the mean follicular diameter measured transvaginally and the volume of follicular fluid aspirated.

A few anatomical structures may look similar to the growing follicle on ultrasound. These include:
• Cross-section of the internal iliac artery and vein
• The cross-section of blood vessels around the uterus and ovary
• The bowel
• Hydrosalpinx
• Ovarian cysts.

Follicle size has long been used as an indicator of oocyte maturity in ovulation induction and

ART. Several ultrasound derived criteria have been measured, including follicular diameter, follicular volume and the surface area of the follicular sphere. In practice, most clinicians estimate the follicular diameter based on the mean of two or more individual readings. Penzias et al[25] found the mean diameter of round and polygonal follicles accurately predicts the total follicular volume. But in cases of follicular crowding as may be seen in ovulation induction, especially with numerous ellipsoid follicles, the correlation between mean diameter and expected follicular volume and presumably, oocyte maturity may be lacking. hMG-stimulated follicles are generally 2 to 4 mm larger than follicles in normally ovulating patients or with CC stimulation.[26]

Prediction of Ovulation

Follicular rupture occurs at a wide range of follicular sizes (13-33 mm) with a mean of 21 mm diameter. The variation in the maximum follicular diameter before ovulation extends the time of ovulation over a 10-day period or more making size a poor indicator of imminent ovulation. After the LH surge, the thecal tissue becomes hypervascular and edematous and the granulosa cell layer begins to separate from the theca layer, seen sonographically as a line of decreased reflectivity around the follicle ("double contour") suggesting impending ovulation in 24 hrs.[27] Within 6 to 10 hrs before ovulation, separation and folding of the granulosa cell layer produces a crenation or irregularity of the lining of the follicle. Echoes have been identified in the follicle before ovulation ascribed to the presence of an expanded cumulus oophorus. Unfortunately, despite the fact that a number of sonographic signs have been described, currently there is no sonographic sign that predicts exactly when ovulation will occur. The signs only give evidence that the time of ovulation is nearing.

Confirmation of Ovulation

Although ultrasound does not allow precise timing or prediction of when ovulation will occur, it is an excellent technique for confirming ovulation once it has occurred. The ultrasound signs of ovulation are:

- Complete disappearance of the follicles
- Decrease in the size of the follicle
- Irregularity of the follicular contour
- Filling of the follicle with echodense structures
- Increased fluid in the cul-de-sac
- Hyperechogenic secretory endometrium.

Confirmation of ovulation is important in performing IUIs in order to maximize the potential for pregnancy. The exact timing of ovulation after the LH surge may vary and when multiple follicles are present, multiple ovulations may occur over a period of time.

Timing of hCG

Human chorionic gonadotropin is used as an LH surrogate to trigger ovulation in gonadotropin induced cycles. hCG is usually administered when there is at least one follicle measuring 16 to 18 mm in diameter (usually three in IVF cycles), estradiol levels of 200 to 300 pg/mL per large follicle and endometrial thickness of at least 8 mm.

Prevention of OHSS

Ovarian hyperstimulation syndrome (OHSS) is the most serious complication after hMG treatment and is characterized by ovarian enlargement secondary to the development of multiple luteal cysts. OHSS has been classified on the basis of the degree of ovarian enlargement and associated clinical findings into mild, moderate and severe. Torsion, rupture and hemorrhage of the ovary may result from ovarian enlargement, and fluid shifts are seen including ascites and hydrothorax. After ovulation induction with gonadotropins, especially for IVF, many patients may have mild OHSS. However careful monitoring can generally limit the incidence of severe OHSS to less than 1 percent.

It is the sensitivity of the ovary that may be the cause of the OHSS, not just the dose and duration of gonadotropin treatment. Withholding hCG is the treatment most widely used for prevention of cases which show huge number of follicles and very high levels of E2. Check[28] suggested withholding hCG if E2 was 500 pg/mL per mature follicle, or more, or more than 2000 pg/mL no matter how many follicles are present. However many cases of OHSS occur with normal or low estrogen whereas high E2 does not always lead to hyperstimulation. Various other methods have been tried like use of recombinant FSH, GnRH-a as ovulatory trigger, etc. Complete prevention of OHSS is not possible with currently available means and even in the most careful hands occasional cases may still occur.

Ultrasonographically, hyperstimulated ovaries contain numerous small and intermediate-sized follicles (Figure 25.1). It is these secondary follicles, rather than the dominant follicle that are a valuable sign of the possible development of OHSS. The secondary follicles (< 16 mm) constitute a heterogenous group with variable endocrine function. Blankenstein et al[29] further divided these secondary follicles into those of 9 to 15 mm and those greater than 5 mm. The number and size of these correlate to the development of OHSS.

Risk of OHSS as per number of secondary follicles:

< 6 : no risk

~ 8 : mild (more intermediate follicles)

> 10 : moderate to severe (more small follicles)

Small follicles continue to grow after hCG administration, thus increasing the estrogen secretion and contributing to the cascade of OHSS. hCG administration is less likely to be followed by clinically significant hyperstimulation if the follicles are subsequently aspirated at oocyte retrieval.

MONITORING OF ENDOMETRIAL DEVELOPMENT

Apart from follicular dynamics, the assessment of endometrial appearance (thickness and echogenic pattern), also plays a role in planning stimulation protocols, monitoring cycles and predicting clinical outcome (Figure 25.2). The endometrium undergoes cyclical changes with typical sonographic patterns during the different phases of natural as well stimulated cycles. Different echogenic patterns have been described such as double layered or "triple-line pattern"— outer echogenic and inner hypoechoic (Figure 25.3), hyperechoic and isoechoic endometrium. The best prognosis is seen when the triple line pattern is present before oocyte retrieval and the endometrial thickness is more than 6 mm.[30] In some studies, endometrial thickness was seen to be greater in conception cycles when compared to

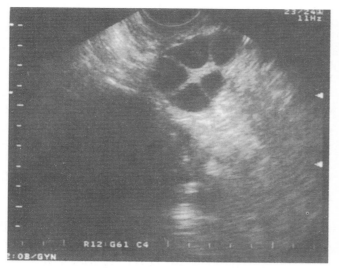

FIGURE 25.1: Ultrasound picture showing follicles in a stimulated ovary

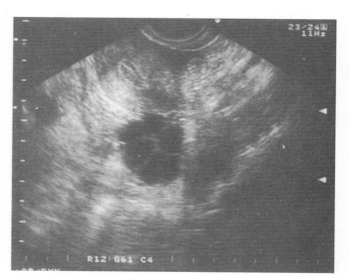

FIGURE 25.2: Ultrasound picture showing both stimulated ovary and corresponding endometrial appearance

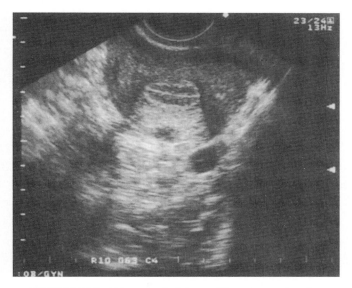

FIGURE 25.3: Ultrasound picture of the uterus showing triple-line appearance of the endometrium

nonconception cycles,[31-33] while in others no significant correlation was found.[34, 35] The endometrial appearance will also vary depending on the stimulation protocol used. The question that needs to be answered is whether an abnormal endometrial pattern reflects an intrinsic impairment of endometrial development and receptivity or simply an abnormal response to the hormonal milieu produced by the stimulation protocol used.

"ULTRASOUND ALONE" MONITORING?

The combination of USG and E2 levels has long been accepted as the optimal monitoring for ovulation induction. The value of ultrasonography lies in its ability to characterize the number, size, growth, location and disappearance of the follicles and to detect changes in uterine size and endometrial thickness. USG follow-up of the leading follicle is important for the determination of the optimal timing of hCG administration. USG follow-up of the secondary follicles along with E2 levels are necessary for the decision to withhold hCG if there is increased risk of OHSS.

It is believed by some that observation of the follicle without concurrent hormone monitoring is equivalent to evaluating the morphology but not the function of the ovary. For this reason, most people use USG in conjunction with hormone monitoring. E2 levels have been shown to correlate well with the diameter of the leading follicle, uterine dimensions and endometrial thickness all of which can be easily measured by ultrasound. These USG indices can therefore be considered as biological assays of estrogen activity.[36] As incidence of early luteinization is minimal with the use GnRH-a, in many IVF protocols, the determination of serum LH and progesterone is also redundant and merely USG without hormone monitoring is adequate especially when the GnRH-a long protocol is used. Moreover, with increasing use of recombinant FSH where estradiol levels are expected to be lower, USG monitoring takes on greater importance. There is no difference in duration of gonadotropins, number of oocytes, number of embryos, pregnancy rates or incidence of OHSS with "USG alone" monitoring.[37-40] Shoham et al[36] found ultrasound alone to be successful in preventing multiple pregnancies and diminishing incidence and severity of OHSS.

Ultrasonographic examination is quick, simple and noninvasive and provides immediate results. Serial USG is as safe and effective as the conventional ultrasonic and hormonal monitoring of ovarian response in controlled ovarian hyperstimulation protocols in general and GnRH-a treated IVF cycles in particular. With the increasing trend towards simplification of IVF and reduction of the costs involved, many centers now use ultrasound alone or combined with minimal hormonal assays for the monitoring of controlled ovarian hyperstimulation.

MONITORING PROTOCOL

Different units follow different protocols for monitoring COH for IVF. A simplified protocol followed in our unit is based on a combination of ultrasound with minimal hormonal monitoring and is as follows:
- Baseline ultrasound scans and serum hormone levels on day 23 of the cycle before starting GnRH-a
- Scan and hormone levels after 10 days of GnRH-a to rule out the presence of ovarian cysts,

ensure endometrial shedding and downregulation with an estradiol level of less than 50 pg/mL. As this stage the GnRH-a dose is halved and stimulation with gonadotropins is commenced

- Hormone levels and USG on Day 5 to 6 of gonadotropin stimulation
- USG on day 8 to 9 and after this every alternate day till a mean follicular diameter of 15 mm is achieved followed thereafter by daily follicular scans till day of hCG administration
- Hormone levels are assessed again on the day of hCG administration. hCG is given when there are at least 3 follicles of 16 to 18 mm mean diameter and E2 of 200 to 300 pg/mL per large follicle.

CONCLUSION

An ideal monitoring system is one which can assess accurately, the quality of the individual growing oocytes and not of the follicles, as is the case with most monitoring systems used today. Such an ideal monitoring system would minimize the chances of retrieving immature or postmature oocytes with their compromised developmental potential. However, no such ideal monitoring system or any index that indicates the true maturity of the oocytes exists. Hence, we have to depend on some indirect means of gauging the quality of oocytes. The most commonly used methods being hormone monitoring and ultrasound measurement of follicular size. Simplification of monitoring by use of ultrasound alone has been found to be no less effective, more convenient and cost-effective than conventional USG and hormonal monitoring and this has been adopted by many ART units.

REFERENCES

1. Yovich JL. Assisted Reproduction. In Grossman A (Ed): Clinical Endocrinology. Blackwell Scientific: Oxford, 1992;773.
2. Phelps JY, Levine As, Hickman TN et al. Day 4 estradiol levels predict pregnancy success in women undergoing controlled ovarian hyperstimulation for IVF. Fertil Steril 1998;69:1015-19.
3. Hershlag A, Asis MC, Diamond MP et al. The predictive value and management of cycles with low initial estradiol levels. Fertil Steril 1990;53:1064-67.
4. Khalaf Y, Taylor A, Braude P. Low serum estradiol concentrations after five days of controlled ovarian hyperstimulation for in vitro fertilization associated with poor outcome. Fertil Steril 2000;74:63-66.
5. Loumaye E, Engrand P, Howles CM et al. Assessment of the role of serum luteinising hormone and estradiol response to follicle stimulating hormone in in vitro fertilisation outcome. Fertil Steril 1997;67:888-99.
6. Haning RV Jr, Lavin RM, Behrman HR et al. Plasma estradiol window and urinary estriol glucouronide determination for monitoring menotropin induction of ovulation. Obstet Gynecol 1982;54:442.
7. Asch RH, Li H, Balmaceda JP et al. Severe ovarian hyperstimulation syndrome in assisted reproductive technologies: Definition of high risk groups. Hum Reprod 1991;6:1395-99.
8. Morris RS, Paulson RJ, Sauer MV et al. Predictive value of serum estradiol concentration and oocyte number in severe ovarian hyperstimulation syndrome. Hum Reprod 1995;10:811-14.
9. Mathur RS, Akanda AV, Keay SD et al. Distinction between early and late hyperstimulation syndrome. Fertil Steril 2000;73:901-07.
10. Sharara FI, McClamrock HD. High estradiol levels and high oocyte yield are not detrimental to in vitro fertilization outcome. Fertil Steril 1999;72:401-05.
11. Ng EHY. What is the threshold value for serum estradiol levels associated with adverse IVF outcome? Letters to the Editor. Fertil Steril 2000;73:1071.
12. Wilson EA, Jawad MJ, Hayden TL. Rates of increase of human estradiol concentration in normal and human menopausal gonadotropin induced cycles. Fertil Steril 1982;37:46.
13. Lopata A. Concepts in human in vitro fertilization and embryo transfer. Fertil Steril 1983;40:289-301.
14. Givens CR, Schriock ED, Dandekar PV et al. Elevated serum progesterone levels on the day of human chorionic gonadotropin administration do not predict outcome in assisted reproduction cycles. Fertil Steril 1994;62:1011-07.
15. Prien SD, Canez MS, Messer RH. Increases in progesterone after human chorionic gonadotropin administration may predict cycle outcome in patients undergoing in vitro fertilization-embryo transfer. Fertil Steril 1994;62:1066-68.
16. Hofmann GE, Bentzein F, Bergh PA et al. Premature luteinisation in controlled ovarian hyperstimulation has no effect on oocyte and embryo quality. Fertil Steril 1993;60:675-79.
17. Mio Y, Sekijima A, Iwabe T et al. Subtle rise in serum progesterone during the follicular phase as a predictor of outcome in vitro fertilization. Fertil Steril 1992;58:159-66.
18. Fritz MA, Speroff L. The endocrinology of the menstrual cycle: Interaction of folliculogenesis and neuroendocrine mechanisms. Fertil Steril 1982;38:509-29.

19. Hodgen GD. Oocyte transfer and fertilization in vitro. In Crosignano PG (Ed): Serono Clinical Colloquia on Reprod No. 4. Academic Press: New York, 1983.

20. Hackeloer BJ, Fleming R, Robinson HP et al: Correlation of ultrasonic and endocrine assessment of human follicular development. Am J Obstet Gynecol 1979;135: 122.

21. Hackeloer BJ, Sallam HN. Ultrasound scanning of ovarian follicles. Clin Obstet Gynecol 1982;10:603-20.

22. Vargyas JM, Marrs RP, Kletzky OA et al. Correlation of ultrasonic measurement of ovarian follicle size and serum estradiol levels in ovulatory patients using clomiphene citrate for in vitro fertilization. Am J Obstet Gynecol 1982;144:569.

23. Marrs RP, Vargyas JM, March CM. Correlation of ultrasonic measurements in human menopausal gonadotropin therapy. Am J Obstet Gynecol 1983;145:417.

24. Pache TD, Wladimiroff JW, De Jong et al. Growth patterns of nondominant follicles during normal menstrual cycle. Fertil Steril 1990;54:638-42.

25. Penzias AM, Emmi AM, Dubey AK et al. Ultrasound prediction of follicular volume: Is mean diameter reflective? Fertil Steril 1994;62:1274-76.

26. Dodson M. Transvaginal Ultrasound Churchill Livingstone: New York, 1991.

27. Picker RH, Smith DH, Tucker MH et al. Ultrasonic signs of imminent ovulation. J Clin Ultrasound 1983;11:1-2.

28. Check JH. Menotropins and sonography. Letters to the Editor. Fertil Steril 1986;46:156-58.

29. Blankstein J, Parente C, Shalev J et al. Ovarian hyperstimulation syndrome: Prediction by number and size of preovulatory follicles. Fertil Steril 1987;47:597-602.

30. Dickey RP, Olar TT, Curole DN et al. Endometrial pattern and thickness associated with pregnancy outcome after assisted reproductive technologies. Hum Reprod 1992;7:418-21.

31. Glissant A, De Mouzon J, Frydman R. Ultrasound study of the endometrium during in vitro fertilization cycles. Fertil Steril 1985;44:786-90.

32. Gonen Y, Casper R, Jacobsen W et al. Endometrial thickness and growth during ovarian stimulation: A possible predictor of implantation in in vitro fertilization. Fertil Steril 1989;52:446-50.

33. Fleishcher AC, Herbert CM, Sack GA et al. Sonography of the endometrium during conception and nonconception cycles of in vitro fertilisation and embryo transfer. Fertil Steril 1986;46:442-47.

34. Rabinowitz R, Laufer N, Lewin A et al. The value of endometrial measurements in the prediction of pregnancy following in vitro fertilization. Fertil Steril 1986;45:824-28.

35. Ueno J, Oehninger S, Bryzski RG et al. Ultrasonographic appearance of the endometrium in natural and stimulated in vitro fertilization cycles and its correlation with outcome. Hum Reprod 1991;6:901-04.

36. Shoham Z, Di Cardo C, Patel A et al. It is possible to run a successful ovulation induction program based solely on ultrasound monitoring? The importance of endometrial measurements. Fertil Steril 1991;56:836-41.

26 *Ovarian Follicular Stimulation Regimens in ART—The Bourn Hall Experience*

HISTORICAL REVIEW OF FOLLICULAR STIMULATION IN ART

Of all the advances that have occurred in the field of assisted reproduction technology (ART) in the 25 years since the birth of Louise Brown,[1] among the most significant must be the development of recombinant technology to produce recombinant follicle stimulating hormone (r-hFSH), recombinant luteinizing hormone (r-LH) and recombinant hCG. These products give to the practitioner of ART the purest and most effective therapeutic agents for the stimulation of ovarian follicles.

During these 22 years we have seen major changes in follicular stimulation protocols. It started with natural cycle in vitro fertilization (IVF) for the birth of Louise Brown, then on to the use of clomiphene in combination with human menopausal gonadotrophin (HMG). In the mid 1980s the LH-RH agonists[2] were introduced and have since been used in a number of different protocols in combination initially with HMG, passing through to the developments of urinary FSH (u-FSH), high purity FSH (HP-FSH) and now to recombinant FSH (r-hFSH). Up until recently, FSH has been combined with LH-RH agonists, but the LH-RH antagonists[3] are now available and are likely to be increasingly used in the future.

The changes at Bourn Hall in the use of gonadotrophins through the 1980s and early 1990s are shown in Table 26.1. As the use of u-FSH and then HP-FSH came about, concerns were expressed that LH was required to achieve adequate

TABLE 26.1: Changes in the use of gonadotrophins at Bourn Hall since 1980

1980—1989	—	hMG
1989—1993	—	u-FSH $\pm$ hMG
1993—1994	—	u-FSH $\rightarrow$ FSH-HP
1994—1995	—	FSH-HP
1995—1996	—	FSH-HP $\rightarrow$ rec-FSH
1996—2000	—	rec-FSH only

follicular stimulation as it is present in HMG, and it was felt that adequate follicular development and the production of mature oocytes could not be achieved without adding some LH to the u-FSH preparations. It has long been known that raised serum LH levels in ART are associated with reduced oocyte fertilization rates[5-8] and reduced embryo implantation rates.[9,10] Further, if a pregnancy did occur, raised LH levels were associated with increased miscarriage rates.[8,10] It was subsequently confirmed that the large majority of women do have sufficient endogenous LH for normal ovarian steroidogenesis, even in "down-regulated" LH-RH analogue cycles for ovulation induction[11-14] or for ART. In the most significant of these papers, a meta-analysis by Daya *et al*,[15] which looked at cycles both with and without LH-RH agonist co-treatment, found that u-FSH alone was more effective than HMG. They stated that the results clearly showed a preference for FSH alone in IVF cycles and that the future role of HMG in ovarian follicular stimulation for IVF should be questioned.

During the time of these changes, Bourn Hall was undertaking trials of different superovulation

TABLE 26.2: Superovulation regimens—changes in analogue protocols
• Clomiphene 50-100 mg. days 2-6 + hMG/FSH-HP/r-FSH from cycle day 5
• Buserelin/Nafarelin cycle days 2-4 + hMG/FSH-HP/r-FSH from day 3
• Buserelin/Nafarelin from day 2 on + hMG/FSH-HP/r-FSH from day 3 on
• Buserelin/Nafarelin from day 21 on + hMG/FSH-HP/r-FSH when downregulated and ready
(Bourn Hall Clinic Protocols)

regimens for ART with different LH-RH agonist regimens. These are shown in Table 26.2. The clomiphene-HMG stimulation regimen was superseded in the mid 1980's by the ultra-short protocol, in which the buserelin or nafarelin was given only for three days, from cycle days 2–4, thus achieving a "flare" effect. However, a clinical trial conducted at Bourn Hall in 1993 by Marcus et al[16] showed that the long luteal phase down-regulation protocol with the LH-RH analogue was superior to the ultra-short protocol. Wikland et al[17] showed the changes that had occurred in their program during the same time that Bourn Hall was experimenting with their different LH-RH analogue protocols, and also reflected the changes in gonadotrophin use at that time. They clearly showed that the change to high-purity FSH alone produced fewer cancelled cycles and better pregnancy rates. They confirmed our own findings that the use of HP-FSH alone was sufficient to achieve improved pregnancy rates and treatment could be considerably simplified–particularly with the self-administration by subcutaneous injection of the HP-FSH preparation.

The Introduction of Recombinant FSH (r-hFSH)

As r-hFSH became available in 1994/1995, so clinical trials began to be conducted using this newer preparation. Bergh et al[18] and Frydman et al[19] were the first to publish large series of patients comparing the use of r-hFSH (Gonal-F) with HP-FSH (Metrodin-HP). In both of these series it was found that significantly fewer numbers of ampoules of r-hFSH were used compared to HP-FSH, significantly more oocytes were recovered and significantly more embryos were available to transfer to the uterus or cryopreserve. The combined results of these two trials are shown in Table 26.3.

Between the years 1993 and 1999, a large number of papers were published comparing the use of r-hFSH against u-FSH. Daya and Gunby[20] reviewed twelve reports that were suitable for inclusion in a meta-analysis. All of the trials except one showed a trend in favor of the use of r-hFSH, but were not individually significant. The common odds ratio, however, showed a significant benefit to the use of r-hFSH over u-FSH in terms of clinical pregnancy (Table 26.4). In addition, this meta-analysis showed benefit of follitropin α (Gonal-F) over follitropin β (Puregon) (Table 26.5).

In a comparative analysis of multifollicular development in IVF and ICSI in different categories of ovarian responders, Oehninger et al[21] found that r-hFSH appeared to be superior in achieving an ongoing pregnancy in IVF and ICSI treatment cycles in intermediate and high responders over the use of HP-FSH or u-FSH. Similarly, Manassiev et al[22] compared the effectiveness of r-hFSH against u-FSH or HP-FSH in five clinical trials and produced similar results to those of Daya et al[20]. All five studies showed improved pregnancy rates with recombinant FSH. As in the Daya study, however, all confidence intervals included 1, but the combined meta-analysis showed significantly improved pregnancy rates, with a common odds ratio of 1.35 and confidence intervals of 1.08–1.74 in favor of r-hFSH.

TABLE 26.3: Results of early trials comparing recombinant-FSH and urinary FSH-high purity				
Study	Treatment	Ampules (75 IU)	Oocytes	Embryos
Bergh et al 1997	Gonal-F® (n = 119)	21.9 ± 5.1	12.2 ± 5.5	8.1 ± 4.2
	Metrodin® HP (n = 102)	31.9 ± 13.4	7.6 ± 4.4	4.7 ± 3.5
Frydman et al 1998	Gonal-F® (n = 130)	27.6 ± 10.2	11.0 ± 5.9	5.0 ± 3.7
	Metrodin® HP (n = 116)	40.7 ± 13.6	8.8 ± 4.8	3.5 ± 2.9

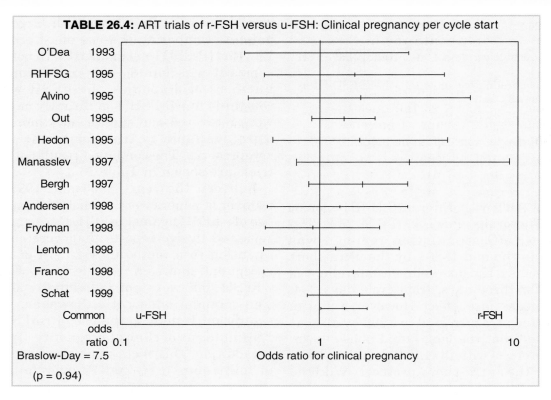

TABLE 26.4: ART trials of r-FSH versus u-FSH: Clinical pregnancy per cycle start

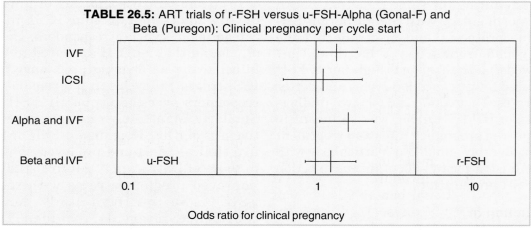

TABLE 26.5: ART trials of r-FSH versus u-FSH-Alpha (Gonal-F) and Beta (Puregon): Clinical pregnancy per cycle start

In a large double blind, randomised study comparing r-hFSH (Gonal-F) with HP-FSH (Metrodin-HP) in women undergoing ART, including ICSI, Frydman et al[23] reported on a series with 139 patients in each group, all in LH-RH analogue long luteal phase down-regulation cycles. The number of oocytes recovered was significantly higher in the Gonal-F group and the number of days of stimulation and the total number of 75 IU ampoules of FSH used were both highly significantly less in the Gonal-F group than in the Metrodin-HP group.

The data from FIVNAT (the French National IVF Register) from 4,338 cases who achieved ovum pick-up between 1994 and 1998 have been analysed.[24] They were an uniform group with tubal disease only, less than 35 years of age with normal ovulatory cycles, all undergoing their first IVF cycle in a long down regulation protocol. The conclusion of the study using this homogeneous group of young women showed that the use of r-hFSH was associated with the highest pregnancy rate for the lowest number of embryos transferred.

As practitioners continued to gain experience with the use of r-hFSH, so the question again arose whether some groups of patients should receive HMG or r-LH to supplement their stimulation protocols. A number of papers have confirmed that the addition of HMG or r-LH does not improve the outcome. The study by Mercan et al[25] of the Jones Institute looked at the use of u-FSH with and without the addition of HMG and found there were significantly more mature oocytes in the FSH alone group (P=0.0001) and a significantly higher pregnancy rate (40% vs 28%; p=0.05) with the FSH alone group. Sills et al[26] found the same, with improved pregnancy rates (64.7% vs 35.7%; ns) when comparing HP-FSH alone against HP-FSH and r-LH combined.

Cohen et al[27] compared the use of HP-FSH with HP-FSH and HMG combined and found that there were significantly worse implantation rates when HMG was added. Similarly, they found that adding HMG to r-hFSH also did not help the implantation rates, which were significantly worse in the added HMG group.

Most recently, Ben Amor[28] in a randomised double blind placebo controlled study looked at the effect of exogenous r-LH being added to r-hFSH in a protocol in which the r-LH was added during the late follicular phase in normo-ovulatory women undergoing stimulation for multiple follicular development. The addition of r-LH did not provide any additional benefit in terms of reducing the number of days of stimulation, reducing the consumption of FSH ampoules, improving the number of oocytes retrieved or the maturity of the oocytes. There was no increase in the number of developing embryos or improvements in the clinical pregnancy rates.

A number of more recent studies have confirmed that follicular stimulation with r-hFSH alone does achieve a more satisfactory follicular response than HP-FSH or u-FSH. Raga et al[29] looked at the effect of r-hFSH use in 30 young infertile women with previous poor responses to stimulation, but who had normal basal concentrations of FSH and estradiol. They prospectively randomised these women to receive either r-hFSH or HP-FSH. They concluded that r-hFSH was more effective than HP-FSH in young previously poor responders with normal serum FSH levels. Similarly, De Placido et al[30] looked at the outcome of "poor responders" to previous stimulation with HP-FSH. There were fewer, but not significant, numbers of days of stimulation and number of ampoules of gonadotrophin used in the r-hFSH group. However the oestradiol levels at three different stages in the cycles were significantly better with r-hFSH and there were significantly more mature oocytes recovered, better fertilization rates and highly significantly more (p=0.007) pre-embryos available for transfer.

An unpublished study by Gearon and Abdalla[31] of the Lister Hospital in London, showed significantly improved pregnancy rates with r-hFSH in a large series (r-hFSH, n=297 vs HP-FSH, n=306), but the most significant finding in this large study is that, although the women under 38 years of age achieved better pregnancy rates in the r-hFSH group, but not significantly so, the older women ($\geq$ 38 years of age) showed a significantly improved pregnancy rate of 32.7 percent vs 13.6 percent (p=0.011) of the r-hFSH group versus the HP-FSH group. They attribute this finding to improved oocyte and embryo quality achieved with r-hFSH over HP-FSH. This is the first study that shows such a significant improvement in the quality of oocytes in older women.

The paper by Loumaye et al,[32] which assessed the role of serum LH and estradiol in response to FSH stimulation and the outcome of in vitro fertilization demonstrated that there was no relation between basal LH levels and outcome. Further, the highest pregnancy rates were achieved when the estradiol per oocyte ratio was between 70 pg/ml–140 pg/ml. When the estradiol levels were below 70 pg/ml per oocyte retrieved the pregnancy rates were very poor (5.3% compared with 31.3 percent in the 70 pg/ml-140 pg/ml group) and the higher the estradiol level per follicle or per oocyte, again, worse results were obtained, with pregnancy rates of 23.9 percent when the estradiol per oocyte ratio was 210 pg/ml-280 pg/ml group.

The conclusions of this study were that the response to FSH is independent of LH levels at the start of the cycle and at the time that hCG is administered; also, that women with undetectable levels of LH will perform as well as women with higher levels of LH. The most significant finding from a clinical viewpoint is that the optimum level of estradiol per large follicle and therefore, on average per oocyte recovered, if maintained at between 70 pg/ml–140 pg/ml will achieve the best results. This has had the effect in our programme of trying to "push" patients with low estradiol levels per follicle into the higher range if possible and also to give hCG earlier if it appears that estradiol levels per follicle will exceed 140 pg/ml. In our own program, therefore, we aim to achieve estradiol levels of approximately 100 pg/ml per follicle, which requires much greater flexibility on the timing of the administration of hCG.

Recombinant LH (Luveris®) is now becoming available to practitioners in many countries. A multicenter, double blind, comparative, parallel group, dose finding, phase II clinical study comparing the safety and efficacy of r-hLH with u-hCG for inducing final follicular maturation and early luteinization in women undergoing super-ovulation with prior to IVF was published by Loumaye et al.[33] They concluded that a single injection of r-LH (Luveris) is effective in inducing final follicular maturation and early luteinization in IVF patients achieving embryo transfer. 5000 IU of r-hLH appeared to be as effective as 5000 IU of u-hCG and was well tolerated in doses up to 30,000 IU administered subcutaneously. Significantly, they found that a single administration of r-hLH was associated with a reduction in moderate ovarian hyperstimulation syndrome (OHSS), especially in patients with estradiol levels in excess of 3,000 pg/ml and/or > 20 follicles on the day of hCG or LH administration.

Management of Stimulation Cycles for ART at Bourn Hall Clinic

The evolution of ovarian follicular stimulation protocols for ART over the past 25 years has been mentioned earlier in this chapter. For the past 8 years at Bourn Hall, all follicular stimulation protocols have involved the use of r-hFSH (Gonal-F®) alone. Our policy is always to check the serum FSH, LH, estradiol and prolactin levels of all women over 35–36 years of age before a treatment cycle and, if they have had a previous treatment, the previous responses to stimulation are reviewed carefully. The starting doses of r-hFSH in first ART cycles are:

Age < 35   :   start 150 IU r-hFSH sc daily
Age 35–39   :   start 225 IU r-hFSH sc daily
Age 40 +   :   start 300 IU r-hFSH sc daily

After 5–7 days of stimulation the dosages may be adjusted upwards or downwards depending on the follicular response. If women have had poor responses or exaggerated responses to treatment using this protocol in previous cycles then the starting dosage will be increased or decreased depending on that experience.[34]

"Downregulation" is achieved with buserelin (Suprecur®) 500 mcg subcutaneously daily or, nafarelin (Synarel®) 400 mcg intranasally, both from menstrual cycle day 21 onwards until the "baseline" evaluation, which takes place in the first few days of menstruation. If "baseline" levels of estradiol (< 50 pg/ml), LH (< 5 iu/l) and progesterone (< 2 pg/ml) have been achieved, then the dose of buserelin is reduced to 200 mcg subcutaneously daily or nafarelin reduced to 200 mcg intranasally daily. The start of follicular stimulation with r-hFSH (Gonal-F®) is timed to start so that the collection of oocytes is programmed for the convenience of the patient and the clinic.

hCG is usually administered when two or more follicles have achieved 18 mm in diameter. However, as discussed earlier, flexibility is exercised with the timing of hCG in order to try and achieve estradiol levels of approximately 100 pg/ml per follicle > 12 mm–14 mm in diameter. 10,000 IU of hCG (Profasi®) is given 34-36 hours before the planned time of oocyte recovery.

Luteal phase support is provided with progesterone only. No luteal hCG has been used for the past 10 years at Bourn Hall, even in patients at low risk of OHSS. Progesterone in the form of

Cyclogest 400 mg PV or PR 12 hourly is given starting on the evening of oocyte collection or, most recently, Crinone® gel 8 percent *per vaginam* has been used. The use of Crinone® with its plastic vaginal applicator is popular with patients. Tests of serum hCG levels on day 15 postoocyte recovery are carried out and, if pregnancy is achieved, a vaginal ultrasound scan is carried out on day 35 following oocyte recovery to confirm a clinical pregnancy.

Is There a Difference between Follitropin α (Gonal-F®) and Follitropin β (Puregon®)?

The meta-analysis of Daya and Gunby[15] was the first to point out that there may be a difference in follicular response and clinical outcome between follitropin α (Gonal-F®) and follitropin β (Puregon®). This meta-analysis showed that there was a significant difference in the outcome when follitropin α was compared with urinary FSH (common odds ratio 1.36: confidence intervals 1.022, 1.80). Follitropin β (Puregon®) did not show a significant difference (common odds ratio of 1.19 and confidence intervals of 0.93, 1.53).

Brinsden *et al*[35] compared the efficacy and tolerability of the α and β preparations of r-hFSH. The study was small as there was not expected to be a significant difference in the end points. The study also set out to document the safety and tolerability of both preparations. The results of the comparison are shown in Table 26.6. There was no significant difference in any of the parameters. Although the clinical pregnancy rates appeared to favor follitropin α, the difference was not significant. However, when the local tolerance of the two preparations was compared, the proportion of injections that led to at least one report of a symptom (itching, swelling, redness, bruising or pain) differed significantly between the α and the β preparations (p=0.014). Similar differences between the two preparations are reported in two other studies.[36, 37]

The Cost Benefit of Recombinant Gonadotrophins

The American Society of Reproductive Medicine (ASRM) in their Practice Committee Report of June 1998[38] states that "Recombinant FSH was more effective for IVF than urinary FSH in stimulating multiple follicular development and, when results from cryopreserved embryos were included, was associated with higher pregnancy rates". Similarly, the Royal College of Obstetricians and Gynecologists in the United Kingdom, in a report "The Management of Infertility in Tertiary Care", Evidence Based Clinical Guidelines No.6, published in January 2000,[39] reported that "Recombinant FSH produces significantly more oocytes in an IVF cycle compared to urinary derived high-purity gonadotrophin preparations, however, pregnancy rates in fresh and embryo replacement cycles are similar" (grade-A evidence) but, "If fresh and frozen embryo replacements are considered, the use of recombinant FSH produces a higher pregnancy rate when compared to urinary derived high-purity gonadotrophin preparations" (grade A evidence). The Report goes on to state that:

TABLE 26.6: Summary of results of comparsion of Gonal-F vs Puregon (Brinsden *et al* 1994[34])

Parameter	Gonal-F®	Puregon®	p-value
Oocytes retrieved (n)	12.14 ± 1.68	12.32 ± 1.83	0.94
Proportion of MII oocytes (%)	81.8	70.3	0.22
Follicles ≥ 11 mm on DhCG (n)	13.27 ± 1.61	14.86 ± 2.09	0.54
Follicles ≥ 14 mm on DhCG (n)	10.05 ± 1.23	10.68 ± 1.18	0.71
2 Pn fertilized oocytes (n)	6.41 ± 1.15	6.09 ± 1.27	0.85
Viable embryos (n)	5.59 ± 1.12	5.14 ± 1.07	0.77
Embryos transferred (n)	2.18 ± 0.13	2.35 + 0.17	0.41
Pregnancy rate (%)	31.8	27.3	0.74
Clinical pregnancy rate (%)	31.8	18.2	0.30
Embryo implantation rate (%)	19.6 ± 0.07	17.6 ± 0.09	0.86

"Because of the small differences in outcome, additional factors should be considered when choosing a gonadotrophin regimen, including patient acceptability, costs and drug availability" (grade C evidence). There is now no doubt about the clinical benefits of recombinant gonado-trophins, which are listed in Table 26.7.[40] The only disadvantage that could be attributed to the use of r-hFSH is the apparent increased cost of treatment. With the increasing awareness of cost benefit analysis, which is being conducted in all treatments in medicine today, it is important to establish any cost benefit in the use of r-hFSH. This has recently been reviewed by Ledger.[41] Using a Markov model and looking at the effectiveness of treatment—i.e. "success", as judged by an ongoing pregnancy beyond 12 weeks gestation, he looked at the cost of an ongoing pregnancy and the mean number of cycles that it takes to achieve an ongoing pregnancy. Using the Markov model with 100,000 "virtual patients", 37,358 successes could be expected with u-FSH and 40,575 successes with r-hFSH. The cost per u-FSH successful pregnancy was £ 6,060 (US $ 9696) and per r-hFSH success was £ 5, 906 (US $ 9,449) (SD = £ 232: p < 0.0001). When assessing the mean number of cycles that it took to achieve a successful pregnancy, u-FSH was 5.25 cycles and r-hFSH 4.59 cycles. This highly sophisticated,

TABLE 26.7: What are the clinical benefits of recombinant gonadotrophins?
Advantages:
• Improved logistics of the pharmaceutical process
• Controlled manufacture
• More homogenous product
• Reduced batch-to-batch variability
• Potentially unlimited supply
• Should never be shortages
• Not reliant on a supply of urine
• No risk of infection
• No risk of contamination with drugs or metabolites
• No sero-conversion to anti-Gn antibodies
• Effective, safe and less traumatic SC administration
• Greater purity and specificity
• ? Smaller doses needed
• ? More predictable responses
Disadvantages:
• Cost (??)
(From: Balen A *et al Hum Reprod and Webtract*, 1999)

but well validated statistical analysis, when applied to model the cost effectiveness of recombinant versus urinary gonadotrophins, demonstrated that the use of recombinant gonadotrophins is associated with a lower cost per pregnancy and a lower number of treatment cycles per success. This finding was further validated by a study by Sykes *et al*,[42] which again used the Markov model with data from the paper by van Out *et al* 1995[43] together with the data from 20 UK IVF clinics and the experience of an expert panel. The authors of this paper confirm the conclusions of Ledger[41] that recombinant FSH is the most cost effective therapy for follicular stimulation for ART.

CONCLUSIONS

The development of recombinant gonadotrophins for follicular stimulation in ART has been one of the most significant advances in ART in the 25 years since the birth of Louise Brown. The purity of the product and the ease of administration for patients are two of the most important factors from the point of view of patients. The evidence from most studies over the last 8 years is that it is superior in effectiveness to HP-FSH, u-FSH and HMG. The single factor that has delayed the more widespread acceptance of r-hFSH has been the apparent increased cost of using it in treatment cycles. The recent evidence that has become available from analysis of the large body of data and use of the Markov model has shown that r-hFSH is the most cost effective preparation for follicular stimulation in ART today.

There is no doubt that the future of follicular stimulation will involve r-hFSH. Very few patients, those who are truly gonadotrophin deficient, will require some additional r-LH to facilitate normal estrogen secretion and follicular development. It is likely that r-LH will be used exclusively in place of u-HCG for the final maturation of oocytes in ART protocols because of the apparent greater safety of r-LH, both from the purity and safety points of view. Present evidence also indicates that the GnRh analogues started in the midluteal phase of the preceding cycle, combined with r-hFSH, give the best pregnancy rates and make more embryos available for cryopreservation.

It is likely that in the near future—the GnRh antagonist will increasingly be used instead of the GnRh agonist, with the advantage of shorter treatment duration, less profound suppression and possibly reduced amounts of r-hFSH required for follicular stimulation.

REFERENCES

1. Steptoe PC, Edwards RG. Birth after reimplantation of a human embryo (letter). Lancet. 1978;2:366.
2. Porter RN, Smith W, Craft IL. Induction of ovulation for in vitro fertilisation using Buserelin and gonadotrophins. Lancet. 1984;2:1284.
3. Klingmuller D, Diedrich K, Sommer L. Effects of the GnRH antagonist Cetrorelix in normal women. Gynecol Endocrinol. 1993;7:2.
4. Diedrich K, Diedrich C, Santos E. Suppression of the endogenous luteinising hormone surge by the gonadotrophin release–releasing hormone antagonist Cetrorelix during ovarian stimulation. Hum Reprod. 1994;9:788-91.
5. Stanger JD, Yovich JL. Reduced in vitro fertilisation of human oocytes from patients with raised basal luteinising hormone levels during the follicular phase. Br J Obstet Gynecol. 1985;92:385-93.
6. Howles CM, Macnamee MC, Edwards RG. Follicular development and early luteal function of conception and non-conceptual cycles after human in vitro fertilisation. Hum Reprod. 1987;2:17-21.
7. Shoham Z, Mannaerts B, Insler V, Coelingh-Bennink H. Induction of follicular growth using recombinant follicle-stimulating hormone in two volunteer women with hypogonadotrophic hypogonadism. Fertil Steril. 1993;59:738-42.
8. Shoham Z, Balen A, Patel A, Jacobs HS. Results of ovulation induction using human menopausal gonadotrophin or purified follicle stimulating hormone in hypogonadotropic hypogonadism patients. Fertil Steril. 1991;56:1048-53.
9. Homberg R, Armar NA, Eshel A, Adams J, Jacobs HS. Influence of serum luteinising hormone concentrations on ovulation, conception, and early pregnancy loss in polycystic ovary syndrome. Br Med J 1988;297:1024-26.
10. Regan L, Owen EJ, Jacobs HS. Hypersecretion of luteinising hormone, infertility and miscarriage. Lancet 1990;336:1141-44.
11. Chappel SC, Howles C. Re-evaluation of the roles of luteinizing hormone and follicle-stimulating hormone in the ovulatory process. Hum Reprod. 1991;6:1206-12.
12. Homburg R, Eshel A, Kilborn J. Combined luteinising hormone releasing hormone analogue and exogenous gonadotrophins for the treatment of infertility associated with polycystic ovaries. Hum Reprod. 1990;5:32-35.
13. Howles C. Do raised serum luteinizing hormone levels during stimulation for in-vitro fertilization predict outcome? Br J Obstet Gynaecol. 1990;97(7):659-60.
14. Wikland M, Borg J, Hamberger L, Svalander P. Simplification of IVF: minimal monitoring and the use of subcutaneous highly purified administration for ovulation induction. Hum Reprod 1994;8:1430-36.
15. Daya S, Gunby J, Hughes EG. Follicle stimulating hormone versus human menopausal gonadotrophin for in vitro fertilisation cycles: A meta-analysis. Fertil Steril 1995;64:347-54.
16. Marcus SF, Brinsden PR, Macnamee MC. A comparative trial between an ultrashort and long stimulation protocol of LH-RH analogue with gonadotrophin for in vitro fertilisation. Hum Reprod 1993;8:238-43.
17. Wikland M, Nilsson L, Bergh C, Hamberger L. Results from in vitro fertilisation and intracytoplasmic sperm injection with purified gonadotrophins (Metrodin-HP). Horm Res 1995;5:238-40.
18. Berg C, Howles CM, Borg K. Recombinant human follicle stimulating hormone (Gonal-F) versus highly purified FSH (Metrodin-HP): results of a randomised comparative study in women undergoing Assisted Reproductive Techniques (ART). Hum Reprod 1997;12:2133-39.
19. Frydman R, Haverell C, Camier B. A double blind, randomised study comparing the efficacy of recombinant human (FSH: Gonal-F) versus highly purified urinary FSH (Metrodin-HP) in inducing superovulation in women undergoing assisted reproductive techniques. Hum Reprod 1998;13:180-85.
20. Daya S, Gunby J. Recombinant versus urinary follicle-stimulating hormone for ovarian stimulation in assisted reproduction. Hum Reprod 1999;14:2207-15.
21. Oehninger S, Barroso G, Jones D, Muasher S. Recombinant and urinary FSH preparations: A comparative analysis of multi-follicular development and IVF/ICSI outcome in different categories of ovarian responder. Mid East Fertil Soc J. 1999;4:114-22.
22. Manassiev NS, Tenekedjier KI, Collins J. Does the use of recombinant follicle-stimulating hormone instead of urinary follicle-stimulating hormone lead to higher pregnancy rates in in vitro fertilisation-embryo transfer cycles? Assist Reprod 1999;9(1):7-12.
23. Frydman R, Howles CM, Truon G (For the French multicentre trialists). A double blind, randomised study to compare recombinant human follicle stimulating hormone (FSH:Gonal-F) with highly-purified FSH (Metrodin-HP) in women undergoing assisted reproductive techniques including intracytoplasmic sperm injection. Hum Reprod 2000;15:520-25.
24. FIVNAT. French IVF/ICSI Register, 1998.
25. Mercan R, Mayer J, Walker D, Jones S, Oehninger S, Toner J, Muasher S. Improved oocyte quality is obtained

with follicle stimulating hormone alone than with follicle stimulating hormone/human menopausal gonadotrophin combination. Hum Reprod 1997;12:1886-89, 1997.

26. Sills ES, Levy D, Moomjy M, McGee M, Rosenwaks Z. A prospective, randomised comparison of ovulation induction using highly purified follicle-stimulating hormone alone and with recombinant human luteinising hormone in in vitro fertilisation. Hum Reprod 1999;14:2230-35.

27. Cohen J. Personal communication and presented at IVF World Congress Serono Symposium, 10 May 1999.

28. Ben Amor. The effect of luteinising hormone administered during luteal follicular phase in normo-ovulatory women undergoing in vitro fertilisation. Hum Reprod 2000;15:(Suppl 1):46, Abstract 0-116.

29. Raga F, Bonilla-Musoles F, Casan E, Bonilla F. Recombinant follicle stimulating hormone stimulation in poor responders with normal basal concentrations of follicle stimulating hormone and oestradiol: Improved reproductive outcome. Hum Reprod 1999;14:1431-34.

30. De Placido G, Alviggi C, Mollo A, Strina I, Varricchio M, Molis M. Recombinant follicle stimulating hormone is effective in poor responders to highly purified follicle stimulating hormone. Hum Reprod 2000;15:17-22.

31. Gearon C, Abdulla H. Personal communication 1999.

32. Loumaye E, Engrand P, Howles CM. Assessment of the role of serum luteinising hormone and oestradiol response to follicle-stimulating hormone on in vitro fertilisation treatment outcome. Fertil Steril 1997; 67:889-99.

33. Loumaye E, Piazzi A, Engrand P. Results of a phase II, dose finding clinical study comparing recombinant human luteinising hormone (r-hLH) with human chorionic gonadotrophin (hCG) to induce final follicular maturation prior to in vitro fertilisation. Fertil Steril (Supplement) 1998;0-236,S88.

34. Macnamee MC, Brinsden P. Superovulation strategies in assisted conception. In PR Brinsden (Ed.): A Textbook of in vitro fertilization and assisted conception.

Parthenon Publishing, Carnforth and New York. 2000;91-102.

35. Brinsden P, Akagbosu F, Gibbons L, Lancaster S, Gourdon D, Engrand P, Loumaye E. A comparison of the efficacy and tolerability of two recombinant human follicle-stimulating hormone preparations in patients undergoing in vitro fertilisation–embryo transfer. Fertil Steril 2000;73:114-16.

36. Sargent S. A study to evaluate the ease of use and tolerability by patients of gonadotrophins old and new. British Fertility Society Annual Meeting: Abstract PO22, 1998.

37. Afnan MA, Kennefick A. Recombinant gonadotrophins: Is there a difference in the tolerability of these products? British Fertility Society Abs book page 1999;75:1.

38. American Society of Reproductive Medicine, Practice Committee Report. Fert and Ster Supplement, June 1998.

39. Guideline development group, Royal College of Obstetricians and Gynaecologists. Management of infertility in tertiary care. Evidence based clinical guideline 2000;6:46.

40. Balen AH, Hayden CJ, Rutherford AJ. What are the clinical benefits of recombinant gonadotrophins? Clinical efficacy of recombinant gonadotrophins. Hum Reprod 1999;14:1411-17.

41. Ledger W. A cost-effective analysis of Gonal-F (follitropin alpha) compared to urinary FSH-HP in ART: results from the UK. Presented at ESHRE 2000 (Serono Symposium).

42. Sykes D, Out HJ, van Loon J. Economic evaluation of recombinant follicle-stimulating hormone (Puregon) in infertile women undergoing IVF in the UK. J Reprod Fert Abstract series 25 for BFS meeting 2000;48:24.

43. Out H, Mannaerts B, Driessen S, Coelingh-Bennink H. A prospective, randomised, assessor blind, multi-centre study comparing recombinant urinary follicle-stimulating hormone (Puregon vs Metrodin) in in vitro fertilisation. Hum Reprod 1995;10:2534-40.

• Hrishikesh D Pai
• Rishma Dhillon Pai • Nandita P Palshetkar

27

Recombinant FSH in Ovulation Induction

INTRODUCTION

Fifteen percent of couples will experience infertility at some time during their reproductive lives. Over the past forty years, injectible gonadotrophins have established a leading role in the treatment of both male and female infertility. Unfortunately, despite major improvements in the purity of the natural gonadotrophin products, the source has always remained the same: the urine of postmenopausal women, which needs to be collected in bulk for processing. Over 60,000,000 liters of urine from approximately 300,000 donors per year needs to be collected to meet the growing demands.

However, difficulties in obtaining enough raw material, together with a rapid increase in demand, led to worldwide shortages of the natural products. In 1996, the introduction of the first recombinant human FSH, Gonal-F-R, then in 2001 the introduction of a recombinant hCG (r-hCG) and a recombinant LH brought about a radical change in the quality, standardization and availability of gonadotrophins.

History

By the early 1960's a purified extract of human menopausal gonadotrophin (hMG) was made available and the first pregnancy was obtained with this product in 1962. Continued improvement in purity resulted initially in the development of products containing only FSH activity.

However, these preparations only contained about 50 percent FSH with as much as 95 percent contaminating protein. With the use of biotechnology processes, highly purified urinary human FSH containing greater than 95 percent pure FSH was developed in 1993.

Finally, in 1995, the final transition to a true drug was made where the starting material and complete manufacture was under vigorous control, and this was the recombinant FSH (r-hFSH).

The objective of recombinant DNA technology is to insert genes into a cell so that it produces a desired protein. Once identified, the gene that codes for the desired protein is isolated by enzymatically cleaving it from the DNA chain.

The isolated gene is then spliced to a larger piece of DNA termed a vector. The section of DNA containing the desired gene, and the vector sequence derived from two different sources, is termed recombinant DNA (r-DNA). The next stage is to insert the r-DNA into a host cell. This is usually carried out by the process of transfection whereby the r-DNA is taken up by the host cell.

The r-DNA utilizes the host cell's own machinery for protein synthesis. Powerful promotor sequences which were also transfected cause the expression of the r-DNA and eventually the desired protein is produced.

The amino acid sequences of the alpha and beta-subunits of r-hFSH are identical to those of natural human FSH. Thus, r-hFSH is the authentic human molecule. There is no LH activity.

Research led to the transfection of the human DNA genes into a mammalian cell line and to the introduction of the first 99.9 percent pure recombinant FSH, Gonal-F ®, to receive a Europe-wide product license in 1995.

Follicle Stimulating Hormone (FSH)

Human follicle stimulating hormone (hFSH) and LH are secreted by the gonadotrophin cells of the pituitary. Structurally, FSH is a glycoprotein dimer consisting of two non-covalently linked protein subunits, alpha and beta. The molecule also contains four asparagines—linked carbohydrate chains, two of which are linked to an alpha-subunit and two to the beta-subunit. The glycosylated molecule has an overall size of 35 to 45 kd.

The amino acid sequence is the same as that of the alpha-subunit of the other glycoprotein hormones-LH, thyroid stimulating hormone (TSH) and human chorionic gonadotrophin (hCG). The beta-subunit is unique and is responsible for the physiological specificity of the hormone.

The primary structure of the alpha-subunit of FSH was one of the first to be reported for a human hormone, in the 1970s. However, the primary sequence of the beta-subunit was not published until 1985. The tertiary structure of the molecule is maintained by six intrachain disulfide bonds which are essential for the full biological activity of the hormone.

Biological Role of FSH

In The Male

FSH plays an important role in both males and females. In the testes, the action of FSH is primarily in seminiferous tubule maturation. The target cells of the hormone are the Sertoli cells. In the presence of a high intratesticular androgen level (which depends upon the steroidogenic activity of LH on Leydig cells) FSH induces spermatogenesis.

In The Female

In the ovary, the target cell of FSH is the granulosa cell. The hormone binds to specific plasma membrane receptors in the granulosa cells and brings about four main effects:

1. Activates the adenylate cyclase system, leading to increased conversion of androgens originating from the theca into the estrogens, estrone and estradiol.
2. Stimulates proliferation of the granulosa cells, resulting in follicular growth.
3. Induces a marked increase in LH and prolactin receptors on the granulosa cells.
4. Causes activation of steroidogenic enzymes necessary for progesterone biosynthesis.

Two Cell, Two Gonadotrophin Theory

Follicular estrogen biosynthesis under the influence of FSH is due to the aromatization of androgens originating in the theca, which subsequently diffuse through the basal lamina into the granulosa cells. Theca cells synthesize androstenedione and testosterone from cholesterol, when stimulated by LH. Thus, both LH and FSH are necessary for follicular estrogen biosynthesis.

However, only very small amounts of LH are required during the gonadotrophin dependent phase of follicular growth.

The LH Ceiling Concept

Elevations in serum tonic LH levels during the follicular phase of controlled ovarian superovulation cycles can lead to poor oocyte quality with a reduced fertilization rate. LH is required to assist FSH to stimulate follicular growth normally, but above a ceiling level it may induce follicular atresia.

Clinical Applications

There are currently two recombinant human FSH preparations available: Gonal F (Ares-Serono), and Recagon (Organon)

FSH preparations are used clinically in:
• The treatment of anovulatory infertility.
• Controlled ovarian hyperstimulation in medically-assisted reproduction programs.
• The treatment of male hypogonadotrophic hypogonadism (in combination with hCG).

Treatment of Anovulatory Infertility

- WHO Group-I patients have hypothalamic-pituitary failure. They are amenorrheic with no evidence of endogenous estrogen production. In order to have optimal follicular development, both LH and FSH must be provided. Recombinant DNA technology means that both these hormones are commercially available and can be individually titrated in order to achieve the optimum response.
- Group-II patients have hypothalamic-pituitary dysfunction and present with a variety of cycle disorders including amenorrhea, oligomenorrhea and luteal phase deficiencies. These patients may respond to clomiphene citrate and FSH therapy is normally reserved for patients who do not respond to clomiphene.

Controlled Ovarian Hyperstimulation

The most important application of FSH is to induce the development of multiple follicles. Superovulation has been of fundamental importance to the success of IVF. The aim of superovulation is to increase the number of mature oocytes available for retrieval, thereby improving pregnancy rates by having more choice in the quality of embryos to replace, and having excess embryos for cryostorage.

Successful superovulation requires precise monitoring and adjustment of the FSH dose in order to maximize oocyte retrieval and minimize the number of abandoned cycles. In 1999, a systematic review of 12 randomized controlled trials of r-FSH versus u-FSH in ART showed r-FSH, to have a superior pregnancy rate over u-FSH in IVF.[1]

FSH Versus Human Menopausal Gonadotrophin (hMG) for ART

In the early days of assisted reproduction techniques (ART), hMG was the primary pharmacological agent used to achieve multiple follicular development prior to embryo transfer. A meta-analysis of eight randomized trials in which FSH was compared with hMG for *in vitro* fertilization cycles, has demonstrated that the use of FSH in IVF cycles is associated with a 50 percent higher clinical pregnancy rate than with hMG.[2] The FIVNAT report for 1999 showed that the pregnancy rates in ART were higher for rFSH compared to hMG.

r-FSH IN ART

All the treatment regimes used in ART necessitate an initial period of superovulation. This requires a sustained increase in serum concentration of FSH which overrides the process of single follicle selection and induces development of multiple follicles, thus permitting the collection of a number of mature oocytes which are available for fertilization or replacement. It also provides excess embryos to be cryopreserved, thus overall increasing the chance of pregnancy per stimulated cycle.

Superovulaton is performed with the use of adjuvant GnRH-agonist therapy. This allows the sustained growth of a large cohort of follicles, whilst preventing the spontaneous LH surge.

Daya and Gunby[3] found that treatment with r-hFSH resulted in significantly higher clinical pregnancy rates compared with u-FSH.

r-FSH and GnRH-Agonist

There are two distinct suppression regimens when FSH is used after pituitary suppression with a GnRH –agonist. In the short-protocol, exogenous FSH stimulation starts a few days after the onset of GnRH-agonist treatment. In the long protocol, stimulation with FSH begins only after suppression of endogenous gonadotrophin release as measured by a lack of ovarian activity.

r-FSH and GnRH Antagonists

Unlike GnRH agonists, which initially cause stimulation of the pituitary followed by suppression, antagonists occupy pituitary GnRH receptors to cause immediate suppression. GnRH antagonists can be used as a single dose however most studies have used a multiple dose regimen. Treatment times are shorter, as a result there are fewer intermediate follicles with a lower incidence of OHSS.

A recent randomized, double-blind study has investigated the clinical efficacy of rFSH compared to u-hFSH HP.[4] The results:

- An improvement in the overall response to stimulation
- A higher number of embryos available
- The use of fewer ampules without any increase in OHSS.

WHO Group I Anovulation

Patients with hypogonadotrophic hypogonadism have abnormally low serum gonadotrophins and negligible levels of circulating estrogens. A daily dose of 75 IU r-hLH was found to be effective in promoting optimal follicular development in the majority of the women, in addition for-FSH.

A negative relationship between body weight and serum FSH concentrations was observed and adjustment of FSH dose in relation to body weight can reduce ovarian response variability. There is no correlation between the blood level of FSH and ovarian response and dose adjustments should be made at intervals of no less than 3 to 5 days.

r-hFSH is effective in stimulating follicular development in WHO group I anovulation, but co-administration of LH is mandatory in order to obtain adequate follicular steroidogenesis, demonstrated by estradiol secretion, endometrial growth and luteal phase progesterone secretion.

r-FSH in WHO Group-II Anovulation

The second indication for r-hFSH to be evaluated is the stimulation of single follicular development in WHO group II anovulatory patients administration of r-hFSH resulted in an exponential rise in serum estradiol and immunoreactive inhibin, showing that exposure to endogenous LH is sufficient to support FSH –induced follicular development in WHO group II anovulation.[5] WHO group II patients who did not have PCOS, were studied by Wiedemann.[6] They confirmed the effectiveness of r-hFSH in inducing a mono-or bifollicular ovarian response in 89 of 107 cycles (83.2%) and the pregnancy rate was good (14% per ovulatory cycle).

Prospective multicenter study, comparing the efficacy of r-hFSH and u-hFSH for three consecutive cycles in patients with normogonadotrophic chronic anovulation demonstrated that r-hFSH is more efficient, as illustrated by a significantly higher number of follicles with diameters of over 12 mm and significantly higher median serum estradiol concentration.[7,8] The total dose needed to reach ovulation and the median treatment duration were significantly lower in r-hFSH treated patients. Differences between r-FSH and u-FSH which might explain this increased effectiveness include the isohormone profile,[9] (44) the percentage of degraded FSH forms present[10] the pharmaceutical formulation, contaminative proteins possibly with FSH- inhibiting activity in u-FSH or small differences in the oligosaccharide structure.

In PCOS patients 'FSH-threshold' concept initially put forward by Brown[11] has gained wide support. It emphasized the narrow range of requirements for FSH to initiate follicular growth and led to advise a stepwise administration of increasing amounts of gonadotrophins (conventional **'step-up' protocol**) until the ovarian response is considered to be sufficient, according to ultrasonography and hormone determinations. Later on, other authors[12] suggested a slower and less pronounced increase in gonadotrophin doses to reduce the incidence of ovarian hyperstimulation further. This **chronic low-dose step-up'regimen** is now widely used to induce ovulation in oligomenorrheic women who are infertile.

Since these patients have normal or elevated serum LH levels, addition of LH to FSH treatment is unnecessary. Using a chronic low-dose protocol starting with 75 IU per day for 14 days, increased by 50 percent every seven days thereafter, in cases of no response, ovulation rates of over 60 percent were achieved by this protocol.[13]

Sequential Low-dose Protocol

Dose of FSH is reduced by half when the leading follicle is > or =14 mm diameter.

A modification of the **step-down protocol**, in which 300 IU was given on day one followed by 3 days free of treatment, then 75 IU daily with stepwise dose increments by Balasch *et al* (68SMALL) used more ampules but had fewer cancelled cycles.

RECOMBINANT VERSUS URINARY FSH IN ART[14]

r-hFSH, at an ovarian level is more effective than urinary gonadotrophins in promoting the process of follicular development.

Recombinant Versus Urinary FSH with a GnRH Agonist in a Long-protocol

Prospective, multicenter study compared r-hFSH with u-hFSH in an IVF-ET program.[15] A total of 981 patients who received intranasal buserelin were randomized to treatment with r-hFSH or u-hFSH given intramuscularly. Among patients receiving the recombinant product, a significantly higher number of oocytes were retreived with a lower total dose of FSH (2138 vs. 2385 IU) over a shorter treatment period (10.7 vs 11.3 days; compared with u-hFSH. The number of high-quality embryos was also significantly higher among those receiving r-hFSH. There were no differences between the two groups in implantation rates or clinical pregnancy rates per attempt and per transfer. More embryos were cryopreserved in the group receiving r-hFSH, reflecting the high number of mature oocytes. When frozen embryo cycles were included in the analysis, ongoing pregnancy rates were significantly in favor of r-hFSH (25.5% with r-hFSH vs 20.4% with u-hFSH). The incidence of the ovarian hyperstimulation syndrome (OHSS) was similar in the two treatment groups.

A meta-analysis of three prospective multi-centers, randomized, comparative trials[16] showed that the ongoing pregnancy rate at least 12 weeks after ET per started cycle was 22.9 percent for r-hFSH and 17.9 percent for urinary gonadotrophins.

Comparison of Recombinant with Highly Purified FSH

Is the recombinant product any more effective in inducing multiple follicular development for ART than highly purified urinary FSH?

Results of the first double-blind, randomized comparison of r-hFSH and u-hFSH HP (Metrodin HP) administered subcutaneously in women undergoing ART have been published.[17] Study included 278 pituitary down-regulated patients and found that, among those treated with r-hFSH, there was a significantly higher mean number of oocytes recovered and embryos obtained. In the r-hFSH group the treatment duration was shorter and fewer 75 IU ampules were required. Incidence of severe OHSS was < 1 percent in both groups.

Recombinant FSH is More Effective than Urine Derived FSH in Superovulation Induction for ART

The overall conclusion was that compared with u-hFSH and u-hFSH HP, the use of r-hFSH to induce superovulation in women undergoing ART is associated with more embryos being obtained after the administration of a lower total FSH dose.

The number of embryos in culture is a major determinant in predicting pregnancy outcome.

Zeilmaker,[18] who replaced blastocytes in 265 sequential transfers, found that the chance of having at least one blastocyte to transfer was significantly increased if the woman had more than four oocytes collected. The use of r-hFSH to stimulate superovulation results in a higher number of embryos than with urinary FSH products, the embryos that are not needed for immediate transfer can be cryopreserved.

Choice of Regimen for Superovlation Induction

There is still some controversy as to the most appropriate method of ovarian stimulation.

Starting dose of FSH in normally ovulating women undergoing ovarian stimulation for IVF is usually between 150 to 225 IU/day FSH, depending on the patient's age or previous ovarian response.

Data from two large multicenter studies using r-hFSH for ovarian stimulation in woman undergoing IVF[19,20] indicate that the response to ovarian stimulation using a fixed starting dose of 150 IU r-FSH was similar to that obtained with 225 IU. Devroey suggested recently that a starting dose of 100 IU r-hFSH may be sufficient.[21]

Other studies show that starting dose of 100 IU is actually suboptimal in an unselected ART population.

Another variable in the protocols is the dosing regimen of GnRH agonist. In patients down regulated by a GnRH agonist depot, the total dose of r-hFSH required was 28.4 × 75 IU ampules whereas, in patients given daily GnRH agonists either subcutaneously or intranasaly, only 20.1 and 20.9 ampules, respectively, were used. Results suggest depot administration of the GnRH agonist should not be the route of choice.

Adverse Effects

Occurrence of **OHSS.** However, it has been shown that rFSH is more effective than u-hFSH HP in inducing multiple follicular developments, without any associated increase in OHSS.

Use of urinary gonadotrophin implies limited product consistency with varying amounts of LH and (hCG).[4] Other disadvantages are the theoretical risk of contamination and the limited purity of the product.

Outcome of Pregnancy

A major problem of high-order multiple pregnancy, resulting in pregnancy complications. Incidence of congenital abnormalities does not indicate any increased risk.

Increased Risk of Premature Delivery

Advantages

- Its local tolerance is good after both intramuscular and subcutaneous injection.[22]
- r-hFSH can be injected subcutaneously leading to voluntary self-administration in about 50 percent of cases, contrasting with less than 10 percent in the u-hFSH group.[23]
- Increased purity
- Batch to batch consistency.

A major advantage of r-hFSH is the ability to titrate the dose precisely as it is supplied in ampules of 37.5, 75 and 150 IU, allowing accurate, precise and flexible dosing in ovulation induction and ART. Injection volumes can reduce injection discomfort and pain. Injection syringes are graduated in International Units (37.5 IU–600 IU). Individual dose adaptation is simple, easy and safe and preloaded syringes are also available.

SUMMARY

- r-FSH is highly consistent from batch to batch.
- It is more potent than urinary gonadotrophins, resulting in the availability of more embryos for replacement and cryopreservation.
- r-FSH is associated with a higher pregnancy rate than u-hFSH..
- It is more cost-effective than u-hFSH..
- It is well-tolerated.

The dosing options are easy, safe, effective and convenient.

The use of recombinant luteinizing hormone, gonadotrophin-releasing hormone agonist or human chorionic gonadotrophin to trigger ovulation.

The midcycle luteinizing hormone (LH) surge is a key event in the menstrual cycle. The surge induces the cumulus oophorus mucinification, allowing the oocyte to be released subsequently from the follicular wall. Second, it provokes the resumption of the oocyte meiosis, that is, from germinal vesicle stage to metaphase II. The LH surge triggers follicular rupture, expelling the oocyte from the follicle and leading to its capture by the fallopian tube. It induces a shift in the granulose cell steroidogenic process, changing it from a chiefly estradiol secretory process to a progesterone secretory one forming an active corpus luteum.

Indications for an Artificial Surge

In WHO group-I anovulation; follicular growth induced by a combined administration of follicle-stimulating hormone (FSH) and LH is usually not followed by a spontaneous LH surge. In WHO group-II anovulation; the restoration of follicular growth by FSH administration does not usually lead to a correct timing and adequate amplitude of the LH surge.[24]

In ovulatory patients undergoing stimulation of multiple follicular development by administration of pharmacological doses of FSH before assisted reproductive technology (ART), it has been shown that feedback mechanisms are often disrupted. This leads to mistimed LH surges that are often also blunted.[25,26] The administration of a surrogate LH surge has therefore become a standard procedure in ART.

A third indication for a LH surge surrogate could be in patients undergoing intrauterine insemination with washed sperm (IUI); in such patients the probability of conception appears to be related to the duration of the spontaneous surge.[27]

The Natural LH Surge

The natural surge lasts for about 2 days and is made-up of an ascending phase, a plateau and a descending phase. LH serum levels, when measured by radioimmunoassay (RIA), are about 10 to 20 times the basal LH levels. Together these differences indicate that administration of an equal dose of LH and hCG (in terms of molarity), assuming all other pharmacokinetic properties to be similar (for example, rate and extent of absorption, distribution), will lead to a higher and more prolonged biological signal with hCG than with LH.

Urinary hCG was easier to obtain than LH. Recently hCG produced *in vitro* by recombinant DNA technology has entered the clinical phase of evaluation (Ovidrel). The pharmacokinetic characteristics of the recombinant hCG are very similar to those of the urinary hCG, its efficacy and its safety. It is anticipated that recombinant hCG will become the reference preparation for inducing a surrogate LH surge in most patients.

The widely accepted dose range for hCG is 5000 to 10000 IU as a single injection. The efficacy and safety of the surrogate hCG surge are well established and to date there are no arguments for questioning its use at least in most patients. In humans, recombinant hLH has been tested for triggering final follicular maturation before IVF-embryo transfer (ET). A first pregnancy has been reported.[28]

A comparison was made of recombinant hLH 5000, 15000 or 30000 IU, or recombinant LH 15000 IU followed by 10000 IU 2 days later, with urinary hCG 5000 IU. The low-dose LH appeared to be as effective as hCG for triggering oocyte nuclear maturity. hCG was more often associated with moderate ovarian hyperstimulation than r-hLH. Repeated administration of r-hLH let to higher incidence of moderate OHSS, confirma-

tion that the duration of exposure to LH/hCG is a determinant for development of OHSS.

Recombinant LH had demonstrated promising results in inducing final follicular maturation and may offer some safety advantages in at-risk populations, as those at risk of ovarian hyperstimulation or multiple pregnancy.

Even more important than such advantages as therapeutic products, is clinical relevance and efficacy of these new drugs. r-hFSH has proved to be more efficacious than urinary FSH for ovulation induction in PCOS patients and inducing multiple follicular development in pituitary suppressed women undergoing ART. r-hFSH in combination with r-hLH has also resulted in effective stimulation of follicular growth in WHO group I anovulation. Interestingly, preliminary data indicate that r-hLH used for induction of follicular maturation and early luteinization in women undergoing superovulation with r-hFSH for ART, is a more physiological surrogate surge than urinary hCG and thus would be beneficial in terms of reducing the risk of OHSS.

Currently, both purity and batch-to-batch consistency make r-hFSH the first choice of treatment in infertile women. r-LH appears to be a drug of choice in WHO group-I patients and in selected patients as an ovulation trigger.

Finally, r-hCG is a safe and effective agent in triggering ovulation and it may prove to be a more reliable ovulation inducing agent than urinary hCG.

REFERENCES

1. Daya S, Gunby J. Recombinant versus urinary follicle stimulating hormone for ovarian stimulation in assisted reproduction cycles (Cochrane Review). In: the Coochrane Library, Isssue 1, 2001. Oxford: Update Software.
2. Daya S, Gunby J, Huges EG, Collins JA, Sagle MA. Follicle-stimulating hormone versus human menopausal gonadotrophin for in vitro fertilization cycles: A meta-analysis. Fertil Steril 1995;64(2):347-54.
3. Daya S, Gunby J. Recombinant versus urinary follicle stimulating hormone for ovarian stimulation in assisted reproduction. Hum Reprod 1999;14(9):2201-15.
4. Frydman R, Howles CM, C Truong F et al. A double-blind, randomized study comparing the efficacy of recombinant human follicle-stimulating hormone (r-hFSH/ Gonal-F®) and highly purified urinary FSH

(uhFSH HP/ Metrodin HP ® in inducing superovulation in women undergoing assisted reproduction techniques (ART). Hum Reprod 2000;15 (3):520-25.

5. Van Dessel HJHM, Donderwinkel PFJ, Coelingh Bennink HJT, Fauser BCJM. First established pregnancy and birth after induction of ovulation with recombinant human follicle-stimulating hormone on polycystic ovary syndrome. Hum Reprod 1994;9:55-56.

6. Wiedemann R, Katzorke TH, Schindler A, et al. Low-dose recombinant human follicle-stimulating hormone therapy in World Health Organization group II anovulatory women. 11th Annual Meeting of the European Society for Human Reproduction and Embryology, Hamburg, 1995;abstract 224.

7. Geurts TBP, Peters MJH, van Bruggen JGC, et al. Puregon (Org 32489): human recombinant FSH. Drugs Today 1997;33 (Suppl 1/F):1-25.

8. White D, Fauser BCJM, Ohbrai M, et al. Recombinant FSH (Puregon) is more efficient than urinary FSH (Metrodin) in clomophene-resistant normogonadotropic chronic anovulatory women: a prospective, multicentre, assessor-blind, randomized, clinical tria. Fertil Steril 1998;(In press).

9. Matikainen T, de Leeuw R, Mannaerts B, Huhtaniemi I. Circulating bioactive and immunoreactive recombinant human follicle stimulating hormone (Org 32489) after administration to gonadotrophin-deficient subjects. Fertil Steril 1994;61:62-69.

10. Bergh C, Howles CM, Borg K, et al. Recombinant human follicle stimulating hormone (r-hFSH; Gonal–F) versus highly purified urinary FSH (Metrodin HP): results of a randomized comparative study in women undergoing assisted reproductive techniques. Hum Reprod 1997;12: 2133-39.

11. Brown JB. Pituitary control of ovarian function- concepts derived from gonadotrophin therapy. Aust NZ J Obset Gynaecol 1978;18:47-54.

12. Buvat JB, Buvat-Herbaut M, Marcollin G, et al. Purified follicle-stimulating hormone in polycystic ovary syndrome: Slow administration is safer and more effective. Fertile Steril 1989;52:553-59.

13. Serono Study 5642, data on file

14. Recombinant Human FSH Study Group. Clinical assessment of recombinant human follicle-stimulating hormone in simulating ovarian follicular development before in vitro fertilization. Fertil Steril 1995;63:77-86.

15. Out HJ. Hum Reprod 1995;10;2534-40.

16. Out HJ. Fertil Steril 1997;68:138-42.

17. Frydman R, Avril C et al. 14th Annual Meeting of the European Society for Human Reproduction and embryology, Gothenburg, 1998;Abstract.

18. Scholtes MCW, Zeilmaker Fertil Steril 1998;69:78-83.

19. Thornton SJ. Hum Reprod 1996;11:104.

20. Camier B. 14th Annual Meeting of the European Society for Human Reproduction and Embryology, 1998.

21. Devroe P. Hum Reprod 1998;13:565-651.

22. Out HJ, Reimitz PE, Coelingh Bennink HJT. A prospective, randomized study toassess the tolerance and efficacy of intramuscular and subcutaneous administration of recombinant follicle-stimulating hormone (Puregon). Fertil Steril 1997;67:278-83.

23. Loumaye E, Martineau I, Piazzi a, et al. Clinical assessment of human gonadotrophins produced by recombinant DNA technology. Hum Reprod 1996; 11(Suppl 1):95-107.

24. Seibel MM, Kamrava MM, McArdle C, Taymor ML. Treatment of polycystic ovary disease with chronic low-dose follicle stimulating hormone: Biochemical changes and ultrasound correlation. Int J Fertil 1984;29:39-43.

25. Glasier A, Hillier SG, Thatcher SS, Baird DT, Wickings EJ. Superovulation with exogenous gonadotrophins does not inhibit the luteinizing hormone surge. Fertil Steril 1988;49:81-85.

26. Loumaye E. The control of endogenous secretion of LH by gonadotrophin-releasing hormone agonists during ovarian hyperstimulation for in vitro fertilization and embryo transfer. Hum Reprod 1990;5:357-76.

27. Cohlen BJ, te Velde ER, Scheffer G, van Kooji RJ, de Brouwer CPM, van Zonneveld P. The pattern of the luteinizing hormone surge in spontaneous cycles is related to the probability of conception. Fertil Steril 1993;60:413.

28. Imthurn B, Piazzi A, Loumaye E. Recombinant human luteinizing hormone to mimic midcycle LH surge. Lancet 1996;248:332-33.

• **Thankam R Varma**

28

Role of GnRH-Agonists as an Ovulation Trigger

INTRODUCTION

Since the mid-1970s several authors have reported the use of native luteinizing hormone releasing hormone (LHRH) for the induction of ovulation, with limited success. The LH surge induced by native LHRH was not always sufficient in terms of amplitude and duration to cause the cascade of events leading to ovulation.

In the normal menstrual cycle, the mid-cycle LH and FSH surge (lasting for 48 hrs) is a complex and carefully orchestrated event elicited in the late follicular phase with persistently elevated estrogen concentrations in combination with a small, but distinct, rise in progesterone.[1]

Until recently human chorionic gonadotrophin (hCG) represents the standard management for the substitution of the endogenous LH surge to induce final stages of oocyte maturation in ovarian hyper-stimulation protocols for *in vitro* fertilization. Unfortunately, now it is evident that hCG does contribute to the occurrence of the OHSS, a potentially life-threatening complication.[2-4]

An alternative to exogenous hCG could be the GnRH analog to induce an endogenous rise in both LH and FSH levels due to the initial flare effect.[5, 6] The induction of an endogenous LH and FSH surge is thought to be more physiological compared to with the administration of hCG and may reduce the incidence of OHSS due to much shorter half-life of LH.[8, 9]

Although effective and useful, GnRH-a usage lost interest during nineties, as ovarian hyper-stimulation protocol included GnRH agonist co-administration to suppress premature LH surge during the follicular phase preventing the endogenous LH surge.

GONADOTROPHIN RELEASING HORMONE (GnRH)

The gonadotrophin releasing hormone (GnRH or LHRH) releasing factor was isolated in 1971 by Schally and Guillemin. GnRH is a decapeptide synthesized by the neurons located in the arcuate nucleus and in the preoptic area of the hypothalamus. Through axons of these neurons, it is transported and released in pulses to the portal system of the pituitary, where it binds to gonadotrophin specific receptor. Bonding of GnRH to its receptor produces the conversion of GTP (guanosine triphosphate) into GDP (guanosine diphosphate) through protein G which provides the energy required to increase the intracellular concentration of calcium and of protein-kinase C. This leads to the release of gonadotrophins from the pituitary.

Gonadotrophin secretion depends on the pulsatile secretion of GnRH by the hypothalamus. The pulsatility varies according to the timing of the menstrual cycle. Soonafter the chemical structure of the GnRH molecule was discovered, GnRH analogs were developed, agonists as well as antagonists. Agonists are powerful stimulants of the secretion of gonadotrophins and antagonists are suppressors of the gonadotrophic function of the pituitary.

GnRH agonists are substances which have great affinity for GnRH receptors in the pituitary and their prolonged half-life, makes them more powerful than the natural GnRH. After the initial stimulation, GnRH agonists release gonadotrophins (flare-up effect), after 1 or 2 weeks of continuous administration, they produce a significant drop in FSH and LH concentrations through a mechanism of down-regulation or desensitization.

The modification of the GnRH molecule responsible for the agonist action of analogs occur in the amino acids located in positions 6 and 10. Substitution of glycine in position 10 with a NH_2 ethyl amide terminal increases the potency of the GnRH.

The endogenous LH surge induced by GnRH-a works through an indirect mechanism that relies on the patient's own pituitary reserve and response to GnRH. The GnRH-a induced LH surge has a sharper profile with a higher peak value but a shorter duration than the natural LH surge.[10]

The efficacy and safety of the LH surge induced by GnRH-a was first investigated in WHO Group II anovulatory PCOS patients. These studies showed that the risks of OHSS and multiple births were not totally blunted and demonstrated a high incidence of luteal phase deficiency. Hence, luteal phase support is likely to be required when GnRH-a is used to trigger ovulation.

HUMAN CHORIONIC GONADOTROPHIN

In patients treated with gonadotrophins, the luteinizing hormone (LH) surge is usually absent or attenuated, therefore the administration of human chorionic gonadotrophins (hCG) is required to induce oocyte maturation and ovulation,[11, 12] whereas acute exposure of hCG may replace the LH Surge for the induction of the periovulatory events, it remains to be determined whether hCG exposure alters the normal patterns of the final stages of follicular development, oocyte maturation and corpus luteum function.[13, 14]

Although similar in action to LH, hCG, because of its longer half-life (> 24 hours versus 60 minutes)[15, 16] does not provide a physiologic stimulus that is identical to the endogenous LH surge.[17, 18] Furthermore, by contrast with the spontaneous normal menstrual cycle, where both LH and FSH are secreted at midcycle, administration of hCG results in an increase in LH activity only.

Because of its longer half-life compared to LH, hCG administration, to hMG-treated patients results in multiple corpora lutea, and supra physiological levels of estradiol (E_2) and progesterone (P) throughout the luteal phase. In patients with excessive responses to gonadotrophin stimulation, this sustained luteotropic stimulation may result in "Ovarian hyperstimulation syndrome" (OHSS), the most serious complication related to gonadotrophin therapy.[19-20] Excessive levels of circulating E_2 have been implicated in the relatively high rates of implantation failure and early embryonic loss in stimulated cycles.

hCG has been shown to effectively induce ovulation, final oocyte maturation, and corpus luteum formation. However, hCG can still be detected in the serum for 10 days after the preovulatory bolus injection. Consequently, continued support of the corpus luteum by hCG, elicits supra physiological luteal phase steroid concentrations. Moreover, hCG in the late follicular phase may stimulate the growth of medium-sized follicles which may subsequently ovulate and may cause OHSS in high risk group.[4, 21, 22]

Hyperresponsiveness of the ovary to stimulation, large late follicular phase number of follicles and very high E_2 levels, both exogenous and endogenous hCG have clearly been associated with OHSS.[23-25]

The raised steroid levels in the luteal phase when hCG was given to trigger ovulation, may suppress the release of endogenous gonadotrophins required to maintain corpus luteum support.[26] This situation may have a negative impact on endometrial receptivity hence luteal phase support is necessary.[27, 28]

Exogenous hCG is implicated in the development of multiple corpora lutea and sustained luteotropic effect due to its prolonged circulating half-life compared with native LH which produces high level of E_2.[5, 16, 29]

Until recently, hCG was the only effective therapy available for the induction of oocyte maturation and ovulation in stimulated cycles. The use of native GnRH to trigger a midcycle. LH surge and ovulation is ineffective because it elicits a transient LH surge for only a few hours, which is physiologically insufficient to initiate meiotic maturation of the oocytes and to trigger ovulation. Previous attempts to trigger ovulation with repeated injections or infusion of GnRH in anovulatory women after hMG treatment yielded variable results. [16, 30-32]

GONADOTROPHIN-RELEASING HORMONE AGONIST

The potent GnRH analog (GnRH-a) induces a sustained release of LH from the pituitary gland that may last for 24 hours. This initial "flare-up" effect is followed by pituitary desensitization to further GnRH-a treatment. [33, 34] In 1988, Lewit et al, in their preliminary reports demonstrated the efficacy of one or two GnRH injections to trigger a sustained preovulatory LH/FSH surge, that effectively induced oocyte maturation in patients undergoing ovarian stimulation for the purpose of IVF/ET. [24, 25] None of the patients developed OHSS.

Moreover, when GnRH is used, luteal phase steroid levels seem closer to normo-ovulatory cycles[35] which may improve endometrial receptivity. [27, 28]

GnRH agonists in patients undergoing ovarian hyperstimulation is believed to be more physiological and of special benefit to high responders with an increased risk of developing OHSS; Fauser et al, in 2002[36] reported very high hCG levels lasted for 24 hours (from 12-36 hours after triggering of oocyte maturation) and clearance of the 10,000 hCG required around 10 days.

The Spontaneous LH/FSH Surge in Ovulatory Spontaneous Cycle

Follicle-enclosed oocytes are arrested in the prophase of the first meiotic division until the midcycle LH/FSH surge. The surge initiates a cascade of events that results in germinal vesicle breakdown and reinitiation of meiosis, luteinization of the follicular wall, and eventually, ovulation.

The duration of the normal midcycle LH surge is 48.7 ± 9.3 hours.[1] It's onset occurs abruptly. The normal LH surge can be divided into three phases, a rapidly ascending limb (14 hours), a peak plateau phase (14 hours) and a long descending phase (20 hours). The rate of increase and decrease in the LH concentration is greater than that of FSH. Serum E_2 levels reach a peak at about the time of the onset of the LH surge and decline rapidly. The circulating P level increases exponentially, beginning 12 hours after the onset of the LH surge. It then plateaus for approximately 24 hours preceding ovulation. After follicular rupture (usually 36 hours after LH surge onset), a second rise in the P level and a continuous fall in the E_2 concentration are observed, reflecting an acute shift in the ovarian steroidogenesis in favor of P and the beginning of the luteal phase.

The temporal relationship between the LH surge and human oocyte maturation *in vivo* throughout the human preovulatory period has been studied by Seibel et al.[37] If an oocyte was harvested more than 18 hours after the onset of the LH surge, resumption of meiosis had occurred. Twenty-eight to 38 hours after the onset of the LH surge, preovulatory oocytes in metaphase II were obtained. The studies in humans and monkeys suggest that the threshold duration for the LH surge levels required to reinitiate meiosis appears to be 14 to 18 hours. To achieve metaphase II, oocytes, at the time of follicle aspiration, a LH surge of more than 28 hours appears to be required.[37]

An endogenous LH/FSH surge occurs infrequently or is attenuated in women treated with gonadotrophins, despite persistently elevated levels of E_2.[11] Therefore, administration of hCG is needed to induce oocyte maturation and ovulation. It has been suggested that nonsteroidal factors, gonadotrophin inhibin surge-inhibiting factor and inhibin, present in follicular fluid, are secreted from the ovary and block the surge mode of LH and FSH secretion induced by either a bolus of E_2 or GnRH.[38, 39] However, GnRH-a injection can overcome the block and elicit a LH/FSH surge in ovarian stimulated patients that is comparable in magnitude to that of the normal menstrual cycle.

The GnRH-a Induced LH/FSH Surge

Several regimens for the induction of a pre-ovulatory LH/FSH surge with GnRH-a have been reported and were found to be effective in triggering oocyte maturation and ovulation. These include single or repeated injection of GnRH-a (100-500 mcg) given either subcutaneously or intranasally.

Pituitary and ovarian responses to mid-cycle GnRH-a injection resulted in an acute release of LH and FSH. The serum LH and FSH levels rose over 4 and 12 hours, respectively, and were elevated for 24 to 36 hours. The amplitude of the surge was similar to that seen in the normal menstrual cycle, but the surge consisted only of two phases: a short ascending limb (> 4 hours) and a long descending limb (> 20 hours).

Despite the presence of supra physiological concentration of E_2 before the GnRH-a injection, the dynamics and pattern of ovarian hormone changes in the periovulatory period in ovarian-stimulated women were qualitatively similar to the changes seen in the normal natural cycle. As in the natural cycle, the LH surge was associated with a rapid rise of P and the attainment of peak E_2 levels for the first 12 hours after the injection of GnRH-a. This was followed by transient suppression of P biosynthesis and gradual decline in E_2 level during the 24 hours preceding follicle aspiration. After oocyte retrieval, a second rapid rise of P and a continuous fall in E_2 were observed, reflecting an apparently normal transition from the follicular to the luteal phase in ovarian steroidogenesis.

The Luteal Phase and GnRH-a

Patients given GnRH-a to trigger endogenous LH surge had an apparently normal follicular-luteal shift in ovarian steroidogenesis but had lower circulating luteal E_2 and P levels than did patients injected with an ovulatory dose of hCG.[40] Some of these patients had early luteolysis and a short luteal phase.[40,41] The longer duration of plasma hCG elevation compared with the briefer GnRH-a induced LH elevation may result in higher luteal phase E_2 and P levels. After ovulation, the corpus luteum is dependent on pituitary LH.[42,43]

Prolonged down regulation of pituitary GnRH receptors after a higher dose GnRH-a in the midcycle may result in reduced LH support for the developing corpora lutea, reduced steroidogenesis and early luteolysis. Currently, patients treated with midcycle GnRH-a are given P and E_2 to support the luteal phase. Currently, the dosage of GnRH-a varies between 0.1 mg to 0.5 mg.

Fauser et al (2002)[36] reported that their recent study showed that antagonist can be used to prevent premature LH surge using ganirelix, then used triptorelin 0.2 mg or leuprorelin 0.5 mg to trigger ovulation. They confirmed the luteal steroids were closer to the physiological range, the duration of LH surge was shorter compared with natural cycle (24 h vs 36-48 h respectively). The oocyte quality was good, 72 to 85 percent of oocytes were in metaphase II with good fertilization and embryo implantation rates. Luteal phase was supported.

Parneix et al in 2001[41] studied 231 treatment cycles, control group received hCG, the study group received different GnRH-agonist. They reported GnRH-a produced shorter inadequate luteal phase in the GnRH-a group compared with hCG group. Pregnancy rates did not differ significantly between GnRH-a groups and hCG group. Luteal phase support is recommended for the GnRH-a groups.

All current protocols use GnRH-a 100 to 500 mcg. The minimal effective dose of GnRH-a required to trigger an endogenous midcycle LH surge sufficient to induce oocyte maturation and ovulation, without affecting the normal development and function of the corpus luteum, remains to be established.

Prevention of OHSS and GnRH-a

An important benefit emerging from the use of GnRH-a, rather than hCG, for ovulation induction, is the ability of this therapeutic regimen to prevent OHSS, the most serious complication related to gonadotrophin therapy. The pathogenesis of OHSS is multifactorial, but it clearly is related to the existence of multiple functioning corpora lutea and to the sustained luteotrophic effects of endogenous or exogenous hCG.

Until recently, there has been no means by

which OHSS could be totally prevented because with holding hCG administration results in failure to ovulate and conceive. Follicle aspiration and elective cryo preservation of all the embryos to minimize the risk of OHSS in IVF patients at high-risk of OHSS does not eliminate the syndrome.[45] In 1998, a report was published which suggested that midcycle injection of GnRH-a, Buserelin 500 mcg one or two doses, 8 hours apart is effective, not only for the induction of oocyte maturation and ovulation, but also for the prevention of OHSS in ovarian-stimulated patients.[6,43] It was found that the supra physiological levels of E_2 did not adversely affect the outcome following GnRH-a administration. The serum luteal E_2 and P were much lower than expected and more comparable with the levels found in normal menstrual cycle. This would suggest that many of luteal cysts in GnRH-a treated patients were hormonally inactive, the OHSS in these patients will not develop unless multiple hormonally active corpora lutea are present.

Lewit et al in 1995[43] reported the outcome of 73 treatment cycles involving 44 high responders with a previous history of OHSS and with high estradiol level (> 13,200 P mol/L) on the day of triggering using GnRH-a—None developed OHSS. Luteal support with progesterone and estradiol valerate was necessary to maintain adequate serum levels of these hormones, without such support, precipitous decline in the levels of estradiol and progesterone was observed.

Itskovitz et al in 2000[44] reported that GnRH-a 0.2 mg of triptorelin effectively triggers an endogenous LH surge for final oocyte maturation after ganirelix treatment in stimulated cycles and it prevents OHSS in high responders with more than 20 follicles and high serum E_2 levels (3000 pg/ml), 83 percent of oocytes were in metaphase II—none developed OHSS.

Shalev et al in 1995[45] studied 45 patients divided into groups randomly divided to receive either a single SC injection of 0.1 mg triptorelin or single I.M injection of 10,000 IU hCG, IUI was performed at 24 and 48 hours following the injection. GnRH agonist was found to be as effective as hCG in achieving pregnancy rate, but

GnRH-a group had lower incidence of OHSS, 4 cycles versus 8 cycles in hCG group.

Dong et al in 1999[46] reported that they used GnRH agonist to trigger oocyte maturation and ovulation in PCOS patients using gonadotrophins with E_2 levels of 8379 ± 2958 P mol/L 83.3 percent ovulated and 22.2 percent became pregnant, only one of the 18 cycles ended in OHSS.

Tay in 2002[47] stated that GnRH-a is able to induce an endogenous surge of LH and FSH and the effect may be more physiological than that of exogenous hCG and the incidence of OHSS appeared to be decreased.

BENEFITS AND LIMITATIONS

The currently available data suggest that GnRH-a is an effective alternative to hCG for use in IVF cycles or for the induction of ovulation in anovulatory women. Pregnancy rates in cycles in which oocyte maturation was induced by GnRH-a are similar to the rates observed in hCG cycles.

The use of GnRH-a instead of hCG for ovulation induction has several potential advantages. We are not certain whether midcycle FSH surge plays any major physiologic role in these periovulatory events in primates. The presence of midcycle FSH surge is not obligatory because normal oocyte maturation and ovulation do occur after administration of hCG. It is not sure whether the use of GnRH-a because of its release of endogenous FSH as it occurs in normal cycle, has any advantage over the use of hCG, which has no FSH-like activity.

A potential advantage for the use of GnRH-a instead of hCG for ovulation induction stems from the short (24-36 hours) duration of the LH surge induced by GnRH-a, which provides a more physiologic ovulatory stimulus than the extended surge (approximately 6 days) associated with hCG. This time-limited stimulus can be restricted to the few follicles that are more mature, and thus a lower frequency of multiple pregnancy could be expected in patients undergoing ovarian stimulation for the purpose of ovulation induction.

GnRH-a induced LH surge is associated with lower luteal E_2 and P than that seen after hCG administration. Luteal support and the desired level of E_2 and P could be managed more accurately, thus avoiding the excessive levels of circulating estrogens and theoretically, improving the chances for implantation and pregnancy rates in stimulated cycles.[27, 48]

GnRH-a would not be effective in triggering an adequate LH surge in women with a low gonadotrophic LH reserve for example, hypothalamic hypogonadism, or in cycles where GnRH-a down regulation was used to prevent a spontaneous LH surge or early luteinization.

Oliveness et al in 1996[49] reported the use of GnRH-a to trigger ovulation in patients pre-treated with a GnRH antagonist. Oliveness et al in 2000[50] reported that GnRH-a is a useful alternative to hCG in triggering ovulation especially in high risk patients for OHSS. Shalev in 1995[51] confirmed the benefits of using GnRH-a, decapeptyl, 0.1 mg for triggering oocyte maturation and ovulation even in non-IVF treatment cycles.

The introduction of gonadotrophin-releasing hormone (GnRH) agonists combined with gonadotrophins is considered to be one of the most significant advances in the development of in vitro fertilization (IVF) treatment. However, ovarian hyperstimulation syndrome (OHSS) remains a significant complication of controlled ovarian hyperstimulation. One possible strategy to reduce the risk of this complication would be the use of GnRH agonists instead of hCG to trigger ovulation.

In 1988, Lewit et al reported that GnRH-a is useful to trigger ovulation in patients undergoing ovarian stimulation. They also stated GnRH-a is useful in preventing OHSS. They used 0.2 mg of decapeptyl to trigger ovulation.

Emperaire and Ruffle in 1991[10] stated that GnRH agonist may be an alternative to conventional hCG to trigger ovulation and also to reduce the risk of OHSS and Multiple pregnancy.

The capacity of GnRH agonists to trigger ovulation after gonadotrophin treatment of anovulatory women[10] or to induce final stages of oocyte maturation after ovarian hyperstimulation for IVF has been well established.[5-7, 40]

Several controlled and uncontrolled clinical studies have confirmed the efficacy of GnRH-a for triggering ovulation, pregnancy rates are comparable to those achieved by hCG. The incidence of OHSS, a life-threatening condition appears to be decreased. The recent introduction of GnRH antagonist has led to the renewed interest in the use of GnRH agonist to induce final oocyte maturation, ovulation and subsequent pregnancy.

SUMMARY

The physiologic basis and clinical applications of the use of GnRH-a, rather than hCG, to induce the final stage of oocyte maturation and ovulation in gonadotrophin-treated cycles were reviewed. A single midcycle dose of GnRH-a is able to trigger a preovulatory LH/.FSH surge, leading to oocyte maturation and pregnancy in women undergoing ovarian stimulation for IVF/ET or induction of ovulation. The number of oocytes in metaphase II, the fertilization rate and subsequent pregnancy rate seem to be the same in GnRH-a and hCG treated groups.

The dosage of GnRH-a to trigger ovulation varies from 0.1 to 0.5 mg either single or multiple doses 8, 12 or 24 hours apart. Majority of clinicians tend to use a single dose of GnRHa 0.1 to 0.2 mg.

The potential clinical advantages of GnRH-a over hCG in gonadotrophin-treated cycles include (1) The ability to titrate the amplitude and duration of the L H surge, (2) Better control of luteal steroid hormone levels, (3) a higher implantation rate, (4) a lower rate of multiple pregnancy and (5) a reduced risk of OHSS-one should advocate the use of GnRH-a to trigger ovulation in patients at high-risk for developing OHSS.

REFERENCES

1. Hoff JD, Quigley ME, Yen SSC. Hormonal Dynamics at Midcycle: a re-evaluation. J Clin Endocrinol Metab 1983;57:792-96.
2. Elchalal U, Schenker JG. The Pathophysiology of Ovarian hyperstimulation syndrome-Views and Ideas; Hum Reprod. 1997;12:1129-37.
3. Fauser BC, Devroey P, Yen SSC, Gosden R, Crowley WF, Baird DT, et al. Minimal Ovarian stimulation for IVF: Appraisal of potential benefits and drawbacks. Human Reprod. 1999;14:2681-86.
4. Whelan JG, Vlahos NF. Ovarian Hyperstimulation syndrome. Fertil Steril 2000;73:883-96.

5. Gonen Y, Balakeir H, Powell W, Casper F. Use of Gonadotrophin-releasing hormone agonist to trigger follicular maturation for *in vitro* fertilization. J Clin Endocrinol Metab. 1990;71:918-22.

6. Itskovitz-Eldor J, Boldes R, Levron J, Yohanan E, Kahana L, Brandes J. Induction of preovulatory luteinizing hormone surge and prevention of ovarian hyperstimulation syndrome by gonadotrophin-releasing hormone agonist. Fertil Steril 1991;56:213-20.

7. Imoedemhe DAG, Chan RC, Sigue RB, Pacpaco EL, Olazo AB. A new approach to the management of patients at risk of hyperstimulation in *in vitro* fertilization program. Hum Reprod. 1991;6:1088-91.

8. Shoham Z, Schachter M, Loumaye E, Weissman A, Macnamee M, Insler V. The luteinizing hormone surge-the final stage in ovulation induction: modern aspects of ovulation triggering. Fertil Steril 1995;64:237-51.

9. Kol S, Lewit N, Itskovitz-Eldor J. Ovarian hyperstimulation syndrome after using gonadotrophin-releasing hormone analogue as a trigger of ovulation: causes and implications. Hum Reprod 1996;11: 1143-44.

10. Emperaire JC, Ruffie A: Triggering ovulation with endogenous luteinizing hormone may prevent the ovarian hyperstimulation syndrome. Hum Reprod 1991;6:506-10.

11. Ferraretti AP, Garcia JE, Accosta AA, Jones GS. Serum luteinizing hormone during ovulation induction with human menopausal gonadotrophin for *in vitro* fertilization in normally menstruating women. Fertil Steril 1983;40:742-47.

12. Schenken RS, Hodgen GD. Follicle-stimulating hormone-induced ovarian hyperstimulation in monkeys: blockage of the luteinizing hormone surge. J Clin Endocrinol Metab 1983;57:50-55.

13. Stouffer RL, Hodgen GD, Graves PE, Danforth DR, Eyster KM, Ottobre JS. Characterization of Corpora Lutea in monkeys after superovulation with human menopausal gonadotrophin or follicle-stimulating hormone. J Clin Endocrinol Metab. 1986;62:833-39.

14. Vande Voort CA, Hess DL, Stouffer RL. Luteal function following ovarian stimulation in rhesus monkeys for *in vitro* fertilization: a typical response to human chorionic gonadotrophin treatment simulating early pregnancy. Fertil Steril 1988;49:1071-75.

15. Yen SSC, Llenera G, Little B, Pearson OH. Disappearance rate of endogenous luteinization hormone and chorionic gonadotrophin in man. J Clin Endocrinol Metab 1968;28:1763-1967.

16. Damewood MD, Shen W, Zacur HA, Schlaff WD, Rock JA, Wallach EE. Disappearance of exogenously administered human chorionic gonadotrophin. Fertil Steril 1989;52:398-400.

17. Strickland TW, Puett D. Contribution of subunits to the function of luteinizing hormone/human chorionic gonadotrophin recombinants. Endocrinology 1981;109: 1933-42.

18. Combarnous Y, Guillou F. Martinat N. Functional status of the luteinizing hormone/chorionic gonadotrophin receptor complex in the rat Leydig cells. J Biol Chem 1986;261:6868-71.

19. Itskovitz-Eldor J, Levron J, Kol S. Use of gonadotrophin releasing hormone agonist to cause ovulation and prevent the ovarian hyperstimulation syndrome. In Clin Obstet Gynecol 1993;36:701-10.

20. Golan A, Ron-El R, Herman A, Soffer Y, Weinraub Z, Caspi E. Ovarian hyperstimulation syndrome: An update review. Obstet Gynecol Survey 1989;44:430-40.

21. Sullivan MW, Stewart-Akers A, Krasnow JS, Berga SL, Zeleznik AJ. Ovarian response to women to recombinant follicle-stimulating hormone and luteinizing hormone: A role for LH in the final stages of follicle maturation. J Clin Endocrinol 1999;84:228-32.

22. Loumaye E, Piazzi A, Engrand P. The use of recombinant LH, GnRH agonist or hCG to trigger ovulation. In Shoham Z, Howles CM, Jacobs HS (Eds.): Female infertility therapy current practice. London Dunitz. 1999;125-35,

23. Dahl Lyons CA, Wheeler CA, Frishman GN, Hackett RJ, Siefer DB, Haning RV. Early and late presentation of the ovarian hyperstimulation syndrome. Hum Reprod 1994;9:792-99.

24. Enskog B, Henriksson M, Unander M, Nilsson L, Brannstrom M. Prospective study of the clinical and laboratory parameters of patients in whom ovarian hyperstimulation syndrome developed during controlled ovarian hyperstimulation for *in vitro* fertilization. Fertil Steril 1999;71:808-14.

25. Mather R, Akande AV, Leay SD, Hunt LP, Jenkins JM. Distinction between early and late hyperstimulation syndrome. Fertil Steril. 2000;73:901-07.

26. Gibson M, Nakajima ST, McAuliffe TL. Short-term modulation of gonadotrophin secretion by progesterone during the luteal phase. Fertil Steril 1991;55:522-28.

27. Forman R, Fries N, Testart J, Belaiseh J, Hazout A, Frydman R. Evidence of an adverse effect of elevated serum estradiol concentrations on embryo implantation. Fertil Steril 1988;49:118-22.

28. Simon C, Garcia Velasco JJ, Valbuena D, Peinado JA, Moreno C, Remohi J, Pellicer C. Increasing uterine receptivity by decreasing estradiol levels during the preimplantation period in high responders with the use of a follicle-stimulating hormone step-down regimen. Fertil Steril. 1998;70:234-39.

29. Beckers NG, Laven JS, Eijkemans MJ, Faucer BC. Follicular and luteal characteristic following early cessation of gonadotrophin-releasing hormone against during ovarian stimulation for in vitro fertilization. Hum Reprod 2000;15:43-49.

30. Nakano R, Mizuno T, Kotsuji F, Katayama K, Washio M, Tojo S. "Triggering" of ovulation after infusion of synthetic luteinizing hormone releasing factor (LRF). Acta Obstet Gynecol Scand 1973;52:269-72.

31. Keller PJ. Treatment of anovulation with synthetic luteinizing hormone-releasing hormone. Am J Obstet Gynecol 1973;116:698-705.

32. Crosignani PG, Trojsi L, Attanasio A, Tonani E, Donini P. Hormonal profiles in anovulatory patients treated with gonadotrophin and synthetic luteinizing hormone-releasing hormone. Obstet Gynecol. 1975;46:15-22.

33. Casper RF, Sheehan KL, Yen SSC. Gonadotrophin-estradiol responses to a superactive luteinizing hormone-releasing hormone agonist in women. J Clin. Endocrinol Metab 1980;50:179-1981.

34. Monroe SE, Henzl MR, Martin MC, et al. Ablation of folliculogenesis in women by a single dose of gonado-trophin-releasing hormone agonist: significance of time in cycle. Fertil Steril 1985;43:361-68.

35. Lanzone A. Fulghesu AM, Apa R, Caruso A, Mancuso S. LH surge induction by GnRH agonist at the time of ovulation. Gynecol Endocrinol 1989;3:213-20.

36. BC Fauser D, De Jong F, Oliveness H, Wramsby C, Tay J, Itskovitz-Eldor J, et al. Endocrine profile after triggering of final oocyte maturation with GnRH agonist after cotreatment with GnRH antagonist Ganirelix during ovarian hyperstimulation for in vitro ferti-lization. Clin Endocrinology Metab 2002;87:709-15.

37. Seibel MM, Smith DM, Levesque L, Borten M, Taymor ML. The temporal relationship between the luteinizing hormone surge and human oocyte maturation. Am J Obstet Gynecol 1982;142:568-72.

38. Danforth DR, Sinosich J, Anderson T, Cheng Y, Bardin CW, Hodgen GD. Identification of gonadotrophin surge-inhibiting factor (GnSIF) in follicular fluid and its differentiation from inhibin-Biol Reprod 1987;37: 1075-82.

39. Danforth DR, Hodgen GD. The regulation of pituitary gonadotrophin secretion by gonadotrophin surge-inhibiting factor (GnSIF) and inhibin. In Hodgen GD, Rosenwaks Z, Spieler JM (Eds.): Non-steroidal gonadal Factors: Physiological roles and possiblities in contraceptive development-Norfolk: Jones Institute Press 1988;221.

40. Segal S, Casper RF. Gonadotrophin-releasing hormone agonist versus human chorionic gonadotrophin for triggering follicular maturation in in vitro fertilization. Fertil Steril. 1992;57:1254-58.

41. Parneix I, Emperaire JC, Ruffie A, Parneix P. Com-parison of different protocols of ovulation induction, by GnRH agonists and chorionic gonadotrophin. Gynecol Obstet Fertil 2001;29(2):100-15.

42. Itskovitz J, Boldes R, Levron J, Erlik Y, Kahana L, Brandes JM. The induction of LH surge and oocyte maturation by GnRH analogue (Buserelin) in women undergoing ovarian stimulation for in vitro fertilization. Gynecol Endocrinol. 1988;2(Suppl 2):165.

43. Lewit N, Kol S, Manor D. Itskovitz-Eldor J. The use of GnRH analogue for induction of the preovulatory gonadotrophin surge in assisted reproduction and prevention of the ovarian hyperstimulation syndrome. Gynecol Endocrinol. 1995;9(Suppl 4):13-17.

44. Itskovitz-Eldor J, Kol S, Mannaerts B. Use of a single bolus of GnRH agonist triptorelin to trigger ovulation after GnRH antagonist ganirelix treatment in women undergoing ovarian stimulation for assisted repro-duction, with special reference to the prevention of ovarian hyperstimulation syndrome. Preliminary report: Short communication. Hum Reprod 2000:15(9).

45. Shalev E, Geslevich Y, Matilsky M, Ben-Ami M. Induction of preovulatory gonadotrophin surge with gonadotrophin-releasing hormone agonist compared to preovulatory injection of human chorionic gonado-trophin for ovulation induction in intrauterine insemination treatment cycles. Hum Reprod. 1995; 10(9):2244-47.

46. Dong H, Chen S, Xing F. Application of gonadotrophin-releasing hormone agonist for triggering ovulation in high-risk gonadotrophin stimulating cycles of infertile polycystic ovary syndrome patients. Zhonghua Fu Chan Ke Za Zhi 1999;34(2):94-96.

47. Tay CC. Use of gonadotrophin-releasing hormone ago-nists to trigger ovulation. Hum Fertil (Camb): 2002; 5(1):G 35-37.

48. Gidley-Baird AA, O' Neill C, Sinosich, MJ Porter RN, Pike IL, Saunders DM. Failure of implantation in human in vitro fertilization and embryo transfer patients; the effects of altered progesterone/estrogen ratios in human and mice. Fertil Steril 1986;45:69-74.

49. Oliveness F, Fanchin R, Bouchard P, Taieb J, Frydman R. Triggering ovulation by a gonadotrophin-releasing hormone (GnRH) agonist inpatients pretreated with a GnRH antagonist. Fertil Steril 1996;66(1):151-53.

50. Oliveness F, Cunha-Filho JS, Fanchin R, Bouchard P, Frydman R: The Use of GnRH antagonist in ovarian stimulation. Hum. Reprod. Update 2002;8(3):279-90.

51. Shalev E. Low-dose decapeptyl used to induce a pre ovulatory gonadotrophin surge in non-IVF treatment cycles. Gynecol. Endocrinol 1995;4(Suppl):19-24.

• Mehroo D Hansotia • Jaydeep D Tank

29

Altering Management Strategies in Women with a Poor Response to Ovarian Stimulation

"Look to the essence of a thing: whether it be a point of doctrine, of interpretation, or of practice"!
—Marcus Aurelius Antonimus

Ovulation induction protocols for *in vitro* fertilization (IVF) are constantly under review and revision in an attempt to decrease gonadotrophin requirements while improving follicular recruitment and pregnancy rates. Attention has begun to turn on women who fail to produce an optimal number of follicles in response to ovulation induction.

DEFINITION

A "poor response" in the context of *in vitro* fertilization (IVF) can be defined as a failure to produce an adequate number of mature follicles, and/or a peak estradiol concentration less than a defined minimum." The cut-off points implied in this definition vary between different centers. Many opt to cancel the IVF cycle when their defined minimum concentrations are not reached despite the lack of evidence of improved outcome in subsequent cycles.

The definition of a poor responder varies between IVF centers, but generally includes women who fail to produce an optimal number of follicles (usually less than or equal to 3, of a diameter greater than or equal to 18 mm) in response to ovulation induction or who have a suboptimal number of oocytes retrieved.

PREDICTING A POOR RESPONSE

Predicting ovarian response to stimulation constitutes a pivotal task in the organization of a successful *in vitro* fertilization (IVF) program. In spite of its importance it remains an inexact science to say the least. Several approaches have been taken and we outline a few of them below.

Age

The age of the patient is crucial for the prognosis of an IVF cycle. There are numerous studies, which show that patients over 35 have a poor IVF outcome. Despite normal fertilization rates, this could be due to the higher cancellation rates and reduced number of oocytes and embryos obtained, for these reasons their chances of achieving a pregnancy are significantly reduced.[1,2]

However, if patients over 35 have a good ovarian reserve they will probably respond well, and if they receive 2 or 3 good quality embryos, their chances of getting pregnant are similar to those of patients under 35.[3]

On the other hand, among the poor responders with fewer than 4 oocytes, the pregnancy rates are higher in the younger group of patients.[4]

Baseline Serum FSH

Besides considering the patient's age, it is very important to measure her early follicular phase (days 3-5) basal plasma FSH levels. In our program FSH levels greater than 15 mIU/mL are classically considered to be a bad prognostic factor for ovarian response. The majority of the studies agree on the importance of FSH to discriminate those patients who will have an adequate response to the stimulation and subsequently have higher chances of achieving a pregnancy.[5-7]

Although the data look convincing, it is true that occasionally a patient with a high basal FSH confounds our expectations and responds well to stimulation. Interpretation of the results of this test should never be regarded as final and the ultimate test is always actually stimulating the patient and assessing her response. Other recently published articles have shown that the results of these FSH measurements could be overinterpreted on their predictive value.[8, 9]

Serum Estradiol

Another important hormonal parameter to be taken into consideration is estradiol. There are several studies which have shown that patients with early follicular levels (days 3-5) of Estradiol greater than 80 pg/mL are most likely to have their IVF cycle cancelled because of a poor response.[10]

Other studies suggest that Estradiol should be evaluated in combination with FSH in order to have clear information on the functional ovarian reserve of a patient.[11,12]

Baseline Serum LH

Low levels of LH have also been related with poor ovarian functional reserve. Day 3 LH levels lower than 3 mIU/mL may mean a bad prognosis for an IVF cycle. The FSH/LH ratio also seems to be important and some authors have shown that values of this quotient greater than 3 were usually associated with high cancellation rates.[13]

Inhibin

It is well known that when the functional pool of ovarian follicles reduces, the ovary loses its ability to restrain the pituitary and there is a clear rise in FSH levels. It was thought that this situation can be diagnosed early by the reduction in the inhibin levels.[14] Nevertheless, other studies

suggest that neither inhibin B nor inhibin A is a good marker to evaluate the ovarian reserve and that other tests should be used.[15]

Dynamic Tests

In the majority of cases, basal hormonal estimations are sufficiently informative but sometimes it is necessary to perform dynamic tests. It is vital to gauge the benefit of the information to be gained from the test and the decision that can be taken after the test is performed, before subjecting the patient to any one of the tests.

In our experience, neither the leuprolide test nor the Efort test are necessary, and only the hMG test and the classic clomiphene test are really useful. According to us these tests have a limited value in actually treating the patient.

Ultrasound

The new high-frequency transvaginal transducers with excellent resolution power allow very accurate studies of ovarian morphology and function to be performed. New 3-D equipment is useful to measure the number of antral follicles[15] as well as specific ovarian characteristics such as its volume and vascular supply.[16]

New Diagnostic Possibilities

Among the poor responders there is a 1.2 percent risk of cancellations due to premature luteinization in stimulated cycles under pituitary suppression with GnRH analogs. It has been suggested that stimulated ovaries produce a substance named "gonadotrophin surge-attenuating/inhibiting factor (GnSAF/IF)" which attenuates the LH surge by reducing GnRH-stimulated LH secretion. Bioactivity ascribed to GnSAF/IF is present in steroid-free human serum and follicular fluid in both spontaneous cycles of normally cycling women and stimulated cycles. The production of this substance is regulated during the cycle by the ovary, and it has been hypothesized that GnSAF/IF could also play a role in preventing premature luteinization in stimulated cycles.[17]

A recent study has shown that lower GnSAF/IF bioactivity is detected amongst women with prior premature luteinization during ovarian stimulation under GnRH compared to normally responding patients. This observation could explain the pituitary escape from GnRH downregulation.[18]

ALTERING STRATEGIES FOR POOR RESPONDERS

In the earlier days of IVF cycles, the ovum pick up was performed in natural cycles. It was soon realized that the extremely limited number of oocytes available in such cycles was a major barrier to success in an IVF program. Assisted reproduction took a new turn when drugs which could stimulate the ovary to produce multiple follicles were introduced. Advances and an explosion of literature on the subject of ovarian stimulation have made it a fascinating and complex subject. It is one of the most important clinical aspects of IVF and reminds us all the time that each patient is different and that management has to be individualized.

GnRH-agonists

GnRH-agonists (GnRH-a) were introduced into IVF superovulation regimens in the late 1980s, and have become established as a component of standard regimens in most centers worldwide. Each style of GnRH-a regimen (long, short or ultrashort) is associated with its particular advantages and disadvantages. In general, the "long protocol" approach tends to be the most widely used. There is however, no firm evidence as yet, that the long protocol is superior to the short one. In fact, controversy still exists over the use of long-term desensitization versus a short-term desensitization. A recent study showed that long-term downregulation does not improve pregnancy rates in a general IVF program.[19] Data from the Cochrane review, however, does corroborate with the general feeling that the long protocol is more effective than the short one.[20] Twenty-six trials met the inclusion criteria for the meta-analysis. The common odds ratio (OR) for clinical pregnancy per cycle started was 1.32 (95% Cl, 1.10-1.57) in favor of the long GnRH-a protocol. The studies were subgrouped, depending on

whether, in the long protocol, the GnRH-a was commenced in the follicular phase (8 trials) or luteal phase (16 trials). The respective ORs were 1.54 (95% Cl, 1.11-2.13) and 1.21 (95% Cl, 0.98-1.51). After excluding the four trials using the ultrashort protocol, the OR for long versus short protocols (22 trials) was 1.27 (95% Cl, 1.04-1.56). A comparison of long versus ultrashort protocols (4 trials) produced an OR of 1.47 (95% Cl, 1.02-2.12). On the basis of clinical pregnancy rate per cycle started, this meta-analysis demonstrates the superiority of the long protocol over the short and ultrashort protocols for GnRH-a use in IVF and GIFT cycles.

However, when we look at the data specific for poor responders we find that controversy over the best protocol looms large. Studies both for and against the long protocol are reported. In a study by Belaisch *et al*, an appreciable benefit was shown for women who were poor responders in previous cycles and then put on the long protocol in the subsequent cycles.[21] On the other hand, in a study by Ben Rafael *et al* no appreciable difference was found.[22]

Apart from a preventive effect on the luteinizing hormone (LH) surge, most of the beneficial effects of these molecules are still only partly known. Great variability between protocols hampers our comprehension of the mechanisms involved in the overall clinical improvement seen with this therapy. The hypophyseal desensitization induced by GnRH-agonists is greatly dependent on the dose and duration of their administration, but the residual gonadotrophin secretion is imperfectly estimated by hormonal measurements using radioimmunometric assays. Moreover, the specific role of GnRH-agonist-induced ovarian quiescence on subsequent ovarian responsiveness to gonadotrophins and on endometrial receptivity deserves further investigation.

Finally, a direct ovarian action of GnRH-agonist on steroidogenesis, folliculogenesis and embryo quality is still controversial in humans. These putative deleterious effects of GnRH-agonists have led some authors to recommend a reduction of both dose and duration of GnRH-agonist administration for women identified by a poor response to gonadotrophins. Using this approach, a few reports have recently shown some clinical advantages for ovarian responsiveness, but no convincing evidence for any improvement in pregnancy rate.[23]

In a study to determine whether a controlled ovarian hyperstimulation (COH) regimen that involves GnRH-agonist discontinuation of downregulation, versus a conventional long GnRH-a protocol the study reported the following: In 31 patients with a basal FSH level that was not persistently high, the new regimen resulted in a significantly higher number of retrieved oocytes compared with the standard protocol (7.6 +/– 1.03 versus 4.0 +/– 0.68, respectively). The authors concluded that whereas for most low responders, the new COH regimen offers no further advantage, future prospective studies may demonstrate whether it can confer a benefit for a subset of patients with a basal FSH level that is not persistently high.[24]

Another group used the administration of microdoses of GnRH-agonist to determine if women who previously had demonstrated poor ovarian responsiveness during ovulation induction for IVF would obtain an improved follicular response. This group reported that ovarian responsiveness was enhanced during the microdose GnRH-a stimulation cycle when compared with the previous stimulation cycle. Specifically, the patients had a more rapid rise in E2 levels, much higher peak E2 levels, the development of more mature follicles, and the recovery of larger number of mature oocytes. None of the patients had premature LH surges as evidenced by a significant rise in LH levels or a significant decline in E2 levels. There were no differences in the fertilization rates.[25]

The Role of Recombinant FSH

The introduction of recombinant products has brought great hope. Their potential is only now being realized and they do certainly represent a breakthrough, in scientific technology.

Studies like the one reported by De Placido *et al*, contend that compared to highly purified FSH the recombinant version of FSH gives a much better outcome in poor responders.[26] This study was carried out using the short protocol of GnRH-a. The use of recombinant FSH resulted in a significant increase ($P < 0.05$) in the mean number of mature oocytes (2.4 +/– 1.4 versus 1.7 +/– 0.8), mean peak estradiol concentration (606 +/– 252 versus 443 +/– 32 pg/mL) and fertilization rate (73.0 versus 53.3%). The authors concluded that rFSH in a GnRH-agonist short protocol improves the ovarian outcome in poor responders to FSH-HP with high basal concentrations of FSH.

Hofmann *et al*, recommend FSH in high doses (6 ampules/day: 6FSH) for ovarian hyperstimulation for IVF in women with a previous poor response to stimulation with the equivalent of "4FSH".[27] Luteinizing hormone levels did not differ between stimulations, but both FSH and estradiol levels were higher in the 6FSH compared to the 4 FSH cycles. There were fewer cancellations in the 6 FSH cycles, but similar numbers of preovulatory oocytes were retrieved, fertilized, and transferred. The pregnancy rates per attempt and retrieval were also higher in the 6 FSH cycles. They concluded that raising and maintaining FSH levels during stimulation in low responders reduced cancellations and improved IVF outcome.

A different approach was taken by Rombauts *et al*.[28] They administered recombinant human FSH before the onset of the menstrual period (experimental group) or in the early follicular phase after the onset of menses (control group). Patients in the experimental group were ready for oocyte retrieval on menstrual cycle day 11 instead of cycle day 14. The number of oocytes retrieved was not significantly different between the two groups. This group concluded that poor responders do not benefit from commencing recombinant human FSH therapy in the late luteal phase.

ALTERNATIVE STRATEGIES

Several other approaches have been taken by other workers for these patients.

The outcome of IVF through natural cycles in poor responders was studied in a prospective manner.[29] Eleven patients in whom oocyte retrieval was cancelled or who failed to conceive because of a poor response were included in the analysis. The data for natural cycles (n = 16) were compared with data obtained during previous stimulated cycles (n = 25) in the same women. Out of 16 natural cycles, 13 (81.3%) were scheduled for oocyte retrieval as compared to 13 out of the 25 stimulated cycles (52%). Eighteen metaphase II oocytes were obtained during stimulated cycles, giving a 66 percent fertilization rate. In natural cycles, 11 metaphase II oocytes were available giving a fertilization rate of 78.6 percent. A mean number of 51.5 +/– 25 ampules of gonadotrophins per cycle were used during ovarian stimulation. Three clinical pregnancies were obtained after embryo transfer in natural cycles (18.8%/started cycle) compared to none in stimulated cycles. Although this is a small study and more work is needed on this aspect it offers an interesting alternative to these patients. This may not be the first approach to be considered in IVF, but it may be considered as an alternative after two ovarian response failures using classical protocols of stimulation.

Awonuga *et al* reviewed their experience with IVF using low-dose clomiphene citrate for stimulation in "non" and "poor" responders.[30]

The treatment outcome in 11 non- and 20 poor responders with clomiphene citrate treatment cycles, were compared with the treatment outcome in the previous long protocol buserelin/hMG cycles. The clinical pregnancy rates per oocyte collection achieved in the first clomiphene citrate cycle in non (9.1%)- and poor (10%) responders were comparable to those achieved by poor responders (11.9%) who had buserelin/hMG protocol. Although the numbers were small, a similar pregnancy rate could still be achieved in poor responders up to the third attempt using clomiphene citrate.

A study was performed to assess the effect of oral contraceptive pills (OCP), administered before the initiation of superovulation, on ovarian response and IVF treatment results in patients with previous "low response" to exogenous gonadotrophin stimulation.[31] Contraceptive pills were administered for 28 to 42 days and were immediately followed by Menotropin treatment. The study group (n = 50 cycles) was compared

with the control group consisting of previous cycles (n = 88) of the same women. Significant differences were noted in peak estradiol levels (983 +/– 739 vs 517 +/– 249 pg/mL, P < 0.01, paired Student's *t* test) and the number of preovulatory follicles between the study and the control groups. Thirty-three of the cycles (66%) reached the stage of ovum pick-up, compared with 22 (25%) of the previous IVF cycles in these women. The mean number of oocytes retrieved was 6.1 +/– 3.0 and 2.4 +/– 1.3 in the study and control groups, respectively (P < 0.01; paired Student's *t* test). Embryo transfer (ET) was performed in 62 percent of the treatment cycles and resulted in five clinical pregnancies (16.1% per ET). No pregnancies were recorded in the control group.

The Role of Growth Hormone Therapy

A growing interest in the effect of growth hormone (GH) on ovulation induction for oligo-ovulation and IVF has been stimulated by various animal studies. These suggest that GH may increase the intraovarian production of insulin like growth factor I (IGF I), which in turn amplifies the granulosa cell response to gonadotrophins. In human granulosa cell preparations, aromatase activity, 17 beta-estradiol and progesterone production have all been augmented by IGF I. The GH receptor gene and GH binding sites have also been found in human granulosa cells.

Although limited by small sample size, the Cochrane review failed to demonstrate statistically or clinically significant differences in clinical pregnancy rate with routine use of GH for IVF ovulation induction.[32] The lack of GH effect on the total number of ampules of hMG required for ovulation induction, and the total number of oocytes retrieved per IVF cycle are consistent with this conclusion. Given the expense of GH, these data do not support the routine use of GH for IVF ovulation induction.

In poor responders, the results are slightly more encouraging. Although confidence intervals are wide and include unity, the common odds ratio for pregnancy per cycle of 2.55 suggests that a benefit may be present. This finding is in keeping with a trend towards reduced gonadotrophin requirements among GH treated women. In a recently published multicenter study of GH augmentation for ovulation induction in hypogonadotrophic women (4098), 64 women undergoing treatment, a dose response effect was seen with increasing amounts of GH (4-24 IU every 2 days × 7 injections) reducing the total gonadotrophin requirement from 37.2 to 22.3 ampules. Although this sample is not directly comparable with the IVF poor responder group, these findings add weight to the hypothesis that GH augmentation may improve oocyte yield when numbers have been low in the past. In unselected patients who generally respond well to stimulation, this effect is unlikely to be meaningful.

In confirmed poor responder IVF patients a multicenter randomized double blinded trial is warranted to investigate the effect of GH augmentation. Key elements of design should include the standardization of GnRH-a/hMG/hCG IVF protocol, dose of GH and the definition of a poor responder—< 4 oocytes retrieved in a previous IVF attempt might be appropriate. The primary outcome of live birth rate or if necessary, clinical pregnancy rate, should be defined and measured. Only by considering such outcomes, can this therapy be truly tested. Given the high cost of treatment, one component of this study should also be an economic evaluation.

CONCLUSION

Although several strategies have been outlined for poor responders, the unfortunate fact remains that as yet we have not been able to effectively formulate a strategy for patients who respond poorly to hyperstimulation. However, hope is on the horizon for these patients with large efforts going on all over the globe to tackle this problem.

REFERENCES

1. Hull MGR, Fleming CF, Hughes AO et al. The age related decline in female fecundity—a quantitative controlled study of implanting capacity and survival of individual embryos after IVF. Fertil Steril 1996;65(4): 783-90.
2. Templeton A, Morris JK, Parslow W. Factors that affect outcome of IVF treatment. Lancet 1996;348:1402-06.
3. Alrayyes S, Fakih H, Khan I. Effect of age and cycle responsiveness in patients undergoing intracytoplasmic sperm injection. Fertil Steril 1997;68(1):123-27.
4. Hanoch J, Lavy Y, Holzer H et al. Young low responders protected from untoward effects of reduced ovarian response. Fertil Steril 1998;69(6):1001-04.
5. Belaisch-Allart J. Evaluation De La Reserve Folliculaire. Contracept Fertil Sex 1999;27(4):259-62.
6. Hedon B. Comment Evaluer La Reserve Ovarienne En 1999.
7. Lashen H, Ledger W, Lopez-Bernal A et al. Poor responders to ovulation induction—is proceeding to in vitro fertilization worthwhile? Hum Reprod 1999;14(4): 964-69.
8. Barnhart K, Osherhoff J. We are overinterpreting the predictive value of serum FSH levels. Fertil Steril 1999;72(1):8-9.
9. Gulekli B, Bulbul Y, Onvural A et al. Accuracy of ovarian reserve tests. Hum Reprod 1999;14(11):2822-26.
10. Smotrich BB, Widra EA, Gindoff PR et al. Prognostic value of day 3 estradiol on in vitro fertilization outcome. Fertil Steril 1995;64(6):1136-40.
11. Buyalos RP, Daneshmand S, Brzchffa PR. Basal estradiol and follicle-stimulating hormone predict fecundity in women of advanced reproductive age undergoing ovulation induction therapy. Fertil Steril 1997;68(2):272-77.
12. Evers JLH, Slaats P, Land JA et al. Elevated levels of basal estradiol predict poor response in patients with normal basal levels of follicle-stimulating hormone undergoing in vitro fertilization. Fertil Steril 1998;69(6): 1010-14.
13. Mukherjee T, Copperman AB, Lapinski R et al. An elevated day 3 FSH/LH ratio in the presence of a normal day 3 FSH predicts a poor response to controlled ovarian stimulation. Fertil Steril 1996;65(3):588-93.
14. Seifer DB, Lambert-Messercian G, Hogan JW et al. Day 3 serum inhibin B is predictive of assisted reproductive technologies outcome. Fertil Steril 1997;67:110-14.
15. Pellicer A, Ardiles G, Neuspiller F et al. Three dimensional ultrasound in low responders. Fertil Steril 1998;70(4):671-75.
16. Syrop CH, Dawson JD, Husman KJ et al. Ovarian volume may predict art outcomes better than FSH concentration on day 3. Hum Reprod 1999;14(7): 1752-56.
17. Fowler PA, Templeton A. The nature and function of putative gonadotrophinsurge attenuating/inhibiting factor (Gnsaf/if). Endocrine Reviews 1996;17:103-20.
18. Martinez F, Fowler P, Knight PG et al. Gnsaf/If in patients with prior premature luteinization and/or spontaneous ovulation in stimulated cycles under GnRH suppression in IVF communication presented at the XXIII congress of the sociedad espanola de fertilidad (sef). Sevilla 2000;24-26.
19. Fabregues F, Balasch J, Creus M et al. Long-term down-regulation does not improve pregnancy rates in an in

vitro fertilization program. Fertil Steril 1998;70(1): 46-51.

20. Daya S. The cochrane library, Issue 1, Oxford: Update Software 1999.

21. Belaisch Allart J, Testart J, Frydman R. Utilization of GnRH agonists for poor responders in an IVF programme. Hum Reprod 1989;4(1):33-34.

22. Ben Rafael Z, Bider D, Dan U et al. Combined gonadotrophin releasing hormone agonist/human menopausal gonadotrophin therapy (GnRH-a/hMG) in normal, high, and poor responders to hMG. J in vitro Fert Embryo Transf 1991;8(1):33-36.

23. Hugues JN. Cedrin durnerin IC revisiting gonadotrophin-releasing hormone agonist protocols and management of poor ovarian responses to gonadotrophins. Hum Reprod 1998;4(1):83-101.

24. Dirnfeld M, Fruchter O, Yshai D et al. Cessation of gonadotrophin-releasing hormone analogue (GnRH-a) upon down-regulation versus conventional long GnRH-a protocol in administration of gonadotrophins would benefit poor responders. Fertil Steril 1999;72(3): 406-11.

25. Cummins JM, Yovich JM, Edirisinghe WR et al. Enhancement of ovarian responsiveness with microdoses of gonadotrophin-releasing hormone agonist during ovulation induction for in vitro fertilization. Fertil Steril 1994;61(5):880-85.

26. De Placido G, Alviggi C, Mollo A et al: Recombinant follicle stimulating hormone is effective in poor responders to highly purified follicle stimulating hormone. Hum Reprod 2000;15(1):17-20.

27. Hofmann GE, Toner JP, Muasher SJ et al. High-dose follicle-stimulating hormone (FSH) ovarian stimulation in low-responder patients for in vitro fertilization. J in vitro Fert Embryo Transf 1989;6(5):285-89.

28. Rombauts L, Suikkari AM, MacLachlan V et al. Recruitment of follicles by recombinant human follicle-stimulating hormone commencing in the luteal phase of the ovarian cycle. Fertil Steril 1998;69(4):665-69.

29. Bassil S, Godin PA, Donnez J. The Outcome of in vitro fertilization through natural cycles in poor responders. Hum Reprod 1999;14(5):1262-65.

30. Awonuga AO, Nabi A. In vitro fertilization with low-dose clomiphene citrate stimulation in women who respond poorly to superovulation. J Assist Reprod Genet 1997;14(9):503-07.

31. Fisch B, Royburt M, Pinkas H et al. Augmentation of low ovarian response to superovulation before in vitro fertilization following priming with contraceptive pills. Isr J Med Sci 1996;32(12):1172-76.

32. Kotarba D, Kotarba J, Hughes E. Growth hormone for in vitro fertilization (Cochrane Review). Oxford: The Cochrane Library, Issue 2000;3.

30

Ovarian Hyper-stimulation Syndrome

Ovarian hyperstimulation syndrome (OHSS) is a potentially life-threatening iatrogenic complication seen in women having induced ovulation. It is an acute, reversible condition characterized by massive extravascular fluid exudation, associated with depletion in the intravascular volume and hemoconcentration with its attendant sequelae.

It has been estimated from data collected through the world registries of assisted reproduction, that of the 100,000 cycles that occur annually, about 100 to 200 of these would be associated with ovarian hyperstimulation syndrome.[1] Mild OHSS is seen in 8 to 23 percent of all stimulated cycles, moderate in about 0.005 to 7 percent and severe in 0.008 to 1.8 percent.

OHSS occurs in 2 distinct forms differentiated by their time of onset.[2] Early OHSS is usually seen within a week of embryo transfer–between day-3 to day-7 post-hCG administration; and is associated with an "excessive" ovarian response. Late OHSS–manifesting between days-12 to 17, is related to pregnancy and can even occur in cycles where the ovarian response has not been very high.

CLASSIFICATION

Various classifications have been proposed to define the syndrome as well as to identify prognostic markers, which would help in the management of this condition.

Schenker and colleagues proposed one of the earliest classifications of OHSS.[3] They based their assessment of the severity of OHSS on both clinical as well as laboratory findings (Table 30.1).

TABLE 30.1: Classification of OHSS (Schenker and Weinstein, 1978)
Mild Hyperstimulation
Grade 1–s. Estrogen > 150 microgms/day
Urinary pregnanediol > 10 mgs /day
Grade 2–Grade 1 with ovarian enlargement/small cysts
Moderate Hyperstimulation
Grade 3–Grade 2 with abdominal distension
Grade 4–Grade 3 with gastrointestinal symptoms–nausea/ vomiting/diarrhea
Severe Hyperstimulation
Grade 5–Grade 4 with large ovarian cysts and ascites or hydrothorax
Grade 6–Grade 5 with hemoconcentration, with or without coagulation defects

Golan *et al* proposed another classification almost 10 years later.[4] They defined 5 grades of the syndrome, classified into mild, moderate and severe OHSS (Table 30.2).

A third classification that was proposed in 1992 by Daniel Navot *et al*,[5] only defined two types of severe hyperstimulation; mild and moderate forms were not considered at all (Table 30.3).

ETIO-PATHOGENESIS

The pathophysiology of ovarian hyperstimulation is very complex and poorly understood.

The basis is an excessive secretion of vasoactive mediators produced by artificially stimulated ovaries. Some of the mediators involved include

TABLE 30.2: Classification of OHSS (Golan *et al*, 1989)

Mild Hyperstimulation
Grade 1–Abdominal distension and discomfort
Grade 2–Grade 1 with gastrointestinal symptoms–nausea, vomiting, diarrhea; ovaries enlarged up to 5 to 12 cms.
Moderate Hyperstimulation
Grade 3–Features of mild hyperstimulation with ultrasonic evidence of ascites.
Severe hyperstimulation
Grade 4–Features of moderate hyperstimulation with clinical ascites and/or hydrothorax and respiratory difficulties.
Grade 5–All of the above with change in blood volume, increased blood viscosity, hemoconcentration, coagulation defects and reduced renal perfusion.

prolactin; prostaglandins; cytokines; prorenin-renin-angiotensin system; VEGF; angiogenin; the Kinin-Kallikrein system; VCAM and ICAM; selections; von Willebrand factor; and endothelin.[6]

Though elevated serum estradiol levels almost always accompany the cascade of events leading to the development of this syndrome, the exact role of estrogen is still debatable. Some studies have suggested that the high serum Estradiol concentration increases endothelial nitric oxide and prostacyclin release; substances that cause vasodilatation, and this contributes a large extent to the circulatory dysfunction that is seen in OHSS.[7-9]

Another theory involves the ovarian renin-angiotensin enzyme system which when activated

TABLE 30.3: Classification of OHSS (Daniel Navot *et al*, 1992)

Severe OHSS
• Clinical ascites, sometimes hydrothorax
• Hemoconcentration–characterized by hematocrit > 45 percent, TC > 15000/ml
• Oliguria with normal serum creatinine
• Liver dysfunction
• Anasarca
• Ovarian size usually > 12 cm
Critical OHSS
• Tense ascites
• Worsening hemoconcentration–hematocrit > 55 percent, TC > 25000/ml
• Oliguria with elevated serum creatinine
• Renal failure
• Thromboembolic phenomena
• Ovarian size > 12 cm

by gonadotrophin stimulation increases vascular permeability.[10]

These basic events, especially the increased capillary permeability and the arteriolar vasodilatation in the enlarged ovaries, leads to extravasation of fluid into the peritoneal cavity, and transmission of these same mediators, which would then produce similar reactions in other parts of the body. But other studies have shown that the ascites may originate from extraovarian sites.[11]

COMPLICATIONS

OHSS is a serious complication of ovarian stimulation with a potentially fatal outcome. Some of the complications seen include adult respiratory distress syndrome, thromboembolic phenomena, prerenal failure, adnexal torsion etc. (Table 30.4).

TABLE 30.4: Complications associated with OHSS

1. Vascular–thromboembolic phenomena, DIC
2. Abnormal liver functions
3. Respiratory–adult respiratory distress syndrome secondary to pleural effusion or massive ascites.
4. Renal–prerenal failure, pressure effects like hydro-ureter due to compression by the enlarged ovaries.
5. Gastrointestinal–ascites, intraperitoneal hemorrhage.
6. Ovarian–torsion, rupture.

MONITORING

Moderate and severe degrees of OHSS require hospitalization for close monitoring and supportive therapy.

This is one of the most important aspects of therapy for OHSS. Proper monitoring will not only help to identify early complications, but will also assess the degree of severity (Table 30.5). This would include vital signs, regular weighing, abdominal girth, urine output, hematocrit, white cell count and liver and renal function tests. In critical cases invasive hemodynamic monitoring may be required. Ultrasonography will help to determine the severity and the progression of the condition. There may be a role for the assessment of plasma prekallikrein levels, as activation of the plasma kinin system may precede the occurrence of thrombosis.[12] Serum cytokine levels correlate with the progression of the disease and may be used for prognosis,[13] but its advantage over traditional prognosticators like hematocrit is yet to be determined.

TABLE 30.5: Monitoring moderate and severe OHSS
• Regular periodic assessment of vital signs (TPR, BP) • Daily weight recording • Daily abdominal girth measurement • I/O chart • Renal and liver function tests • Hematocrit • Total and differential counts • Coagulation profile • Ultrasound abdomen/pelvis

SUPPORTIVE THERAPY FOR OHSS

Supportive management of OHSS is usually medical, and only very rarely is surgery required.

Medical treatment is based on the maintenance of the intravascular volume and the prevention or/and treatment of any coagulation defects.

Fluid Balance

Correction of the intravascular volume depletion is initially done using intravenous normal saline. Colloidal solutions including 20 percent albumin have also been widely used. However, a recent study published by the Cochrane group suggested that the use of albumin in critically ill-patients– with burns and hypovolemia was associated with increased mortality. However, the significance of this statement in relation to the use of albumin in OHSS is still unclear.[14] The restriction of salt and water is not advocated.

Anticoagulants

Heparin may be administered if there is an abnormal clotting profile to reduce the risk of thromboembolism.

Ionotropes

Dopamine infusion may become necessary if there is renal hypoperfusion, as indicted by oliguria.

Diuretics

The routine use of diuretics is not advised as further depletion of the intravascular volume could only worsen the hypotension and its sequelae. These drugs are to be used in only two clinical conditions associated with OHSS–if there is pulmonary edema and if there is persistent oliguria despite adequate expansion of the intravascular volume.[15, 16]

Other drugs that have been used, though with questionable efficacy include prostaglandin synthetase inhibitors, danazol, antihistamines etc.

Paracentesis

The aspiration of ascitic fluid may be necessary in certain situations; especially when the ascites is the cause of respiratory distress; is associated with pain abdomen; or, when it is the cause of reduced renal perfusion leading to oliguria despite intravascular volume maintenance.[17] More often, in current practice, paracentesis is offered only when OHSS is unresponsive to medical therapy.

The procedure may be carried out either transabdominally or transvaginally,[18] with adequate monitoring, asepsis and fluid replacement. Ascitic fluid in OHSS not only contains large quantities of proteins, but also proinflammatory cytokines.[19] While the removal of the latter accelerates recovery, removal of the former may lead to severe hypoproteinemia. Some studies have suggested autotransfusion of the ascitic fluid to replace the lost protein. This however must be must be viewed rather cautiously as there will be a distinct possibility of transfusing vasoactive mediators into the general circulation.

An acceptable alternative treatment for the ascites associated with OHSS is the percutaneous placement of a pigtail catheter; its main advantage is that it removes the need for multiple abdominal or vaginal paracentesis in severe OHSS.[20]

Ovarian mutilating surgery is not an option for the treatment of OHSS, except when there is evidence of tissue necrosis after torsion. Some of the other indications for surgery in OHSS would include intraperitoneal hemorrhage, rupture of an ovarian cyst or when the OHSS is associated with an ectopic pregnancy. Laparotomy or laparoscopy may be attempted in these cases depending upon the situation and the condition of the patient.

PREDICTING OHSS

Identifying risk factors for OHSS is very important, as it would help to direct or target preventive measures to those high-risk cycles. Some of the pretreatment risk factors are listed in Table 30.6.

TABLE 30.6: Pretreatment risk factors for OHSS
• Young women—less than 35 years of age
• Thin women with a low body mass index
• Polycystic ovarian disease
• Oligomenorrheic anovulation

In addition to the above-mentioned factors are those that become apparent during the treatment cycle (Table 30.7). These would include the type of drugs used; for example, a higher incidence of OHSS has been noted with the use of human menopausal gonadotrophin than with FSH or the recombinant gonadotrophins. A rapid rise in plasma estradiol (E2) levels, 'high' peak plasma E2 levels and 'large' numbers of ovarian follicles and oocytes retrieved have traditionally been used to identify cycles at risk of OHSS. However, the criteria used here are mostly arbitrary and have yielded variable results in predicting OHSS.[21]

TABLE 30.7: Risk factors during the treatment cycle
1. Type of drug used—hMG
2. Absolute serum estradiol concentration- > 2500 pg/ml
3. D9 serum estradiol concentration > 800 pg/ml
4. Rise in serum estradiol concentration by 50 percent or more over 24 hours
5. Ultrasound appearance of the ovary on the day of hCG administration
6. Serum cytokines
7. Serum vascular endothelial growth factor

Plasma estradiol concentrations on the day of hCG administration have been used to predict the risk of OHSS; the risk is supposed to be higher when the estradiol levels are more than 2500 pg/ml, and lower when the level is less than 1000 pg/ml. However, serial monitoring of E2 concentrations has not proven to be infallible, as OHSS has also been reported with E2 levels of 1500 pg/ml. But, a factor that can be considered to be a little more accurate is the rate of rise in E2 concentration; the risk increasing if the values rise by more that 50 percent in 24 hrs.

More recently estradiol assessment on the Day 9 of the menstrual cycle has been found to have a better predictive value. An E2 level of more than 800 pg/ml suggests an increased risk of an exaggerated ovarian response, but does not correlate with implantation or pregnancy rates.[22]

The ultrasound appearance of the ovaries on the day of hCG administration is another parameter used to predict the risk of developing OHSS. Mild OHSS is seen when there are a large number of intermediate follicles (9 to 15 mm), while severe OHSS is seen when there are more small follicles (5 to 8 mm).[23]

Recent trends involve the measurement of the serum cytokines and the vascular endothelial growth factor {VEGF} after administration of the ovulatory hCG.[24, 25]

Accurately predicting OHSS continues to remain one of the major obstacles in prevention of this catastrophe.

Prevention

As there is no definite treatment for OHSS, prevention is the most important aspect of management.[26] Accurate prediction of risk can target the preventive measures to specific cycles. And while various methods have been studied for the prevention of OHSS, the ideal one remains elusive. Till then, reproductive biologists over the world constantly develop, study and refine these techniques (Table 30.8).

TABLE 30.8: Prevention of OHSS
1. Cycle cancellation
2. Coasting or controlled drift
3. Drugs— • GnRH analogs
• GnRH antagonists
• Recombinant LH
• Insulin sensitizers—metformin
• i.v albumin 20 percent
• ACE inhibitors + angiotensin II receptor blocker
• Glucocorticoids
• Progestogens
4. Ultrasound guided follicular aspiration
5. Elective embryo cryopreservation and transfer in subsequent cycle

Prevention of OHSS can be attempted either before administration of the ovulatory hCG or after. While prevention before the ovulatory trigger may reduce the incidence of both early and late onset OHSS, measures adopted after the ovulatory trigger may not be very efficacious for early onset OHSS.

Prior to the administration of hCG, if a definite risk has been identified, one option would be to cancel the treatment cycle by withholding the hCG. This would however mean that the cycle would be "wasted", and involve additional emotional and financial trauma to the patient. Also it must be remembered that spontaneous LH surges could still result in ovulation and the subsequent development of OHSS. This method is rarely used nowadays.

Another option would be "controlled drift" or "coasting"–here further gonadotrophin stimulation is stopped and administration of the ovulatory trigger is deferred till the estradiol concentration has returned to "safe" levels. While there is growing evidence to support this method, there is no clear criteria on when coasting should be started and when it should be stopped. Based on collected data, the general consensus is that coasting should be initiated when the serum estradiol levels exceed 3000 pg/ml but not unless the leading follicles are 15 to 18 mm in diameter; the duration should not exceed 4 days as reduced implantation and pregnancy rates are seen when the coasting is done for longer periods of time. Along with this the hCG administration should be withheld till the serum estradiol levels fall below 3000 pg/ml. These guidelines result in an acceptably low incidence of severe OHSS (< 2%) and provide satisfactory fertilization and pregnancy rates (55-71 and 36.5-63% respectively).[27]

GnRh analogs have been used to trigger ovulation by initiating the "flare" response. This reduces the incidence of OHSS without any deleterious effects on fertilization, implantation or pregnancy rates. However, this method is applicable in gonadotrophin only cycles or when GnRH antagonists are used.

Even the continued administration of GnRH analog for 1 week after the hCG trigger was found to significantly reduce the incidence of "early"

OHSS in cycles where the embryos were electively cryopreserved. This protocol, apart from being very effective, is also safe and cheap.[28]

GnRH antagonists have also been studied in their capacity to reduce the incidence of OHSS. Interestingly, it was found that while Ganirelix did not increase the incidence of OHSS, Cetrorelix had a definite beneficial effect in reducing the incidence.[29]

A single dose of recombinant LH has also been used successfully to trigger ovulation and reduce the incidence of OHSS when compared to hCG.[30]

A recent study conducted by Visnova H et al indicated that the use of insulin sensitizers along with the stimulation protocol in women with polycystic ovarian disease significantly reduces the incidence of hyperstimulation without affecting the quality of oocytes by reducing the intraovarian estrogen levels.[31]

Prevention at the time of oocyte recovery would mean aspiration of all the follicles present. Though this can cause intrafollicular hemorrhage, which can affect ovarian response in subsequent cycles.

20 percent albumin infusion at the time of oocyte recovery has been used with considerable success in preventing OHSS. This will not only maintain the intravascular volume, but also help to sequester the vasoactive substances released by the corpora lutea. The cochrane review carried out in 2002 also shows a clear benefit of administration of IV albumin at the time of oocyte retrieval.[32]

A combination of angiotensin converting enzyme inhibitor (ACEI) and angiotensin II receptor blocker has also successfully been used to prevent OHSS. These drugs are administered for 8 days starting just after oocyte retrieval. While the incidence of early OHSS was significantly reduced, further studies are needed to prove the clinical efficacy of this combination.[33]

Embryo cryopreservation and transfer in subsequent cycles is an accepted method of avoiding the "late" onset OHSS.

I.V. glucocorticoids given at the time of oocyte recovery has also been tried as a preventive measure, albeit without much success. A more recent study assessed the effect of oral

Methylprednisolone on the incidence of OHSS in women with PCOS undergoing COH. OHSS was seen in a significantly lower proportion of Methylprednisolone recipients than in untreated patients (10.0% vs 43.9%). Treatment recipients also had more oocytes retrieved and more embryos fertilized than did untreated participants.[34]

Progestogens for luteal support rather than hCG has been found to reduce the incidence of OHSS.

Comparative studies have been carried out between some of the popular methods of preventing OHSS that are in vogue today. One study compared–IV albumin and "coasting". Coasting was found to be as effective as i.v. albumin in preventing OHSS in high-risk patients but yielded inferior pregnancy rates. Early coasting is as successful as late coasting in preventing OHSS with similar IVF outcome.[35] A Cochrane review carried out in 2002, assessed and found no difference in the incidence of OHSS when the embryos were electively cryopreserved or IV albumin was given at the time of oocyte retrieval.[36]

What must be remembered is that despite the innumerable drugs/protocols that have been proposed for the prevention of OHSS, large scale multicentric randomized trials are necessary to prove their efficacy and safety. However, from the available techniques, it does appear that reducing the risk of OHSS prior to the administration of hCG is best done by coasting or the use of alternative ovulatory triggers such as GnRH analogs or recombinant LH. After the administration of hCG probably the best methods available today are the i.v. infusion of 20 percent albumin and elective cryopreservation of embryos.

REFERENCES

1. Schenker J G, Ezra Y. Fertil Steril 1994;61:411-22.
2. Dahl Lyons CA. Wheeler CA, Frishman GN et al. Early and late presentation of the ovarian hyperstimulation syndrome: Two distinct entities with different risk factors. Hum. Reprod 1994;9:792-99.
3. Schenker and Weinstein: Fertil Steril 1978;30:255-68.
4. Golan A et al. Ovarian hyperstimulation syndrome–an update review. Obstet Gynecol Surv 1989;44: 430-40.
5. Daniel Navot et al. Ovarian hyperstimulation syndrome in novel reproductive technologies: Prevention and treatment. Fertil. Steril 1992;58:249-61.
6. Delvigne A, Rozenberg S. Systematic review of data concerning etiopathology of ovarian hyperstimulation syndrome. Int J Fertil Womens Med 2002;47(5): 211-26.
7. Hayashi T, Fukuto JM, Ignarro LJ, Chaudhuri G. Basal release of nitric oxide from aortic rings is greater in female rabbits than in male rabbits: Implications for atherosclerosis. Proc Natl Acad Sci USA. 1992;89: 11259-63.
8. Karpati L, Chow FP, Woollard ML, Hutton RA, Dandona P. Prostacyclin-like activity in the female rat thoracic aorta and the inferior vena cava after ethinyl estradiol and norethisterone. Clin Sci. 1980;59:369-72.
9. Conrad KP, Joffe GM, Kruszyna H, Kruszyna R, Rochelle LG, Smith RP et al. Identification of increased nitric oxide biosynthesis during pregnancy in rats. FASEB J 1993;7:566-71.
10. Bergh PA, Navot D. Ovarian hyperstimulation syndrome: A review of pathophysiology. J Assist Reprod Genet 1992;9:429-38.
11. Yarali H, Fleige-Zahradka BG, Yuen BH, McComb PF. The ascites in the ovarian hyperstimulation syndrome does not originate from the ovary. Fertil Steril 1993;59:657-61.
12. Kodama H, Takeda S, Fukuda J et al. Activation of plasma kinin system correlates with severe coagulation system disorders in patients with ovarian hyperstimulation syndrome. Hum Reprod. 1997;12:891-95.
13. Abramov Y, Schenker JG, Lewin A et al. Plasma inflammatory cytokines correlate to the ovarian hyperstimulation syndrome. Hum. Reprod 1996;11: 1381-86.
14. Abramov Y, Schenker JG, Lewin A et al. Plasma inflammatory cytokines correlate to the ovarian hyperstimulation syndrome. Hum. Reprod. 1996;11: 1381-86.
15. Balasch J, Fabregues F, Arroyo V et al. Treatment of severe ovarian hyperstimulation syndrome by a conservative medical approach. Acta Obstet Gynecol Scand 1996;75:662-67.
16. Navot D, Bergh PA, Laufer N.Ovarian hyperstimulation syndrome in novel reproductive technologies: prevention and treatment. Fertil Steril 1992;58:249-61.
17. Jenkins JM, Mathur RS, Cooke ID. The management of severe ovarian hyperstimulation syndrome. Br J Obstet Gynaecol 1995;102:2-5.
18. Aboulghar MA et al. Ultrasonically guided vaginal aspiration of ascites in the treatment of severe OHSS. Fertil Steril 1990;53:933.
19. Revel A, Barak V, Lavy Y et al. Characterization of intraperitoneal cytokines and nitrites in women with severe ovarian hyperstimulation syndrome. Fertil Steril 1996;66:66-71.
20. Abuzeid MI, Nassar Z, Massaad Z, Weiss M, Ashraf M, Fakih M. Pigtail catheter for the treatment of ascites

associated with ovarian hyperstimulation syndrome. Hum Reprod 2003;18(2):370-73.

21. Mathur RS, Joels LA, Akande AV et al. The prevention of ovarian hyperstimulation syndrome. Br. J. Obstet. Gynaecol 1996;103:740-46.

22. HO HY, Lee RK, Lin MH, HwuYM. Estradiol level on day 9 as a predictor of risk for ovarian hyper response during controlled ovarian hyperstimulation. J Assist Reprod Genet 2003;20(6):222-26.

23. Blankstein J et al. OHSS prediction by the number and size of preovulatory follicles. Fertil Steril 1987;47:597.

24. Mathur RS, Bansal AS, Jenkins JM. The possible role of the immune system in the etopathogenesis of ovarian hyperstimulation syndrome. Hum Reprod 1997;12:2629-34.

25. Wang Q, Yang G, Yang C, Zhan B, Yang R. The predictive role of vascular endothelial growth factor and estradiol in infertile patients with ovarian hyperstimulation syndrome. Sichuan Da Xue Xue Bao Yi Xue Ban. 2003;34(3):565-67.

26. Navot D et al. OHSS in novel reproductive technologies. Prevention and treatment. Fertil Steril 1992;58:249.

27. Levinsohn-Tavor O, Friedler S, Schachter M, Raziel A, Strassburger D, Ron-El R.Coasting-what is the best formula? Hum Reprod. 2003;18(5):937-40.

28. Endo T, Honnma H, Hayashi T, Chida M, Yamazaki K, Kitajima Y, et al. Continuation of GnRH agonist administration for 1 week, after hCG injection, prevents ovarian hyperstimulation syndrome following elective cryopreservation of all pronucleate embryos. Hum Reprod 2002; 17(10):2548-51.

29. Ludwig M, Katalinic A, Felberbaum RE, Diedrich K. Safety aspects of gonadotrophin-releasing hormone antagonists in ovarian stimulation procedures: Ovarian hyperstimulation syndrome and health of children born. Reprod Biomed Online 2002;5(Suppl 1)(3):61-67.

30. Aboulghar MA, Mansour RT. Ovarian hyperstimulation syndrome: Classifications and critical analysis of preventive measures. Hum Reprod Update. 2003; 9(3):275-89.

31. Visnova H, Ventruba P, Crha I, Zakova J. Importance of sensitization of insulin receptors in the prevention of ovarian hyperstimulation syndrome). Ceska Gynekol. 2003;68(3):155-62.

32. Aboulghar M, Evers JH, Al-Inany H. Intravenous albumin for preventing severe ovarian hyperstimulation syndrome: A Cochrane review. Hum Reprod 2002; 17(12): 3027-32.

33. Aboulghar M, Evers JH, Al-Inany H. Intravenous albumin for preventing severe ovarian hyperstimulation syndrome: A Cochrane review. Hum Reprod 2002; 17(12): 3027-32.

34. Lainas T, Petsas G, Stavropoulou G, Alexopoulou E, Iliadis G, Minaretzis D. Administration of methylprednisolone to prevent severe ovarian hyperstimulation syndrome in patients undergoing *in vitro* fertilization. Fertil Steril 2002;78(3):529-33.

35. Chen CD, Chao KH, Yang JH, Chen SU, Ho HN, Yang YS. Comparison of coasting and intravenous albumin in the prevention of ovarian hyperstimulation syndrome. Fertil Steril 2003;80(1):86-90.

36. D'Angelo A, Amso NN. Embryo freezing for preventing ovarian hyperstimulation syndrome: A Cochrane review. Hum Reprod. 2002;17(11):2787-94.

• Manish Banker • Pravin Patel
• Bharat Joshi • Riddhi Marfatia

31

Ovulation Induction and Ovarian Malignancy

INTRODUCTION

There have been quite a few reports in recent literature raising concern over the possible association between superovulation and ovarian cancer. Most of these reports, however, are isolated case reports. Moreover, the established relation between infertility, low parity and ovarian cancer has made it very difficult to confirm an association. Such an association, if confirmed, will have far-reaching repercussions. Several questions need to be answered before any conclusions can be drawn.

• Is there an independent association between the use of fertility medications and ovarian cancer?
• Are there other factors that can contribute to this ?
• Is there any evidence to the contrary ?

CASE REPORTS

The first case of invasive epithelial ovarian cancer associated with ovulation induction was described by Bamford and Steel[1] in 1982. Since then many other reports have been published describing an association between infertility medication and ovarian cancer or tumors of low malignant potential (Tables 31.1 and 31.2). Both clomiphene and hMG have been found to be associated with the occurrence of ovarian cancer. These are isolated case reports and not controlled studies. The patient population, duration of treatment and the dose of drugs are, however, variable in all these reports.

HYPOTHESES FOR OCCURRENCE OF OVARIAN CANCER

Incessant Ovulation

Fathalla,[11] in 1971, proposed that the etiology of ovarian cancer was related to "incessant ovulation". The ovarian surface epithelium is subject to minor injury during each ovulation. The cumulative effect of repetitive surface injury was thought to contribute to the development of ovarian neoplasm.

TABLE 31.1: Clomiphene citrate and ovarian tumors			
Author	*Year*	*Drug*	*Pathology*
Atlas and Menczer[2]	1982	Clomiphene citrate "repeatedly"	Serous, low malignant potential
Ben-Hur et al[3]	1986	Clomiphene citrate "repeatedly"	Serous, low malignant potential
Ben-Hur et al[3]	1986	Clomiphene citrate 3 cycles	Serous
Kulkarni and McGarry[4]	1989	Clomiphene citrate 3 cycles	Serous
Diett[5]	1991	Clomiphene citrate 1 year	Serous
Balasch and Barri[6]	1993	Clomiphene citrate 6 cycles	Serous, low malignant potential
Karlan[7]	1994	Clomiphene citrate 5 cycles	Serous

TABLE 31.2: Gonadotrophins and ovarian tumors			
Author	*Year*	*Drug*	*Pathology*
Goldberg and Runowicz[8]	1992	hMG (IVF 2 cycles)	Serous, low malignant potential
Goldberg and Runowicz[8]	1992	hMG (IVF 3 cycles)	Serous, low malignant potential
Goldberg and Runowicz[8]	1992	hMG 2 cycles	Serous, low malignant potential
Nijman *et al*[9]	1992	hMG (IVF 2 cycles)	Serous, low malignant potential
Grimbizis *et al*[10]	1995	hMG (IVF 7 cycles)	Serous, low malignant potential

Inclusion Cysts

Zajicak[12] postulated that with ovulation, epithelial inclusion cysts developed in the ovarian surface epithelium. These inclusion cysts may be the source of neoplasia.

Ovulatory Age

Casagrande *et al*[13] in 1979, proposed a relationship between ovarian cancer risk and "ovulatory age". This was based on the theory that the number of ovulatory cycles between menarche and menopause is directly proportional to a woman's risk of ovarian cancer. Any period of anovulation, either due to oral contraceptive pills or pregnancy, is considered "protected time" and is subtracted from the menarche to menopause time interval to yield a woman's ovulatory age.

Stimulation of Epithelial Inclusion Cyst

Cramer and Welch[14] synthesized these theories to propose a model in which epithelial inclusion cysts are thought to be stimulated by elevated gonadotrophins either directly or indirectly through their effect on steroidogenesis, to include malignant transformation. Ovulation inducing agents, which promote multiple ovulation in a single cycle, theoretically could increase the risk of ovarian cancer.

FURTHER EVIDENCE

Publications by Whittemore *et al*[15,16] from the Collaborative ovarian cancer group contributed to the positive association between the use of fertility drugs and the risk of ovarian cancer. They reported on the findings from a combined analysis of 12 United States case control studies, and found that:
• Infertile women using fertility drugs had almost three times the risk for invasive epithelial ovarian cancer, as women without a history of infertility. Infertile women not using fertility drugs were found to have no increased risk
• Parity was protective in that infertile women who used fertility drugs and became pregnant did not have a significantly increased risk of ovarian cancer
• Infertile women using fertility drugs and remaining nulliparous experienced a 27-fold increased risk of ovarian cancer compared with nulligravid controls.

However, the study has numerous drawbacks in the form of selection bias, wide confidence intervals, lack of a uniform etiology of infertility and temporal incompatibility between treatment for infertility and licensing of modern fertility drugs in the subjects reported. Hence, any conclusion linking fertility drugs and ovarian cancer cannot be drawn from this study.

Rossing *et al*[17] studied the risk of ovarian tumors in a cohort of 3837 women evaluated for infertility between 1974 and 1985 in Seattle USA. The risk of ovarian tumors associated with exposure to ovulation inducing medications was assessed through an age-standardized comparison with the rate of ovarian tumors in the general population. The results of this study were:
• There were 11 cases of invasive or borderline ovarian tumors, as compared with an expected number of 4.4
• Nine of the women in whom ovarian tumors developed had taken clomiphene, the adjusted relative risk among these women, as compared with that of among infertile women who had not taken this drug, was 2.3
• Five of the nine women had taken the drug during 12 or more monthly cycles. This period of treatment was associated with an increased risk of ovarian tumors among both women with ovarian abnormalities and those without

apparent abnormalities, whereas treatment with the drug for less than one year was not associated with an increased risk. They concluded that prolonged use of clomiphene might increase the risk of a borderline or invasive ovarian tumor.

There are however, quite a few inconsistencies in their report. Infertile gravid women using clomiphene for more than 12 cycles had a relative risk of 17 for developing an ovarian tumor, whereas infertile nulligravid clomiphene users had a relative risk of 10.8. The higher relative risk in gravid women is difficult to explain, as parity is known to give a protective effect. Secondly, this effect was seen only with prolonged use of clomiphene for 12 cycles or more and not with use for less than 12 cycles. If this relationship were causal, there would be a more consistent dose-dependent relationship. In addition, the small numbers (only 11) especially in those cases using clomiphene for more than 12 cycles (5), limits the precision of risk estimates for this group.

Is the Increased Risk due to Ovulation Induction or due to Infertility Independently?

Multiple studies have found infertility to be an independent risk factor for ovarian cancer.

Joly et al[18] concluded that women who developed ovarian cancer had a gonadal status that predisposed to both ovarian cancer and low fertility.

In 1989, Booth et al[19] found that women who had not conceived after more than 10 years of unprotected intercourse, had 6.5 times the risk of developing ovarian cancer as nulligravid women reporting with less than 3 months of unprotected intercourse. Whittemore found that the ovarian cancer risk to women having more than or equal to 10 years of unprotected intercourse was 1 to 8 times that of women reporting fewer years' worth.

The Other Side of the Coin: Do Fertility Drugs Really Increase the Risk of Ovarian Cancer?

Mosgaard et al[20] studied all Danish women (below the age of 60 years) with ovarian cancer during the period from 1989 to 1994 and twice the number of age-matched controls. Included in the analysis were 684 cases and 1721 controls. The results of this study were
- Nulliparous women had an increased risk of ovarian cancer when compared to parous women (odds ratio 1.5 to 2)
- Infertile, untreated nulliparous women had an odds ratio of 2.7 when compared to fertile nulliparous women
- The odds ratio of ovarian cancer was 0.8 and among treated parous 0.6, compared to non-treated nulliparous and parous infertile women, respectively. They concluded that
  i. Nulliparity implies a 1.5 to 2 fold risk of ovarian cancer.
  ii. Infertility without medical treatment among these women increased the risk further.
  iii. Among parous as well as nulliparous women, treatment with fertility drugs did not increase the ovarian cancer risk compared to nontreated infertile women.

Risk of Cancer after Use of Fertility Drugs with *in vitro* Fertilization

A. Venn A et al[21] investigated the incidence of invasive cancer of the breast, ovary and uterus in a cohort of patients undergoing IVF treatment and examined whether cause of infertility or exposure to fertility drugs to induce superovulation was associated with an increased cancer risk. Ten Australian IVF clinics provided data for women who had been referred for IVF before Jan 1, 1994. The cohort consisted of 29,700 women—20,656 were exposed to fertility drugs and 9,044 were not. Their interpretation of the data was:
   - Women who have been exposed to fertility drugs and IVF seem to have a transient increase in the risk of having breast or uterine cancer diagnosed in the first year after treatment though the overall incidence is no greater than expected
   - Unexplained infertility was associated with an increased risk of the diagnosis of ovarian or uterine cancer.
B. Leila Unkila-Kallio et al[22] analyzed the occurrence of granulosa cell tumor (GCT) in

the whole of Finland from 1965 to 1994, the period when ovulation inducers and oral contraceptives became available. All women with GCT were traced from the Finnish Cancer Registry. The number of courses of clomiphene and gonadotrophins and the number of courses of oral contraceptives used in Finland during the same period were calculated from the sales statistics of these agents. The incidence of GCT declined by nearly 40 percent from 0.74/100000 in 1965 to 1994, a fall occurring at the same time that the use of clomiphene increased 13-fold, that of gonadotrophins 200-fold and that of oral contraceptives 5-fold. This nation wide data on the incidence of GCT falling concomitantly with increasing use of ovulation inducers probably suggest that ovulation inducers are unlikely to cause GCT.

WOMEN'S PERCEPTION OF RISKS AND BENEFITS OF THERAPY IN RELATION TO OVARIAN CANCER RISK

Barry Rosen *et al*[23] asked women undergoing fertility treatment the maximum increased risk of ovarian cancer they would be willing to tolerate in order to take ovulation inducing drugs. It was a prospective study of women attending fertility clinics in Toronto:61 women were approached and 52 were enrolled. What they found was as follows.

Benefits

69 percent estimated that less than 50 percent of women receiving fertility treatment would have a successful pregnancy. Only 14 percent thought it would be more than 50 percent.

Risks

67 percent indicated an awareness of a possible relationship between fertility drugs and ovarian cancer. When explained that the average lifetime risk of ovarian cancer was 1.5 percent, 50 percent said they would accept a risk of 4 to 10 percent and 6 percent would accept risk of 10 percent.

6 percent did not know whether treatment for ovarian cancer was curative, 49 percent believed that the risk could be reduced a great deal by following physician's advice (screening, prevention, lifestyle change).

As a summary, all but one individual thought that the benefits outweighed the risks.

SUMMARY

The etiology of ovarian cancer is probably multi-factorial with genetic, environmental and endocrinological factors either directly or indirectly related to carcinogenesis. The recent observations that infertile women who are on fertility drugs might experience an increased risk for the development of ovarian cancer are difficult to assess because of small numbers and multiple compounding factors.

To summarize:

• There is the risk of a consistent relationship between the number of stimulated cycles and risk of ovarian cancer
• The latency period between exposure and detection of neoplasm is highly variable which raises questions about the biological plausibility of a cause and effect relationship
• The most commonly used fertility medications gained widespread use in 1960s and 1970s. The population of early infertility drug users is just now reaching the age of greatest ovarian cancer incidence (50 to 60 years)
• Large well-designed case controlled studies are needed before definite conclusions can be drawn. Till such results are available, it is the duty of every clinician to:
  • Counsel and educate the patients properly
  • Stop unindicated, unmonitored and prolonged use of fertility drugs
  • Perform careful clinical and investigative evaluation of patients before, during, and after treatment
  • Keep abreast of scientific development.

REFERENCES

1. Bamford PM, Steel SJ. Uterine and ovarian carcinoma in a patient receiving gonadotrophin therapy—a case report. Br J Obstet Gynaecol 1982;89:962-64.
2. Atlas M, Menczer J. Massive hyperstimulation and borderline carcinoma of the ovary—a possible association. Acta Obstet Gynaecol Scand 1982;61:261-63.

3. Ben-Hur H et al. Ovarian carcinoma masquerading as ovarian hyperstimulation syndrome. Acta Obstet Gynaecol Scand 1986;65:813-14.
4. Kulkarni R, McGarry JM. Follicular stimulation and ovarian cancer. Br Med J 1989;299:740.
5. Diett J. Ovulation and ovarian cancer. Lancet 1991;338:445.
6. Balasch J, Barri PN. Follicular stimulation and ovarian cancer. Hum Reprod 1993;8:990-96.
7. Karlan BY et al. Advanced-stage ovarian carcinoma presenting during infertility evaluation. Am J Obstet Gynecol 1994;171:1377-78.
8. Goldberg GL, Runowicz CD. Ovarian carcinoma of low malignant potential, infertility and induction of ovulation—is there a link? Am J Obstet Gynecol 1992;166:853-54.
9. Nijman HW et al. Borderline malignant of the ovary and controlled hyperstimulation—a report of 2 cases. Eur J Cancer 1992;28A:1971-73.
10. Grimbizis G, Tarlatzis BC et al. Two cases of ovarian tumors in women who had undergone multiple ovarian stimulation attempts. Hum Reprod 1995;10:520-23.
11. Fathalla MF. Incessant ovulation—a factor in ovarian neoplasia? Lancet 1971;2:163.
12. Zajicak J. Prevention of ovarian cystomas by inhibition of ovulation—a new concept. J Reprod Med 1978;2:11.
13. Casagrande JT, Pike ML, Ross RK et al. Incessant ovulation and ovarian cancer. Lancet 1979;2:170-72.
14. Cramer DW, Welch WR. Determinants of ovarian cancer risk II—information regarding pathogenesis. J Natl Cancer Int 1983;71:717-21.
15. Whittemore et al. The Collaborative Ovarian Cancer Group Characteristics relating to ovarian cancer risk—collaborative analysis of 12 US case-control studies. 1 Methods. Am J Epidemiol 1993;136:1175-83.
16. Whittemore et al. II Invasive epithelial ovarian cancers in White women. Am J Epidemiol 1992;136:1184-203.
17. Rossing MA, Daling JR, Weiss NS et al. Ovarian tumors in a cohort of infertile women. N Engl J Med 1994;331(12):771-76.
18. Joly DJ et al. An epidemiologic study of the relationship of reproductive experience to cancer of the ovary. Am J Epidemiol 1974;99:190-209.
19. Booth M, Beral V, Smith P. Risk factors for ovarian cancer—a case control study. Br J Cancer 1989;60:592-98.
20. Mosgaard BJ et al. Infertility, fertility drugs and invasive ovarian cancer—a case controlled study. Fertil Steril 1997;67:1005-12.
21. Venn A, Watson L, Bruinsma F et al. Risk of cancer use of fertility drugs with in vitro fertilization. Lancet 1999;354(9190):1586-90.
22. Unkila-Kallio L, Leminen A, Titinen A et al. Nationwide data on falling increase of ovarian granulosa cell tumors concomitant with increasing use of ovulation induces. Hum Reprod 1998;13(10):2828-30.
23. Rosen B et al. The feasibility of assessing women's perceptions of the risks and benefits of fertility drug therapy in relation to ovarian cancer risk. Fertil Steril 1997;68:90-94.

• Michael F Costello
• Peter Sjoblom • Sanu Maiya Shrestha

32

Use of Doppler Ultrasound Imaging of the Ovary during IVF Treatment as a Predictor of Success

INTRODUCTION

It is estimated that approximately one in six couples experiences problems with their fertility at some point in their reproductive lives. Moreover, the number of women experiencing infertility is expected to increase in the next 20 years due to women delaying childbearing. An increase in demand for infertility treatment is anticipated as a consequence.[1]

In vitro fertilization (IVF) has the ultimate aim of assisting the 'infertile' patient to become pregnant and deliver a live infant. Continued improvements to treatment protocols and refinements in the embryology laboratory have resulted in steadily increasing success rates for IVF. Current rates of success are now often quoted as being in excess of 30 percent per cycle depending on variables such as age and previous history of fertility treatment.[2]

There are many factors that determine the success of IVF. These prognostic factors include advanced maternal age and various biochemical and ultrasound markers. Biochemical markers include basal follicular phase FSH, E2, and inhibin B levels in addition to dynamic tests such as the clomiphene citrate challenge test and the gonadotrophin agonist stimulation test. Ultrasound markers that have been shown to correlate with IVF success include ovarian volume and antral follicle count.[3]

Transvaginal conventional ultrasound or B-mode imaging during IVF therapy has significantly enhanced the accuracy of monitoring folliculogenesis during IVF. A mean follicular diameter greater than 18 mm is generally accepted as a criterion of preovulatory status, but ultrasound studies of spontaneous cycles have demonstrated that ovulation can occur with a leading follicle ranging from 15 to 29 mm. However, other than follicle size, this type of ultrasound assessment cannot indicate whether there are differences between follicles that could influence treatment outcome. More recently, transvaginal Doppler ultrasound assessment of the ovaries has been evaluated in an attempt to identify successful IVF cycles.

Doppler Ultrasound: Color Doppler Imaging (CDI) and Power Doppler Imaging (PDI)

Doppler ultrasound is based on the Doppler principle that sound and light waves change in frequency or wavelength when either the source or the receiver is moving away from or towards each other. Doppler-shifted echoes are generated when blood is in motion. These waveforms are familiar as sounds of pulsatile flow of blood through vessels. The frequency of sound waves is expressed in Hertz, where 1 Hertz (Hz) is one sound wave cycle or pulse occurring in 1 second. Sound with a frequency of $\geq 20,000$ Hz is called ultrasound, because it is beyond the frequency range of human hearing. Pulsed-Doppler systems have an advantage over continuous wave Doppler in having the ability to select the depth from which Doppler information is received, thus allowing analysis of blood flow within a segment of a single vessel. Color flow Doppler instruments provide 2-dimensional, color-coded Doppler information superimposed on the real time anatomical display.[4]

Conventional color Doppler imaging (CDI) is based on the mean frequency shift Doppler, and is limited by both angle dependency (dependence on the angle of insonation) that reduces sensitivity to blood flow perpendicular to the sound field and a difficulty in separating background noise from true blood flow. Recently, a variation of conventional CDI which maps the amplitude (energy or power) of the Doppler signal or frequency shift to produce a color image has become available, termed color Doppler energy (CDE) or power Doppler imaging (PDI). The major advantage of PDI over CDI is its increased sensitivity for detecting blood flow through irregular coursed and small vessels with low blood flow. This is because PDI can easily distinguish noise from true blood flow and is angle independent.[5]

However, PDI has the disadvantage of not being able to provide information about speed or direction of flow, and thus, in contrast to CDI, cannot distinguish between arteries and veins which show flow in different directions. Nevertheless, the principal aim of color Doppler is to determine the position of vessels and the presence or absence of flow; thus a lack of information regarding velocity and direction could not interfere with the data obtained by PDI.[6]

Both CDI and PDI are incorporated with software packages, which allows the analysis of Doppler blood flow by calculation of resistance indices, such as pulsatility index (PI) and resistance index (RI), and velocity, such as peak systolic velocity (PSV). Pulsatility index and RI are the measure of resistance to blood flow. Pulsatility index is derived from the difference between the peak systolic velocity (S) and minimal or end diastolic velocity (D) divided by mean maximum velocity over one cardiac cycle (S–D/

Mean). Resistance index is the difference between the peak systolic velocity and end diastolic velocity divided by peak systolic velocity (S–D/S). The PI is not as accurate as RI because of the variability inherent in measurement of mean velocity with present day software programs. The principal reason for using resistance indices is that they cancel out errors caused by the Doppler angle, machine gain, and hypo-or hypertension. They are, however, affected by the heart rate. The measurement of PSV is highly unreliable because it is dependent on the angle of insonation, it displays a high degree of variability on repeat examination, and it cannot describe blood flow over the entire cardiac cycle.[4]

Ovarian Perifollicular Blood Flow (PFBF)

Ovarian PFBF or follicular vascularity can be assessed by CDI, but attempts to quantify the vascularity would be limited because any blood flow at 90° to the ultrasound probe would not be displayed. The recent introduction of the more sensitive PDI overcomes this problem and enables flows with lower volumes and velocities to be displayed leading to improved visualization of small vessels.

There have been four studies published assessing ovarian PFBF in patients undergoing IVF treatment, three of which used PDI[7-9] and one using CDI.[10] All studies were cross-sectional studies, with ovarian PFBF being assessed on the day of, but prior to, human chorionic gonadotrophin (hCG) trigger in the CDI study and on the day of oocyte retrieval in the PDI studies. All four studies demonstrated that ovarian PFBF may be a predictor of pregnancy in IVF.

The PDI and CDI studies will be discussed separately, given the concerns regarding the reduced sensitivity of CDI in detecting small vessel blood flow. The PDI studies assessed the vascularity of the ovarian follicles on the day of oocyte retrieval using a subjective grading system according to the percentage of follicular circumference in which most flow was identified from a single cross-sectional slice. The grading system was as follows:

Grade 1 being < 25 percent of follicular circumference in which flow was identified, grade 2 being

26 to 50 percent of follicular circumference in which flow was identified, grade 3 being 51 to 75 percent of follicular circumference in which flow was identified, and grade 4 being 76 to 100 percent of follicular circumference in which flow was identified.

The results of these PDI studies during IVF are summarized in Table 32.1. Each individual study showed a significant improvement in cycle pregnancy rate (CPR) if embryos resulting from the fertilization of eggs from grade 3 or 4 follicles are used. In addition, we have performed a meta-analysis of the individual studies as shown in Table 32.1. The meta-analysis demonstrates that the CPR is significantly improved by almost 5-fold if embryos resulting from the fertilization of eggs from grade 3 or 4 follicles are transferred during IVF.

The CDI study assessed ovarian PFBF in women at high-risk for IVF treatment failure and also used the same ovarian PFBF grading system. In this CDI study by Coulam et al[10] all pregnancies occurred in women with grade 3 or 4 follicular blood flow on the day of, but prior to, hCG trigger.

The mechanism underlying the link between follicular vascularity and implantation outcome remains unclear at present. However, possibilities include a link between ovarian follicular blood flow and both oocyte quality and corpus luteum function. Oocytes derived from follicles with low oxygen content have been shown to have a significantly higher frequency of defects in chromosome number, spindle organization, and cytoplasmic structure as well as a significantly reduced ability to develop to the 6 to 8 cell stage embryo *in vitro* when fertilized.[11] Such a hypoxic intrafollicular environment could result from a failure of an appropriate microvasculature to develop around the growing or preovulatory follicle.

TABLE 32.1: Summary of published studies comparing clinical CPRs in IVF according to the PDU PFBF grade of the embryos transferred

Reference and site of study	Study design	n age[†]	Ovarian stimulation protocol	Intervention
Chui DKC et al 1997 Cardiff, Wales	Prospective cohort	38 32.5 years (range 25-40)	Ultrashort	PDU of PFBF 32-33 hours post-hCG trigger
Bhal PS et al 1999 Cardiff, Wales	Prospective cohort	179 32.5 years (range NS)	Ultrashort, short or long down regulation	PDU of PFBF 34 hours post-hCG trigger
Borini A et al 2001 Bologna, Italy Meta-analysis	Prospective cohort	75 < 39 years (mean and range NS)	NS	PDU of PFBF (on day of egg collection, exact time NS)

Results (cycle pregnancy rate)				Notes
Grade 1 or 2	Grade 3 or 4	p value[‡]	Or (95% CI)	
0/9 (0%)	10/29 (34%)	0.042	not estimable	
3/41 (7%)	44/153 (29%)	0.002	5.1 (1.5-17.4)	
4/34 (14%)	14/41 (34%)	0.035	3.5 (1.02-12.0)	
7/84 (8.3%)	68/223 (30%)	< 0.001	4.8 (2.1-11.0)	Breslow-Day test for homogeneity c^2 = 1.13, df = 2, p = 0.57

† mean and range of women when available; ‡ Chi-Square or Fisher's exact test as appropriate
CPR, cycle pregnancy rate; IVF, *in vitro* fertilization; PDU, power Doppler ultrasound; PFBF, perifollicular blood flow; n, number of women; hCG, human chorionic gonadotrophin; OR, odds ratio; CI, confidence interval; NS, not stated; <, less than.

Therefore, transvaginal PDI assessment of ovarian PFBF on the day of oocyte collection may be used to improve the outcome of IVF and embryo transfer treatment cycles, by identifying follicles with high-grade (grade 3 or 4) vascularity. In addition, ovarian PFBF has the potential to be used as an additional marker in the process of embryo selection for transfer, enabling the transfer of fewer embryos with a better potential for implantation, and reducing the incidence of multiple gestation without reducing the pregnancy rate. Identifying low-grade ovarian PFBF, preferably before hCG administration, may also allow a more efficient selection of patients completing IVF treatments. Patients with mostly low-grade vascular follicles could be counselled about the poor outcome and given the option to cancel the treatment cycle prior to oocyte retrieval. However, more data would be needed before such prospective management of IVF treatment cycles could be applied in clinical practice.[8]

Interestingly, there has been a prospective study published assessing the use of PDU in stimulated intra-uterine insemination (IUI) cycles. Bhal and colleagues measured the PFBF of all follicles greater than 15 mm diameter on the day of IUI (36 hours after hCG administration) in 182 women undergoing stimulated IUI using the same grading system described in the IVF studies above. These authors found that high-grade (grade 3 or 4) perifollicular vascularity correlated with pregnancy rates and concluded that PDU has the potential to refine the management of stimulated IUI treatment cycles.[12]

Ovarian Stromal Flow Index (FI)

There have been a number of published studies assessing ovarian stromal blood flow index (FI) using 3-dimensional (3D) PDU in the IVF setting, but only one such study examined the relationship between ovarian stromal FI and IVF cycle outcome. Kupesic *et al* prospectively performed transvaginal 3-D PDU in 56 women undergoing IVF with the long GnRH agonist protocol and found a significantly higher mean ovarian FI after pituitary suppression in pregnant cycles compared to nonpregnant cycles. Flow index reflects

the intensity of blood flow and was calculated automatically by a built in computer.[13]

Ovarian Perifollicular Artery PI, RI or PSV

It has been demonstrated that oocytes derived from ovarian follicles with a higher follicular PSV on either the day of hCG trigger (but before the injection) or day of egg collection have a better potential for producing high-grade embryos, with no such association observed with follicular PI.[14, 15] In these studies by the same author, the chance of producing a high-grade embryo was 75 percent if the follicular PSV was $\geq$ 10 cm on the day of hCG trigger compared to 40 percent if PSV was < 10 cm. Likewise, the chance of producing a high-grade embryo was 70 percent if the follicular PSV was $\geq$ 10 cm/s on the day of egg retrieval compared to 14 percent if PSV was < 10 cm/s.

In another prospective study in the IVF setting, Ozaki and colleagues demonstrated a significant correlation between the dominant follicle PSV and both the number of oocytes retrieved and the number of mature oocytes obtained. However, there was no such correlation with the dominant follicle RI or PI. In addition, there was no association between the dominant follicle PSV, RI or PI and the fertilization rate or the ratio of good quality embryos.[16] Huey *et al* found a significant and negative correlation between ovarian perifollicular artery PI and RI on the day before oocyte collection (morning after hCG injection) and embryo cleavage but not embryo morphology in 16 women undergoing IVF.[17] In addition, a significant and negative correlation was found between ovarian perifollicular artery RI and oocyte diploid fertilization rate.

Both the perifollicular PSV and RI were found to have no predictive value for IVF outcome in a prospective study by Balakier *et al.*[18] This study showed no difference in perifollicular blood flow indices PSV or RI between pregnant and nonpregnant cycles in 52 women undergoing IVF.

Therefore, the limited data on ovarian perifollicular blood flow using the qualitative measurement PSV, RI or PI as a predictor of IVF success has demonstrated PSV, but not RI or PI, to be correlated with surrogate markers of IVF success such as number of oocytes retrieved and embryo quality. However, ovarian perifollicular RI and PI has been shown to be correlated with embryo cleavage. Neither ovarian perifollicular PSV, RI nor PI appears to be predictive for the primary outcome measure of pregnancy in IVF.

Ovarian Stromal or Intra-ovarian Artery (IOA) PI or RI or PSV

It appears that, generally, blood flow resistance in the intra-ovarian vessels is low, with a PI of around 1. The blood flow indices vary slightly over the cycle and seem to be lowest midcycle in both natural and IVF treatment cycles.[19-22] A relationship has been observed between intra-ovarian blood flow early in the cycle and the number of follicles growing in the ovary, and low responders appear to have poorer blood flow.[19, 23-25] This is suggestive of angiogenetic activity as a prerequisite for development of healthy follicles.

No relationship has been seen between IOA PI on the day of oocyte collection and the probability of pregnancy after IVF.[7, 8] However, a higher clinical pregnancy rate was observed when the IOA PSV was greater than 10 cm/sec on the day of pituitary down-regulation preceding IVF stimulation.[24]

Tekay *et al*[26] compared intra-ovarian blood flow in women who developed the ovarian hyperstimulation syndrome (OHSS) and women who did not develop this condition, and found no differences in this regard. Pinkas *et al*[21] found no difference in intra-ovarian blood flow between women with PCOS and those without.

CONCLUSIONS

From the available literature, it seems that the most promising Doppler ultrasound imaging of the ovary as a predictor of IVF success is the quantitative assessment of ovarian follicular blood flow using PDU. Further research is required to define its role in the management of IVF treatment cycles, especially in regard to its potential in clinical practice to lower the multiple pregnancy rate without adversely affecting the pregnancy rate by transferring fewer high-quality embryos with a higher implantation potential selected on the basis of ovarian PFBF.

REFERENCES

1. Stephen EH, Chandra A. Updated projection of infertility in the United States: 1995–2025. Fertil. Steril 1998;70:30-34.
2. Toner JP. Progress we can be proud of: U.S. trends in assisted reproduction over the first 20 years. Fertil Steril 2002;78:943-50.
3. Bancsi LF, Broekmans FJ, Eijkemans MJ, de Jong FH, Habbema JD, te Velde ER: Predictors of poor ovarian response in in vitro fertilization: a prospective study comparing basal markers of ovarian reserve. Fertil Steril 2002;77:328-36.
4. RP Dickey. Doppler ultrasound investigation of uterine and ovarian blood flow in infertility and early pregnancy. Hum Reprod Update 1997;3:467-503.
5. Rubin JM, Bude RO, Carson PL, Bree RL, Adler RS. Power Doppler US: A potentially useful alternative to mean frequency-based color Doppler US. Radiol 1994; 190:853-56.
6. Guerriero S, Ajossa S, Lai MP, Risalvato A, Paoletti AM, Melis GB: Clinical applications of colour Doppler energy imaging in the female reproductive tract and pregnancy. Hum Reprod Update 1999;5:515-29.
7. Chui DK, Pugh ND, Walker SM, Gregory L, Shaw RW: Follicular vascularity-the predictive value of transvaginal power Doppler ultrasonography in an in vitro fertilization programme: A preliminary study. Hum Reprod 1997;12:191-96.
8. Bhal PS, Pugh ND, Chui DK, Gregory L, Walker SM, Shaw RW. The use of transvaginal power Doppler ultrasonography to evaluate the relationship between perifollicular vascularity and outcome in in vitro fertilization treatment cycles. Hum Reprod 1999;14: 939-45.
9. Borini A, Maccolini A, Tallarini A, Bonu MA, Sciajno R, Flamigni C: Perifollicular vascularity and its relationship with oocyte maturity and IVF outcome. Ann. NY Acad. Sci. 2001;943:64-67.
10. Coulam CB, Goodman C, Rinehart JS. Colour Doppler indices of follicular blood flow as predictors of pregnancy after in vitro fertilization and embryo transfer (Journal Article) Hum Reprod 1999;14:1979-82.
11. Van Blerkom J, Antczak M, Schrader R. The developmental potential of the human oocyte is related to the dissolved oxygen content of follicular fluid: Association with vascular endothelial growth factor levels and perifollicular blood flow characteristics. Hum Reprod 1997;12:1047-55.
12. Bhal PS, Pugh ND, Gregory L, O'Brien S, Shaw RW. Perifollicular vascularity as a potential variable affecting outcome in stimulated intrauterine

insemination treatment cycles: A study using trans-vaginal power Doppler. Hum Reprod 2001;16:1682-89.

13. Kupesic S, Kurjak A. Predictors of IVF outcome by 3-dimensional ultrasound. Hum Reprod 2002;17: 950-55.

14. Nargund G, Bourne T, Doyle P, Parsons J, Cheng W, Campbell S, et al. Associations between ultrasound indices of follicular blood flow, oocyte recovery and preimplantation embryo quality. Hum Reprod 1996; 11:109-13.

15. Nargund G, Doyle PE, Bourne TH, Parsons JH, Cheng WC, Campbell S, et al. Ultrasound derived indices of follicular blood flow before hCG administration and the prediction of oocyte recovery and preimplantation embryo quality. Hum Reprod 1996;11: 2512-17.

16. Ozaki T, Hata K, Xie H, Takahashi K, Miyazaki K. Utility of color Doppler indices of dominant follicular blood flow for prediction of clinical factors in *in vitro* fertilization-embryo transfer cycles. Ultrasound Obstet Gynecol 2002;20:592-96.

17. Huey S, Abuhamad A, Barroso G, Hsu MI, Kolm P, Mayer J, et al. Perifollicular blood flow Doppler indices, but not follicular pO$_2$, pCO$_2$, or pH, predict oocyte developmental competence in in vitro fertilization. Fertil Steril 1999;72:707-12.

18. Balakier H, Stronell RD. Color Doppler assessment of folliculogenesis in in vitro fertilization patients. Fertil Steril 1994;62:1211-16.

19. Weiner Z, Thaler I, Levron J, Lewit N, Itskowitz-Eldor J. Assessment of ovarian and uterine blood flow by transvaginal color Doppler in ovarian-stimulated women: Correlation with the number of follicles and steroid hormone levels. Fertil Steril 1993;59:743-49.

20. Tan SL, Zaidi J, Campbell S, Doyle P, Collins W. Blood flow in the ovarian and uterine arteries during the normal menstrual cycle. Am J Obstet Gynecol 1996; 175:625-31.

21. Pinkas H, Mashiach R, Rabinerson D, Avrech OM, Royburt M, Rufas O, et al. Doppler parameters of uterine and ovarian stromal blood flow in women with polycystic ovaries and normally ovulating women undergoing controlled ovarian stimulation. Ultrasound Obstet Gynecol 1998;12:197-200.

22. Lunenfeld E, Schwartz I, Meizner I, Potashnik G, Glezerman M. Intra-ovarian blood flow during sponta-neous and stimulated cycles. Hum Reprod 1996;11: 2481-83.

23. Zaidi J, Barber J, Kyei-Mensah A, Bekir J, Campbell S, Tan SL. Relationship of ovarian stromal blood flow at baseline ultrasound scan to subsequent follicular response in an in vitro fertilization program Obstet Gynecol 1996;88:779-84.

24. Engman L, Sladkevicius P, Agrawal R, Bekir JS, Campbell S, Tan SL. Value of ovarian stromal blood flow velocity measurement after pituitary suppression in the prediction of ovarian responsiveness and outcome of in vitro fertilization treatment. Fertil Steril 1999;71:22-29.

25. Altundag M, Levi R, Adakan S, Tavmergen-Goker, EN, Killi R, et al. Intra-ovarian stromal artery Doppler indices in predicting ovarian response. J Reprod Med 2002;47:886-90.

26. Tekay A, Martikainen H, Jouppila P. Doppler para-meters of the ovarian and uterine blood circulation in ovarian hyperstimulation syndrome. Ultrasound Obstet Gynecol 1995;6:50-53.

Section 6

Assisted
Reproductive Techniques

• Meena Chimote • Natchandra Chimote

33

Intrauterine Insemination

INTRODUCTION

Involuntary subfertility is a common problem, affecting up to 15 percent of couples,[1] and the demand for medical treatment is increasing. In an attempt to improve conception rates, artificial insemination techniques in various forms have been practiced for almost 200 years.[2] Recently the most refined of these, intrauterine insemination, alone or in combination with controlled ovarian hyperstimulation (COH), has been the focus of a substantial amount of research.

The rationale of IUI performed using either husband/donor spermatozoa is to overcome problems of vaginal acidity, cervical mucus hostility and deposit adequately good number of highly motile and morphologically normal sperm near the fundal region of uterus at the anticipated time of ovulation. The usefulness of IUI procedures particularly in bypassing cervical barriers in cases of cervical factor has been evidenced by many workers.[3] In the presence of normal sperm and patent tubes the majority of infertility centers routinely offer IUI as first-line treatment.

There is good evidence in the literature in favour of intrauterine insemination[4] as the most cost-effective treatment for unexplained and moderate male factor subfertility. It is also evidenced by a few workers that in cases of subnormal semen samples, deposition of sperm into the uterine cavity prevents intravaginal and intracervical loss of sperm, resulting in increased number of sperm available for fertilization.[5]

However, there is no published data on whether this evidence is being translated into clinical practice.

Against this backdrop, the aim of this chapter is to compare the patterns of use of IUI within fertility units with variable results and emerge out with the best possible IUI protocol, considering female and male factors together, to improve pregnancy rate.

INVESTIGATIONS

Many infertile couples have more than one contributory' cause which should be identified early. Hence, a scientific approach is warranted for efficient and complete evaluation of the female and male factors.

Apart from detailed menstrual history, and physical examination, followed by routine investigations such as blood sugar levels, sickle cell disease, blood counts and sexually transmitted diseases (HIV and VDRL in particular), certain important investigations to be earned out are given in Table 33.1 and 33.2 for female and male partners respectively.

It is essential to have respective normal control values of various parameters by evaluating normal cycling, non PCOS subjects so that even regularly menstruating (eumenorrheic) women with slight menstrual aberrations like regular scanty periods (hypomenorrhea) and oligomenorrhea, with or without PCOS states can be classified. These criteria of classification of the

TABLE 33.1: Evaluation of female partner

Physical parameters	Clinical parameters	Endocrinological parameters
Anthropometric: Weight (kg) Height (meters) Body Mass Index (BMI) Waist girth (cm) Hip girth (cm) W : H Ratio	**Trans vaginal Sonography:** Evaluation of uterus and Ut. Cavity Measurements of ovarian volume, no. of follicles and evaluation of texture to classify non PCOS and PCOS states **HSG:** (if necessary) **Diagnostic Laparoscopy and hysteroscopy:** (if necessary) For evaluation ot cervical tubal, uterine and ovarian factors	**Day 3 Hormones:** LH. FSH. Estradiol, Testosterone, Prolactin SHBG, TSH, Insulin, (when menstrual aberrations are observed) **Day 21 Hormones:** Progesterone.

women undergoing IUI procedure enable to determine ovulation induction protocol.

Anthropometric parameters such as BMI and WHR differentiate non-obese from obese subjects with degree of central adiposity. These essential parameters, if found abnormal, may require further evaluation of hyperandrogenism in terms of hyperinsulinemia and hyperleptinemia that may bring about aberrations in ovulation and cause luteal phase deficiency despite medication.[7] It is also beneficial to evaluate free estradiol index (FEI) and free testosterone index (FTI) in hyperandrogenism with/without clinical evidences and in PCOS states.[8]

Diagnostic evaluation of the uterus to detect disorders are limited to organic rather than functional abnormalities. Ullrasonography is helpful in detecting intrauterine adhesions, septa, polyps, and uterine myomas. Normal and abnormal endometrial growth can also be evaluated.[9, 10] Combination of TVS, HSG, laparoscopy, and hysteroscopy provide excellent information regarding uterine, tubal, and ovarian condition with/without endometriosis, tuberculosis, and adhesions to a clinician and help to plan the therapeutic approach.

Endocrine evaluation of menstruaily aberrated women (hypomenorrheic and oligomenorrheic) plays an important role in deciding the stimulation protocol. Baseline serum concentrations of LH, FSH and LH: FSH ratios sometimes are decisive factors to select stimulation protocol to avoid hyperstimulation or poor response. A ratio of estradiol and testosterone concentrations

TABLE 33.2: Evaluation of male partner

Clinical Parameters	Laboratory parameters	Investigations
Detailed history and examination	Semen analysis as per WHO "criteria	
Hair distribution scoring, physical examination of testis, epididymis and vas deference, measurement of volume of testis in case ofazoo-spermia	Normospcrmia:	No further investigations unless indicated
	Asthcno/necrospcrmia:	Antisperm antibody test
	Teratospermia:	Check for presence ot DM
	Oligospcrmia: (moderate)	Sperm function tests
	Severe oligospermia	Vasogram, thermogram. Doppler study for vancocele
	Azoospermia:	Vasogram. thermogram. Testicular biopsy or fine needle aspiration of testis. Endocrine evaluation of LH, FSH, testosterone. PRL, TSH & insulin

depits the degree of aromatase activity in the developing follicle.

As the first-line management, not only for idiopathic and mild/moderate male factor infertility, but also for so-called normozoospermia, it is imperative to consider male factor evaluation in a very meticulous manner. Therefore, an andrology laboratory should be a part of the IUI program in infertility treating centers. Only after extensive study and evaluation of semen sample, it becomes easier, to choose treatment protocol, method of sperm preparation for IUI, and to counsel the couple with respect to donor sperm if required.

INDICATIONS

The initial indications for IUI were failure of sperm to penetrate cervical mucus and male infertility. During the past decade the indications for IUI have been liberalized and now it is frequently employed, often in conjugation with the woman's use of clomiphene citrate or gonadotrophins. The current controversies resolve around issues of techniques and those of efficacy. Indications for therapeutic insemination with husband/donor sperm are varied and are presented in Table 33.3.

COUNSELING

Even though the cumulative pregnancy rates in normocyclic women undergoing IUI with donor sperm (TDI) due to their partner's infertility (azoospermia) are proof of the efficacy of artificial insemination as such, though results of IUI with husband's sperm are variable. A survey of the literature published over the past 20 years shows a wide variation in the probability of conception per cycle after conventional IUI. This applies even to prospective randomized studies, which break down the pregnancies achieved according to causes of subfertility (male factor, cervical factor, endocrine factor or idiopathic factor) where pregnancy rates range between 3 and 15 percent.[12, 13] Despite presence of sperm (though subnormal) in male or slight clinical and endocrinological aberrations in females, a couple usually is reluctant to undergo IUI treatment with lot of confusion about success rate of the procedure. Hence, at this point before starting the treatment, a trusting working relationship should be established between the two partners to the treatment agreement, and the patient and a clinician, as this is indispensable on the road to success.

TABLE 33.3: Indications of intrauterine insemination

Insemination by husband's sperm	Insemination by donor sperm
1. **Female factors** • Anatomic defects of vagina or cervix • Hostile cervical mucus • Sexual dysfunction • Mild to moderate endometriosis • Endocrine anomalies • Chronic anovulatory cycles	1. **Male factors** • Azoospermia • Severe oligospermia • Severe Astheno/necrospermia • Failure in at least six IUI cycles with oligospermia • Sterility due to disease or vasectomy, orchidectomy, chemical or radiation exposure
2. **Male factor** • Anatomic defect of penis e.g. hypospadias • Sexual/ejaculatory dysfunction • Retrograde ejaculation • Semen volume in excess or deficit • Immunologiocal factor • Male subfertility-oligospermia, asthenospermia, teratospcrmia	• Sexual/ejaculatorv dysfunction • Genetic considerations (e.g. hemophilia. Huntigton's chorea) • Rh- incompatibility
3. **Other factors** • Idiopathic poor post coital test • Combined infertility factors • Unexplained infertility	

Fertility counseling, which can be described as the process of assisting individuals or couples to make informed decisions about their bioreproductive state should be provided at several different stages of treatment.[11] Specially, in donor sperm insemination, complete confidentiality should be assured. The screening of donor sperm, selection of donor, method of sperm preparation and anticipated success rate in the individual cases with possibilities of complications should be informed. In recent years, introduction of intra cytoplasmic sperm injection (ICSI), first reported by Palermo et al in 1992, has improved results of IVF-ET in severe male factor and in couples with previous IVF failures. Testicular Extraction of sperm along with ICSI allow the development of viable embryos and viable pregnancy in azoospermic (obstructive/non obstructive) men.[15-19]

In, the most recent times, men with congenital absence of vas deference can still be the genetic fathers opting out of donor insemination protocol.[20] However, the cost factor has deprived many couples of these techniques and therefore, the first aim is to subject the selected couple with subnormal male factor to the most cost effective and non invasive treatment protocol of IUI with either husband's or donor sperm, if the couple gives consent after counseling. Donor inseminations are useful in azoospermia, severe oligospermia, or Astheno/necrospermia refractory to treatment. They also are useful for the rare woman who has a history of fetal loss due to Rh sensitization. Genetic diseases may, on occasion, be an indication for donor insemination.

INDUCTION OF OVULATION

There has been extensive progress in infertility management by IUI alone or in combination with controlled ovarian stimulation. Ovarian stimulation with clomiphene citrate (CC) alone has been used for induction of ovulation for more than three decades,[21] however; various combinations with CC are also in practice in the recent years.

1. C. C. (50/100/150 mg) daily from D3 to D7 and injection hCG (5000 IU) at the time of LH surge. (Most commonly practised)

2. C.C. (50/100/150 mg) daily from D3 to D7 + inj. HMG (75 IU) from D8 to D10, followed by inj. HCG at the time of LH surge.

3. HMG/highly purified FSH/rec. FSH +inj. hCG

The rationale behind using clomiphene citrate is that it has a desirable central action of stimulating a transient increase in gonadotrophin secretion.[22] Superovulation increases the number of oocytes available for insemination, thereby increasing the chances of fertilization. Superovulation also increases the number of female gametes in the fallopian tube and IUI reduces obstacles to sperm migration by shortening the distance of male gametes to reach the site of fertilization. In addition to this, subtle ovulatory defects, disorders in endometrial development or borderline aberrations in corpus luteum function can be corrected by gonadotrophin therapy. Occult seminal defects are treated by various methods of sperm washing which also may be a major instrumental process to enhance fecundity.[23]

In spite of the high ovulation rate with the use of clomiphene citrate, the pregnancy rate is much lower (Franks S et al., 1985). It is believed that, due to, antiestrogenic effect of CC at the level of cervical mucus and endometrium, fertilization and embryo development, the pregnancy rates are low. Besides this, about 20-25 percent anovulatory women are resistant to CC and fail to ovulate at doses up to 150 mg daily. With gonadotrophins, the risk of multiple pregnancies as well as hyperstimulation increases. Hence, recently aromatase inhibitors have been introduced in induction and augmentation of ovulation such as Letrozole.

PREDICTION OF OVULATION

An accurate prediction of the time of ovulation is the utmost important factor for the success of IUI procedure, because it informs the optimal timing for insemination. Usually, insemination is done after 36 hours of administration of hCG injection. Therefore, decision of the day of administration of hCG injection is the most crucial part of IUI program.

Measurement of basal body temperature (BBT), commonly practiced method earlier, has a drawback of its retrospective diagnosis of ovulation and thus becomes an inappropriate method. Similarly, changes in cervical mucus are unreliable because, the interval between appearance of preovulatory type of mucus and the ovulation itself is variable.

The measurements of number, growth and rupture of Graflfian follicle, the measurement of endometrial pattern have proven to be more accurate method in monitoring the cycle.[24] The endometrial proliferation and proper differentiation during follicular and subsequent luteal phase are directly influenced by the circulating estrogen and progesterone levels.[25] Several guidelines have been suggested such as estradiol concentration of 250-400 pg/ml per mature Graffian follicle and the mean follicular diameter of at least 14 mm as determined by ultrasonography may predict the time of ovulation.[27] Ultrasonography monitoring and detection of the beginning of LH surge by hormonal assays of serum estradiol, LH, progesterone, and 17-alpha hydroxy progesterone may be the most precise method.

SPERM PARAMETERS FOR THE OUTCOME IN IUI

It is almost impossible to predict the fertilizing potential of a semen sample in individual cases.[28] Though, normal values of semen variables are given by WHO, numerous prospective studies have shown that routine semen analysis is only a weak predictor of male fertility.[29] Men with relatively low count in the semen sample (oligospermia) can show normal fertility potential and vice versa, when subjected to sperm function tests.[30] Hence, sperm function tests (SFT) have come to stay for the diagnosis of 'male factor' in normal as well as subnormal semen samples.

Because sperm is concentrated, introduced past the cervical mucus barrier, and have immotile and abnormal forms removed by processing, (The initial quality necessary for achieving pregnancy may be lower for IUI than the WHO normal values. Many workers have evidenced in their studies that, with sperm count > 5 million/ml, motility > 30 percent and normal morphology > 14 percent in the given semen sample, pregnancies were achieved in IUI programme with variable pregnancy rate.[31-33] It is highly improbable that pregnancy can be achieved after homologous insemination of less than 1 million spermatozoa.[34-36] When more than 15 million motile sperm are inseminated, there is no increase in the pregnancy rate; however, there is an increase in multiple pregnancies when the inseminate exceeds 20 million motile sperm.[37] Some workers also have reported that pregnancy rates were substantially higher when more than 10 million motile sperm were inseminated compared with inseminations of less than 10 million sperm.[38]

SPERM PREPARATION

There are a variety of methods that allow the separation of a more promising population of sperm. Sperm preparation technique is a very crucial step in the success of IUI. Semen processing in the laboratory not only separates highly motile functional sperm with normal morphology in high percentage, but also removes seminal plasma, which contains prostaglandins and cytokines, as well as possible antigenic or infectious matter along with defective and non-vital sperm and debris.

Current techniques of sperm preparation for intrauterine insemination require centriftigation of human semen to separate spermatozoa from the seminal plasma. Centrifugation increases reactive oxygen species (ROS) formation in semen. Moreover, high levels of ROS are associated with sperm membrane injury through spontaneous lipid peroxidation, which may alter sperm function.[39] Hence, regardless of technique used, a shorter centrifugation period in the preparation of sperm for IUI has been recommended to avail better quality of sperm for insemination.[10]

Several methods of sperm preparation for IUI such as centrifugation and washing, Swim up and swim down methods, Density gradient separation systems (Percoll, Ficoll, Sil-Select), and Glass wool filtration have been described. Each of these techniques has its specific advantages and shortcomings, and all methods may be suitable for normal semen samples. However, semen samples with subnormal parameters have always been a challenging job and it can be carried out successfully with improvisation in the prevailing techniques.

All sperm separation methods produce specimens with better motility and more uniform morphology; this improvement may not necessarily translate into increased pregnancy rates.

INTRAUTERINE SPERMTRANSFER

Sperm prepared by using any preparatory technique, are highly concentrated in number and therefore about 0.4 to 0.5 ml of prepared sperm are deposited in fundal region of uterus with the help of non toxic, flexible yet, stiff catheters which are available commercially. The reason to inseminate small volumes of sperm sample is to avoid reflux through the cervix into the vagina, or efflux through the tubes into the peritoneal cavity. The patient is placed in lithotomy position so that the cervix is visualized with the help of a speculum. The sperm sample then is withdrawn into the catheter, which is plugged to the tuberculin syringe. The catheter now containing sperm sample, is manipulated through to the cervix into the uterine cavity taking precaution of not damaging endometrium and then the sperm sample is released slowly with minimal compression into the uterine cavity. After the transfer, catheter is kept in its place for a while to avoid a suction effect and prevent reflux. After the procedure the patient should rest for 20-25 minutes. Though, the procedure seems to be very easy however, poorly performed technique is frequently responsible for low pregnancy rate.

LUTEAL PHASE SUPPORT

Day 21 monitoring of ultrasound and serum progesterone and 17α-Hydroxy progesterone levels, can confirm the completion of ovulatory process. It is usually at the discretion of an infertility center to determine the cut-off values of these hormonal levels. However, formation of corpus luteum may give a positive indication of ovulation. Depending on the levels of the aforementioned hormones, clinician can take the decision to give luteal phase support either with progesterone containing suppositories or injections.

The earliest indication of pregnancy can be obtained by monitoring the patient on Day 28 for serum beta hCG levels. More than 25 mlU/ml of hCG level can be considered as positive indication for pregnancy. Further support with hCG injections is usually suggested for a better result.

EXPERIENCE AT VACC

The authors of this chapter carried out a study of 1468 IUI cycles in 606 women (mean age 29.4 ± 0.3 years) at Vaunshdhara Assisted Conception Centre, Nagpur, with an average infertility interval of 8.3 ± 0.7 years, in the span of last three years, averaging 2.42 ± 0.45 IUI cycles per subject. The subjects were classified as eumenorrheic with/without PCOS, hypomenorrheic with/without PCOS and oligomenorrheic with/without PCOS based on the their menstrual history and ultrasound study. Their anthropometric, clinical, biochemical and metabolic parameters along with diagnostic or operative laparoscopy and hysteroscopy findings were evaluated to enable them to

TABLE 33.4: Results ofIUI in women withArithout menstrual aberrations				
Group	*Preg/No. of cycles*	*Husband with Normospermia*	*Husband with subnormal sperm*	*Donor sperm*
Eumcnorrhcic Non PCO	58/303	12/76	7/80	39/147
Eumcnorrhcic PCOS	66/362	24/142	11/103	31/117
H vpomcnorrhcic Non PCOS	14/126	06/67	02/26	06/33
H vpomcnorrhcic PCOS	54/319	21/148	03/28	30/143
Oligomenorrheic Non PCOS	07/132	03/74	00/14	04/44
Oligomenorrheic PCOS	32/226	12/94	02/27	18/105
Total no. Preg/cycle	**231/1468**	**78/601**	**25/278**	**128/589**

	TABLE 33.5: Results of Hormonal monitoring					
Groups: range of P ng/ml	No. of Cycles	E2 pg/ml	LH mIU/ml	17-OHP ng/ml	No. of Preg	% PR
A: 0.2 to 0.5	142	140 ± 23[***]	8.7 ± 2.4	2.4 ± 0.4[*]	03	21
B: 0.6 to 2.5	769	246 ± 36	11.4 ± 1.8	1.8 ± 0.2	189	24.6
C: > 2.5	557	124 ± 12[***]	7.8 ± 2.8	2.4 ± 0.2[*]	39	7.0
Total	**1468**	**196 ± 27**	**8.4 ± 1.7**	**2.0 ± 0.4**	**231**	**15.7**

[*]Indicates P value < 0.05,
[***]Indicates P value < 0.0005

enroll in IUI procedure. The results of 1468 IUI cycles are given in Table 33.4.

It is observed from Table 33.4 that, the overall pregnancy rate per IUI cycle was 15.74 percent with test controls (eumenorrheic non PCOS) giving higher PR of 19.14 as against 18.23 percent in eumenorrheic PCOS. PCOS with menstrual aberrations (hypomenorrheic and oligomenorrheic) in each group showed quite enhanced PR as compared to non-PCOS with/without menstrual aberrations (16.93, and 14.16% vs. 11.11, 5.3% PR respectively).

Therefore it may be stated that, PCOS with/without menstrual aberrations give a better pregnancy rate as compared to non-PCOS with/without menstrual aberrations if IUI cycles are monitored for E2, LH, P and 17-OHP.

The PR in IUI with husband's normal sperm was found to be low when compared with IUI with donor sperm (12.98 vs 21.73%). Others also have reported increased pregnancy rates when higher number of donor sperm were inseminated.[41] PR in IUI with subnormal husband's sperm (count 12.3 ± 4.7 million with average good motile sperm > 30 percent, and normal morphology 21.6 ± 3.2%) was found to be even lower than that with husband's normal sperm (8.99 Vs. 12.98%). Several workers have reported similar results ranging from 2 to 10 percent in IUI with subnormal sperm.[42, 43]

MONITORING CYCLES TO TIME HCG ADMINISTRATION

In the present study, IUI was performed in CC + hCG (857 cycles), CC + HMG + hCG (329 cycles), HMG + hCG (163 cycles), and FSH + hCG (119 cycles) stimulated cycles. When ultrasound scan and E2 levels suggested no more than three ovulatory follicles in both ovaries, monitoring was performed at regular intervals. When the lead follicle reached 18-20 mm in diameter, serum E2, LH and progesterone and sometimes 17-OHP concentrations were measured to decide administration of hCG. The results of hormonally monitored cycles are given in Table 33.5.

It is quite evident that, progesterone, 17-OHP levels are the most decisive factor and not the elevated LH levels, for the administration of hCG so as to achieve better pregnancy rate. This finding is in concurrence with a study of smaller group done earlier by the same author.[44]

Monitoring of estradiol especially in PCOS, enabled to avoid risk of ovarian hyperstimulation syndrome (OHSS). It also helped when lead follicle displayed an abnormal rate of growth, either too fast or too slow. When there were excessive number of small follicles associated with 3-4 leading follicles, a high E2 level (approx. 1500 pg/ml) indicated an increased risk of hyperstimulation, hence before hCG administration, cycles were cancelled.

Despite linear growth throughout the follicular phase, follicle size was not a reliable parameter for the accurate timing of the onset of ovulation. Therefore it is suggested that, hormone measurements along with ultrasound are the best predictors of ovulation.

Insemination was performed 36 to 40 hours after hCG administration. With endogenous LH surge noted by double fold LH levels on the day of hCG administration, insemination was performed after 24 hrs of hCG. Only one

TABLE 33.6: Pregnancies in various sperm preparation techniques

Semen quality	Direct Layering Preg/Cycle	Swim Up Gradients Preg/Cycle	Percoll Gradients Preg/Cycle	HSA Preg/Cycle	Total Preg/Cycle
Normal sperm	24/182	14/122	9/88	31/209	78/601
Subnormal sperm	2/32	2/34	9/107	12/105	25/278
Donor sperm	35/169	33/179	12/56	48/185	128/589
Total	**61/383**	**49/335**	**30/251**	**91/499**	**231/1468**

insemination was performed to avoid the risk of endometrial damage due to second insemination.

SPERM PREPARATION

Apart from routine techniques of sperm preparation, a two-layered human serum albumin (HSA) gradients technique was in particularly, used in subnormal semen samples. The results are given in Table 33.6.

It was observed that, pregnancy rate in HSA gradient technique (18.24%) was highest amongst rest of the techniques irrespective of semen quality. It may be noted that, PR of 11.4 percent with subnormal sperm, scored over rest of the techniques used for the same. Hence, it may be suggested that HSA gradients sperm preparation technique can be used for IUI procedures, especially in cases of subnormal semen quality. The authors of the present study earlier[15] observed similar findings with a smaller number of IUI cycles.

COMPLICATIONS

Very few complications may occur after IUI:
• Uterine cramps have been reported after IUI with apparently no further consequences
• Although, there is a theoretical risk of transporting bacteria with insemination pelvic infections reported are very rare.[46] Salpingitis has been reported after IUI.[47] Chances of pelvic infections are 1:800 inseminations.[48]
• OHSS may occur after IUI with super stimulation.
• Chances of multiple pregnancies with superovulation ranges from 7.5 to 29 percent per couple.[49]
• Multiple pregnancies are associated with maternal and fetal complications.[50]

CONCLUSION

Intrauterine insemination after ovarian stimulation with/without gonadotrophins is an undoubtedly successful and efficacious therapy of involuntary childlessness. It is a relatively simple, non-invasive, cheap and cost effective technique. Pregnancy rates of approximately 18-20 percent in couples with cervical factor, unexplained infertility or severe male factor seem to be quite realistic. IUI can be performed even without the facilities of an IVF center. However, a clinic with IVF facilities offers a better place in case, complications such as OHSS occurs. The cycle can be converted into an IVF cycle, and if necessary; cryopreservation of embryos may be possible.

Even though various techniques such as IVF-ET or ICSI to treat male factor infertility are available, they are not easily available or out of financial reach for many couples. Hence, male factor evaluation particularly in case of oligospermia, asthenospermia, teratospermia and subsequent selection of sperm preparation are crucial steps to offer relatively inexpensive and less rigorous treatment of IUI, with husband's sperm to achieve pregnancy though with relatively lower pregnancy rate or with donor sperm with higher pregnancy rate.

REFERENCES

1. Templeton A, Fraser C, Thompson B. The epidemiology of infertility in Aberdeen. Brit Med J 1990;301:148-52.
2. Brinsden R, Marcus S. An overview of intrauterine insemination. In Meniru GI(Ed.): A Handbook of Intrauterine Insemination. Cambridge University Press, Cambridge, 1997;1-8.
3. Confine E et al. Fertil Steril 1986;46:55.
4. Toffle RC et al, Fertil Steril 1985;43:743.

5. Natchilgall RD et al., Artificial insemination of husband's sperm. Fertil Steril 1979;32:141.

6. Tariq Miskry et al. The use of intra uterine insemination in Australia and New Zealand. Human Reproduction 2002;17(4):956.

7. Peiris AN et al. The relationship of insulin to sex hormone binding globulin: role of adiposity. Fertil Steril 1989;52:69.

8. Kirschner MA et al. Androgen-estrogen metabolism in women with upper versus lower body adiposity. J.Clin Kndocrinol Metab 1990;70:473.

9. Randolph JR et al. Comparison of real time ultrasonography, hysterosalpyngography, Laparoscopy/hysteroscopy in the evaluation of uterine abnormalities. Fertil Steril 1986;46:828.

10. Valdos E et al. Ultrasound evaluation of female genital anomalies. Am J Obstet Gynaecol 1984;149:285.

11. World Health Organization (WHO): Practical manual for semen analysis 1992.

12. Arici A et al. Evaluation of clomiphen citrate and human choriconic gonadotrophin treatment: a prospective randomized, crossover study during intrauterine insemination cycles. Fertil Steril 1994;61:314-18.

13. Balasch J et al. Late low dose pure follicle stimulating hormone for ovarian stimulation in intrauterine insemination cycles. Hum Reprod 1994;9:1863-66.

14. Raeburn AR, Meniru MO. Fertility counseling In: Meniru GI, Brinsden PR, Craft IL(Eds.): A handbook of intrauterine insemination. Cambridge University Press, Cambridge: 1997 ;46-55.

15. Schoysman D,Vanderwlmen P, Nij's et al. Pregnancy after fertilization with human testicular spermatozoa (letter). Lancet 1993;342:1237.

16. Devroey P, Tourney H, Liu J. Fertilization of human oocytes after testicular sperm extraction and intracytoplasmic sperm injections. Fertil Steril 1994;62:639-64.

17. Silber SJ, van Steirteghen AC, Liu J. High fertilization and pregnancy rate after intracytoplasmic sperm injection with spermatozoa obtained from testicular biopsy. Hum Reprod 1995;10:148-52.

18. Tourney H, Devroey P, Liu J. Microsurgical epididymal sperm aspirations and intracytoplasmic sperm injection: a new effective approach to infertility as a result of bilateral absence of vas deferens. Fertil Steril 1994;61:1045-51.

19. Calderon G, Belil I, Aran B. Outcome of intracytoplasmic sperm injection and testicular spermatozoa in the treatment of azoospermic patients. References en Gynaecologic Obstetrique 1997;5:199-202.

20. Devroey P, Nagy Z, Gossens A. Pregnancies after testicular sperm extaction and intracytoplasmic spenn injection in non-obstructive azoospermia. Hum Reprod 1995;6:1457-60.

21. Clark JH, Guthrie SC. Agonistic and antagonistic effects of climiphen citrate and its isomers. Biol Repro 1981;25:667-72.

22. Steven L Young, Opsahi MS, Fritz MA. Serum concentrations of enclomiphene and zuclomiphene across consecutive cycles of clomiphene citrate therapy in anovulatory infertile women. Fertil Steril 1999;71:639-44.

23. Wallach EE. Gonadotrophin treatment of ovulatory patients: The pros and cons of empiric therapy for infertility. Fertil Stenl 1991;55:478-80.

24. Sakamoto C, Yoshimitsu K, Nakamura G. Sonographic study of endometrial responses to ovarian hormones in patients receiving ovarian stimulation. IntJGynaecol Obstet 1988;27:407-14

25. Fleisher AC, Herbert CM, Hill GA. Transvaginal sonography of the endometrium during induced cycles. J Ultrasound Med 1991;10:93-95.

26. Sher G, Herbert C, Massarani G. Assessment of late proliferative phase endometrium by ultrasonography in patients undergoing in vitro fertilization and embryo transfer (IVF-ET). Hum Reprod 1991;6:232-37.

27. Ritchie WGM. Ultrasound in evaluation of normal and induced ovulation. Fertil Stenl 1985;43:167.

28. Devroey P et al. Do we treat the male or his gamete? Hum Reprod 1988;13(Suppl 1):175-85.

29. Jouannetn P et al. Male factors and the likelihood of pregnancy in infertile couples. 1. Study of sperm characteristics. Int J Androl 1988;11:379-94.

30. Hull MGR et al. Infertility treatment: Relative effectiveness of conventional and assisted conception methods. Hum Reprod 1992;7:785-96.

31. Dickey RP et al. Comparison of sperm quality necessary for successful intrauterine insemination with World Health Organization threshold values for normal sperm. Fertil Steril 1999;71:684-89.

32. Matorras R et al, Sperm morphology analysis (strict criteria) in male infertility is not a prognostic factor in intrauterine insemination with husband's sperm. Fertil Stenl 1995;63:608-11.

33. Huang HY et al. The impact of the total motile sperm count on the success of intrauterine insemination with husband's spermatozoa. J Assist Reprod Genet 1996;13:56-63.

34. Byrd W et al. A prospective randomized study of pregnancy rates folloeing intrauterine and intracervical insemination using frozen donor sperm. Fertil Steril 1990;53:521-27.

35. Dodson WC and Haney AF, Controlled ovarian hyperstimulation and intrauterine insemination for treatment of infertility. Fertil Steril 1991;55:457-67.

36. Campana A et al. Intrauterine insemination: evaluation of results according to the woman's age, sperm quality, sperm count per insemination and life-table analysis. Hum Reprod 1996;11:732-36.

37. Kerin J, Byrd W. Supracervical replacement of spermatozoa. Iir.Soules MR (Ed.): Controversies in Reproductive Endocrinology* and infertility, Elsevier, Amsterdam, 1989.

38. Van Voorhis BJ et al., Cost effectiveness of infertility treatments: a cohort study. Fertil Steril 1997;67:830.

39. Iwasaki A, Gagnon C. Formation of reactive oxygen species in spermatozoa of infertile patients. Fertil Steril 1992;57:409-16.

40. Shekarriz M et al. A method of human semen centrifugation to minimize the iatrogenic sperm injuries caused by reactive oxygen species. I: Eur Urol 1995;28(l):31-35.

41. Shapiro SS. Strategies to improve efficiency of therapeutic donor insemination. Infertil ReprodMed Clin North Am 1992;3:469.

42. Kerin JFP et al., Improved conception rates after intrauterine insemination of washed spermatozoa from men with poor quality semen. Lancet 1984;1:533-34.

43. Arid A et al. Evaluation of clomiphen citrate and human chorionic gonadotrophins treatment: A prospective, randomized crossover study during intrauterine insemination cycles. Fertil Steril 1994;61:314-18.

44. Chimote M et al. Serum progesterone at the time of hCG and pregnancy outcome. 11th World congress on in vitro fertilization and Human reproductive genetics. Monduzzi Editors- International Proceeding Division, Sydney, Australia 1999;115-19.

45. Chimote N et al. Can HSA gradient sperm preparation replaces Percoll gradient method in intrauterine insemination? 11th World Congress on in vitro fertilization and reproductive genetics. Mondussi (Ed.): International proceedings division Sydney, Australia 1999;47-51.

46. Stone SC et al. Recovery of microorganisms from pelvic cavity after intracervical or intrauterine artificial insemination. Fertil Steril 1986;46:61

47. Gorson SL, Batzer FR, Gocial B. Intrauterine insemination and ovulation stimulation as treatment of infertility. J Reprod Medi 1989;34:397.

48. Dodson WC, Haney AF. Controlled ovarian hyperstimulation and intrauterine insemination for infertility. Fertil Steril 1991;55:457-67.

49. Goldfarb JM, Peskin B, Austin C. Evaluation of predictive factors for multiple pregnancies during gonadotrophin/lUI treatment. J Assist Reprod Genet 1991;14:88-91.

50. Gleicher N, Campbell DP,Chan CHL. The desire for multiple births in couples with infertility problems contradicts present practice patterns. Hum Reprod 1995;10:1079-84.

• Pankaj Shrivastav

34

Oocyte Retrieval and Embryo Transfer for in vitro Fertilization

In the last decade major advances have been made in the fields of ovarian stimulation and embryo culture. However, the techniques of oocyte retrieval and embryo transfer have remained substantially the same during this period. Oocyte retrieval during the early days of IVF was performed using a laparoscopic approach. This route is very rarely used now. During the late 1980's, vaginal ultrasound scanning became routinely available and it became possible to retrieve oocytes vaginally. The major advantage of this route over the laparoscopic route was that the procedure could be performed without general anesthesia and the patient suffers minimal post-operative discomfort. The laparoscopic route is still used when the patient is undergoing the Gamete Intrafallopian Transfer (GIFT) treatment, but has largely been superseded by ultrasound guided techniques. In the days of laparoscopic oocyte retrieval when the pelvis was found to be "frozen", ultrasound guided percutaneous oocyte retrieval was performed. This too is very rarely used now. However, in situations where one of the ovaries is very high due to pelvic or abdominal adhesions, or the ovaries are so large that the follicles situated at the superior pole of the ovary cannot be reached, we still resort to percutaneous oocyte retrieval using abdominal ultrasound guidance.

The technique of ultrasound guided vaginal oocyte retrieval is fairly standard, but minor variations do exist from center to center. The patient is encouraged to void urine prior to her being brought into the operation theatre. Most centers perform this procedure under sedation and para-cervical analgesia and the patient suffers almost no discomfort at all. Until recently our center performed the procedure using Midazolan (Dormicum, Roche SA) and Fentanyl (Janssen Pharmaceuticals). The patient under the influence of these drugs is arousable, but remains drowsy for an hour or two following the procedure. At present, we use Remifentanil (Ultiva, Glaxo Wellcome, UK) which is delivered using a IVAC-TIVA (Alaris Systems, UK) pump. The major advantage of Remifentanil is its extremely short duration of action. As soon as the medication is stopped, the patient awakens and is able to leave the center shortly thereafter. Early reports had suggested that Propofol (Diprivan, Zeneca, UK) accumulates in the follicular fluid (Coetsier *et al*[1]) and it was recommended that as the drug may exert a negative effect on the oocyte, the procedure should be kept as short as possible. However, recent studies have shown that detrimental effect of Propofol on fertilization, cleavage, implantation and pregnancy rates (Christiaens *et al*[2]).

Once the patient has been sedated, she is put in the lithotomy position and the skin of the lower abdomen, perineum and upper thighs cleaned using Betadine (Povidone-Iodine solution). A sterile speculum is then inserted into the vagina to visualize the cervix. The vagina is cleaned by repeatedly flushing it with sterile saline. Fears that cleaning the vagina with saline may not provide adequate vaginal disinfection have been unfounded (Van Os, et al[3]). In their study they report that when Betadine was used instead of normal saline to disinfect the vagina, the fertilization and cleavage rates remain unchanged. However, the pregnancy rate was significantly higher when saline was used to clean the vagina and this without an increase in the rate of infection.

At the Dubai Gynaecology and Fertility Centre we then administer a para-cervical block using 10 ml of 1 percent Xylocaine, the drug being administered at the 3 and 9 O'clock positions. The use of the para-cervical block decreases the requirement of intravenous analgesia.

The needle used to retrieve oocytes depends on whether the operator favors flushing the follicles or not. Proponents of single lumen needles point to the lower perception of pain when the needle diameter is smaller and at the reduced operative time when no flushing is performed (Aziz et al[4]). At the Dubai Gynaecology and Fertility Centre we use a double lumen needle so as to enable us to flush the follicles when no oocyte is visualized in the initial aspirate. Kingsland et al[5] found no difference in the number of oocyte retrieved, the fertilization, or the pregnancy rate whether the follicles were flushed, or not. However, in our own experience there appears to be a 33 percent enhancement in the oocyte retrieval when flushing is utilized. We retrieve the oocytes using a Craft suction device (Rocket, London, UK) and do not use pressures above 180 mm of mercury to aspirate the follicular contents, for fear of damaging the oocyte.

Once the oocyte retrieval has been completed care is taken to ensure that there is no oozing from the puncture site in the vaginal vault. If any oozing is present it is easily controlled by using pressure with a cotton swab. In rare instances a single suture may be required to arrest a persistent ooze. We routinely cover all oocyte retrieval procedure with antibiotics. If the patient is not allergic to Penicillin, a single intravenous dose (600 mg) of Augmentin is given at the time of the retrieval and the antibiotic is continued orally for 3 days, i.e. till 12 hours after the embryo transfer.

If the patient is allergic to Penicillin, two doses (80 mg) of intravenous Gentamicin are used, one at the time of oocyte retrieval and the second an hour before embryo transfer.

Very rarely no oocytes are retrieved from the follicles despite repeated flushing. While this may be an age related feature in women over the age of 40 years, it sometimes occurs in young women too. Awonuga et al[6] have reported that there may be a lack of bioavailability of hCG which may lead to non-retrieval of the oocytes.

Though ultrasound guided vaginal oocyte retrieval is relatively safe and easy procedure, complications may sometimes arise. Rarely infections from the vagina can be introduced into the pelvic cavity. In our own experience of approximately 3500 oocyte retrievals performed in Dubai over the last 9 years, we have come across only 1 case of pelvic infection following oocyte retrieval. The patient presented 3 days after oocyte retrieval with high grade fever and throbbing pelvic pain. After examination a diagnosis of an ovarian abscess was made and this was aspirated vaginally. The pus retrieved from the abscess, grew E. coli which was also present in the vaginal swabs. She was given the appropriate antibiotic and the condition resolved within 48 hours.

Damage to the blood vessels can occur especially in procedures performed by junior staff during the early part of the learning curve. The illiac vessels can look suspiciously like follicles and it is important that operators under training inspect each follicle in two dimensions before advancing the needle. Rare complication has been reported by Coccia et al;[7] one of their patients returned with an acute abdomen following the puncture of a dermoid cyst at the time of oocyte retrieval. All these complications are thankfully rare.

Following the procedure we advise patients to rest in bed or in an easy chair for an hour or two prior to returning home. They are advised to continue the antibiotic till after the embryos are transferred and paracetamol is given to ease any postoperative discomfort.

Women with polycystic ovaries who produce a large number of follicles and who have large ovaries are at risk of developing the ovarian hyperstimulation syndrome (OHSS). We transfuse 5 percent Albumin or Hespan (Hetastarch 6%, Sodium Chloride 0.9%) during the oocyte retrieval and this minimizes the risk of OHSS.

More recently immature oocyte retrieval from unstimulated women with Polycystic Ovarian Syndrome has been reported. The retrieval is performed 10 to 14 days after the patients period and the women is primed with 10,000 IU of hCG prior to the retrieval. Immature oocytes are cultured in medium supplemented with Follicular Stimulating Hormone and Luteinising Hormone. Intracytoplasmic sperm injection (ICSI) can then be performed on the mature oocytes to generate embryos, which have resulted in clinical pregnancies. The advantage of this technique is that it avoids the problem of hyperstimulation in women who have polycystic ovarian disease (Chian et al [8]).

EMBRYO TRANSFER

Following oocyte retrieval, the oocytes are inseminated, fertilization checked for 24 hours later and the embryos are further cultured for another 24 or 48 hours (in case of blastocyst transfer, 96 hours) before they are ready to be transferred into the uterine cavity. I will first detail how embryo transfer procedures are performed at the Dubai Gynaecology and Fertility Centre and follow this with a discussion of the various factors that may affect the outcome of the embryo transfer.

The patient is asked to ring up early in the morning on the day of the embryo transfer to ascertain what time she needs to come into the Centre. She is instructed not to pass any urine for an hour before the appointed time of the embryo transfer. Additionally, she is asked to drink 2 glasses of water an hour before she comes in. On the morning of the embryo transfer, she is instructed not to use the Cyclogest (Shire Pharmaceuticals, UK) pessaries vaginally and instead to use the rectal route. Once she is at the Centre she is placed on the operating table and put in the lithotomy position. Prior to the speculum being inserted, a quick transabdominal ultrasound examination is performed to check whether the bladder is reasonably full and whether the endometrium can be easily visualized. The cervix is then visualized and any excess discharge or cervical mucous wiped away by means of a swab moistened with culture medium. The speculum is then adjusted so as to provide the most appropriate angle of the cervical canal for the introduction of the catheter. The ultrasound probe is then placed on the abdominal wall to obtain a longitudinal view of the uterine cavity and cervical canal. The embryos are loaded in 10 to 15 µl of culture medium at the tip of a Wallace catheter, a small air bubble being positioned on either side of the embryos. The catheter is gently introduced into the cervical canal taking care to avoid touching the vaginal wall. Once the tip of the catheter is seen (on scan) to have negotiated the internal os, it is gently advanced to about 1-1½ cm from the fundus. If difficulty is experienced in negotiating the internal os, the hub of the guiding catheter is advanced to the level of the internal os to stiffen the tip of the transfer catheter. The transfer catheter is then gently manipulated past the internal os. Only if difficulty is still experienced in negotiating the internal os, is a malleable stillet used to enter the uterine cavity. Once the cavity has been entered, the malleable stillet is removed and the transfer catheter advanced into the uterine cavity. The embryos are then expelled very gently. The movement of the embryos into the uterine cavity can be easily visualized on the ultrasound screen as the tiny bubbles on either side of the culture medium can be seen entering the uterine cavity. If difficulty is experienced in entering the uterine cavity in spite of using the malleable stillet, the cervix is held with a tenaculum to try and straighten the uterocervical axis. In these situations, we have found that using a paracervical block, whereby 5 ml of 2 percent Xylocaine is injected at 3 and 9 O'clock positions, helps in easing the transfer procedure. If entry of the catheter fails despite all these measures, cervical dilatation under ultrasound guidance is carried out.

Some centers have suggested that a mock embryo transfer be performed either prior to starting the cycle, or just prior to the real transfer

(Sharif et al [9]). The advocates of a mock embryo transfer suggest that the length of the uterus cervical canal can be measured at this time so as to allow replacement of the embryos without touching the uterine fundus. We ourselves do not practice mock embryo transfers. As we routinely conduct embryo transfer under ultrasound guidance, it is easy to ascertain the direction of the uterus cervical canal and to determine exactly where the embryos should be replaced without having to touch the uterine fundus.

It is important that the embryo transfer be performed in as atraumatic a way as possible, as this will effect the eventual pregnancy outcome. Junctional zone contractions have been demonstrated in the uterine cavity and these are stimulated by excessive cervical and uterine manipulations. Use of a tenaculum is also thought to increase these contractions. Junctional zone contractions could cause the embryos to relocate either to the Fallopian tube (and may be responsible for the 2.1 to 9.4% reported incidence of ectopic pregnancy following IVF and ET) or the cervix. Junctional zone contractions are stimulated during difficult transfers and can be seen as strong endometrial waves in the fundal area (Ijland et al [10]). These authors have shown that the overall risk of ectopic pregnancy is 1.5 to 10 times higher when the embryo transfer procedure is difficult, than when the procedure is easy. Lesny et al [11] have shown that a difficult transfer procedure generated strong random waves in the fundal area and waves from the fundus to the cervix, which could be responsible for expelling the embryos into the cervical canal or into the fallopian tubes. Fanchin et al [12] have reported a stepwise decrease in clinical and ongoing pregnancy rates as well as implantation rates, with increasing frequency of uterine contractions.

Many units perform embryo transfer by means of the touch technique. In this technique the catheter is introduced into the uterine cavity till the tip is felt to encounter the fundus. The catheter is then withdrawn 1-2 cm and the embryos are deposited at this level. It is now being realized that visualization of the uterine cavity by means of an abdominal ultrasound is of great importance.

Apart from indicating the utero cervical axis, it enables transfer of embryos at a point 2 cm below the fundus without having to touch the fundus at all. Wood et al [13] have shown that embryo transfer using a soft catheter under good ultrasound visualization results in a significant increase in clinical pregnancy rates.

There are contradictory opinions as to whether the choice of catheter effects the outcome of the embryo transfer procedure. While some authors,[14] report that the choice of catheter does not effect the pregnancy rate, it is reasonable to expect that the less traumatic the procedure the more likely is it to be successful. A stiff catheter which either traumatizes the cervical canal or endometrium and may lead to bleeding, is likely to compromise results. For this various authors [16] have shown a preference for one type of catheter over others. We ourselves prefer to use the Wallace catheter, as the inner transfer catheter is very soft and very rarely causes bleeding from trauma to the cervical canal or endometrium.

After embryo transfer patients are kept horizontal for about 15–20 minutes after which they are encouraged to empty their bladders. Following this they are free to travel back home and no restrictions are placed on their movements. Botta and Grudzinskas [17] have shown that prolonged bed rest following embryo transfer is not associated with a better outcome of the IVF procedure as compared with a 20 minute rest. Similarly, Woolcott and Stanger [18] have shown that standing upright shortly after embryo transfer does not affect the position of the embryos transferred into the uterine cavity.

Neither the vagina nor the ectocervix can be considered sterile areas and endocervical swabs and embryo transfer catheter tips have tested positive for microbial growths.[19] The clinical pregnancy rate per transfer is 57 percent in a group of patients without any microbial growth as compared to 29.6 percent in a group with positive microbial growth from the catheter tip. The tip of the catheter should not be allowed to touch the vaginal wall or the ectocervix at the time of the transfer. In our practice, we continue the antibiotic started at the time of the oocyte retrieval till 12 hours have elapsed after the embryo transfer.

While the transcervical transfer of embryos into the uterine cavity is the most commonly used techniques, other techniques do exist. Zygote or embryo, intrafallopian transfer using either the laparoscopic route or the retrograde transcervical route have been advocated. However, no advantage of these techniques over the traditional transcervical intrauterine transfer have been reported and they are not commonly used. Gestaldi et al[20] reported an intraendometrial embryo transfer using a modified Monash catheter, but it was Kato et al[21] who first reported a transmyometrial embryo transfer. The latter author replaced the embryos into the uterine cavity using a Tovaco needle and catheter. Pregnancies were reported with both these techniques. Light sedation was required for the procedure. Asaad and Carver-Ward[22] reported transmyometrial, subendometrial transfer for a patient who had repeatedly failed to conceive using traditional embryo transfer techniques. The patient conceived and was delivered of healthy twin girls vaginally. Anttila et al[23] report a case of transmyometrial embryo transfer in a patient with cervical atresia. Another option in patients with cervical atresia would be to do a laparoscopic zygote intrafallopian transfer.

Over the last decade, the procedures for oocyte retrieval and embryo transfer have been standardized. Any future improvement in the success rate of IVF will probably be due to an improvement in ovarian stimulation or embryo culture techniques.

REFERENCES

1. Coetsier T, Dhont M, Sutter P De, Merchiers E, Versichelen L, Rosseel MT. Propofol anaesthesia for ultrasound guided oocyte retrieval: Accumulation of the anaesthetic agent in follicular fluid. Hum Reprod 1992;7:1422-24.
2. Christiaens F, Janssenswillen C, Van Steirteghem AC, Devroey P, Verborgh C, Camu F. Comparison of assisted reproductive technology performance after oocyte retrieval under general anaesthesia (propofol) versus paracervical local anaesthetic block: a contolled study. Hum Reprod 1998;13:2456-60.
3. Van Os HC, BJ Roozenburg HC, Janssen-Caspers HA, Leerentveld RA, Scholtes MC, Zeilmaker GH, Alberda AT. Vaginal disinfection with povidon iodine and the outcome of in-vitro fertilisation. Hum Reprod 1992; 7:349-50.
4. Aziz N, Biljan MM, Taylor CT, Manasse PR, Kingsland CR. Effect of aspirating needle calibre on outcome of in vitro fertilisation. Hum Reprod 1993;8:1098-1100.
5. Kingsland CR, Taylor CT, Aziz N, Bickerton N. Is follicular flushing necessary for oocyte retrieval? A randomised trial. Hum Reprod 1991;6:382-83.
6. Awonuga A, Govindbhai J, Zierke S, Schnauffer K. Continuing the debate on empty follicle syndrome: Can it be associated with normal bioavailability of beta-human chorionic gonadotrophin on the day of oocyte recovery? Hum Reprod 1998;13:1281-84.
7. Coccia ME, Becattini C, Bracco GL, Scarselli G. Acute abdomen following dermoid cyst rupture during transvaginal ultrasonographically guided retrieval of oocytes. Hum Reprod 1996;11:1897-99.
8. Chian RC, Buckett WM, Tulandi T, Tan SL. Prospective randomized study of human chorionic gonadotrophin priming before immature oocyte retrieval from unstimulated women with polycystic ovarian syndrome. Hum Reprod 2000;15:165-70.
9. Sharif K, Afnan M, Lenton W. Mock embryo transfer with a full bladder immediately before the real transfer for in vitro fertilisation treatment: the Birmingham experience of 113 cases. Hum Reprod 1995;10:1715-18.
10. Ijland MM, Hoogland HJ, Dunselman GAJ, Lo CR, Evers JLH. Endometrial wave direction switch and the outcome of in vitro fertilisation. Fertility Sterility 1999;71: 476-81.
11. Lesny P, Killick SR, Tetlow RL, Robinson J, Maguiness SD. Embryo transfer–can we learn anything new from the observation of junctional zone contractions ? Hum Reprod 1998;13:1540-46.
12. Fanchin R, Righini C, Olivennes F, Taylor S, Ziegler D de, Frydman R. Uterine contractions at the time of embryo transfer alter pregnancy rates after in vitro fertilisation. Hum Reprod 1998;13:1968-74.
13. Wood EG, Batzer FR, Go KJ, Gutmann JN, Corson SL. Ultrasound-guided soft catheter embryo transfers will improve pregnancy rates in in vitro fertilisation. Hum Reprod 2000;15(1):107-12.
14. Diedrich K, van der Ven H, al-Hasani S, Krebs D. Establishment of pregnancy related to embryo transfer techniques after in vitro fertilisation. Hum Reprod 1989;4:111-14.
15. Ghazzawi IM, Al-Hasani S, Karaki R, Souso S. Transfer technique and catheter choice influence the incidence of transcervical embryo expulsion and the outcome of IVF. Hum Reprod 1999;14:677-82.
16. Gonen Y, Dirnfeld M, Goldman S, Koifman M, Abramovici H. Does the choice of catheter for embryo transfer influence the success rate of in vitro fertilisation? Hum Reprod 1991;6:1092-94.
17. Botta G, Grudzinskas G. Is a prolonged bed rest following embryo transfer useful? Hum Reprod 1997;12:2489-92.

18. Woolcott R, Stanger J. Ultrasound tracking of the movement of embryo associated air bubbles on standing after transfer. Hum Reprod 1998;13:2107-09.

19. Egbase PE, al-Sharhan M, al-Othman S, al-Mutawa M, Udo EE, Grudzinskas JG. Incidence of microbial growth from the tip of the embryo transfer catheter after embryo transfer in relation to clinical pregnancy rate following in vitro fertilisation and embryo transfer. Hum Reprod 1996;11:1687-89.

20. Gastaldi C, Loda G, Salvi R et al. Preliminary report on intra-endometrial embryo transfer (IET). Hum Reprod 1993;8(Suppl 1):37.

21. Kato O, Takatsuka R, Asch RH. Transvaginal-transmyometrial embryo transfer; the Towako method; experience of 104 cases. Fertil Steril 1993;59:51-53.

22. Asaad M, Carver-Ward JA. Twin pregnancy following transmyometrial-subendometrial embryo transfer for repeated implantation failure. Hum Reprod 1997;12:2824-25.

23. Anttila L, Penttila TA, Suikkari AM. Successful pregnancy after in vitro fertilisation and trans-myometrial embryo transfer in a patient with congenital atresia cervix: Case report. Hum Reprod 1999;14:1647-49.

• Kamini A Rao

35

Prognostic Markers in in vitro Fertilization— Embryo Transfer

INTRODUCTION

In the complex technology of IVF-ET, we deal with a number of variables right from screening stage to the stage of establishing viable pregnancy and a successful term delivery thereafter. These variables, singly or in combination with others, contribute largely to the success of this maneuver. Correct understanding of these variables, in turn could serve as milestones on the road to success. These variables or milestones could then be translated quantitatively and/or qualitatively and defined with greater precision. The observation of these variables, alternately described as markers, may help to predict success or failure of the procedure in terms of the desired results and may further contribute to achievement of higher success rates.

These milestones or the markers, which indicate the prognosis, to be called hereafter as prognostic markers, can be broadly divided into two categories—clinical and laboratory. The clinical markers are dealt with during such procedures as the initial screening of the patients (both female and male), indication for which the patients are being taken up for IVF-ET, controlled ovarian hyperstimulation (COH), ultrasound (US) studies during COH, follicular aspiration, follicular flushing, embryo transfer and nature and quantum of luteal support provided. The laboratory markers constitute gonadotrophin and steroidal levels, and assessment of basic seminal parameters during the screening procedure, gonadotrophin and steroidal levels during COH, examination of oocyte quality, sperm preparation, the insemination procedure, the embryonic development in vitro, and post-transfer monitoring.

In the interest of lucidity of presentation and easy comprehension, these prognostic markers are dealt with under each procedure during the IVF program.

INITIAL SCREENING BEFORE RECRUITMENT

Indication

The indication for which the patient is being taken up for IVF-ET has an important bearing on success or failure. Women with PCO, endometriosis, associated male factor, male factor alone, are known to respond poorly in terms of pregnancy rates, whereas women with tubal factor, unexplained infertility (> 80% fertilization rates), recipient women with donated oocytes are known to yield optimal pregnancy rates.

The question whether bilateral salpingectomy compromises ovarian function has remained unsettled. The analysis of our data indicates that in women having undergone bilateral salpingectomy, the ovarian response to stimulation in an IVF program does not appear to get compromised.

About 25 percent of women with PCOD are known to go for alternate procedures like IVF-ET. The outcome of these patients with IVF treatment is highly erratic, they are known for either under-response or over-response. Fertilization rates and implantation rates are rather disappointing in spite of normal sperm parameters—probably because of poor oocyte quality, consequently the clinical pregnancy rates are not so encouraging. The use of LHRH analogs during COH with the objective of keeping high basal LH low, has certainly improved the success rates in this class of patients.

Ovarian Status

Though most women recruited in standard IVF program are ovulatory or perhaps in some cases oligoovulatory, it is prudent to confirm their ovulation status. Further, their ovarian status is assessed by carrying out basal FSH on day 3. If the level is less than 15 mIU/mL, she is likely to be a good responder, if however, it is more than 15 mIU/mL, she is likely to be a poor responder during COH. Pregnancy rates are also better in the former than in the latter.

Endometrial Status

Assessment of endometrial status routinely during screening, especially in women with secondary infertility and repeated GIFT/IVF failures has been rewarding. Even in women with long-standing primary infertility with suggestive pelvic factor, this must be carried out in view of the high incidence of tuberculosis infection. This assessment can be made by hysterosalpingography and/or hysteroscopy.

Midluteal endometrial biopsy and/or progesterone may yield useful information regarding possible existence of luteal phase defects. In our center, we routinely perform midluteal progesterone as part of the screening process and if the level is more than 10 ng/mL, the patient is regarded as having no luteal problem. If less, appropriate screening is carried out and the fault corrected.

Basic Seminal Parameters

Assessment of semen parameters before and after wash, provides useful guidelines to the likely course of the IVF treatment cycle. From our experience, it can be said that postwash parameters give definite indication of the likely fertilization rate, the possible number of pre-ovulatory, oocytes that one should target at, and the number of embryos one would require for transfer depending upon the availability and the need for freezing of the embryos. This exercise enables the clinician to chalk out appropriate strategy for COH to achieve the targetted number of oocytes and good quality embryos, which ultimately reflect on the outcome of the IVF maneuver.

CONTROLLED OVARIAN HYPERSTIMULATION (COH)

Selection of the Stimulation Protocol

In the author's well considered and candid opinion, this is the most vital part of the IVF program, once the patient is selected and informed consent obtained. There are two important objectives, *viz* obtain the required number of good quality oocytes to produce optimal rate of fertilization and consequently the required number of good quality embryos for transfer, and generate the most ideal endometrial status at the time of oocyte recovery for effective implantation. Achievement of both these objectives to run concurrently, demands a high degree of precision in adopting the right strategy for stimulation, monitoring of the patient and judgement for timing of hCG injection prior to oocyte recovery. Needless to say, therefore, that the stimulation protocol so selected, individualized for each patient, is likely to reflect the success or failure of the procedure in each patient.

In the author's experience, five important considerations such as the age, the basal endocrine profile (FSH, LH), indication for which the patient is being treated by IVF-ET, presence of absence of associated endometriosis and presence of absence of associated male factor determine the final option out of several stimulation protocols at the disposal of the clinician. Cysts, if present, may be aspirated, as per guidelines given later and stimulation regimen started. The importance of age, basal FSH, indication for IVF-ET and associated endometriosis and male factor has been dealt with. The importance of basal LH is dealt with below.

Basal LH on day 3 gives yet another useful marker which helps in deciding the right strategy for COH. This is regardless of whether the patient has ultrasonically proven PCO or not. Women with day 3 LH more than 8 mlU/mL need a different strategy during COH employing LHRHa in short or long protocol. The need in these patients is to keep the LH low and less than 8 mlU during COH. LH is thus controlled during periovulatory phase through the use of suitable combination of hMG and FSH, while continuing LHRHa in a suitable dosage. It has been adequately demonstrated that in women with high LH levels (> 8 mlU/mL) during periovulatory phase, the oocyte recovery rates, fertilization rates, and implantation rates are low.

Basal ultrasound scan helps in detecting the presence of cysts. It is our experience, that if the cyst is of more than 25 mm and if estradiol is less than 25 pg/mL, it interferes with the ovarian response to stimulation. Hence, aspiration of such a cyst prior to stimulation is known to entail a better ovarian response to the stimulation protocol in our center.

The secret of reaching four important benchmarks, *viz* the targetted number of oocytes for recovery, targetted fertilization rate, targetted number of good quality embryos and effective implantation, lies in touching four vital milestones during COH and these are—synchronization of follicular growth with endometrial maturity, correct timing of hCG administration, selection of the right embryos for transfer, and creating the right hormonal mileu in the endometrium in terms of optimal $P:E_2$ ratio at the time of transfer. These four milestones represent the markers for prognosis. Whilst the first three are controllable to a large extent, the fourth one is difficult as we still do not know what is the right ratio. But it is certainly known that the ratio of $P:E_2$ is important and not the levels of each hormone for effective implantation. Synchronization of follicular and endometrial maturity demands very high degree of precision and understanding of endocrinological

aspects from the specialist and it is possible to achieve, though difficult in many cases. For selection of the right embryos, we follow the concept of embryo scoring in our center and this helps us in deciding, which embryos to transfer and which to freeze for donor programs. For achieving the optimal $P:E_2$ ratio at the time of transfer, a great deal will depend on the E_2 and P levels at the time of hCG administration, P administered during oocyte recovery or not, and type and degree of luteal support provided.

The adequacy of laboratory support by way of optimal culture conditions, sperm preparation techniques adopted to get maximum morphologically normal motile sperm yield, satisfactory fertilization rates and embryo development cannot be overemphasized. These are equally important requirements for optimal pregnancy rates. Reinsemination of unfertilized oocytes, in our opinion, does not help and is not being practised at our center. It may include polypronuclear fertilization and embryos cleaving thereby, do not implant.

ASSOCIATED MISCELLANEOUS MARKERS

Clinical

Hydrosalpinx

Women with hydrosalpinx have an associated risk for ectopic pregnancy and postaspiration infection. Repeated IVF attempts fail to result in pregnancy but salpingectomy followed by IVF-ET is known to yield pregnancy. Hence hydrosalpinx in a woman is known to be associated with failure of IVF program.

Chlamydial Antibodies

Chlamydia trachomatis microorganism commonly infects the tubes and is asymptomatic in 75 percent of the women infected producing chronic salpingitis. These women remain infertile. There is very little data on the outcome of IVF-ET in this class of women. Reports about the future of these patients after treatment with IVF-ET are controversial. Our own experience in our center, though limited, indicates that the presence of these antibodies does not adversely influence the outcome of IVF-ET.

Encounters in Stimulation Phase

There is much controversy regarding the levels of LH, P, and E_2 during the stimulation phase. There is data for and against high levels of E_2 and P. Majority of workers regard elevated levels of LH after D_9 of stimulation as being derogatory to the outcome. In our center we assay LH and P daily from D_9 of stimulation. Our own data analysis confirms the derogatory effects of raised LH and raised progesterone during the periovulatory phase. Regarding E_2, we have not made any study but we are inclined to believe that high E_2 levels (say > 400 pg/mL/mean follicular volume) on the day of hCG may adversely affect prospects of implantation. Hence, we try and maintain E_2 levels on the day of hCG at around 250 pg/mL/ mean follicular volume.

Prolactin has been known to get elevated during the stimulation phase and it has been reported that this elevation of prolactin has no impact on the outcome of IVF. We have no experience in this regard as we do not assay prolactin during stimulation phase.

Follicular flushing has been shown to be associated with reduced pregnancy rates. Indeed it has been demonstrated to reduce granulosa cell mass, thereby warranting greater luteal support. In fact, the utility of flushing itself has been questioned. In our center, flushing is occasionally done, though we have no analysis of data to say one way or the other.

Endometrium and the Implantation Window

In spite of replacing good quality embryos, 85 to 90 percent of these embryos get rejected. Obviously, the endometrium is not receptive to these so-called good embryos. Though, we have lots to do still in improving the quality of embryos, in the present state of technology there is much more to do for improving the endometrial receptivity.

Identification of the most important published studies through MEDLINE involving different stimulation protocols reveals the following.
- The relative importance of receptive endometrium has been adequately demonstrated in agonadal women receiving embryos from donated eggs.
- Widely used stimulation protocols frequently result in endometrial imbalance, the specific reason being unknown. It is speculated that supraphysiologic E_2 and progesterone levels may be responsible for the aberrant endometrium.
- The data gathered are indicative of compromised capacity of the endometrium to permit implantation at the time of embryo transfer.
- Experience gained in agonadal women, with artificial endometrial cycles with hormone replacement therapy (HRT) has been rewarding.

THE DAY OF EMBRYO TRANSFER

In the spontaneous pregnancy, implantation is known to take place about 5 to 7 days after fertilization, i.e. on day 17 to day 19. Attempts have been made to transfer embryos during this period. Retrospective data analysis has demonstrated that maximum clinical pregnancies are obtained when embryos are replaced during this period. Further evidence to this effect has been obtained from studies on recipients of egg donation programs. Many workers prefer to replace the embryos in the recipients on day 3 to 5 of progesterone administration during HRT.

The Window of Implantation

Delayed rise in hCG in some GnRHa/hMG pregnancies is a known observation and it is suggestive of a delay in implantation. hCG, which appears in maternal serum only after implantation, is the earliest reliable detectable marker for implantation. Implantation time *in vivo* and the time of implantation after IVF, have been evaluated by many using serial hCG measurements. It has been shown that the GnRHa/hMG protocol widens the implantation window, which in part, may explain the improved pregnancy rates reported with GnRHa protocols.

Laboratory

A number of factors during processes of sperm preparation, fertilization, embryo development and cryopreservation of embryos are known to influence pregnancy rates. We shall deal with important factors only.

Sperm Morphology

A number of workers have noticed a correlation between fertilizing ability and sperm parameters. There is good evidence to demonstrate that morphologically normal sperm offer the best fertilizing potential, whereas increased morphologically abnormal sperm give reduced fertilizing capacity. Hence, the method employed to recover the highest density of morphologically normal sperm is likely to determine the fertilization rate which in turn may influence the pregnancy rates.

Oocyte Quality

Oocyte quality is a very important prognostic marker to determine the pregnancy rates. Different qualities of oocytes are recovered in the follicular aspirates—immature, mature, post-mature. It is the mature oocyte which has the highest pregnancy potential. Immature oocytes recovered, on prolonged preincubation period do fertilize, these embryos whether they give pregnancies is not yet known, because whenever embryos developed out of immature oocytes have been replaced, they are transferred along with other good quality embryos developed out of mature oocytes. Hence, it is difficult to say which embryo has implanted and given the pregnancy. Immaturity and chromosomal abnormalities in oocytes have been widely reported. Oocyte quality is vastly a result of stimulation protocol. Post-mature oocytes, though fertilized, do not implant. Optimal oocyte quality, by traditional criteria, as defined by Lucinda Veek, are known to develop into good quality embryos and cleavage rate.

Fertilization

Fertilization can be influenced by a number of male factors, besides oocyte quality and zona pellucida antibodies, such as morphology, presence of antisperm antibodies, sperm acrosin activity, etc. Standard semen analysis has never been proven to be a useful parameter for deter-

mining sperm fertility potential. Sperm fertilizing ability has received attention from clinicians and scientists alike. The development of bioassays to assess sperm function at fertilization level has enhanced our knowledge of the interaction between the sperm and the egg. A number of tests have been in use. Sperm binding capacity to zona pellucida reduced in couples with male factor has been well documented.

Acrosin, a constituent of the acrosome is involved in sperm-oocyte interaction. Sperm devoid of acrosin have no fertilizing potential, and acrosin levels have been shown to be higher in fertile men than in infertile men. Acrosin activity, has been shown to be correlated with the proportion of mature oocytes fertilized and transferred as cleaving embryos. The higher the acrosin activity, the greater is the likelihood of potential success in IVF.

Female antisperm antibodies have been well implicated in female infertility and females with high titers of these antibodies have proven to be failures even in IVF-ET. Incubating the oocytes of these females, *in vitro*, even with albumin instead of using maternal serum has proved to be insufficient. It appears that there may be greater complexity to the problem of antisperm antibodies than the simple contamination of the serum and the follicular fluid. This remains an area for further research.

EMBRYO DEVELOPMENT

Attempts are being made to improve the embryo quality. Platelet activating factor (PAF-acether, as is known now) or an analog substance has been proposed as an early embryonic signal to indicate embryo viability. Mild thrombocytopenia has been a known phenomenon during early pregnancy in the normal fertile population. PAF is secreted by the growing embryo immediately after insemination. Many studies have shown that PAF produced by early embryonic development plays a significant role in the implantation. PAF has also been measured in the embryo culture media. However, this concept has yet to find its place in the practical laboratory setting, and hence it calls for further research.

CONCLUSION

The practice of IVF-ET, both standard and applied, calls for standardized equipment, experience and above all dedication on the part of the staff. Systematic data recording and retrospective data analysis are invaluable and pave the way for further improvements. Various well-defined milestones in this rapidly developing technology have been dealt with through the world literature survey and my own experience in our center in India and abroad. These variables, singly or in combination with others contribute in a large measure to the success of the procedure. Current understanding of these variables could serve as milestones on the road to success.

FURTHER READINGS

1. Cohen J. A review of clinical microsurgical fertilisation. In Cohen J, Malter HE, Talansky BE, et al (Eds): Micromanipulation of Human Gametes and Embryos 1991;163-90.
2. Confino E et al. The predictive value of hCG beta-subunit levels in pregnancies achieved by in vitro fertilization and embryo transfer: An international collaborative study. Fertil Steril 1986;45:526.
3. Dimitry ES et al. Beneficial effects of a 24 hour delay in human chorionic gonadotrophin administration during in vitro fertilization treatment cycles. Human Reproduction 1991;6(7):944-46.
4. FIVNAT (French in vitro National), French national IVF registry: Analysis of 1986 to 1990 data. Fertil Steril 1993;59(3):587-95.
5. Frydman R, Eibschitz I. Uterine evaluation by microhystoscopy. Human Reproduction 1987;2:481-87.
6. Glass RH, Gollus MS. Habitual abortion. Fertil Steril 1978;29:257-65.
7. Hann G et al. Results of IVF from a prospective multicentre study. Human Reprod 1991;6(6):805-10.
8. Kingsland CR et al. Is follicular flushing necessary for oocyte retrieval? A randomised trial. Human Reprodn 1991;6(3):382-83.
9. Leeton EA et al. Plasma concentrations of human chorionic gonadotrophin from the time of implantation until the second week of pregnancy. Fertil Steril 1982;37:773.
10. Mortime D et al. Morphological selection of human spermatozoa 'in vivo' and 'in vitro'. J Reprodn Fertil 1982;64:391-99.
11. Moss TR. Chlamyda trachomatis: Importance in in vitro fertilization: J Soc Med 1984;77:40.
12. Pattinson HA et al. Transient hyperprolactinemia has no effect on endocrine response and outcome in in vitro fertilization (IVF). J in vitro fert and Embryo Transfer 1990;7(2):89-93.
13. Pousette A et al. Increase in progressive motility and improved morphology of human spermatozoa following their migration through Percoll gradients. Int J Androl 1986;9:1-13.
14. Rowland GF et al. Failure of in vitro fertilization and embryo replacement following infection with Chlamydia trachomatis. J in vitro Fert Embryo Transfer 1985;2:51.
15. Scott R et al. Follicle stimulating hormone levels on cycle day 3 are predictive of in vitro fertilization outcome. Fertil Steril 1989;51(4):651-54.
16. Society for Assisted Reproductive Technology, The American Fertility Society, Assisted reproductive technology in the United States and Canada: 1993 results from the Society for Assisted Reproductive Technology generated from the American Fertility Society Registry. Fertil Steril 1993;59(5):956-62.
17. Standell A et al. Hydrosalpinx reduces in vitro fertilisation/embryo transfer pregnancy rates. Human Reproduction 1994;9(5):861-63.
18. Tadir Y. Microsurgical fertilization: World survey 1993. J of Asst Reprodn and Genetics 1994;11(1):5-13.
19. Tasdamir I et al. Effect of chlamydial antibodies on the outcome of in vitro fertilization (IVF) treatment. J Asst Reprodn and Genetics 1994;11(2):104-06.
20. Torode HW et al. The role of chlamydial antibodies in an in vitro fertilization programme. Fertil Steril 1987;48:987.
21. Tur-Kaspa I et al. Ovarian stimulation protocol for in vitro fertilisation with gonadotrophin-releasing hormone agonist widens the implantation window. Fertil Steril 1990;53(5):859-64.
22. Verhulst G, van der Steen N, van Steirteghem AC, Devroey P. Bilateral salpingectomy does not compromise ovarian stimulation in an in vitro fertilisation/embryo transfer programme. Human Reproduction 1994;9(4):624-28.

36

• **Kamini A Rao**

Semen Intrafallopian Transfer

INTRODUCTION

Treatment of infertility using Assisted Reproductive Techniques (ARTs) has gained popularity over the last two decades. There are different methods of treatment such as gamete intrafallopian transfer (GIFT), zygote intrafallopian transfer (ZIFT), *in vitro* fertilization-embryo transfer (IVF-ET) or intracytoplasmic sperm injection (ICSI). All these methods of assisted reproduction in induced cycles increase the chance of fertilization because there are more oocytes, the semen is artificially improved and the sperm's path is shortened.

Jansen and Anderson (1987) reported on the catheterization of the fallopian tubes through the vagina under ultrasound guidance, using a specially designed device.[1] Catheterization and transfer of capacitated spermatoza to the oviduct resulted in a few normal pregnancies. Later transvaginal intrafallopian semen transfer was successfully attempted by Holst and Forsdahl (1988) employing blind catheterization of the fallopian tubes transvaginally using a specially designed catheter.[2] Ten women with unexplained infertility who underwent this procedure resulted in four normal singleton pregnancies.

At our center, we have reported a simplified cost-effective technique called the translaparoscopic semen intrafallopian transfer (SIFT). In this technique prepared semen is directly introduced into one or both fallopian tubes timing with ovulation. The causes of infertility in selected patients are often due to cervical hostility, tubal (single patent tube), male and unexplained factors.

The investigations include a hysterosalpingography and a diagnostic laparoscopy to confirm patency of the tubes, rule out endometriosis and adhesions of the tubes with other pelvic structures. The semen sample is analyzed and its processability also assessed. The minimum criteria for inclusion into the SIFT program is a total count not less than 10 million/mL with a motility of 50 percent or more with less than 20 percent abnormal forms. A semen culture and sensitivity test is done prior to the procedure and any infection present is appropriately treated.

INDUCTION OF OVULATION

Ovulation is induced by using clomiphene citrate (CC—100 mg/day) alone from day 2 to 6 of the cycle, or in combination with individually tailored doses of human menopausal gonadotrophin (hMG) from day 4 depending on the results of follicle growth, monitored daily ultrasonographically. A dose of 5000 IU of human chorionic gonadotrophin (hCG) is given 34 to 40 hours prior to the procedure.

SPERM PREPARATION

Semen is obtained by masturbation in a sterile container and prepared by the swim-up technique, which has been modified from the technique reported by Mahadevan and Baker (1984).[3] For swim-up, 2 mL of culture medium is added to 1 mL of semen and centrifuged at 800 to 1000 rpm for 6 minutes. The supernatant is decanted and 2 mL of Earle's bicarbonate culture medium is added to the sperm pellet and the pellet thoroughly mixed with the culture medium using a 1 mL syringe. Centrifugation is then repeated. The supernatant layer is decanted off and the culture medium is stratified over the sperm pellet and incubated at 37°C for 30 minutes. Active sperms move up into the culture medium and only the supernatnt is used for insemination.

SIFT TECHNIQUE

The SIFT technique is a simple laparoscopic procedure, which is done 34 to 40 hours after administration of hCG. The procedure is done under IV sedation (Diazepam 10 mg + Pethidine 100 mg). The patient is placed in a supine position and the abdomen painted with spirit. Local anesthesia (1% Xylocaine) is infiltrated around the umbilicus. Pneumoperitoneum is created by passing a 12 cm long (Veres) cannula. About 1.5 to 2 liters of carbon dioxide gas is insufflated into the peritoneal cavity through the cannula. An incision of 0.25 to 0.5 cm is made below the umbilicus to pass the 6 mm trocar cannula, through which the double puncture laparoscope is introduced. A second incision 0.25 to 0.5 cm is made in the left lateral region 3 to 4" away from the midline to inset a 4 mm trocar cannula. A Semm's grasping forceps is passed through this to grasp the fallopian tube at the fimbrial end. A puncture is made at the right lateral region 2" away from the midline, to pass another needle (16G 18 CM) with stilette. The fallopian tube is held firmly to the fimbrial end and cannulated to the lateral one-third portion. The stilette is removed and the GIFT catheter loaded with 0.3 to 0.5 mL of processed semen is fed into the cannula. The cannula is slowly withdrawn and with the GIFT catheter *in situ*, 0.1 to 0.2 mL of the processed sample is slowly injected. The same is done to the other fallopian tube. After insemination both the trocars are removed, pneumoperotoneum reduced and the two incisions sutured using linen. The SIFT technique is an out-patient procedure and the patient can be sent home within 2 to 2½ hours, after the procedure.

In our clinic we have shown a 32 percent success rate with the SIFT technique. Out of these, patients stimulated with clomiphene citrate and hMG showed a better success rate of 18 percent compared to those who were stimulated with clomiphene citrate alone who showed a success rate of 14 percent. Success rates are 20 to 25 percent in IVF-ET and GIFT procedures.[4,56] Our success rate of 32 percent compares favorably with other ARTs.

CONCLUSION

In a developing country like India, the cost involved in procedures like IVF-ET, GIFT or ZIFT which includes hormonal and ultrasound monitoring of the case can be very time-consuming, costly and hence prohibitive for infertile couples to take up treatment. SIFT is a simple, cost-effective procedure. This technique eliminates the use of expensive equipment required for IVF or GIFT. Though a fairly successful technique the advent of newer advanced techniques does not qualify or validate the continued use of GIFT, making it more or less obsolete as time goes by.

REFERENCES

1. Jansen RRS, Anderson JC. Lancet 1987;11:309-10.
2. Holst N, Forsdahl F. Acta Obstet Gynaecol Scand 1988;67:471-72.
3. Mahadevan M, Baker G. Assessment and preparation of semen for in-vitro fertilisation. In Wood C, Trouson AO (Eds): Clinical in-viro Fertilisation Springer Verlag: Berlin 1984;83-97.
4. Hurley VA, Osborn JC, Leonei MA et al. Fertil Steril 1991;55(3):559-62.
5. Tabert LM, Hammond M, Bailey L, et al. Fertil Steril 1991;55(3):555-58.
6. Corsan GH, Kammann E. Fertil Steril 1991;55(3):468-77.

• Korula George • Herman A Fernandes

37

Gamete Intrafallopian Transfer

INTRODUCTION

Introduction of *in-vitro* fertilization and embryo transfer (IVF-ET) in 1978 by Steptoe and Edwards was a major breakthrough in the treatment of the infertile couple. Originally introduced to circumvent the problem of tubal damage, IVF-ET was soon utilized in other situations like endometriosis, unexplained infertility and even for male factor problems. In an attempt to improve the pregnancy rates, modifications of IVF were introduced in select situations. Gamete intrafallopian transfer (GIFT) was introduced in 1984 by Asch *et al*[1] to solve the problem of unexplained infertility. Later indications for GIFT expanded to include endometriosis and male factor infertility.

As with most treatment protocols in infertility, newer methods are introduced based on theoretical principles and are frequently not subjected to rigorous scrutiny of randomized controlled trial. With the passage of time, some of these procedures have become established, without their efficacy having been fully tested. Unfortunately, in infertility, randomized controlled trials are few and often involve small numbers, but when available should influence practice.

Ovulation induction with clomiphene citrate combined with hCG and intrauterine insemination (IUI) is used to treat infertility in nontubal situations. In these procedures, an assumption is made that ovulation occurs followed by ovum pickup and that a good concentration of motile sperms are present in the tube for fertilization to occur.

With GIFT one is able to ensure that this ideal situation occurs by placing the gametes directly into the fallopian tube. Tournay *et al*[2] have looked at the various aspects of tubal transfers and raised some very interesting issues.

Placement of gametes in the fallopian tubes takes advantage of the protective tubal environment, assuming that the oviduct milieu is beneficial. The tubal environment enhances oocyte maturation and sperm function allowing for better embryo development. The other major advantage of GIFT is better synchronization between the developing embryo and the uterine endometrium as it enters the uterine cavity only by day 5 or 6 as compared to a day 2 or 3 transfer in an IVF cycle.

In unexplained infertility, one is always worried about the "egg factor". Perhaps continued intratubal existence will help in an improvement as compared to *in vitro* culture systems.

In GIFT, uterine trauma and hypermotility of the uterus can be avoided and this would be especially advantageous if a difficult embryo transfer through the cervix is anticipated.

In the older age group patient, exposure of oocytes to *in vitro* culture systems may be associated with a hardening of the zona pellucida. The intratubal environment encountered in GIFT may possibly prevent this from occurring.

The difficulties with GIFT are that it is technically more difficult and the patient has to undergo a laparoscopy at the time of a transvaginal oocyte retrieval (TVOR), necessitating general anesthesia. Selection of gametes for transfer is based on an assessment of the cumulus oocyte complex and no proper evaluation of actual quality of the oocyte is taken into account. In IVF, one is able to assess or detect problems of fertilization as well as make a selection of good quality embryos for transfer.

In the earlier years, the results with GIFT were better than those with IVF perhaps indicating that *in vitro* culture systems were suboptimal. The development and introduction of better culture systems, especially blastocyst culture media, has resulted in the policy of extended culture. Blastocyst transfer allows selection of high quality embryos which when transferred will result in excellent pregnancy rates.

INDICATIONS

Nontubal etiological factors like:
- Unexplained infertility
- Mild male factor problems although intra-cytoplasmic sperm injection (ICSI) is more commonly used
- Endometriosis—early disease
- Anovulation
- Cervical factor
- Oocyte donation in premature menopause.

SCREENING

All men should have a semen analysis and an estimation of the total motile fraction. Ideally, sperm antibodies and immunobead tests should be done.

Screening for HIV and hepatitis B is recommended.

In the female routine blood chemistry is required prior to an anesthetic procedure, HIV, hepatitis B, physical examination and a prior assessment of pelvic organs by a laparoscopy and hysteroscopy is essential. At routine diagnostic laparoscopy, it is a good practice to make an assessment about suitability for GIFT.

LABORATORY FACILITIES REQUIRED

Facilities for IVF/ICSI and embryo freezing should be available so that excess oocytes collected are not discarded. They should be run through the process of IVF so that an assessment of fertilization can be made. These embryos can be frozen either on day 2 or 3 or even be allowed to go to the blastocyst stage prior to freezing. A frozen embryo transfer cycle can be initiated, if required, at a later date.

OVULATION INDUCTION

Controlled ovarian hyperstimulation using gonadotrophins after downregulation with GnRH-analogs is the standard procedure. Once oocyte development is optimal, (3 or more oocytes of $\geq$ 18 mm size) maturation is induced with 10,000 units of hCG and an ultrasound-guided TVOR performed 34 hours later. The procedure is preferably done under a general anesthetic, as a laparoscopy for GIFT will also need to be carried out.

THE EMBRYOLOGIST'S ROLE

Sperm Preparation

A total motile fraction of at least 500,000 sperms is required for GIFT. The semen is collected at least 2 hours before TVOR. Abstinence for 3 days but not more than 7 days is advised and the semen is collected in a non-toxic, wide mouthed sterile plastic container. It is advisable to freeze at least 2 semen samples prior to the procedure to ensure availability of a sample if problems with collection occur.

The semen is allowed to liquefy before it is examined microscopically to quantify the concentration and percentage of progressively motile sperms. Liquefied semen is washed with HEPES-based culture medium (HTF—human tubal fluid medium) supplemented with 8 percent maternal serum. Motile sperms are isolated either by the standard swim-up procedure or by 1 mL Percoll gradient of each 40:70:90 percent overlaid with 1 mL of fresh semen. The motile fraction obtained is incubated till the time of transfer.

Oocyte Selection

Oocyte cumulus complex (OCC) is identified from the TVOR aspirates under a stereomicroscope. With the help of pasture pipettes, the OCC is washed twice in HTFM (HEPES-HTF) and is graded based on the cellular morphology of the cumulus and coronal cells and is then transferred to culture tubes containing 1 mL HTF. OCC with well spread-out cumulus, loosely packed corona cells and with partial or clear visibility of the oocyte are selected for transfer. All oocytes retrieved are incubated at 37°C in an atmosphere of 5 percent CO_2.

Loading

In a Petri dish three droplets are prepared: the first contains 100,000 to 200,000 sperm per oocyte, the second contains the selected oocytes, while the third is a drop of medium. The embryologist, using a 1 mL syringe attached to the GIFT catheter (e.g. COOK IVF, K-GIFT-1010, 5.0 FR, 50 cm length), loads the catheter under the vision of a stereomicroscope in the following order: medium drop, air-gap, oocyte drop, air-gap and finally sperm drop followed by an air-gap (Figure 37.1). The total volume should not exceed 100 µL. When the transfer procedure is ready, the loaded catheter is brought into the operating room and the clinician guides the catheter through the GIFT trocar into the selected fallopian tube till the double marked line on the catheter. Correct placement of the catheter needs to be verified. The embryologist then injects the contents and confirms flow by the movement of the air-gaps. After transferring the gametes, the catheter is slowly withdrawn and examined in the laboratory to confirm transfer.

| AIR | SPERM | AIR | OOCYTES | AIR | MEDIUM |

FIGURE 37.1: Loading sequence of GIFT catheter

Excess oocytes retrieved undergo the conventional IVF culture procedure and embryos obtained are either frozen at the 4 to 8 cell stage of the culture are is extended to the blastocyst stage and good quality blastocysts are frozen for subsequent frozen embryo transfer. Problems in fertilization can be detected by this procedure.

Procedure

The exact positioning of the equipment and personnel should be worked out in advance. It is important to ensure that there is no breakdown in sterile techniques.

Carbon dioxide is the preferred gas used, although air is an option.[3] Better pregnancy rates have been reported with the use of halogen light as compared to xenon light source.[4] Standard double puncture laparoscopy technique is used with a third puncture being made for the GIFT trocar. Peritoneal suctioning to remove blood, often found after a TVOR procedure, is followed by selection of the tube for transfer. The ovaries are heavy and tend to drop into the POD making access to the fimbrial end of the tube difficult. Care should be taken to avoid trauma, and the tube handled gently with an atraumatic grasper. The GIFT trocar should be inserted carefully so that its axis lies in line with the ostial opening, ensuring easy cannulation of the tube.

The question of whether both tubes should be cannulated and injected as compared to one tube has been resolved with the literature suggesting that a single tube transfer will be adequate. This makes the procedure quick and easy to perform.[5]

It has been suggested that pregnancy rates would be better if the tube on the side of the dominant ovary (from which the maximum number of oocytes were retrieved) was chosen for transfer.[6] Driscoll et al[7] have investigated this aspect, suggest transfer to the most convenient tube.

Most transfers occur on the right tube partly because the majority of surgeons are right handed as also due to the presence of the sigmoid colon on the left. Left sided transfers usually occur when there is a specific indication like a better tube or easier access.

In many countries, not more than three oocytes can be legally transferred assuming a similar pregnancy potential in women of all ages. Fertility in the older women is reduced and this must be taken into account. Moreover, in GIFT, unfertilized oocytes are transferred as compared to IVF where a limit can be set on the number of embryos returned. Nadkarni et al[8] recommend a more flexible approach suggesting women of more than 40 have all the retrieved oocytes transferred, while caution is exercised in women of less than 30 years of age. With this policy no multiple pregnancies occurred in the above 40 age group.

Laparoscopy versus Nonsurgical Transfer

Ultrasound-guided transcervical tubal transfer, tactile dependent transcervical tubal transfer, hysteroscopic tubal cannulation with transfer, and falloposcopic transfer of gametes have all been advocated as an alternatives to laparoscopic transfers. Proponents of these procedures imply safe, easy and quick procedures with avoidance of a full-blown anesthetic.

Jansen and Anderson[9] in a case controlled study reported a 20 percent pregnancy rate with ultrasound-guided transfer as compared to 35 percent with the laparoscopic approach.

Seraccholi et al[10] commenting on to hysteroscopic versus laparoscopic replacement were said to obtain pregnancy and implantation rates of 29.8 percent and 9 percent with hysteroscopy and 43.3 percent and 14 percent with laparoscopic replacement.

Carbon dioxide insufflation is used for hysteroscopy and prior to actual injection of gametes, insufflation is discontinued and the hysteroscope removed leaving the transfer catheter in place. The hysteroscopic appoach has also been advocated when a laparoscopy is reckoned to be difficult, although this seems questionable. Alternatives to laparoscopic cannulation of the tubes for transfer of gametes warrants further evaluation.

RESULTS

In the largest single-center study involving 2941 consecutive GIFT cycles Healy et al[11] reported cumulative pregnancy and live birth rates of 49.6 percent and 38.8 percent respectively with three cycles of GIFT. They found advancing age to be a major negative factor.

Guzick et al[12] recommended ovulation induction with clomiphene citrate combined with IUI as a first line of therapy for unexplained infertility based primarily on cost-effectiveness. They, however, obtained a 27 percent GIFT pregnancy rate as compared to 20.7 percent with IVF and

recommend these procedures as second line therapy. Ranieri et al[13] in the only randomized trial that compared GIFT versus IVF following failed ovulation induction and IUI for unexplained infertility, obtained a clinical pregnancy rate of 34 percent with GIFT as compared to 50 percent with IVF and ET. No statistical difference between the two groups was obtained implying that no real differences exist, as suggested by the earlier nonrandomized reports.

CONCLUSION

Gamete intrafallopian transfer was introduced for the treatment of nontubal infertility. It has been a popular procedure especially as initial reports suggested better pregnancy rates as compared to regular IVF. Suboptimal in vitro culture conditions may have been responsible for these initial reports. Recent data suggest equality between IVF and GIFT techniques, and there is a tendency among clinicians to forsake the latter procedure. The introduction of more physiological and better culture media allows development of gametes to the blastocyst stage, allowing better selection of embryos for replacement with excellent pregnancy rates. With this changing scenario the role for GIFT may soon become questionable.

REFERENCES

1. Asch et al. Pregnancy after translaparoscopic gamete intrafallopian transfer (GIFT). Lancet 2: 1034-35, 1984.
2. Tournay et al: Tubal transfer—a forgotten ART. Hum Reprod 1996;11:1815-22.
3. Milki AA, Tazuki SI. Comparison of carbon dioxide and air pneumoperitoneum for gamete intrafallopian transfer under conscious sedation and local anaesthesia. Fertil Steril 1998;69:552-54.
4. Evans J, Wells C, Hood K. A possible effect of different light sources on pregnancy rates following gamete intrafallopian transfer. Hum Reprod 1999;14:80-82.
5. Haines CJ, Land O'Shea RT. Effect of unilateral versus bilateral tubal cannulation and the number of oocytes transferred on the outcome of GIFT. Fertil Steril 1991;55:423-25.
6. Ransom et al. Tubal selection for GIFT. Fertil Steril 1994;61:386-89.
7. Driscol et al. Transfer of gametes into the fallopian tubes—is choice of side important? Hum Reprod 1996;11:1881-83.

8. Nadkarni et al. What factors predetermine the risk of having a high-order multiple pregnancy with gameter intrafallopian transfer? Hum Reprod 1996;11:655-59.

9. Jansen Anderson. Transvaginal versus laparoscopic gameter intrafallopian transfer—a case-controlled retrospective comparison. Fertil Steril 1993;59:836-40.

10. Seraccholi et al. Gamete intrafallopian transfer—prospective randomized comparison between hysteroscopic and laparoscopic transfer techniques. Fertil Steril 1995;64:355-59.

11. Healy et al. Cumulative pregnancy and live birth rates after gamete intrafallopian transfer. Hum Reprod 1997;12:1338-42.

12. Guzick et al. Efficacy of treatment for unexplained infertility. Fertil Steril 1998;70:207-13.

13. Ranieri et al. Gamete intrafallopian transfer or in-vitro fertilization after failed ovarian stimulation and intra-uterine insemination in unexplained infertility? Hum Reprod 1995;10:2023.

• Ameet Patki
• Shailaja Gada Saxena • Firuza R Parikh

38

Oocyte Donation

INTRODUCTION

Oocyte donation, unlike its male counterpart of sperm donation, which has been a routine clinical treatment for male infertility for many years, has only become feasible since the widespread introduction of *in vitro* fertilization (IVF). Prior to the advent of IVF there was neither a source of oocytes for donation nor the laboratory or clinical techniques available to ensure successful fertilization and transfer of the resulting embryo. Oocyte donation has now become a widely used treatment modality for infertility due to premature menopause. Preliminary work in the monkeys demonstrated that it was possible to maintain pregnancy artificially, after ovariectomy, using exogenous hormones (Salat-Baroux *et al* 1988). There are several reports in literature of successful pregnancies following oocyte donation (Lutjen *et al* 1984; Devroey *et al* 1987).

Donor oocytes are being used more and more as a means to create a family in couples where the female partner no longer possesses the biologic ability to create a child due to hypergonadotrophic hypogonadism or inheritable genetic disorders. Oocyte donation also provides unique opportunity for the study and understanding of the steroid replacement parameters necessary to induce uterine receptivity, the synchronization of embryo development with uterine receptivity prior to implantation and the endocrinology of pregnancy in the absence of ovarian function. In addition, oocyte donation affords a scientific opportunity to study the unique biologic participation of the uterus in the process of human embryo implantation.

Indications for Donor Oocyte

The patients requiring donor oocyte can be divided into two main groups:

Women with Non Functioning Ovaries

a. Premature ovarian failure
b. Ovarian agenesis
c. Bilateral oophorectomy
d. Menopause

Women with Functioning Ovaries

a. Risk of inheritable genetic disease in children
b. Failed IVF due to poor quality oocytes
c. Inaccessible ovaries

Female fertility begins to decline years before the onset of menopause, despite continued regular ovulatory cycles. The age-associated decline in female fecundity and increased risk of spontaneous abortions are largely attributable to abnormalities in the oocyte. There is a growing demand for oocyte donation from women, in their early forties, who fail to conceive after several cycles of IVF with their own oocytes (Rosenwaks, 1987). Recent data suggests that women after 40 years of age have better pregnancy rate with donor oocytes. There are also a small but growing number of postmenopausal women desiring pregnancy through oocyte donation. Pregnancy rates appear to be comparable in this group to younger age groups and depend upon the age of the donor and not the recipient (Legro et al 1995).

Evaluation of Oocyte Recipients

- A routine medical and reproductive history along with a general physical examination and pelvic examination is mandatory.
- Standard preconception testing in form of blood type and Rh factor and rubella immunity should be confirmed.
- Serologic test for syphilis and serum testing for hepatitis B (HBV) surface antigen, hepatitis C (HCV) antibody, cytomegalovirus (CMV) antibody and human immunodeficiency virus 1 (HIV-1)
- All recipient couples undergo a counseling session to check for possible psychological factors. In cases of known donor oocyte treatment, it is important to rule out possible repercussions on the child by either the donor or recipient couples. In cases of unknown oocyte donors, the counseling should also stress the confidentiality of the oocyte donor. Anonymity is maintained between donor and recipient couples, although non-identifying Information is available to both on request. In both known and unknown donors, the counselor should assess the recipient couple's attitudes concerning telling the child about the conception at an appropriate time. A consent form outlining the success rates, risks, and implications of the donor oocyte program must be signed by the recipient couple.
- Hormonal profile to assess ovulatory functions.
- Vaginal sonographic assessment to evaluate the endometrium for its appearance, measurement and response to hormonal therapy. Sonography can also rule out any pelvic pathology.
- Clinical evaluation for any uterine abnormality, hysterosalpingography (HSG) or other suitable procedure should be performed.
- Screening for possible medical conditions for heart disease, diabetes, hypertension, pap smear, mammography especially in those over 40 years of age to avoid possible future complications in pregnancy.

Evaluation of the Partner of the Oocyte Recipient

- Laboratory tests like semen analysis, blood type and Rh factor, serologic test for syphilis and serum testing for hepatitis B (HBV) surface antigen, hepatitis C (HCV) antibody, cytomegalovirus (CMV) antibody and human immunodeficiency virus 1 (HIV-1) and appropriate genetic screening.
- Psychological counseling of the partner is also essential.

Selection of the Donor

- Because of shortage of oocyte donors, some recipients seek their own donor, either a close friend or a relative. This is done for altruistic motivation. In case of known donor, related issue such as the potential impact of the relationship between the donor and recipient should be explored.
- Sharing of oocytes from an assisted reproduction cycle where a patient undergoing IVF treatment donates her excess oocytes.
- Now a days professional donors are also available although at a price.
- Pragmatic considerations such as the difficulty in recruiting suitable donors support the use of known oocyte donors. Psychological evaluation and counseling of the donor and her partner is essential.
- According to the new ICMR guidelines, which will come into force soon, known donors are to be discouraged. Only professional donors or shared oocyte donation is to be considered.
- An ideal donor is a woman between the ages of 21 to 35, with previous successful pregnancies, in a stable relationship and completed her family. All these factors may not be mandatory since they are infrequently found in these women but age is the most critical.

The efforts, commitment, discomfort and risk derived from ovarian stimulation and oocyte retrieval limits the donor availability (Ahuja et al 1997). Donor recruitment is a difficult endeavor, taking into account that a considerable number of potential donors may have a positive finding on medical, genetic or psychological testing that prohibits donation.

Providing oocyte donation to two recipients from a single cohort of eggs obtained from a single donor has the theoretic advantage of permitting a greater number of fresh ETs (Moomj'y *et al* 2000). Historically, shared donation involves IVF patients willing to donate half of their oocytes to a recipient, for reduction in the cost of the treatment cycle (Ahuja *et al* 1997; Peskin *et al* 1996). Moomj'y *et al* have noticed that shared anonymous oocyte donation provides high pregnancy rates per donor retrieval. It also helps in cost reduction of the treatment. For anonymous oocyte donation, sharing of oocytes between two phenotypically matched recipients provides a good opportunity for the recipient to experience pregnancy, while keeping medical risks and discomforts to an absolute minimum for the donor group. Precious human oocytes are well utilized in shared oocyte donation.

Sapndorfer *et al* (2000) in their study of 354 cycles in 267 patients noted no statistically significant difference in the pregnancy success between the first, second and third oocyte donation attempts. However, failure in the first cycle was noted to be associated with compromised outcome in the second attempt compared with success on the first attempt. Patients who had a successful delivery after a single attempt were twice as likely to have a successful delivery after a second attempt, which implies that previous delivery is a positive predictor of a successful second attempt at oocyte donation.

Shared oocyte donation model is widely used and it is regarded as a well-established process in the treatment of infertility among women. It offers the advantage of increasing the availability of donated eggs without putting a third party inadvertently at risk. Additionally, it provides the possibility to study the contribution of different clinical and laboratory factors to establishment of pregnancy.

Screening and Testing of Oocyte Donors

- A personal and sexual history of the donor should be obtained to exclude donors who may be at a high-risk of HIV or other sexually transmitted diseases.

- Serologic test for syphilis and serum testing for hepatitis B (HBV) surface antigen, hepatitis C (HCV) antibody, cytomegalovirus (CMV) antibody and human immunodeficiency virus 1 (HIV-1)

- Appropriate genetic evaluation of the donor should be performed. Genetic screening of the donor for various autosomal dominant and recessive disorders, X-linked disorders and single gene disorders is important. Family history is an effective screening tool for many genetic disorders and should be used routinely to exclude certain genetic disorders.

- If the donor oocyte creates a potential for Rh incompatibility, couples should be informed about the obstetrical significance of the condition.

- Vaginal USG to confirm ovulation and ovarian size and morphology. These tests should also include accessibility for oocyte collection.

- Hormonal profile to confirm ovulatory cycles.

- In some centers, it is mandatory to quarantine the resulting embryos for atleast 6 months in view of a small but potential risk of HIV infection.

- The possibility of genetic risk factors depends on the medical and family history of the donors. Hence detailed history is of utmost importance not only of the donor but also of the first-degree relatives.

- Routine cytogenetic testing is not feasible but must be offered to those specific ethnic groups with a high frequency.

Success of Oocyte Donation

The success of oocyte donation is reportedly influenced by multiple factors including the age of the oocyte donor and recipient, the embryo quality and the reproductive status and endometrial receptivity of the recipient.

- Donor's age is one of the most significant factors as the oocyte age is one of the primary contributors to IVF outcome (Stolwijk *et al* 1997).

- It has also been reported that recipient's age is inversely proportional to the success of oocyte donation (Borini *et al* 1996; Yaron *et al* 1998). However, Noyes *et al* (2001) suggest that the age of the recipient is not necessarily a poor prognosticator to the success of oocyte donation cycle.

- Endometrial thickness and pattern have been implicated as predictors of success in oocyte donation cycles (Abdalla *et al* 1994; Gonen *et al* 1997)
- According to a three years retrospective analysis for the prediction of success of oocyte donation by Noyes *et al* (2001), the most reliable predictive factor for pregnancy in oocyte donation cycles are the quality of the embryos transferred and recipient's mid-cycle endometrial thickness.

Reasons for High Pregnancy Rates in Ovum Donation Program

- Lack of endometrial hyperstimulation.
- No risk of hyperestrogenism.
- No premature luteinization.
- Better control of window of receptivity.

In donor oocyte program there are 3 main principles:

- Preparation of recipient endometrium.
- Window for embryo transfer.
- Early pregnancy management with exogenous hormones.

Preparation of Recipient Endometrium

The value of endometrial thickness as a prediction of a successful IVF cycle is controversial (Gonen *et al* 1989). A trend towards pregnancy with increasing endometrial thickness exists, but a lower limit for successful implantation has yet to be defined. In donor oocyte program, significantly higher pregnancy rates have been reported by some workers when the endometrial thickness was more than 10 mm (Check, 1994). However, the ideal endometrial development for successful donor oocyte transfer has yet to be defined.

Hormone Replacement

An important point in deciding the dose and route of administration of exogenous steroid hormones for endometrial preparation lies in the difference between peripheral plasma verses the uterine circulation. Studies in the rhesus monkey have shown that there is an existence of a counter current flow exchange mechanism between the uterine arteries and the ovarian veins (Ginther *et al* 1974). This counter current mechanism raises the uterine blood progesterone (P4) atleast 10 times higher than in peripheral circulation. These and other studies have suggested that monitoring of peripheral plasma E2 and P4 levels does not necessarily give an accurate indication of their levels in the uterine environment. A concomitant ultrasound scan of the endometrial maturation should be carried out at the same time as the hormone assay, as USG gives a more accurate picture of the endometrial development.

Nowadays there is great variation in both the dose and route of hormone therapy. Serhal and Craft (1987) introduced a constant regimen with a variable length of follicular phase. Estradiol valerate 6 to 8 mg daily with progesterone added a day before the oocyte retrieval from the donor. This enables adjustment of the follicular phase to synchronize the donor and recipient cycles before adding progesterone.

Most donor oocyte programs employ estrogen replacement therapy in the form of estradiol valorate 4 to 8 mg daily. Progesterone replacement is usually in the form of either progesterone pessaries 200 to 300 mg daily or injectables 50 to 100 mg daily. Although few studies are available for transdermal estrogen, it has shown comparable results as oral route (Steingold K, Matt D *et al* 1991).

In ovulating women inducted for donor oocyte programs, it has been noted that there is significant degree of break-through ovulation and bleeding with decreased pregnancy rates compared to women with ovarian failure. Hence it is now accepted that ovulatory cycles should be initially down regulated with GnRH followed by HRT. In menopausal patients, a reduced implantation rate has been reported (Flamigni *et al* 1993).

These studies suggest an aging effect on endometrial receptivity with regards to supporting the nidation and continuation of a pregnancy. The delay in secretory maturation is overcome with increased dosages of progesterone, preferably injectables 50 to 100 mg daily.

Window for Embryo Transfer

The window for donor oocyte transfer is wide and not strictly defined. Rosenwaks (1987) has defined the window for a 2 day embryo from days 17 to 19 of an ideal 28 day cycle or 3 to 5 days after P4 administration. Several research groups have failed to identify any distinctive features or histopathological appearances, which need to be present for successful implantation. Hence this suggests that endometrial conditions may not be tightly controlled in the humans for successful implantation. However, it is observed that the embryos need to be at an earlier stage of development than that of the endometrium.

Pregnancies in Oocyte Recipient

Successful pregnancy in women without ovarian function can be achieved with the addition of exogenous estrogen and progesterone only. Placental steroidogenesis is found as early as 2 weeks following embryo transfer (Calderon 1991). Significant levels of endogenous E2, P4 and β-HCG are found by the 8th gestational week and hence HRT at this stage would appear of little benefit.

Results of Donor Oocyte Programs

Many factors are involved in pregnancy rates achieved through donor oocyte programs. Though a wide range of pregnancy rates exists among different donor oocyte clinics, several conclusions can be drawn from their results.

1. Pregnancy rates of donor oocyte procedures are equal to or possibly higher than routine IVF programs.
2. Transfer of fresh embryos has a higher pregnancy rate than that of frozen- thawed embryos.
3. The age of the donor is an important factor in achieving good pregnancy rate.
4. The age of the recipient is not significant, since any decrease in endometrial receptivity can be overcome by increasing HRT dosages.
5. Pregnancy rates are directly related to the number of embryos transferred.

Donor oocyte program Jaslok Hospital and Reliance Life Sciences:

	Pregnancy Rate (n = 55)	Miscarriage Rate (n = 20)	Take home Baby rate (n = 33)
No. of Patients: 3 or more cleaving embryos + endo-metrium > 8 mm (n = 110)	50% 55/110	36.3% 20/55	30% 33/110

Legal implications of Donor Oocyte Program

Donor oocyte programs have revolutionized thinking in human reproduction. There no longer exists a finite age for women to become pregnant. In several Western countries and Australia, it is accepted legally that the gamete recipient as the legal parent and the gamete donor as having no legal right or responsibilities towards the resulting child.

REFERENCES

1. Abdalla H, Brooks A, Johnson M, Kirkland A, Thomas A, Studd J. Endometrial thickness: A predictor of implantation in ovum recipients. Hum Reprod 1994;9:363-65.
2. Ahuja KK, Mostyn BJ, Simons EG. Egg sharing and egg donation: Attitudes of British egg donors and recipients. Hum Reprod 1997;12:2845-52.
3. Borini A, Bianchi L, Violini F, Maccolini A, Cattoli M, Flamigni C. Oocyte donation program: Pregnancy and implantation rates in women of different ages sharing oocytes from single donor. Fertil Steril 1996;65:94-97.
4. Calderon I, Me Clure N, Azuma K, Mac Lachlan V, Leeton J, de Kretser D, Sapiro M, Healy D. The endocrinology of early donor oocyte program in patients with no ovarian function. Endocrine Soc. Aust. Sydney 1991;68.
5. Check JH. The use of the donor oocyte program to evaluate embryo implantation. Ann, NY Acad. Sci. 1994;734:198.
6. Devroey P, Smitz J, Wisanto A. Primary ovarian failure: Embryodonation after substitution therapy. 5th World Congress on IVF and ET Norfolk, Virginia, 5-10 April (Abstract. No OC : 427) 1987.
7. Flamigni CF, Borini A, Violini F, Bianchi L, Serrao L. Oocyte donation: Comparison between recipients of different age groups. Hum Reprod. 1993;8(12):2088.
8. Ginther O, Dierschke D, Walsh S, Del Campo C. Anatomy of arteries and veins of uterus and ovaries in rhesus monkeys. Biol. Reprod. 1974;11:205.

9. Gonen Y, Casper R. Prediction of implantation by the sonographic appearance of the endometrium during controlled ovarian stimulation for in vitro fertilization (IVF). J in vitro Fertil Embryo Transf 1990;7:146-52.

10. Gonen Y, Casper R, FF Jacobson W, Blaukier J Endometrial thickness and growth during ovarian stimulation: A possible predictor of implantation in in vitro fertilization. Fertil Steril 1989;52:446.

11. Legro RS, Wong IL, Paulson RJ, Lobo RA, Sauer MVC. Recipient's age does not adversely affect pregnancy outcome after oocyte donation. Am J Obstet Gynaecol 1995;172:96.

12. Lutjen P, Trounson A, Leeton J, Findlay J, Wood E, Renou P. The establishment and maintenance of pregnancy using in vitro fertilization and embryo donation in a patient with primary ovarian failure. Nature 1984;307:174-75.

13. Moomjy M, Mangieri R, Beltramone F, Cholst I, Veeck L, Rosenwaks Z. Shared oocyte donation: Society's benefits. Fertil Steril 2000;73(6):1165-69.

14. Noyes N, Hampton BS, Berkeley A, Licciardi F, Grifo J, Krey L. Factors useful in predicting the success of oocyte donation: A 3-year retrospective analysis. Fertil Steril 2001;76(1):92-97.

15. Peskin BD, Austin C, Lisbona H, Goldfarb JM. Cost analysis of shared oocyte in vitro fertilization. Obstet Gynecol 1996;88:428-30.

16. Rosenwaks Z. Donor eggs: their application in modern reproductive technologies. Fertl Steril 1987;47(6): 895.

17. Salat-Baroux J, Cornet D, Alvarez S. Pregnancies after replacement of frozen thawed embryos in a donation program. Fertil Steril 1988;49:817-21.

18. Serhal PF, Craft IL. Ovum donation: A simplified approach. Fertil Steril 1987;48:265-69.

19. Steingold K, Matt D, De Ziepler D. Comparison of transdermal to oral estradiol administration on hormonal and hepatic parameters in women with premature ovarian failure. J Clin Endocrinol Metab 1991;73:275.

20. Stolwijk A, Zielhuis G, Sauer M, Hamilton C, Paulson R. The impact of the woman's age on the success of standard and donor in vitro fertilization. Fertil Steril 1997;67:702-10.

21. Yaron, Y, Ochshorn Y, Amit A, Kogosowski A, Yovel I, Lessing J. Oocyte donation in Israel: A study of 1001 initiated treatment cycles. Hum Reprod 1998;13: 1819-24.

• Nalini Mahajan

39

Alternatives to ART

INTRODUCTION

Assisted reproduction technology (ART) has helped to fulfill the dreams of many an infertile couple. Innovative techniques have been introduced to achieve pregnancies in various types of infertility and also to improve existing pregnancy rates. However, pregnancy rates are still unacceptably low and the cost of technology very high.

Alternative techniques in ART have been introduced from time to time with the intent of achieving pregnancy while avoiding the high cost of ART. Some techniques have an acceptable pregnancy rate while others do not. In countries like India the social pressures on a couple to reproduce are very high, the per capita income is low and no funding is available for treatment, hence the use of these measures where indicated, is very relevant. This chapter is an attempt to look at these techniques in the Indian context and to see which of these procedures can or should be used where *in vitro* fertilization is not available or affordable.

Alternative techniques in ART are defined as procedures which assist reproduction but do not involve *in vitro* fertilization.

The procedures advocated can be divided into two broad groups
• Techniques involving handling of sperm/alternatives to intrauterine insemination (IUI)
• Techniques involving handling of sperm and oocyte/alternatives to *in vitro* fertilization (IVF).

Alternatives to IUI

• Direct intraperitoneal insemination (DIPI)
• Direct intrafollicular insemination (DIFI)
• Intrafallopian insemination (IFI)
• Fallopian tube sperm perfusion (FSP)
   Tubal patency in at least one tube is an important prerequisite for these methods.

Alternatives to IVF

• Peritoneal oocyte sperm transfer (POST)
• Follicular aspiration, sperm injection and assisted rupture (FASIAR)
• Direct oocyte transfer (DOT)
• Intravaginal culture (IVC)
• Gamete intrafallopian transfer (GIFT).

INDICATIONS

Indications for the use of these procedures are as follows:
• Unexplained infertility
• Male subfertility
• Endometriosis
• Ovulatory dysfunction
• Cervical hostility
• Tubal infertility.

TREATMENT PROTOCOL

Certain basic steps of management remain the same for all the procedures. The patient has to undergo:
• Ovarian stimulation

- Follicular monitoring
- Administration of human chorionic gonadotrophin (hCG) trigger
- Sperm preparation
- Oocyte aspiration
- Luteal phase support.

Ovarian Stimulation

Evidence-based medicine suggests that controlled ovarian hyperstimulation (COH) significantly improves the pregnancy rate by increasing the number of potential oocytes available for fertilization. It would be prudent therefore, to achieve superovulation prior to performing any of these procedures.

Drugs commonly used for ovarian stimulation are:
- Clomiphene citrate (CC)
- Clomiphene citrate in combination with human menopausal gonadotrophin (hMG)
- hMG or FSH
- Gonadotrophin-releasing hormone-agonist (GnRH-a) or antagonist for pituitary downregulation and gonadotrophins for ovarian stimulation.

Pregnancy rates improve with a follicular recruitment of at least six follicles. However, due to the risk of high order multiple pregnancies, the attempt should be to achieve two or three good follicles in procedures where oocyte aspiration is not being carried out. In patients of PCOS however, this is easier said than done!

Follicular Monitoring and hCG Administration

Transvaginal ultrasound has added a new dimension to the monitoring of follicular and endometrial growth. A baseline ultrasound is performed on day 2 or 3 of the menstrual cycle, prior to stimulation to look for the presence of ovarian cysts. Ovarian stimulation is withheld in the presence of a cyst of 15 mm diameter or more. Further monitoring is carried out from day 8 onwards, the frequency depending on the ovarian response.

Follicles should be measured in two planes and the follicular growth recorded serially. Endometrial thickness is measured and character of the endometrium noted. If Doppler is available a look at the uterine and ovarian blood flow is helpful in assessing uterine receptivity and oocyte quality.

When the average diameter of the largest follicle reaches 17 to 18 mm, 5000 IU or 10,000 IU hCG should be administered to trigger the LH surge. The exact dose of hCG required for achieving second meiosis/follicular rupture has not been determined, but it would be wise to use a smaller dose to avoid the risk of OHSS. It should be noted that giving high doses of hCG does not overcome the problem of LUF and such temptations are better avoided.

Procedures are carried out 34 to 36 hours after the hCG trigger. The problem of a premature surge leading to an early rupture of the follicle exists in non-downregulated cycles. In these cycles, it would be sensible to monitor the patient twice a day once the follicle is 15 to 16 mm in size.

Sperm Preparation

Semen preparation can be carried out by the "swim-up" technique or by the use of a discontinuous density gradient. The latter gives better results in the presence of a compromised semen sample. The final pellet is diluted in 0.3 to 0.5 mL of medium.

Oocyte Aspiration

Ovum pick-up is done 34 to 36 hours after the hCG trigger. The patient is put in a lithotomy position. A thorough vaginal toilet is performed with IL of saline. A 16 G ovum pick-up needle is passed into the follicle, through a biopsy guide attached to the transvaginal ultrasound probe. Aspiration is done using a low suction pressure of about 100 mmHg. The aspirate containing the oocyte is collected in a sterile Falcon tube.

ALTERNATIVES TO IUI

The overall success rate of IUI is still between 10 and 15 percent. Higher success rates are seen with different stimulation protocols/different etiologies of infertility but as a whole results are depressingly low. The presumed reasons being:
- Insufficient sperm migration[1]

• Partial tubal obstruction due to narrowing of the endometrial glandular lumen during midfollicular phase and collection of debris.[2]

Over the years a number of techniques have been introduced to overcome these problems and improve conception rates.

Direct Intraperitoneal Insemination (DIPI)

A prepared sample of semen is placed in the pouch of Douglas under ultrasound guidance at the time of ovulation.

Procedure

The patient is placed in a "sitting lithotomy position" to ensure that the peritoneal fluid gravitates to the pouch of Douglas. After cleaning the vagina with an antiseptic solution a transvaginal ultrasound scan is performed to identify the fluid. Once the site is determined, a 19 G disposable needle is passed through the ultrasound biopsy guide into the peritoneal fluid with a single rapid movement (Figure 39.1). The patient should be warned that she would feel a sharp pain. Once the needle tip is identified within the fluid a small amount of peritoneal fluid is aspirated to confirm correct placement. The prepared semen sample is then injected into the pouch of Douglas. If the patient is apprehensive a mild analgesic or sedative may be given.

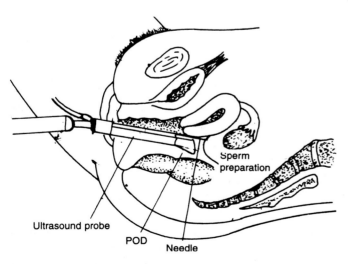

FIGURE 39.1: Direct intraperitoneal insemination, POD—Pouch of Douglas

In theory the procedure is very simple but in practice it can be quite cumbersome. Identification of a good pocket of fluid may be difficult at times because only a small quantity of fluid is present and it is hidden between loops of bowel. Excessive bowel movement further adds to the problem.

Results

Pregnancy rates vary from 7 to 20 percent[3] per cycle. There is no increase in the multiple or ectopic pregnancy rate. Amongst the ovarian stimulation regimes used the pituitary down-regulation and COH gives a significantly better result.[4] A comparison of DIPI versus IUI has shown that there is no significant difference in the pregnancy rates.[5] Conception rate in the different categories of subfertility also remains the same for both procedures.[6]

Drawbacks

• Invasive
• Blood in the peritoneal cavity can compromise results
• Risk of infection
• Risk of bowel injury.

Conclusion

The invasiveness of the procedure coupled with no improvement in pregnancy rates has led to a low popularity. However, the one indication for which it has a degree of merit is severe cervical stenosis where IUI is sometimes not possible even under ultrasound guidance.

Direct Intrafollicular Insemination (DIFI)

A prepared sample of semen is injected directly into the preovulatory follicles under ultrasound guidance.

Procedure

With the patient in lithotomy position a transvaginal scan is done to identify the preovulatory follicles. After cleaning the vagina a 16 G needle is introduced into the follicle and the prepared semen sample is injected into it. Generally the procedure is well tolerated and does not require anesthesia or analgesia. However, if there are more than one or two follicles the patient may be given light sedatives.

Results

The first successful pregnancy was reported by Lucena et al in 1991.[7] Since then many centers have tried the procedure. Success rates vary from 2 to 20 percent.

Conclusion

The logic of this procedure defies understanding. In addition there remains a theoretical risk of an ovarian ectopic pregnancy in case the fertilized oocyte fails to extrude. No recommendations can be made for the use of this technique.

Intrafallopian Insemination (IFI)

Success of transcervical tubal cannulation prompted the use of tubal cannulation for intrafallopian insemination. Jansen and Anderson in 1987 reported the first procedure.[8] Tubal cannulation is carried out under ultrasound guidance, hysteroscopic control or using a tactile technique.

A coaxial catheter system (Cook OB/GYN) is used to enter the tube. The outer catheter is guided toward the tubal ostia, the inner catheter loaded with the prepared sperm in 0.3 mL of medium is moved through the outer catheter into the tube and the sperm is delivered 2 to 4 cm distal to the tubal ostium. Insemination can be done on the side with the greater number of mature ovarian follicles or bilaterally.

Results

Results vary with operator expertise. Pregnancy rates of 7 to 23.8 percent have been reported.

Disadvantages

- Highly invasive
- Trauma to endometrium and tube
- May induce abnormal myosalpingeal contractions
- Vasovagal syncope
- Infection.

Conclusion

The procedure never gained acceptance. The potential for increased risk from complications and no improvement in pregnancy rates does not justify its use.

Fallopian Tube Sperm Perfusion (FSP)

Fallopian tube sperm perfusion (FSP) is being dealt with in detail elsewhere in the book. In short and to complete the overall picture, Kahn et al introduced FSP in 1992.[9] The procedure involves the perfusion of the fallopian tube with a prepared sample of semen diluted in 4 mL of medium. Sperm reflux is prevented by obstructing the internal os with an Allis forceps, a pediatric Foley's catheter[10] or specially designed systems. Apart from ensuring sperm delivery, it helps to overcome partial obstruction of the tube.

Initial reports of the procedure were very encouraging[11] but as more studies were carried out it was realized that PR's were no better than with IUI. It was Trout and Kemmann in 1999,[12] who revived the interest in this procedure. In a randomized controlled trial and a meta-analysis of literature, they reported that FSP did indeed increase the pregnancy rate significantly in patients with unexplained infertility. However, pregnancy rates did not differ between the two procedures for all other etiologies of infertility.

ALTERNATIVES TO IVF

These procedures can be used in women with bilateral tubal block.

Peritoneal Oocyte Sperm Transfer (POST)

Peritoneal oocyte sperm transfer (POST) was described by Coulam et al in 1989.[13]

Procedure

Following ovum pick-up, the pouch of Douglas is repeatedly rinsed with culture medium until the aspirate is clear. The aspiration needle is left in position and a maximum of 4 oocytes and 4 million motile spermatozoa in 1 mL Earl's medium are drawn into a long embryo transfer catheter. The catheter is passed through the aspiration needle and the oocyte-sperm mixture injected into the pouch of Douglas. The catheter and needle are then withdrawn simultaneously. The procedure is carried out on an outpatient basis (Figure 39.2).

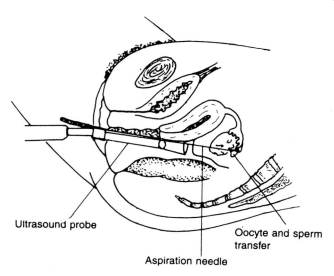

FIGURE 39.2: Peritoneal oocyte and sperm transfer

Advantages

• Office procedure
• Avoids the laboratory costs of IVF-ET
• Avoids the surgical costs and risks of GIFT.

Disadvantages

• Blood in the POD may compromise results
• For complete aspiration of fluid in the POD, the needle may have to be withdrawn and reinserted a number of times, thus increasing the risk of trauma and infection.

Results

Pregnancy rates of 3 to 26 percent per cycle have been reported.

Conclusion

This procedure has limited application. It can be used to reduce the risk of high order multiple pregnancy in patients stimulated for IUI who exhibit multifolliculogenesis, when facilities for IVF are not available.

Follicular Aspiration Sperm Injection and Assisted Rupture (FASIAR)

Follicular aspiration sperm injection and assisted rupture combines the concept of COH, IUI and POST. The preovulatory follicle(s) is punctured under ultrasound guidance. 2 mL of follicular fluid is aspirated into a syringe containing 2 mL of sperm suspension. The sperm concentration used is 10 million motile sperms. This fluid is then injected around the ovary ensuring that the needle has been withdrawn from the follicle.[14] In the original technique as described by Paulson and Thornton, an IUI was performed in addition.[15]

Advantage

• Does not require embryological expertise.

Drawbacks

• It has the same drawbacks as DIPI and POST. In addition, there is only a presumption of the oocyte having been recovered from the follicle, since oocyte identification is not done.

Recommendation

This procedure may be of benefit in patients who show a luteinized unruptured follicle. It, however, requires validation through proper randomized controlled trials.

Direct Oocyte Transfer (DOT)

Oocytes with sperm are transferred directly into the uterine cavity. This technique was first described by Craft et al in 1982 and later modified by Bucktt and Tan.[16]

Procedure

After oocyte recovery, the oocytes are incubated for 6 hours in culture medium prior to insemination and then incubated for a further hour. Four to six oocytes and about 20,000 sperm are then transferred into the uterine cavity in 20 mL culture medium with a normal embryo transfer catheter, 7 hours after pick-up. In the modified technique, the cumulus cells are mechanically stripped off the oocytes. Insemination is done

3 hours after retrieval. A maximum of four oocytes with tightly bound sperm are then transferred into the uterine cavity, 5 hours after pick-up. Further simplification of the procedure entailed transfer of the gametes into the uterine cavity without preincubation.[17]

Results

Pregnancy rates of 6.5 percent per cycle were reported with the original technique and 18.6 percent per cycle with the modification.

Conclusion

Since this procedure involves culture of gametes *in vitro* it defeats the very purpose of the alternative techniques, which is to avoid the expensive laboratory set-up. With excellent culture media being available commercially and improved culture conditions there is no place for this technique today.

Intravaginal Culture (IVC)

Ranoux *et al*[18] came up with the novel idea of using the vagina as an incubator.

Procedure

A small 3 mL polypropylene tube is filled with culture medium . One to four oocytes and 10 to 20,000 motile sperm are added to the tube. The tube is hermetically sealed making sure that no air is trapped inside and placed in the posterior vaginal fornix. Usually a tampon or contraceptive diaphragm is used to keep the tube(s) in place.

After 48 to 50 hours, the tube is removed and transferred to the laboratory. The resultant embryos are then identified and transferred using standard embryo transfer techniques. Spare embryos may be cryopreserved.

A fertilization rate of 60 percent and PR of 15 to 22 percent have been achieved. Initial results claimed this technique to be comparable to IVF. However, conventional IVF results are superior.

Advantages

- Avoids the detrimental effects of light exposure and temperature variation on gametes seen in IVF.

- Psychological comfort to the patient that she is actively participating.

Disadvantages

- Lost cryotubes
- Embryo yeast infection
- Unacceptable to some patients.

Gamete Intrafallopian Transfer (GIFT)

Since the procedure is being dealt with in another chapter only a brief mention of this very important alternative technique will be made here.

Of all the alternatives developed to overcome the limitations of IVF, GIFT is perhaps the one most widely used. Numerous trials have been carried out to assess its efficacy and various modifications introduced to improve the technique and make it less invasive. GIFT was introduced[19] in an era when oocyte recovery was done laparoscopically and therefore delivering gametes into the fallopian tube did not involve any extrasurgical procedure.

Transvaginal GIFT was introduced to combine the advantage of *in vivo* fertilization and transvaginal ultrasound-guided follicular puncture.

Results

The success rate of GIFT equals that of IVF. An average pregnancy rate of 25 percent has been reported. SART (Science for Assisted Reproduction Technology) results for 1996,[20] in an assessment of, 44,647 cycles of IVF and 2,879 of GIFT showed that for IVF the pregnancy rate per transfer was 33.3 percent and delivery rate per transfer 27.9 percent. For GIFT the pregnancy rate per transfer was 35.1 percent and delivery rate per transfer was 29.3 percent.

Transcervical GIFT did not enhance the pregnancy rate when compared to IVF-ET.[21]

Recommendation

Efforts to simplify GIFT by developing transcervical methods of transfer have not translated into higher pregnancy rates than those of IVF-ET. Tubal cannulation, either laparoscopic or transvaginal, is more difficult to learn than simple intrauterine embryo transfer. However, compared to IVF this method requires less laboratory equipment and renders *in vivo* fertilization possible.

Since pregnancy rates are similar, it is logical that one would opt for a simpler and less invasive method of gamete delivery. The use of this procedure is justified in cases where the possibility for IVF does not exist, or for patients who refuse IVF.

Transvaginal GIFT offers an acceptable pregnancy rate for patients who cannot be treated with laparoscopic GIFT. Results of transvaginal GIFT are lower than laparoscopic GIFT.[22] Therefore recommendations for its routine use become questionable.

CONCLUSION

The large numbers of alternative techniques that have cropped up over the years are testimony to the fact that we have not yet optimized ART.

A number of these techniques have been validated and may be applied where indicated. Others need to be relegated to history. They came up in an era when there were a lot of limitations in culture media, culture techniques and our very understanding of reproduction.

While using these procedures, one has to weigh the cost of IVF against the lower success rates achieved with many of these techniques. Wasting time, money and effort not to mention the emotional stress associated with failure to achieve pregnancy is not justified. Referral to an ART center is definitely a better option. New developments are an important facet of science, however, there is the need to evaluate each technique and compare it to the existing well-established reproductive technologies through well-controlled prospective randomized controlled trials.

REFERENCES

1. Mamas L. Higher pregnancy rates with a simple method for fallopian tube sperm perfusion, using the cervical clamp double nut bivalve speculum in the treatment of unexplained infertility—a prospective randomized study. Hum Reprod 1996;11(12):2618-22.
2. Amso NN, Crow J, Lewin J et al. A comparative morphological and ultrastructural study of endometrial gland and fallopian tube epithelia at different stages of the menstrual cycle and the menopause. Hum Reprod 1994;9:2234-41.
3. Seracchioli R, Melega C, Maccolini A et al. Pregnancy after direct intraperitoneal insemination. Hum Reprod 1991;6:533-36.
4. Minoura H, Takeuchi S, Shen X et al. GnRH agonist—increasing the pregnancy rate after combined treatment with hMG/hCG and direct intraperitoneal insemination. J Reprod Med 1999;44(1):18-22.
5. Gregoriou O, Papadias C, Konidaris S et al. A randomized comparison of intrauterine and intraperitoneal insemination in the treatment of infertility. Int J Gynaecol Obstet 1993;42(1):33-36.
6. Tiemessen CH, Bots RS, Peeters MF et al. Direct intraperitoneal insemination compared to intrauterine insemination in superovulated cycles—a randomized cross-over study. Gynecol Obstet Invest 1997;44(3):149-52.
7. Lucena E, Ruiz JA, Mendoza JC et al. Direct intrafollicular insemination—a case report. J Reprod Med 1991;36(7):525-26.
8. Oei LM, Surrey ES, McCaleb B et al. A prospective randomized study of pregnancy rates after trans-uterotubal and intrauterine insemination. Fertil Steril 1992;58:167-71.
9. Kahn JA, Von Durin V, Sunde A et al. Fallopian tube sperm perfusion: First clinical experience. Hum Reprod 1992;7(Suppl 1):19-24.
10. Li TC. A simple, non-invasive method of fallopian tube sperm perfusion. Hum Reprod 1993;8:1848-50.
11. Fanchin R, Olivennes F, Righini C et al. A new system for fallopian tube perfusion leads to pregnancy rates twice as high as standard intrauterine insemination. Fertil Steril 1995;64:505-10.
12. Trout SW and Kemmann E. Fallopian sperm perfusion versus intrauterine insemination: A randomized controlled trial and metaanalysis of the literature. Fertil Steril 1999;7(5):881-85.
13. Coulam CB, Peters AJ, Genting M et al. Pregnancy rates after peritoneal ovum-sperm transfer. Am J Obstet Gynaecol 1991;164(6Pt 1):1447-49.
14. Lin CP, D'Amico JF, Nakajima ST. Initial experience with a modification of the follicle aspiration, sperm injection, and assisted rupture technique. Fertil Steril 2000;73:855-58.
15. Paulson RJ, Thornton MH. Follicle aspiration, sperm injection, and assisted rupture (FASIAR): A simple new assisted reproductive technique. Fertil Steril 1997;68:1148-51.
16. Bucktt WM, Tan SL: Alternative assisted conception techniques. In Brinsden PR (Ed): A Textbook of In vitro Fertilization and Assisted Reproduction 1999;(2nd edn):243-55.
17. Ransom MX, Garcia AJ, Doherty K et al. Direct gamete uterine transfer in patients with tubal absence or occlusion. J Assist Reprod Genet 1997;14(1):35-38.

18. Ranoux C, Aubriot FX, Dubuisson JB et al. A new in vitro fertilization technique: Intravaginal culture. Fertil Steril 1988;49:654-57.

19. Asch RH, Ellsworth LR, Balmaceda JP et al. Pregnancies after translaparoscopic gamete intrafallopian transfer. Lancet 1984;II:1034-103.

20. Assisted reproductive technology in the United States: 1996 results generated from the American Society for Reproductive Medicine/Science for Assisted Reproductive Technology Registry. Fertil Steril 1999;71:798-807.

21. Hurst BS, Tucker KE, Guadagnoli S et al. Transcervical gamete and zygote intrafallopian transfer. Does it enhance pregnancy rates in an assisted reproduction program? J Reprod Med 1996;41(11):867-70.

22. Strowtzki T, Korell M, Seehaus D et al. 'Bland' transvaginal gamete intra-fallopian transfer in distal tubal and peritubal pathology—an evaluation in respect to the laparoscopic approach. Hum Reprod 1993; 8(10):1703-07.

• Jaideep Malhotra
• Narendra Malhotra • Shivani Chaturvedi

40

Surrogacy and Adoption

SURROGACY

INTRODUCTION

Surrogacy is a new word for India while adoption is as old as time. The reasons which make adoption a more prevalent palliation to refractory sterility are plenty. In our epics, adoption is glorified by citing example of Lord Krishna and *Maa* Yashoda and is not a taboo in any sense. Secondly, the prevalent form of adoption in India is interfamily adoption, i.e. adopting a nephew or a niece. This does increase the feasibility since such nephews and nieces are a plenty due to unrestrained fertility. Also, the legal situation is easy to handle and the child remains within the family. This is a type of "Indianized surrogacy" and can be seen in many homes and often works for everyone's benefit.

Addressing the all important financial constraints which may make surrogacy a pipe dream for the common man. An infertile couple resorting to surrogacy may have tried a few cycles of IVF, or perhaps ICSI-ET which may have drained their resources. The surrogate mother has to be downregulated according to the natural mother's ovarian cycle and her endometrium prepared to receive the embryo all of which amounts to additional expense. Also significant is the issue of payment to the surrogate mother. On the other hand, an adoption may not cost much, is painless and quick.

The important question is; Is not an adopted baby somebody else's baby! Does not his or her face remind you of someone else?

Though the mother has a big heart, the question of acceptability does arise. Would the adopted child always be someone else's, while a baby through surrogacy could still be your very own? Specially the "gene-savvy" younger generation would rather accept a baby born out of their own ovaries and testes rather than a stranger's baby with an unknown genetic make-up. Also important are the concerns regarding genetically transmitted diseases and limitations, which may plague a well-educated couple. Would not they want a child who takes after her granny?

Not to be ignored is the psychological make-up of the natural mother. She may perceive surrogacy as her own personal failure. Since the father any way contributes the sperms, the mother may face feelings of inadequacy and may end up developing "guilt-jealousy complex" for the surrogate mother. It is like having your own egg in somebody else's basket and may lead to emotional complications if counseling is not provided.

The legal situation concerning surrogacy is still not transparent in India and issues of rights and inheritance may arise. Also has any one paid any concern to the all important baby? Should he or she know about his/her conception?

These questions have yet to be answered, but the future holds promise. With oocyte selling right at the click of the mouse on the net, it is not far when you may log on to "uterus.com" or "rent-a-uterus.com" and get instant access to willing surrogates. Whatever the future holds, Shakespeare did say it right: "What is in a name for which you call a rose, would smell as sweet".

GESTATIONAL SURROGACY

Gestational surrogacy (as distinct from traditional surrogacy, where the egg belongs to the female carrying the pregnancy) is a complex and unique medical procedure that is now an established and successful treatment alternative. The first pregnancy following *in vitro* fertilization (IVF) and the subsequent transfer of embryos to an unrelated surrogate was reported in 1985. This type of treatment has evolved rather slowly, and regretfully is still not accepted by the Society for Assisted Reproductive Technology (SART) as a reportable event in our specialty. Furthermore, in many parts of the world both traditional and gestational surrogacy remain unacceptable and illegal as a treatment option.

Issues that need to be comprehensively addressed include the following:

- The particulars of the medical process, including management of failed cycles and how many cycles a couple will try with the same surrogate. It is imperative that realistic expectations are set for all parties
- Potential complications of pregnancy that might commit the surrogate to periods of prolonged bed rest or absence from work
- Establishment of parameters of acceptable conduct by the parties throughout the arrangement inclusive of nutrition, smoking, alcohol ingestion, travel during pregnancy, attendance and involvement of the commissioning parents at prenatal visits and the delivery
- Chorionic villus sampling (CVS) or amniocentesis and what to do in the event of an unfavorable result

- Multifetal reduction in cases of multiple pregnancy
- Ownership and disposition of any remaining embryos
- When, what and how to involve children of either the gestational carrier or the commissioning parents
- Life, medical and disability insurance—It is important that coverage is in place for any catastrophic illness and/or medical consequences of the treatments. Also, the possibility of obtaining insurance or adjusting the payment to the surrogate in the event of prolonged absence from work because of bed rest necessitated by the pregnancy
- Management of the delivery, the inevitability of postpartum depression, suppression of lactation in the gestational surrogate and the prospects of drug-induced lactation in the intended mother
- Legal matters—Identifying the mechanisms to be utilized to finalize parental rights and to ensure that the surrogate mother understands that she will have no rights to the child should she decide to change her mind. The laws of each country differ and it is essential that an attorney familiar with reproductive law is involved. Passport issues for overseas couples need to be addressed and arrangements need to be made for the issuing of expedited birth certificates
- Financial matters—The establishment of trust accounts need to be discussed along with the apportioning of finances, billing, etc.
- Psychological—This is arguably the most important issue. Factors that influence a potential gestational surrogate mother to enter to the program, her expectations, her ability to "walk away" after the delivery, the involvement of her partner and/or their children. We have found it necessary to provide intercurrent adjunctive psychological support throughout the process, which can go a long way to avoiding escalation of problems should they arise. While the reality is that gestational surrogate mothers are providing the proverbial "womb for rent", it is imperative that at all times they be treated with the respect, dignity and compassion that

they deserve. They constantly need to be acknowledged and appreciated. This is particularly so when they may be experiencing severe nausea and vomiting in the early stages of the pregnancy, or there is a spontaneous early pregnancy loss.

One can clearly see from the above list that gestational surrogacy is an extremely complex process and involves knowledge and expertise in many different areas. For this reason, teamwork is fundamental and essential for successful outcomes. It is the opinion of the authors that when problems arise in surrogacy it is usually because of a breakdown in communication or counseling, with consequent unrealistic expectations by any members of the unit.

SCREENING

After completion of the orientation process and the selection of a surrogate, a comprehensive screening of all parties is undertaken. A physician needs to evaluate the intended parents for suitability for controlled ovarian hyperstimulation and egg retrieval. Several patients who have undergone a hysterectomy for malignancy have also had their ovaries moved high out of the pelvis to avoid harmful effects of radiation. In such cases, transabdominal ultrasound-guided egg harvesting is the preferred method. Screening for sexually transmitted diseases (human immunodeficiency virus, hepatitis, herpes, cytomegalovirus and toxoplasma) is undertaken on all parties. When screening a potential surrogate, the physician is concerned with regularity of menstrual cycles, normalcy of the uterine cavity (assessed by hysterosalpingography), concomitant medical problems and ease of conception in prior pregnancies. Hypertension, diabetes mellitus and thyroid disorders are relative contraindications for admission into the program, as is a past history of infertility problems in the gestational carrier.

At the completion of the screening procedure, the nurse coordinator will meet with all parties to ensure all contracts are in place and discuss specific cycle coordination with the individuals. The nurse will also address transportation of frozen embryos, which may have been generated elsewhere. This can be quite complex, especially when working with couples from other countries, as it is quite difficult to arrange for embryos to travel unaccompanied. Arrangements need to be made for out-of-town monitoring and methods of communication with the patients and/or physician. While the internet and fax machines have facilitated this process, it is essential that the issue be discussed in person.

"With respect to cycle coordination, it should be attempted, to minimize the stay of all parties in the said place. Also, because of the unpredictable responses of some patients to controlled ovarian hyperstimulation, natural cycle endometrial preparation in the gestational carrier is unsuitable.

Standard controlled ovarian hyperstimulation protocols are used for the genetic parents/egg donors. We suggest that they come to the center on day 6 or 7 of stimulation (to enable them to get over travel fatigue and to acclimatize for the final stages of egg development). The gestational carrier is suppressed with gonadotrophin-releasing hormone-analog-therapy and she commences estrogen administration (estradiol valerate 2 mg every 3 days, increased as required, dependent upon ultrasound and serum estradiol levels) prior to or no later than the start of the gonadotrophin therapy in the genetic mother. The aim is for an endometrial thickness of greater than or equal to 8 mm, along with serum estradiol levels of greater than or equal to 300 pg/mL.

SURROGACY MODEL

The Health Care Surrogate Act (HCSA) in Illinois has been proposed as a model for state laws naming surrogate medical decision-makers for those without advance directives (ADs). Our objective was to determine if the HCSA identifies the same surrogate as older persons would choose for themselves. If not, is the discrepancy between legally identified surrogate and preferred surrogate troublesome to respondents? Because it is documented that Black Americans have a variety of family structures, some of which may not be reflected in the HCSA list, we also wished to determine if discrepancies between surrogates named by the law and those desired by patients are associated with black or white race.

Design, Setting and Participants

A convenience sample of 144 patients aged 65 and older, without cognitive impairment, were interviewed at the geriatrics clinic of an academic medical center.

Main Outcome Measures

Respondents without ADs who had a different stated choice for surrogate medical decision-maker than the surrogate defined by the Illinois HCSA, based on their existing family.

Results

26 percent of respondents without ADs chose a surrogate that differed from the surrogate defined by the HCSA. However, 67 percent of those with a different choice for surrogate than defined by law, were not troubled by the discrepancy. The proportion of black subjects (25%) and white subjects (31%), who had surrogate discrepancies, was not significantly different (P = .6). Because the Illinois HCSA named surrogates who would be agreeable to the majority of our respondents, it appears that it may be a useful model for state surrogacy laws. Fortunately in India this problem is not marked by color.

UK Experience

In the UK, in the mid-1980s, profound concern was expressed by the media and professional bodies when Mrs Kim Cotton said that she planned to have a child for another couple and be paid for it. Outrage was expressed by many who felt that Mrs Cotton was "selling her baby", while others saw this as a new form of exploitation of women. It was predicted that career women would in the future bring pressure upon other women to have their children, and that babies would become mere commodities in an increasingly consumeristic society.

Only since the mid-1980s has natural surrogacy and IVF surrogacy (IVF-S) become a generally accepted treatment option for infertile women with certain clearly defined problems. In the UK, it has only been since 1990, following a report by the British Medical Association (BMA), that the medical profession was allowed to become involved in this form of treatment. Earlier, the BMA had issued a statement in 1987, that it was "unethical for a doctor to become involved in techniques and procedures leading to surrogate motherhood". In 1985, following the birth of a child conceived in the surrogacy arrangement by Mrs Cotton, the Surrogacy Arrangements Act (1985) was hurriedly passed through Parliament. This prohibited agencies or individuals (other than the potential surrogate or commissioning parents) from acting on a commercial basis to initiate, negotiate or compile information toward the making of a surrogacy arrangement. Finally, in 1990, the BMA published a report entitled "Surrogacy: Ethical Considerations Report of the Working Party on Human Infertility Services", concluding that, "It would not be possible or desirable to seek to prevent all involvement of doctors in surrogacy arrangements, especially as the Government does not intend to make the practice illegal". Guidelines were proposed and it was recommended that surrogacy should only be used as the last resort.

While this extended debate by the BMA, Parliament and other concerned groups was proceeding, Mr Patrick Steptoe and Professor Robert Edwards at Bourn Hall Clinic were having discussions with their Ethics Committee to allow a case of IVF-Surrogacy to proceed. Following extensive discussion over several months, the Committee finally gave permission for a couple to undergo treatment in 1988. Embryos created from the commissioning couple, were transferred to the sister of the woman, and a child was born to them in 1989 (Table 40.1).

Since the birth of this child, Bourne Hall Clinic has continued to operate a limited IVF-surrogacy (IVF-S) program, and during these 8 years more than 50 couples requesting treatment have been interviewed. The experience of this program is described and some of the ethical and legal issues discussed.

INDICATIONS FOR TREATMENT BY SURROGACY

The principal indications for treatment by IVF-S are clear, but there are other less obvious indications which some may consider as contentious (Figure 40.1):

TABLE 40.1: Results of treatment by IVF surrogacy at Bourn Hall Clinic, 1990-1998

Genetic couples' cycles	
No of started treatment cycles	37
Mean age (yrs) at start of treatment	32.7 (Range = 22-40)
Total stimulation cycles	61 (Mean = 1.6, Range = 1-5)
Mean no oocytes recovered	10 (Range = 2-24)
Mean no embryos frozen/cycle	5.4 (Range = 0-13)
Host surrogate cycles	
No started cycles	75
No cycles to embryo transfer	66 (88%)
Mean no embryos transferred	2.2
Final outcome	
Clinical pregnancies per genetic couple	24/37 (65.8%)
Clinical pregnancies per host surrogate	24/41 (58.5%)
Delivered/ongoing pregnancies per genetic couple	16/37 (43.2%)
Delivered/ongoing pregnancies per host surrogate	16/41 (39.0%)

1. Women without a uterus, but with one or both ovaries functioning, are the most obvious group that may be suitable for treatment by IVF-S. These include:
   - Women with congenital absence of the uterus
   - Women who have had a hysterectomy for cancer or uterine fibroids
   - Women who have had a hysterectomy for severe hemorrhage or ruptured uterus.
2. Women who suffer repeated miscarriage and for whom the prospect of carrying a baby to term is very remote. Also considered within this group are women who have repeatedly failed to achieve a pregnancy following several IVF treatment cycles, and who appear to be unable to implant normal embryos.
3. Women with certain medical conditions which may make pregnancy life-threatening, but for whom long-term prospects for health are good. These include severe heart disease or kidney disease.

SURROGACY AND THE LAW

IVF surrogacy is arguably the most contentious area of infertility treatment. It is the practice, whereby one woman carries a child for another with the intention that the child should be handed over to the commissioning couple after birth. The surrogate is effectively a host for a couple's embryo. No genetic material of the embryo is derived from the surrogate or her partner.

Such emotive and contentious treatment is regulated by the law. The Surrogacy Arrangements Act 1985 combines with sections of the Human Fertilization and Embryology Act, 1990 to provide a workable framework within which such arrangements can take place. One area of particular concern relates to the financial reward a surrogate may receive. The Surrogacy Arrangements Act makes it a criminal offense for commercial surrogacy to be arranged, punishable by a fine and/or up to three months in prison. No offense is committed by a woman wishing to become a surrogate, nor is an offense committed by a couple seeking to persuade a surrogate to carry a child. It is an offense under the Adoption Act 1976, punishable by a fine or up to six months in prison, to give or receive any payment in relation to the adoption of a child, the grant or consent to adoption or the handing over of a child with a view to its adoption, unless that payment is authorized by a court. If a fee paid to a surrogate is found to include a sum in payment for agreement to adoption and handing over a child, the surrogate and the prospective adopters may face prosecution. However, reasonable expenses to compensate a surrogate for her travel, clinic visits and so on, are acceptable; but this fluid arrangement highlights inadequacies in the law. What is considered reasonable? What, if the

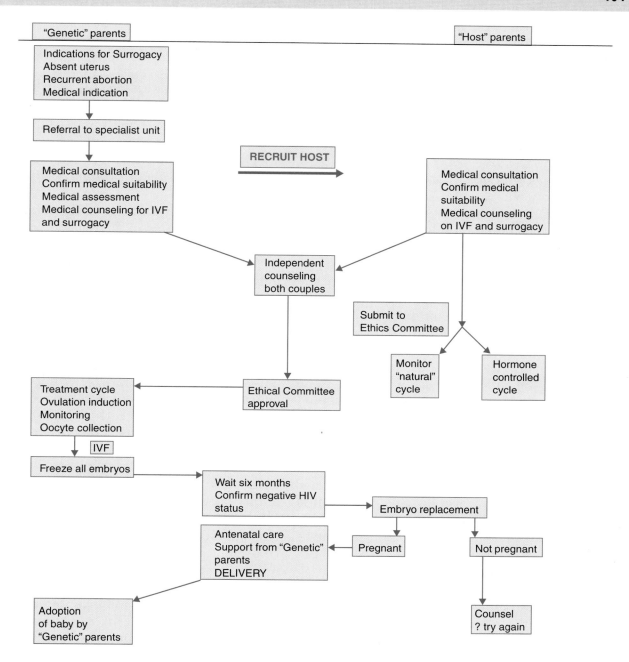

FIGURE 40.1: Algorithm for treatment by IVF surrogacy

surrogate perceives her compensation as inadequate? What recourse does the commissioning couple have within the law? The simple answer is none! In Britain, no contractual agreement can be upheld in law. It seems that couples who enter into surrogacy agreements have to understand that, if all goes well and they end up with a baby, they should be relieved that the arrangements succeeded. For those who experience traumatic events, the law does not uphold any contractual agreements—the commissioning couple cannot sue for breach of contract, nor can the surrogate sue, if she did not receive any agreed payments. If all goes well in a surrogacy arrangement, the couple will have "their" baby; if not, the law will not assist them to win a battle with the surrogate.

In Autumn 1998, the government appointed a review body which tried to address issues of particular concerns. Their recommendations include:

- Payments to surrogates should cover only genuine expenses, documentation of which is required
- Agencies involved in surrogacy arrangements should be required to be registered by the Department of Health, and have a Code of Practice
- A new Surrogacy Act should replace existing legislation and incorporate the new recommendations
- Parental orders will be granted as before, but the commissioning couple will be required to have been resident in the United Kingdom for a period of 12 months prior to application for an order.

Pivotal to the legal situation is the status of the child. Section 27 of the Human Fertilization and Embryology Act stipulates that the woman who carries the child, no other woman, is to be treated as the mother of the child. Hence, should a surrogate choose not to "give" the baby to its genetic parents, it is within her legal rights not to do so.

However, should the arrangement proceed successfully, once the baby is born, legal parentage has to be established. Section 30 of the Human Fertilization and Embryology Act gives the court power to order that the commissioning couple be treated by law as the parents of the child, but only in a limited number of circumstances.

- The couple must be married
- The child must have been conceived from either the placing of an embryo (IVF) or sperm and eggs (GIFT) in the woman, or by artificial insemination. The eggs or sperm or both must come from the commissioning couple
- At the time of the parental order, the child must be living with the couple, and the surrogate must have given full and free consent not less than six weeks after the birth
- No payments (other than for expenses reasonably incurred) must have been made

to the surrogate unless authorized by the court.

Outside of these conditions, "natural" parentage does not apply. However, surrogacy is fraught with dangers. What if the resultant child is disabled? What, if the commissioning couple divorce prior to the birth, or even worse, predecease the birth? Independent legal advice by all parties, including the possibility of taking insurance by the genetic couple, would appear to be prudent.

It is no wonder that, given the complexities of the law pertaining to surrogacy, some professionals shy away from surrogacy arrangements. At Bourn Hall Clinic a scheme is about to be initiated, whereby a named nurse will be allocated to each case, who will have a sound knowledge of law and ethical issues pertaining to surrogacy. This will facilitate continuity of care and allow close relationships to develop, thereby enabling the nurse to be aware of any arising conflicts or potential areas of concern. It will give both the genetic couple and the surrogate opportunities to discuss their case directly with someone who knows them, thus reducing repetition and the risk of misunderstanding.

Trust, confidence and reassurance will be gained by the nurse specialist approach and ability to help. Guidance throughout the intricate infertility program, plus individual care during the emotive embryo transfer phase of the treatment, ensure that the optimal levels of care will be given to the surrogate and the genetic couple. The nurse's coordinating role provides a liaison between the medical team and those receiving treatment. This is an intrinsic factor towards successful treatment outcome.

The frustration and despondency felt by couples unable to have their own children without professional help is unimaginable. Those who require surrogacy do not undertake this treatment lightly, nor do assisted conception units consider surrogacy an option unless it is the only possible course of treatment.

A high standard of professional diplomacy and patience is needed to steer couples through ethical dilemmas, practical disappointments and legal minefields. The allocation of an experienced named nurse, fully conversant with the law and appreciative of the difficulties that can arise, will reduce stress and maximize the chances of an effective treatment and successful outcome.

Infertility still carries an unwarranted stigma in society. It would be naive to believe that informal surrogacy arrangements have not been undertaken for many years. However, it is the formal arrangements and the law surrounding this particularly emotive issue that concerns healthcare professionals. By the provision of high standards of expert, informed nursing care, surrogacy cases can proceed smoothly, with positive benefits to the genetic couple, the surrogate, and most importantly, the child.

ADOPTION

Adoption has always been a child-centered and highly regulated area of family building, with agencies or facilitators charged with the multiple responsibilities of serving the interests of the child, birth parent and adoptive parent. While there are significant differences between gametes and embryos donated to create a child conceived through ART treatments and the children resulting from unintended and unwanted pregnancies, there are also startling similarities and lessons to be learned.

For decades, as with sperm donation, the norm was secrecy—adoptions were "closed" procedures. The prevailing wisdom was that birth parents should not see, and therefore would not think about, their children; adoptive families should not tell, and thus would not remember, that their children were not their biological offspring. Babies were taken from hospitals without good-byes, placements were made only after home studies and criminal record checks confirmed parental fitness of adoptive families. Court records regarding those families were sealed from all involved and for all time. Medical information was sometimes scanty or nonexistent. And no thought was given to placing biological siblings together.

That model has slowly disintegrated over time, as the concept of openness in the adoption process has evolved. At this point, the majority of domestic adoptions in the United States are at least partially open, with birth parents significantly involved in selecting, if not meeting or continuing a relationship with, their chosen adoptive family. A growing movement to open adoption records has resulted in mutual registries in almost half of the states wherein adult adoptees and birth parents link up with one another, and court orders are increasingly sought and obtained by adoptees seeking identifying birth information. Legislative efforts to establish a federal adoption registry are ongoing. A recently enacted (1999) law in the state of Oregon allows adoptees to obtain their original birth certificates directly from the birth register without the need for either a mutual registry or a court order. In India, the procedure of adoption is one's own prerogative. Most of the couples end up adopting a child from within the family which is good and bad especially in a joint family system where a sense of belonging does not come. Secondly, the legal problems concerning wealth and property which come up later on are not for been. There are no clearcut laws or agencies, if available are very few in number and the problem is enormous which just does not get enough mention considering India as one of the most populous country.

Some of the issues that need mentioning include:
• Discussion with the couple about adoption. Its benefits and acceptability
• Referring them to a proper agency either public or private for a systematic and legal procedure
• Educating the adoptive parents about requirements for adoption
• Financial aspect of adoption
• Legal aspects of adoption
• Counseling regarding the health and upkeep of the adopted child. Our customs are such that there have been many incidences where I have seen couples reverting back to ART treatments in spite of adopting a child, especially now, since, awareness about ART treatments and number of clinics offering them has gained a lot of momentum, proper counseling is very important.

Despite wide variation in current adoption laws, certain central principles are common: buying or selling babies is strictly prohibited (although birth parent expenses are frequently permitted); consent to adoption may not be given before birth (with a few exceptions); home studies and criminal record checks of potential parents are commonplace; registries or agency policies for exchange of both identifying and nonidentifying information are in place; legally recognized birth fathers must consent or have their rights terminated; consideration must be given to placement of genetic siblings together; and any promises to place a baby for adoption prior to birth or for financial consideration is illegal.

While there are clear differences between gamete or embryo donors and birth parents, as has been repeatedly explored in the mental health literature, the historical trends in adoption sketched out above present relevant analogies and lessons for ART law and policy makers. Taken together with international developments in the area of donor registries, (which are beyond the scope of the chapter), I suggest that future ART policies and regulation in any country need not necessarily or beneficially follow the historical, medical model of secrecy-based, anonymous donor insemination.

Instead, the future of the ART could benefit from a more open model—one that recognizes the legitimate concerns of donors and acknowledges the privacy of the needs and interests not of the adult parents but of the recipient children.

Adoption and medically assisted reproduction are alternative options for childless parents to fulfill their wish for having a child. In both situations, there is a necessity for the future parents to mourn the loss of their imagined child, which could have been conceived without a third party (adoption agency or medically assisted reproduction). Adoption always represents for the child, a loss of emotional ties with birth parents and the development of new attachments with adoptive parents. Adoption can be considered as a lifetime process of the members involved in the adoption triangle, that is birth parents, adoptive parents and the child. The article dicusses the loss of emotional bonds from primary caretakers as a psychological trauma and addresses mourning difficulties in adoptees. Problems with the development of new attachments with adoptive parents such as loyalty conflicts and the revelation of the adoption are described. Family romance fantasy in adoption and aspects of family dynamics as well as the specific difficulties adoptive parents encounter are explored.

IVF, ADOPTION AND SURROGACY IN ANCIENT TIMES

IVF, adoption and surrogacy was known and practised in ancient times. In the *Mahabharata*, Gandhari, wife of king Dhritarashtra, conceived but the pregnancy went on for nearly two years; after which she delivered a mass (mole). Bhagwan Vyasa found that there were 101 cells which were normal in the mass. These cells were put in a nutrient medium and were grown *in vitro* of full term of these, 100 developed into male children (Duryodhana, Duhshasana and the other Kauravas) and one as a female child (Duhsheela).

There are other well quoted examples which refer to not only IVF but that a male can produce a child without the help of a female. Sage Gautama produced two children from his own semen- a son Kripa and a daughter Kripi, who were both test tube babies. Likewise, Sage Bharadwaj produced Drona, later to be the teacher of the Pandavas and Kauravas. The story relating to the birth of Drishtadyumna and Draupadi is even more interesting and reflects the supernatural powers of the great Rishis. King Drupada had enmity with Dronacharya and desired to have a son strong enough to kill Drona. He was given a medicine by a Rishi and after collection of his semen, processed it and suggested that AIH should be done for his wife, who however refused. The Rishi then put the semen in a yajnyakunda from which Dhrishtadyumna and Draupadi were born. While the above are quoted as examples of IVF and parthenogenesis, there is another story which refers to embryo transfer. This was regarding the seventh pregnancy of Devaki, by the will of the Lord, the embryo was transferred to the womb of Rohini, the first wife of Vasudev, to prevent the baby being killed by Kansa.

THE FUTURE OF THIRD-PARTY REPRODUCTION: WHERE TO FROM HERE?

The existing model of reproductive medicine, where patients with their physicians make private and unfettered decisions about their family building efforts, is beginning to show the strains of modern times. Compared with medical infertility treatment decisions involving biological parents, the legal tensions reflect in recent court battles illustrate that adding anonymous or known gamete or embryo donation in an effort to enable patients to have a child, raises a multitude of questions. As physicians, brokers and patients themselves move into the realm of recruiting, screening and compensating donors and offering or even creating embryos for donation or adoption, major new societal, ethical and legal questions are being raised.

One very recent example is the imbalance between supply and demand for donor eggs, which will almost certainly lead to renewed concerns about commercialization of gamete donation, coercion of donors and the inadequacy of existing voluntary guidelines. Current professional guidelines for egg donor payments do not set a dollar cap, but suggest only that payments should be for the time and effort involved in creating the eggs and not be "so excessive as to constitute coercion or exploitation. A 1995 report of that organization's Ovum *Donor Task Force*, which was composed of mental health professionals, recommended compensation in the range of $1000-3000, suggesting that, "compensation above $3000 may be construed as coercive."

Ironically, one of the tall, smart college students who initially considered answering the $50,000 donor and said she first had "big, ethical discussions" with her friends and ultimately chose not to pursue donation, likening it to prostitution. It would be prudent if such discussions were happening at the level of national policy, and not just on undergraduate campuses.

It remains to be seen if providers or separate entities now moving eagerly into embryo donation will attempt to pay donors for their embryos, even though they were originally created for their own use. Such payments would be difficult to justify and are not recommended under current professional guidelines. Embryo donation also presents a clear need to legally define how parenthood is relinquished and obtained and what duties, if any, are owed to embryo donor with respect to their embryos and the children created from them. Courts called upon to settle individual disputes look to precedent, and, in the absence of specific laws to guide them, may well look to adoption analogies rather than donor insemination laws.

While the debate within the medical profession as to the need for, and scope of, outside regulation will probably continue for some time, there appears to be a growing interdisciplinary consensus' that some outside policies and regulation are both justified and necessary. Few federal laws are currently in place governing the ARTs (the Wyden Act addresses statistical reporting requirements by ART programs). The lessons of Florida and its attempt at legislation should be instructive to others.

Significant efforts are underway by a large variety of policy groups to revisit existing laws and to develop additional legislation aimed at protecting families being created through ART treatment. Included amongst such groups are the American Bar Association, which is drafting a model law addressing numerous issues of the ARTs, the National Conference of Commissioners of Uniform State Laws (NCCUSL), which is updating its Uniform Parentage Act, and the New York State Task Force on Life and the Law, which issued a comprehensive report and suggestions for specific legislation in *The Assisted Reproductive Technologies*: *Analysis and Recommendations for Public Policy* in 1998. Efforts at proposed policy and legislative consensus have identified numerous legal trouble spots in the ARTs, including clarification of both maternity and paternity for children born from donor gametes embryos, and surrogates; embryo status including clarification of disposition options, inheritance and posthumous reproduction; the establishment, content and accessibility of a donor registry; standardized informed consent requirement; restrictions on multiple gestations; the scope of insurance coverage; and the appropriate standard of care owed to and by all involved in creating these brave new families. A number of these groups are beginning to collaborate as they attempt to reach policy consensus on some of these issues.

As the ARTs continue to develop, particularly in their use of donor, the law needs to at least address and define the rights and responsibilities of all involved. The incentive is great to avoid large-scale transgressions (as occurred recently at the University of California in Irvine) or contested custody disputes over children without established parentage. Legal cases such as Lucas, Buzzanca, and Huddleston are serving as wake-up calls for courts, legislatures and policy makers alike.

Ethical Issues Relating to Reproduction Control and Women's Health

There are many ethical aspects which arise from the application of reproduction control in women's health. Women's health can be enhanced, if women are given the opportunity to make their own reproductive choices about sex, contraception, abortion and application of reproductive techno logies. The main issues that raise ethical dilemmas following the development of assisted reproduction techniques are: the right to procreate or reproduce; the process of *in vitro* fertilization itself—is it morally acceptable to interfere in the reproduction process; the moral status of the embryo; the involvement of a third party in the reproductive process by genetic material donation; the practice of surrogacy, cryopreservation of pre-embryos; genetic manipulation; experiments on pre-embryos, etc? Induced abortion raises further issues related to the rights of the woman versus the rights of the fetus. For those who consider life to begin at conception, abortion always equals murder and is therefore forbidden. Those who believe in the absolute autonomy of the woman over her body take the other extreme approach. The discussion surrounding abortion usually centers on whether it should be legal or illegal. Access to safe abortion is critical to the health of women and to their autonomy. The development of new, effective contraceptive methods has a profound impact on women's lives. By the use of contraception, it is possible to lessen maternal, infant and child mortality and to reduce the prevalence of sexually transmitted diseases. Research and development of new, effective, reversible contraceptives for women and men is needed. Dissemination of information about the safety and effectiveness of contraceptive methods is of great importance. Female genital mutilation is still practiced worldwide due to customs and tradition among various ethnic groups. The procedure is considered to be medically detrimental to the physical and mental health of women and girls, and is considered by many as oppression of women. The practice has to be stopped. Recognition of the fetus as a 'patient' has a potential effect on women's right for autonomy;

they have no legal obligation to undergo invasive procedures and to risk their health for the sake of their fetuses. The woman carries ethical obligations toward her fetus. This obligation should not be enforced by the law. At present, women bear most of the burden of reproductive health. All of them have a right of access to fertility regulation. Government and society must ensure the women's equal rights to healthcare just as men have in the regulation of their fertility.

CONCLUSION

In today's era of gene manipulation, the day of designer babies, wombs for hire, animal wombs, plastic wombs is not far away but there will be a price tag attached. The couple, the society and the ART service provider has to decide what price to pay to have a child. Both science and the scientist will go ahead and do whatever can be done.

Lets make families out of couples.

FURTHER READING

1. Brinsden PR. Oocyte recovery and embryo transfer techniques for in vitro fertilization. In Brinsden PR, Rainsbury PA (Eds): A Textbook of in vitro Fertilization and assisted Reproduction. Parthenon Publishers: Carnforth, 1992;139-54.
2. British Medical Association. Changing Conceptions of Motherhood: The Practice of Surrogacy in Britain. BMA Publications: London, 1996.
3. British Medical Association. Surrogacy: Ethical Considerations. Report of the Working Party on Human Infertility Services. BMA Publications, 1990.
4. British Medical Association. Surrogate Motherhood. Report of the Board of Science and Education. BMA Publications, 1987.
5. Human Fertilisation and Embryology Act 1990. Her Majesty's Stationery Office, London, 1990.
6. Human Fertilisation and Embryology Act (s. 27). Her Majesty's Stationery Office, London, 1980.
7. Marrs RP, Ringler GE, Stein AL et al. The use of surrogate gestational carriers for assisted reproductive technology. Am J Obstet Gynecol 1993;168:1858-63.
8. Sathanandan M, Macnamee MC, Wick K et al. Clinical aspects of human embryo cryopreservation. In Brinsden PR, Rainsbury PA (Eds): A Textbook of in vitro Fertilization and Assisted Reproduction. Parthenon Publishers, Carnforth, 1992;251-64.
9. Utian WF, Goldfarb JM, Kiwi R et al. Preliminary experience with in vitro fertilization-surrogate gestational pregnancy. Ferti Steril 1989;52:633-38.

Section 7

Laboratory Management

41

Setting-up of an IVF Laboratory

Infertility is not a disease that if untreated can fulminate to a point of no return. Inability to conceive, subjects couples to lot of frustrations and anguish thereby causing severe psychological stress. This is further aggravated by so-called norms of our culture and society stigmatizing infertile women as "Barren".

The initial assessment visit of the couples should therefore not only focus on infertility investigations, past treatments, ventilating frustration but also planning the next step effectively. Therefore in a good program a caring attitude should be shown towards patients and each couple treated with dignity and respect they deserve. When the patient's welfare is the guiding principle and attention to detail is the "Modus Operandi", the result is a high take home baby rate. It is essential therefore that patient's waiting rooms, consultation chambers and Counselling rooms should have ambience conducive to making couple relaxed. This chapter will discuss the more typical purpose built all-inclusive laboratory with oocyte retrieval and embryo transfer facilities, with special emphasis on problems of construction.

Today's laboratories are commonly placed in city centers in order to serve larger population. Recent development of assays for scanning content of air combined with the awareness that some buildings could be harmful to tissue cultures makes the choice of a laboratory site very important in any new program.

IVF UNIT

The IVF unit consists of:

"Out Patient Area" (OPD)

1. *OPD:* Effective programs require close communication between doctor, patient, nurse, lab director, all office and surgical staff and hence best achieved if all these facilities are located together. This area should have facilities for Doctor's consultation rooms, Counselling room, room for giving injections or drawing of blood, a good spacious patient waiting area and wash room.
2. Preferable to have the USG room also in OPD area. A vaginal probe of 5-7mHZ preferred over an abdominal probe. There should be a free access from here to Out Patient Department. As the OPD would be a crowded area it should be away from main culture area and hence ground floor of the building is preferred.

A brief description of setting up of an IVF lab with a modest budget is discussed:

Laboratory Area

A laboratory design should be based on the anticipated case load and any subspecialty. When commissioning the laboratory, thought should be given to the most recent developments in equipment and facilities. Consideration should also be given to local health and safety requirements. The Endocrinology, Andrology and Embryology laboratories should be housed in this area. IVF programs, no matter how large or small, require concreted efforts of several people; no one person can do it all. The staff should be fully competent, dedicated to perfection, constantly seeking improvement and willing to measure quality of their performance. The laboratory location, equipments and its placement, good protocols and overall maintenance need careful organization.

Location of IVF Lab

1. 2nd floor of building is ideal. Should be a strictly restricted area for the lab staff, OT staff and patients undergoing procedure of ovum pick-ups or embryo transfers. An area of 30-40 sq. mts is sufficient.

2. Air borne contaminants can be detrimental to human gametes and embryos. They can be best controlled by "Clean Room" methods. Particle up to 0.3 μ can be filtered from entering the room. Particulates can be removed by HEPA filters, volatile organics can be scrubbed out of the air by activated carbon filters. Pressurizing the clean areas could control entry of dirty air into it. The air supplying clean room should be separated from rest of the building. The humidity within the culture room should also be completely controlled according to climatic and seasonal variations. The final air handling system must be capable of supplying the space with air, with a temperature of 30-35°C at less than 40 percent relative humidity. Air inlets and outlets should be carefully spaced.[1]

3. The walls of the lab should be non-glossy, non-porous to avoid dust, bacteria and insects from lodging. Paint used for the walls should be aged before use and be non-toxic and water based, formulated for low VOC potential (Acrylic, Vinyl Acrylic, Alkyde, or Acrylic latex polymers).[2] Paints that can influence the air quality should be emission tested. Wallpapers should be avoided. The floor made of non-slippery, non-porous material like vinyl flooring is preferred. Door width should be framed slightly larger than standard to allow bulky instruments to pass through. Only a Hatch as a connecting pass between lab and operation theatre to pass follicular flushing, should be present.

4. The workbenches should have a height (0.75 mts) permissible to work comfortably. Sturdy bench tops, Stabilizers and antivibration tables should be used for micro manipulative equipment to be placed. This is essential for them to function with precision. Drawers, cabinets and tables should be made of stainless steel and glass.[3] Light can be detrimental to embryos. Good to have dimmers in the lab. Outside windows should be fully covered or removed. Special tissue culture filters, designed to fit into fluorescent fixtures over interior windows, or into microscope paths, can remove the high-energy UV and blue parts of the spectrum. UV lighting can be used only in Laminar hoods and more so non – ozone generating UV lights are ideal.[2] Compressed medical grade gases should supply the incubators in which embryos are grown.

5. Lastly but not the least the personal cleanliness of staff in the lab is important. They should only wear antistatic clothing, special head, foot and hand covering, wash hands before entering culture rooms, and follow sterile techniques.[3]

6. A backup power system for important instruments like incubators, freezing machine, micromanipulators, and refrigerators is mandatory.[3] An air conditioning system should be opted for. Emergency exit should open into a separate fire zone and have a separate internal pathway.

7. It is important that there is no eating-place/ cafeteria in the adjoining premises.

8. The study of pollutants and their effect on IVF is not complete, but taken together; the environmental control measures can make a difference in pregnancy rates. Spraying of insecticides, pesticides or any chemicals including room fresheners should be prohibited in and around the laboratory area.

Requirements of an IVF Lab

Equipments and consumables should be of proven quality; with easy availability of maintenance services so that their cost factor is within the projected budget. There factors should be considered during planning and commissioning of the instruments. Appropriate modular placements of incubator, laminar floor units and micromanipulator stations will minimize distances that cultured dishes and tubes need to be moved. Ideally an embryologist should be able to finish one complete procedure without moving more than 3 meters in any direction.[4] The critical items of equipment, including incubators and frozen embryo storage facilities should be appropriately alarmed and monitored. A minimum of 2 incubators is recommended. This should not be considered as excessive, as lack of spare equipment could jeopardize patient care at times of malfunctioning of equipments.[2] Gas cylinders should be preferably placed outside in a separate room and only pipes and tubes should enter the laboratory. Medical gases can be directed into the laboratory using pre-washed Vinyl/Teflon lined tubing or solid manifolds made of stainless steel with suitable compression fittings.

Operation Theatre

This should be located adjoining the IVF lab. Special air filters should be fitted here also. This is a place where Ovum pick-ups and embryo transfers are performed. As mentioned earlier, a hatch should be the only communication to the lab from here. The necessary equipments like hot air oven, suction pump, USG scanner with vaginal probe, all other general equipments required in any theatre including Boyle's apparatus should be present.

Washing Area

For scrubbing and cleaning of lab, ware should be kept dry.

Changing Room

Should be located just before entering the main culture room, enabling staff to change into special lab outfits.

Cryopreservation Room

Good to have a separate freezing room to avoid exposure of oocytes/embryos to cold air from freezing machine. This room should be well ventilated and bench height should be able to accommodate liquid N_2 containers (Storage). Liquid Nitrogen level alarms, with remote notification capability, should be contemplated for all Dewars.[3]

Storage Room

Ample storage spaces should always be planned for IVF laboratories. In the absence of this, laboratory space would be wrongly used which could create havoc. Storage material should be stocked in sufficient quantity to maintain steady supply as long storage of even the sterilized disposal items can release multiple compounds, which could pollute the air.[4] All storage materials should be kept in clean containers (preferably steel) and placed in steel racks.

Masterbatorium

A semen collection room to allow the patient to collect semen is to be placed adjacent to Andrology laboratory. Facility to allow the patient to wash after collection should be available in this area. The room should be spacious, sound proofed not too, large but with all the necessary arrangements to make the couple comfortable for semen collection. This area should be accessible to the concerned patients only and preferably be located at the end of hallway with its own exit.[4]

Record Room

This is a room where records of all patients both clinical and lab details are stored in an order.

Burning In

Construction and renovation can introduce a variety of compounds into the environment, which can have adverse effects like delayed or abnormal embryonic development, absence of fertilization to complete reproductive failure.[5]

Hence Burning in of the finished laboratory is very important before actual operations are started. A typical burn in consists of increasing the temperature of the new area by 10-20°C and increase in ventilation rate will aid in the removal of volatile organics. This period can range from 10-28 days during which time, lighting and auxiliary equipments particularly air exchange module should be kept running in order to repeatedly purge the air. After the burn in is complete the particulate levels should be determined to verify the functioning capacity of HEPA filtration system (using USA Federal Standard 209E).[6] Microbial sampling for aerobic bacteria and fungi is done in new facilities using Andersen sampler followed by microbiological culturing and identification.[6]

QUALITY ASSURANCE

An IVF lab obtains its supply of materials from the clinic and patients, processes it and then returns it to the clinic. Hence the quality system of the lab is closely related to the clinic.[7] Results should be evaluated on a regular basis because percentage of quality pregnancies is the only criteria, which speaks of the quality of the lab.[7] An internal audit checks the procedures introduced and aids us to achieve better success.

PERSONNEL

The optimal ratio of the laboratory staff to the contemplated number of procedure is debatable, and hence economics is the enemy. The ratio should be high, only then the embryologist can devote greater time on quality control, training, and procedural details.[4] Across all these duties the following five job positions can be clearly defined.

1. *Lab Director:* It is ideal to have a person with a medical background with a D.Sc/Ph.D./MCE and at least 3 years experience in the field of embryology.
2. *Clinicians:* With subspecialty in Reproductive medicine/subfertility with sufficient exposure to IVF cases.
3. *Embryologist:* Personnel with a science background, B.Sc/M.Sc. with training or experience in embryology.
4. *Technicians:* With a B.Sc./Diploma in Medical Lab Technology with experience in any medical laboratory.

5. *Nurses/Counsellors:* With experience in dealing with IVF patients and assisting in Ovum Retrieval/embryo replacement.

All the above must have commitment, dedication, ethical know-how and care for sub fertile patients. A complete overall knowledge of the state of the ART is essential.

PROTOCOLS

Standard Operating Protocols giving good persistent results over a period of time should be drafted and strictly followed by the lab personnel. Any changes regarding the same should be discussed and implemented by the concerned people. It is a good practice to maintain a lab protocol book, giving the details of each procedure.

INFORMED CONSENT

As with all medical procedures and treatments, the patients must make the final decision as to what is appropriate and acceptable treatment in their particular situation. Hence it is necessary that every couple be provided with full written informed consent and the forms should indicate all the data concerning the IVF cycle.[4]

ETHICAL CONSIDERATION

Assisted Reproductive Technique (ART) treatments are rapidly evolving thereby increasing the need to formulate an ethics committee. Because of the ethical concerns involved in the treatments, which involve the laboratory handling and manipulation of human gametes and embryos, it is presumed that all ART procedures will be performed in accordance with the recommendation contained in that report.[8] Various societies have been motivated to produce good IVF laboratory practice.

CONCLUSION

This chapter can provide guidance to those medical professionals aspiring to be independent in the world of ART. Best possible attempt has been made to provide useful suggestions and concepts that have been learned from practical experience for the wide variety of problems.

REFERENCES

1. Cohen J, Gilligan et al. ambient air and its potential effects on conception Invitro. Human reproduction 1997;12:1742-49.
2. Simplicity & success in IVF by Beth Anne Ary ND.
3. ESHRE guidelines for good practice in IVF laboratories, Luca Gianoraoli et al; Human Reproduction, 2000; 15(10):2241-46.
4. Textbook of Assisted reproduction techniques by Gardner, Weiss man reprint 2001.
5. Boone WR, Johnson JE et al. Control of air quality in an assisted reproductive technology laboratory. Fertil Steril 1999;71:150-54.
6. Federal Standard 209E. General services administration U.S.A Federal Government, Washington, DC 1992.
7. The Ethical Committee of the American Fertility Society. Ethical consideration of assisted reproductive technologies Fertil Steril 1994;62:1-125.
8. van WG. Inzen about "Model Quality Manual" Tilburey, Fertinet Dec 1999.

• Herman A Fernandes • Korula George

42

Quality Control in IVF Laboratory

INTRODUCTION

In vitro fertilization and gamete manipulation is a highly technical and exacting science. Although pregnancy results are constantly improving, they largely remain below the 50 percent mark and efforts to improve upon these rates are ongoing. The awareness that gametes and embryo's are fragile and susceptible to extraneous insults of diverse origin, led scientists to evolve mechanisms to ensure a stable environment. It was soon realized that consistency of quality was a key factor, thus leading to the establishment of written protocols of practice and conduct in the laboratory.

Ackerman *et al* (1985) were the first to realize the importance of testing for embryo toxicity. Any of the components used for IVF can impair the growth of human embryos. These components, be they media, disposable items, change in lab environment or minor equipment error: they all play a vital role in the success of the program. Generally termed as "embryo toxic substances" they need to be identified and removed for a successful procedure to occur.

Numerous attempts have been made to introduce measures of check but most have been expensive, impractical or difficult to implement. However, the importance of these is well recognized and today formal, well designed quality assurance programs, consisting of internal quality control (QC) and external quality assurance (EQA) are being introduced in the better laboratories globally.

In this chapter we shall discuss the role of QC and QA and the different bioassays available, in an attempt to provide some insight in identifying potential hazards that can affect successful outcome.

QUALITY CONTROL

Quality control can be defined as group of activities routinely performed to identify errors during monitoring of all-important operational aspects that are directly or indirectly involved with performing IVF. In addition to testing of culture media QC should be applied to instruments, culturewares (plasticwares), chemicals and solutions as well as to the influences of the laboratory environment. The activities in an internal QC program can be, for example, daily monitoring of incubators, a weekly check on the Milli-Q water system, temperature appraisal of all test tube heaters, stage warmers and water bath. We, therefore, recommend designing a systematic group of activities to monitor everything that is utilized in an IVF program.

Equipment Monitoring

A monitoring system for all laboratory equipment has been found to be essential as reliable functioning can play an important role in maintaining high standards of care. We recommend daily monitoring of incubators: the CO_2 content verified with a fyrite analyzer and temperature checked with a reliable thermometer. The readings are logged and values extrapolated onto graphs (plot day *vs.* temperature or CO_2 content) everyday. The slightest of variations can be easily identified and acted upon. Similarly test tube heaters, microscope stage warmers and water baths are monitored and readings are recorded. Pipetting devices can be a major source of contamination and hence should be cleaned, serviced and calibrated. Similarly instruments such as pH meters, osmometer, balances and centrifuge should be cleaned and calibrated on a routine basis depending on their use. These formal programs of maintenance and evaluation need to be documented and they represent a form of QC.

Cytotoxic Contaminants

Contaminants and potentially cytotoxic substances that enter the culture system may find their way through glassware, plasticware, chemicals used for media preparation, oils or through the laboratory environment. We have introduced the human sperm survival test as the bioassay to check out the contact materials and culture medium. Motile sperms at a concentration of 5×10^6 per ml are incubated in test and control media in the presence or absence of serum albumin according to the protocol outlined by Claassens *et al,* 2000. To minimize the introduction of cytotoxic substances we follow precautionary measures, such as, all glassware are rinsed thoroughly and soaked in Milli-Q water overnight, then rinsed ten times in Milli-Q water and dried in a dry heat oven. Finally they are packaged and sterilized for a minimum of 2 hours at 200°C in a hot air oven. These procedures minimize the potential presence of endotoxin on glassware.

Plasticware introduced into the culture system is tested against cultureware which has already passed the human sperm survival QC test (negative control). These include test tubes, petri dishes, syringes and filters. Similarly every new batch of culture medium/oil is routinely subjected to QC using the human sperm survival assay.

Moreover, the continuous assessment of supernumerary embryos indirectly allows us to evaluate the performance of these products.

Water

A common source of problems is the water used in preparation of the culture medium. Water constitutes greater than 95 percent of the total volume and hence it needs to be quality controlled. The options available to IVF laboratories is to purchase commercially available culture medium, constitute culture medium from a ready-made powdered media mix or to prepare their own culture medium by purchasing the ingredients from a reliable source (with an assurance certificate that all chemicals are cell culture or embryo tested). Each of these options has their own advantages and disadvantages. Commercial media have a short shelf life, the user has no control over quality and none whatsoever on purity of water used. Batch to batch variations in quality are possible. Maintaining the cold chain from the source of manufacture to the user can be a major problem.

Powdered media have a longer shelf life, but here again the user has no control on the purity of water, which has to be purchased for reconstitution. Inhouse media preparation is a time consuming venture and few laboratories have the expertise, financial resources, facilities or technical experience to embark on the tedious task. However, preparation of medium on site allows the user to ensure batch to batch consistency and provides an opportunity to quality control each and every aspect of media making.

For those who prepare culture medium on site or wish to do so, it is recommended that they should monitor the input and output parameters of the Milli-Q system on a daily basis. In addition, routine test for the presence of chlorines, chloromines, silica, total organic carbons (TOC) and endotoxins must be performed. Increased embryonic fragmentation in the laboratory is the direct reflection of the presence of endotoxin in the culture medium and the most common source is the water. We believe that the initial source of water plays an important role in the final quality of water produced by the Milli-Q system. We, therefore, utilize pharmacy grade double distilled water as feed water into our Milli-Q PF system. This ensures, high purity of water, decreases vigorous sanitization schedules and lengthens the life-span of the filtration cartridge, which makes the system economical to utilize.

Air Quality

Over and above the extensive quality control measures mentioned, one must consider environmental hazards. Chemical air contamination (CAC) has been studied and their effects on the embryo quality and pregnancy rates have been documented (Cohen *et al*, 1997). These authors have not only identified the sources of volatile organic compounds (VOC) in their laboratories, but have suggested ways to reduce and eradicate them from the laboratory air.

The incubator is the heart of the IVF laboratory and chamber environment should be of top quality. A mixture of gases from the cylinders and the laboratory air creates the chamber environment. Gases expelled from the cylinders contain fine particles of rust and hence most incubators have 0.22 μm filters to reduce the possibility of particulate contamination. In addition, we have incorporated charcoal filters to absorb VOC that may exist within the cylinders. Incubators also breathe in 95 percent of air, which may carry CAC and as a further precautionary measure we have installed a VOC-HEPA filter unit within the incubator. This measure has shown remarkable beneficial effects on embryo quality. Gametes and embryos do spend time outside the incubator for manipulation or morphological assessment. An attempt should be made to decrease or eradicate CAC from the circulating air within the laboratory. In our laboratory we have a VAC (ventilation and air conditioning) system, where the air is blown through pre-HEPA filter of 20 micron followed by 5 micron filter panels and finally through HEPA filter into the laboratory. We are currently designing and installing gas phase filters (activated carbon filters) for removal of CAC contamination.

ROLE OF BIOASSAYS

Bioassay is a popular method of quality control and bodies like the ESHRE have issued guidelines that state "laboratory protocol should include in-house quality control procedures using an appropriate bioassay system" (Gianaroli *et al*, 2000). They are objective, reliable and independent of clinical factors. Although several assay methods are available for testing supplies, procedures and environmental influences, debate exists regarding the most appropriate method to be employed in the IVF laboratory.

Bioassays available for testing gametes and embryo contact material include human sperm motility assay (Edwards *et al*, 1980), hamster sperm motility (Bavister and Andrews 1988), and culture of 1-cell (Quinn *et al*, 1984) and 2-cell (Ackerman *et al*, 1984, Parinaud *et al*, 1986) mouse embryos, zona free mouse embryo (Fleming *et al*, 1987), and mouse hybridoma cells (Bertheussen *et al*, 1989).

Sperm Motility Assay

Human or hamster sperm have been used to perform this test. Several investigators have shown that the sperm bioassay meets the criteria for a reliable bioassay and is useful in detecting embryo toxic substances in the IVF program. Bavister and Andrews (1988) first reported the simplicity and reliability of the hamster sperm motility assay. It has high sensitivity in discriminating between water qualities used for preparation of culture medium (Rinehart *et al*, 1988), and later Gorill and co-workers (1991) found this test to be highly reproducible. A comparative study on the diagnostic sensitivity of rodent sperm and embryos by Esterhuizen *et al*, (1994), found mouse sperm more effective at detecting low levels of endotoxin in short periods of time (4-6 hours) compared to mouse embryos, or to human and hamster sperm. On the other hand, it was shown that human sperm could, in fact, detect similar levels of toxicity in surgical gloves (Critchlow *et al*, 1989). Later Morimoto *et al*, (1997) reported that human sperm survival tests could also detect toxins in all contact materials and culture medium. In a more recent study Claassens *et al*, (2000) further demonstrated that human sperm could detect toxins in serum albumin and that the test was comparable to mouse embryo testing in predicting embryo toxicity. Items identified to be sperm toxic within 8 hours by the human sperm motility assay were considered to be clinically significant. Human sperm motility assay has also been used as a predictor of fertilization (Stovall *et al*, 1994) and pregnancy outcome (Alvarez *et al*, 1996).

Cell Lines

There is not much published regarding cell types other than the mouse hybridoma cell for quality control in IVF (Bertheussen *et al*, 1989). Hybritest (Medicult) is a commercially available cell line for testing culture medium. This is a rapidly growing cell line in a defined serum-free culture medium and is also known as 1E6 (mouse hybridoma cell line). As culture medium is serum-free, there is an absence of binding proteins, thus it greatly increases the sensitivity of these cells to toxic substances. The greatest drawback of using this cell line is that it may not be as sensitive as claimed when testing complete culture medium, including those containing serum or serum components.

Mouse Embryo Assay

The mouse embryo bioassay (MEBA) is probably the most widely used test in IVF laboratories and most reports refer to its use in quality assurance of culture medium. Numerous reports have been published regarding the beneficial effects of the assay as a means of QC in IVF (Ackerman *et al*, 1984; Quinn *et al*, 1984; Fleming *et al*, 1987), but it is also extensively criticized as being irrelevant, ineffective and cumbersome (Fleetham *et al*, 1993; George *et al*, 1989). There are a number of factors that can affect the QC outcome of MEBA viz. the mouse strain used as the source of embryos, the stage of development or culture medium.

It has recently been reported that mouse embryos developed by nuclear transfer techniques are much more sensitive to culture conditions than normal ones (Heindryckx *et al*, 2001). This was confirmed by Chung *et al*, (2002). The introduction of such demanding technology for developing embryos by nuclear transfer is not a practical option.

The major reason why IVF laboratories falter in employing the use of animal models (mouse) is because of a lack of access to the facilities of an animal house or a separate mouse embryo laboratory. Investing in such a labor-intensive system seems impractical as the test has been shown to have limited sensitivity. *Secondly,* tests performed in a separate laboratory, using different incubators do not give a true picture of the status of the laboratory where human gametes and embryos are to be cultured.

QUALITY ASSURANCE

Quality assurance comprises of an analysis and evaluation of the quality control procedures in place. QA involves evaluation of the protocols as a means of identifying problems, and it facilitates in establishing policies to improve the overall quality of the laboratory. QA along with QC provides evidence, based on which conclusions can be drawn. There is interdependence between the two.

In our unit we have established policies to evaluate the overall performance of the IVF program. We have introduced weekly discussion of cases, quarterly audit and yearly statistics review. In the weekly meetings, the clinical and laboratory management of each case performed in the past week is critically evaluated. Decisions regarding changes in protocol for a future cycle are formally entered.

At the end of the meeting the overall laboratory data for the week is presented and evaluated to identify subtle changes. If warning signs are detected they need to be investigated and acted upon.

To detect the early warning signs we have set-up base line limits and specific minimum standards for all outcomes (Table 42.1) in the laboratory.

TABLE 42.1: Minimum standards and base line limit measurement

Observation stage		Minimum standard	Base line limit
Denuded oocytes	MII	> 60	≥ 70%
Fertilisation	2PN (normal)	> 60%	≥ 70%
Early Cleavage	2PN	< 50%	> 40%
	1 Cell stage	> 20%	≥ 30%
	> 2 Cell stage	> 20%	≥ 30%
Cleavage	4 Cell stage	> 60%	≥ 70%
	< 4 cell stage	< 40%	< 30%
Embryo Grades	I	> 40%	≥ 50%
	II	> 20%	≥ 30%
Pregnancy rates		> 25%	≥ 35%
Implantation rates		> 15%	≥ 20%

Minimum standards of outcome need to be laid down and can vary between individual laboratories.

The system of surveillance we have introduced consists of:

1. Minor Intervention
2. Major Intervention

If a solitary case shows a drop below the baseline in outcome parameters we conduct a minor intervention which involves a recheck of the batch of media used in terms of pH and osmolarity. In addition incubators are reevaluated for temperature, humidity and CO_2 content, while the temperature of all heating equipment is recorded.

If two consecutive cases or more than one case over the week shows a poor outcome major intervention is indicated. In addition to the minor intervention, in all subsequent cases, the gametes and embryos are cultured in parallel with a new batch of cultureware, media and oil, in an attempt to identify the responsible factor. Implementation of this policy has been invaluable in detecting problems and has resulted in quick amendments being made.

We also have a quarterly and yearly audit report that is presented to the department of obstetrics and gynaecology which further strengthens our evaluation process and enables us to review protocols and make necessary changes.

Appropriate and meaningful procedures help to maintain quality and consistency, thus guaranteeing embryo quality and good pregnancy rates. A simple bioassay like the human sperm survival test can be introduced without any additional expertise or investment. To be effective bioassay procedures must be repeated at regular intervals. We recommend introduction of a weekly review of cases and introduction of a program of minor and major interventions to anticipate and identify potential problems. This will allow immediate action preventing a decline in the quality of the program.

The success of any ART program is greatly dependent on the quality of its IVF laboratory. A reliable laboratory with the capability and competence to maintain high standards as well as the ability to consistently reproduce a good outcome ensures excellent pregnancy rates. Quality control and assurance helps in establishing good laboratory practices, early identification of problems and permits scientifically based conclusions to be drawn. The art of trouble shooting in an IVF laboratory has now become scientific and evidence based.

BIBLIOGRAPHY

1. Ackerman SB, Stokes GL, Swanson RJ, Taylor SP, Fenwick L. Toxicity testing for human in vitro fertilization programs. J In Vitro Fert Embryo Transf Sep 1985;2(3):132-37.
2. Ackerman SB, Taylor SP, Swanson RJ, Laurell LH. Mouse embryo culture for screening in human IVF. Arch Androl 1984;12(Suppl)129-36.
3. Alvarez JG, Minaretzis D, Barrett CB, Mortola JF, Thompson IE. The sperm stress test: a novel test that predicts pregnancy in assisted reproductive technologies. Fertil Steril 1996;65(2):400-05.
4. Bavister BD, Andrews JC. A rapid sperm motility bioassay procedure for quality-control testing of water and culture media. J In Vitro Fert Embryo Transf. 1988;5(2):67-75.
5. Bertheussen K, Holst N, Forsdahl F, Hoie KE. A new cell culture assay for quality control in IVF. Hum Reprod 1989;4(5):531-35.
6. Chung YG, Mann MR, Bartolomei MS, Latham KE. Nuclear-cytoplasmic "tug of war" during cloning: effects of somatic cell nuclei on culture medium preferences of preimplantation cloned mouse embryos. Biol Reprod 2002;66(4):1178-84.
7. Claassens OE, Wehr JB, Harrison KL. Optimizing sensitivity of the human sperm motility assay for

embryo toxicity testing. Hum Reprod 2000;15(7): 1586-91.

8. Critchlow JD, Matson PL, Newman MC, Horne G, Troup SA, Lieberman BA. Quality control in an in-vitro fertilization laboratory: use of human sperm survival studies. Hum Reprod 1989;4(5):545-49.

9. Esterhuizen AD, Bosman E, Botes AD, Groenewald OA, Giesteira MV, Labuschagne GP, Lindeque HW, Rodriques FA, van Rensburg JJ, van Schouwenburg JA. A comparative study on the diagnostic sensitivity of rodent sperm and embryos in the detection of endotoxin in Earle's balanced salt solution. J Assist Reprod Genet 1994;11(1):38-42.

10. Fleetham JA, Pattinson HA, Mortimer D. The mouse embryo culture system: improving the sensitivity for use as a quality control assay for human in vitro fertilization. Fertil Steril 1993;59(1):192-96.

11. Fleming TP, Pratt HP, Braude PR. The use of mouse preimplantation embryos for quality control of culture reagents in human in vitro fertilization programs: a cautionary note. Fertil Steril 1987;47(5):858-60.

12. George MA, Braude PR, Johnson MH, Sweetnam DG. Quality control in the IVF laboratory: in-vitro and in-vivo development of mouse embryos is unaffected by the quality of water used in culture media. Hum Reprod 1989;4(7):826-31.

13. Gianaroli L, Plachot M, van Kooij R, Al-Hasani S, Dawson K, DeVos A, Magli MC, Mandelbaum J, Selva J, van Inzen W. ESHRE guidelines for good practice in IVF laboratories. Committee of the Special Interest Group on Embryology of the European Society of Human Reproduction and Embryology. Hum Reprod 2000; 15(10):2241-46.

14. Gorrill MJ, Rinehart JS, Tamhane AC, Gerrity M. Comparison of the hamster sperm motility assay to the mouse one-cell and two-cell embryo bioassays as quality control tests for in vitro fertilization. Fertil Steril 1991;55(2):345-54.

15. Heindryckx B, Rybouchkin A, Van Der Elst J, Dhont M. Effect of culture media on in vitro development of cloned mouse embryos. Cloning 2001;3(2):41-50.

16. Morimoto Y, Hayashi E, Ohno T, Kawata A, Horikoshi Y, Kanzaki H. Quality control of human IVF/ICSI program using endotoxin measurement and sperm survival test. Hum Cell 1997;10(4):271-76.

17. Parinaud J, Reme JM, Monrozies X, Favrin S, Sarramon MF, Pontonnier G. Mouse system quality control is necessary before the use of new material for in vitro fertilization and embryo transfer. J In Vitro Fert Embryo Transf 1987;4(1):56-58.

18. Quinn P, Warnes GM, Kerin JF, Kirby C. Culture factors in relation to the success of human in vitro fertilization and embryo transfer. Fertil Steril 1984;41(2):202-09.

19. Quinn P, Horstman FC. Is the mouse a good model for the human with respect to the development of the preimplantation embryo in vitro? Hum Reprod 1998;13(Suppl 4):173-83.

20. Rinehart JS, Bavister BD, Gerrity M. Quality control in the in vitro fertilization laboratory: comparison of bioassay systems for water quality. J In Vitro Fert Embryo Transf 1988;5(6):335-42.

21. Stovall DW, Guzick DS, Berga SL, Krasnow JS, Zeleznik AJ. Sperm recovery and survival: two tests that predict in vitro fertilization outcome: Fertil Steril 1994;62(6): 1244-49.

• Sulochana Gunasheela • Varsha Samson Roy

43

In vitro Maturation of Immature Oocytes and their use in Assisted Reproductive Technology

In vitro maturation of immature oocytes retrieved from unstimulated or partially stimulated ovaries and using them for ART is now drawing great interest as an alternative mode of treatment.

Controlled Ovarian Hyperstimulation (COH) is the prerequisite for collection of oocytes in conventional IVF cycles. However, the quality of individual sibling oocytes may vary in the grade of development in each cohort. While a percentage of them show optimum maturity of metaphase II, there are many, which show the presence of Germinal Vesicle or signs of post-maturity or atresia. Even the mature oocyte may show the varying degree of vaculation, pitting of the cytoplasm, or debris in the perivitelline space etc., all suggestive of compromised developmental competence.

The so-called COH practised during induction of ovulation frequently goes out of control leading to the most dreaded complication of Ovarian Hyperstimulation Syndrome with all its manifestation of fluid accumulation in the 3rd compartment, hyper coagulability and pulmonary complications.

Natural cycle IVF is an acceptable alternative but for the fact, that the pregnancy rates are low and the requirement of intense monitoring can be burdensome. The next alternative available is to collect immature oocytes from unstimulated or partially stimulated ovaries.

Immature oocytes retrieved from unstimulated or partially stimulated ovaries display a state of uniform immaturity and a good percentage of them mature to metaphase II. Immature oocytes obtained as a part of the cohort from ovaries stimulated for standard IVF perform poorly as compared to the immature oocytes obtained from unstimulated or partially stimulated ovaries entirely for the purpose of immature oocyte retrieval and maturation.

Why IVM?—Benefits of IVM

The potential benefits of developing an effective IVM program as an alternative clinical strategy to conventional IVF are many: it would not only substantially reduce both the costs of drug treatment and biochemical and ultrasound monitoring, but would also reduce the wastage of immature eggs collected during standard IVF. IVM protocols are much more patient friendly. The use of natural cycle IVM and IVM in partially stimulated ovaries could also lessen the risk of Ovarian Hyperstimulation syndrome and, more controversially ovarian carcinoma. Additionally, IVM may provide a valuable model for investigating the causes of meiotic aberrations and aneuploidy, which are remarkably common in mature human oocytes. In view of all these advantages, IVM deserves greater attention, rigorous experimental evaluation followed by controlled clinical trial to determine whether it is practicable in reproductive medicine.

Transplantation of immature ovarian follicles collected from surgically removed ovaries to patients with Premature Ovarian Failure may be a possibility.

Immature oocytes may be used for GIFT procedures regardless of the age of the recipient, followed by IUI with husband's sperm 48 hours later.

Source of Immature Oocytes

Immature oocytes have been aspirated from specimens obtained after oophorectomy in women of age group varying from 21-50 yrs. Patients undergoing tubectomy or caesarian section can also be motivated to donate their immature oocytes, which can be retrieved during the surgery from *in situ* ovaries. A wedge of the ovary can be excised and oocyte collected thereof. The number of immature oocytes collected does not appear to change whether the collection is made in follicular or Luteal phase or during pregnancy. KY Cha[3] showed an equal number of healthy and degenerated oocytes retrieved at equal rates in either phase of the cycle. Cha collected 275 immature oocytes from 23-oophorectomy specimens at the rate of 11 oocytes/ovary with the number of oocytes significantly falling with the age of the patient. Edward[6] reported a retrieval of 0-62 oocytes from a single ovary from 16-43 yr old patients.

PCO and IVM

One can obtain immature oocytes from resting ovaries of PCOs patients. The ovaries of PCOs patients are characterized by the presence of numerous antral follicles in a state of suspended animation. These have the potential of undergoing the normal growing pattern if they are rescued. This category forms an excellent group for obtaining immature oocytes in large number. These patients are usually anovulatory. They have long irregular cycles with periods of amenorrhea lasting from months to years. PCOs patients when stimulated respond in a phenomenal fashion with sprouting of several follicles uniformly grown. The stimulation can be stopped when follicles are 10-11 mm and aspirated for obtaining immature oocytes.

Oocyte Retrieval Technique

Oocyte retrieval from partially stimulated ovaries is very similar to that used for traditional IVF. Some ovaries are ready for aspiration even after 4-5 days of HMG administration, but in some patients, particularly in PCOs, the follicles go on increasing in number during the course of stimulation, instead of increasing in size. So one can just stop stimulation when there is a substantial number of 10-12 follicles of 10 mm each available for aspiration. HCG 10000 IU is given 36 hrs prior to OPU. Administration of HCG produces a sudden increase in the size of the follicle. Chian *et al*,[6] reported that HCG primed group of patients produced the same number of oocytes as the non-HCG group but the former produced a higher maturation rate (83.4%) as compared to non-HCG primed group (69.1%). They also observed that oocyte maturation occurred much earlier in the HCG primed group. Approximately 78 percent matured in 24 hrs in the HCG primed group whereas, only 5 percent matured in the non-HCG group in the same time interval. Similar was our experience in the HCG primed and the non-primed group.

Immature Oocyte—Identification and Culture

The immature oocytes (Figure 43.1) were identified under a dissecting microscope. Immature oocytes have a varying quantity of

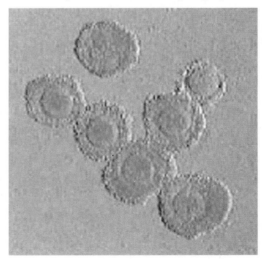

FIGURE 43.1: Immature oocytes at retrieval

cumulus cells surrounding them and it is not a rare phenomenon to see some of them completely naked without a cumulus layer. Some workers prefer using a 50-70 µm filter through which the follicular aspirates are passed. The filter redundant is then checked for the presence of immature oocytes. It is our experience that the filter is not an essential item, with experience one can identify all oocytes fairly rapidly without causing any undue exposure to the oocytes.

Immature oocytes are cultured in Tissue Culture Media (TCM–199) supplemented with 10 percent Human Serum Albumin (HSA), 50 percent Follicular Fluid (FF) and 0.075 IU/ml HMG and 0.5 IU/ml HCG at 37°C in an atmosphere of 5 percent CO_2. They are inspected every 12 hours for assessment of maturity. The *in vitro* maturation culture period might extend from 22-48 hours (Figure 43.2). The oocytes are then denuded to remove the cumulus cells (Figure 43.3), and mature oocytes identified by the presence of first polar body in the Perivitelline Space (PVS). These mature oocytes are then micro-injected with a single spermatozoan (ICSI).

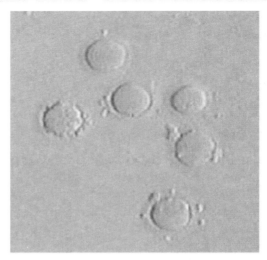

FIGURE 43.3: Denuded oocytes

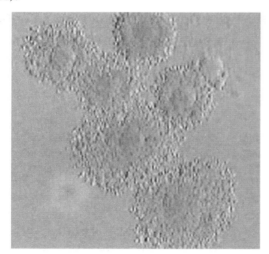

FIGURE 43.2: Expanded cumulus 24 hrs culture

Fertilization is assessed 18 hours after ICSI for the appearance of 2 distinct PN and 2 PB. These zygotes are further cultured and transferred on D2 after performing Laser Assisted Hatching (LAH) 30-45 minutes prior to ET. The

in vitro culture is much more protracted in this program than in the standard IVF cycles. Prolonged culture is known to cause zona hardening and hence we recommend Assisted Hatching to overcome this barrier in all cases of IVM. Women who have had short period of follicular stimulation or no stimulation at all, may require supplementary estrogen therapy in order to prepare the endometrium. Micronised estrogen in the form of oestrodial valerate may be given at a dose of 2 to 6 mg per day depending upon the thickness of endometrium. One must ensure that on the day of embryo transfer the endometrium should be of the thickness of 8-10 mm. Luteal support is given as endovaginal micronised progesterone at a dose of 200 mg twice daily starting on the day of ICSI; E2 and P support will be continued to 12 wks of gestation.

Culture Conditions for IVM

Fairly successful culture conditions have been devised for IVM in bovine and some other species. However, inter-species differences in the physiology of oocyte maturation, especially in its final stages do not allow their direct extrapolation to the human system. Therefore, it is very important that appropriate culture conditions, specifically applicable for human oocytes, be streamlined. The technique of IVM has been applied clinically with some limited success: most of these culture systems employ complex media, supplemented with serum and follicular fluid. Defining these culture conditions is difficult since serum and follicular fluid may contain many unknown substances in addition to albumin, such as amino acids and certain other factors including growth factors.

A variety of medias like Hams F10, EMEN, TCM 199, Menozo 2 etc, have been used by different workers. These medias have been supplemented with gonadotrophins (PMSG, FSH, r-FSH, HCG). Some have also supplemented the media with estradiol (Trounson et al,[12] Russell et al[9]). A protein source in the form of FCS, FBS, BSA, HSA, PPS have been used. Serum when added to the culture acts as a source of albumin, which balances osmolarity and scavenges potentially harmful molecules like metal ions that can act as a source of free oxygen radicals. Cha and co-workers[4] have obtained good results by supplementing TCM 199 with follicular fluid, which contains many undefined factors. Addition of pyruvate as a source of nutrition both to the oocyte and cumulus cells has been tried. Epidermal growth factor (EGF) has been found to play a positive role in various mammalian *in vitro* systems of oocyte maturation. A similar benefit of EGF has also been suggested in humans.

Cryopreservation

The protection given by the nuclear membrane to the DNA contents of the GV oocytes is thought to prevent the disruption caused by thermal or osmotic stress. Such protection is not available in the M2 oocytes where the chromosomes have condensed to form the meiotic spindle, exposing itself to an increase in the risk of spindle damage and aneuploidy. Jagiallo G[7] and associates found that less than 1 percent of 600 human GV oocytes that matured to M2 *in vitro* showed chromosomal abnormalities. Hence, cryopreservation of GV oocyte is more practicable than preserving oocytes in M2 stage.

GIVF Experience in IVM

Our work on IVM for IVF was started for patient service from June 2002 (Table 43.1 to 43.3). Our preliminary experience was obtained by

TABLE 43.1: Preliminary study at GIVF

Parameter	Result
Total patients	22
Total oocytes	185
Oocytes/pt	8.4
No. Matured (M2)	137 (74%)
Fertilized	82 (59.8%)
Cleaved	73 (89%)
Total Emb. Trans.	67
Total ET	19
No. of Emb./Trans	3.5
Pregnancies	2 (ongoing) 1 (Clinical) 1 (Bio)

Notes: 1. Figures in ( ) indicate percentages
2. All patients were stimulated with 10,000 units HCG at follicle size 10-12 mm.

TABLE 43.2: Comparative study

Authors/ Year	Mean No. Oocytes	Mat. rate	Fert. rate	Cleav. rate
Cha et al (1999)	15.2	63%	77% (ICSI)	89%
Trounson et al[10] (1994)	13.1	81%	34% (IVF)	56%
Barnes et al[1] (1996)	–	67%	32% (IVF)	62%
Russell et al[9] (1997)	–	40.62%	75-76% (ICSI)	64-92%
Suikkari et al[10] (2000)	11.2-11.5	64–78%	57-72% (ICSI)	72.7%
GIVF (June 02-Feb 03)	6.8	71.5%	64.3% (ICSI)	85%

recovering oocytes from ovaries of patients undergoing Caesarean Section. The identification of immature oocytes was initially difficult as there was very little cumulus surrounding them; blood clots and fluid blood completely masked the presence of these tiny OCC complex. Soon the method of aspiration was improved and the collection tubes were changed even if there was 2-3 ml fluid or when the tubing showed blood contamination. Almost from the beginning of our experimental stage a

TABLE 43.3: Comparative IVM outcome

Author	No. of pts.	No. of cycles	No. of emb/trans.	No. of preg.	No aborted	No. ong/del
Cha et al[5] (2000)	65	85	3.9 ± 2.2 (Ut.ET) 6.3 ± 2.2 (ZIFT + ET)	8/39 (20.5%) (Ut. ET) 15/40 (37.5) (ZIFT + ET)	6 (26%)	17 (20%)
Chian et al[6] (2000)	17	24	2.6 ± 1.0	8/24 (33%)	2 (25%)	6 (25%)
Tim Child et al[11] (2001)	95	121	—	32/119 (26.8)	13 (39%)	19 (16%)

Note: Figures in ( ) indicate percentages

good percentage of oocyte matured, fertilized and cleaved. This gave us the confidence to introduce this service to our IVF patients.

The incidence of PCO in our hospital group of infertile women has been around 65 percent. Among these nearly 4-5 percent of patients who undergo stimulation for IUI develop fairly severe degree of OHSS requiring hospitalization, and repeated aspiration of ascitic fluid. The incidence of OHSS in patients of similar group undergoing IVF and ET has been much less because in the latter group one has the advantage of freezing all the embryos and deferring the ET to a cold cycle.

The concept of IVM appeared to give the answer for total prevention of OHSS in the vulnerable patients particularly the PCOs patients.

The experimental period also showed that in patients who had HCG given to them at the end of a short period of Gonadotrophin therapy, follicular aspiration was easy. The follicular walls were fragile and easy to break through, thus allowing free maneuver of the needle through the ovary. Gonadotrophin was given as daily injections until the follicle grew to 10-12 mm. At this stage 10,000 units of HCG was given, USG guided aspiration of follicles was done 36 hrs later.

There were also a group of PCO patients who started in the growth velocity during HMG injection for IUI or IVF. The observation was with increase in days of stimulation the number of follicles increased exponentially while the size remained the same. This kind of patients cause anxiety in several ways—Are they going to produce mature oocytes at all? Or will the oocytes just perish inside with continued stimulation? Does this behaviour prognosticate an impending onset of OHSS? These types of patients were also taken up for early aspiration and IVM by termination of induction protocol by injection of HCG 10,000 units and aspiration of follicles 36 hrs later. One group of patients who are likely to benefit from this procedure are women in incipient failure.[2] When such women are stimulated, one usually sees a cohort of follicles of the size 8-9 mm. When stimulation protocol is continued for the sake of achieving a better growth of follicles; they usually end up in having only one or two follicles of 17 to 18 mm. Such patients can be aspirated at an earlier stage and immature oocytes obtained. Our observation has been that immature oocytes appear uniformly immature. One does not see varieties of oocytes that are seen in standard IVF; like, for example pre-ovulatory oocytes are often seen mixed with immature, intermediate, postmature and atretic ones.

DISCUSSION

Normally in monovular species like the human, the follicular development is characterized by a group of primordial follicles getting into the growth trajectory resulting in a selection of one dominant follicle with atresia of the remaining cohort. The antral follicle grows from a size of 1-2 mm to 15-20 mm and the oocytes within grow from a diameter of 35 μm to 120 μm over several months.

In a natural cycle 1-2 follicles become dominant in the final growth phase leading to an increase in the E_2/A ratio of the dominant follicle. The remaining follicles of the cohort continue to be dominated by androgen and undergo atresia. Wittmaack et al,[11] studied a large number of gonadotrophin-stimulated cycles and reported that the ability for fertilization and cleavage of oocytes from smaller size follicles was not different from follicles of >1.5 cm, but the general observation is that there is a dramatic decrease in the rate of maturation, fertilization and cleavage of oocytes retrieved from follicles <14 mm when other follicles of the same cohort are >14 mm.

In vivo immature oocytes (Germinal Vesicle stage) resume meiosis, with the break down of Germinal Vesicle (GV) and extrusion of first polar body under the influence of the leutinizing hormone surge. Without the LH surge, immature oocytes in vivo cannot reach the stage of metaphase II (MII) and ovulate. Normally the pre ovulatory LH surge occurs in the middle of the menstrual cycle around D12 to D14 of a normal 28 day cycle. However, when immature oocytes are isolated from small antral follicles and cultured in vitro with FSH and LH in the culture media, they resume meiosis within 48 to 54 hours (Trounson et al[10]). Two possible mechanisms might account for this. Firstly, follicular fluid in small antral follicles contains maturation inhibiting factors (MIF). When these immature oocytes are liberated from this follicular environment, the effect of the MIF signals is reduced and hence the immature oocytes may undergo spontaneous maturation in vitro. Secondly, certain supplements in the maturation media like gonadotrophins or growth factors may induce maturation in vitro. This mechanism involves the production of a positive stimulatory factor by the cumulus cells that act on the oocyte to trigger off maturation. This mechanism bypasses the negative influence of the meiosis arresting pathway. High concentrations of FSH and LH in the culture media may act like the LH surge and induce resumption of meiosis in immature oocytes in vitro within 48 hours of culture.

CONCLUSION

In vitro maturation of immature oocytes is a newly adopted program in our setup; it is not possible to make any conclusions to prove or disprove any controversy. As mentioned earlier we do believe that there is a sub-set of patient population like the PCOs who stand to benefit the most by IVM. It is very important to form a protocol regarding the selection, stimulation and monitoring of cycles and the optimum culture conditions for IVM.

The success of the procedure depends mostly on the ability to retrieve large number of oocytes. The fertilization rate and cleavage rate of the IVM oocytes are almost similar to that of the in vivo matured oocytes obtained during conventional IVF / ICSI cycles. The high foetal loss rate noticed in every study appears to be related to the choice of PCO patients, but if these patients are properly programed and pre-treated before taking up for this procedure it is quite likely that the foetal loss rate would reduce.

REFERENCES

1. Barnes F, Kauche A, Tiglias J, Wood C, Wilton L, Trounson A. Production of embryos from invitro matured primary human oocytes. Fertility and Sterility 1996;65:1151-56.
2. Behrman SJ, Grant W, Patton Jr. Progress in infertility, 4th edn. Little Brown and Company Inc. 1988;100-12(Fig. 7-7).
3. Cha KK, KOO JJ, KO JJ, Choi DH, Han SY, Yoon TK Pregnancy after Invitro fertilization of human follicular Oocytes collected from non-stimulated cycles, their culture Invitro and their transfer in a donor oocyte programme. Fertility and Sterility 1991;55:109-13.
4. Cha KY, Chung HM, Lim JM, et al. Clinical experience with In Vitro oocyte maturation. In Jansen R, Mortimer D (Eds.): Towards Reproductive Certainty. Proceedings of the 11th World Congress on In Vitro Fertilization and Human Reproductive Genetics. Parthenon Publishing Group, Lancaster, UK, 1999;210-17.
5. Cha KY, Se Y, Han Hyung M, Chung, Dong H, Choi Jeong M, Lim Woo S, Lee Jung J Ko, Tae K Yoon. Pregnancies and deliveries after Invitro maturation

culture followed by in vitro fertilization and embryo transfer without stimulation in women with polycystic ovary syndrome. Fertility and Sterility 2000;73: 978-83.

6. Chian RC, Buckett WM, Tulandi T, Tan SL. Prospective randomized study of human chorionic gonadotrophins priming before immature oocyte retrieval from unstimulated women with polycystic ovarian syndrome. Human Reproduction 2000;15:165-70.

7. Edward RG. Maturation Invitro of human Oocytes. Lancet 1965;2:926.

8. Jagiallo G, et al. Chromosomes today 1979;43.

9. Russell JB, Knezerich KM, Fabian KF, Dick JA. Unstimulated immature oocyte retrieval: early versus midfollicular endometrial priming. Fertility and Sterility 1997;67:616-20.

10. Suikkari A, Tulppala M, Turri T, Hovatta O, Barnes F. Luteal phase start of low dose FSH priming of follicles results in an efficient recovery, maturation and fertilization of immature human oocytes. Human Reproduction 2000;15:747-51.

11. Tim J, Child Ahmad Kamal Abdul-Jalil, Bulent Gulekli, Seang Lin Tan. Invitro maturation and fertilization of oocytes from unstimulated normal ovaries, polycystic ovaries, and women with polycystic ovary syndrome. Fertility and Sterility 2001;79:936-42.

12. Trounson A, Wood C, Kausche A. Invitro maturation and the fertilization and developmental competence of Oocytes recovered from untreated polycystic ovarian patients. Fertility and Sterility 1994;62:323-62.

13. Wittmaack FM, Kreger DO, Blascol, Tureck RW, Mastroiannil Jr, Lessey BA. Effect of follicular size on Oocyte retrieval, fertilization, cleavage and embryo quality in Invitro fertilization cycles: a.6–year data collection Fertility and Sterility: 1994;62: 1205-10.

• J Menezes • P Sjoblom
• L Cummins • B Mathiyalagan • J Lukic

44

Assessment of Embryo Quality as a Predictor of IVF Outcome

INTRODUCTION

During the last decade IVF laboratory procedures have undergone revolutionary changes. These include the introduction of intracytoplasmic sperm injection, (ICSI), in 1992, changes in the formulation of culture media and the increased use of sequential media to extend embryo development to the point where the embryonic genome switches on, right up to the blastocyst stage (Quinn, 2002).[1]

However as a consequence of transferring multiple embryos,multiple gestations have become commonplace. With twins and triplets accounting for 30 percent of all ongoing pregnancies, more than half of all IVF/ICSI children belong to a set of multiples. Health economists, obstetricians and neonatologists have deplored the epidemic of multiple births after ART (De Sutter *et al,* 2002).[2] Multiple pregnancy has been identified as the most important risk factor contributing to the multiple birth defects and neurological and psychological sequelae observed in children conceived by IVF and ICSI (Lambert, 2002).[3] Very high long-term costs result from the increased morbidity of twins after birth and even more so from higher order pregnancies. Among patients themselves, there is a growing awareness of the risks involved in a twin pregnancy, especially those undergoing IVF/ICSI treatment for second or third pregnancies. The high incidence of iatrogenic twins is no longer considered as an unavoidable price to be paid in order to achieve an acceptable ongoing pregnancy rate.

The only strategy to reduce the incidence of multiple pregnancies following ART is to resort to elective single embryo transfer (eSET). Health economic analysis has found that since single embryo transfer allows the avoidance of twins and thus reduces pregnancy related and neonatal care costs, there is no difference between single and double embryo transfer in regards to the cost per child born.[2] Achieving an acceptable pregnancy rate with eSET poses a huge challenge to the entire IVF program and in particular to the embryologist, to successfully select the one embryo with the highest implantation potential as well as to efficiently cryopreserve the remaining viable embryos.

BLASTOCYST CULTURE

In order to achieve this goal, progressive efforts are being made worldwide to identify embryos with high implantation potential at various stages of development. There are two options available. *In vivo* embryos enter the uterus at the morula stage and implantation of the embryo occurs only when the blastocyst stage is reached. The shift of control from the maternal genome to the embryonic genome is a requirement for progressing through the next cell cycle from the four cell stage on Day 2. During recent years sequential culture media have been developed which specifically cater to the changing metabolic requirements of the embryo from the zygote to the blastocyst stage. Using these media which are now commercially available namely Quinn's Advantage Cleavage and blastocyst culture media (Sage IVF, USA), EBSS/M2 (Medicult, Denmark),G1/G2 (Scandinavian IVF Science, Sweden)etc, culture to the blastocyst stage and blastocyst transfer is now feasible (Gardner and Lane,1998[4]; Coates *et al,* 1999).[5] Transfer of one or two blastocysts results in fewer multiple pregnancies and only the most competent embryos are cryopreserved.

When selecting blastocysts for transfer, they are graded initially on a scale of 1 to 6 with regard to blastocoele development (Gardner *et al,* 2000).[6] This numbering is based on the degree of expansion as well as hatching status

• Early, blastocoele less than half the volume of the embryo
• Blastocoele greater than half the volume of the embryo
• Full blastocyst–blastocoele completely fills the embryo
• Expanded blastocyst–blastocoele volume is larger than that of early embryo with zona thinning
• Hatching
• Hatched

The second step in scoring the blastocysts assesses the development of the inner cell mass (ICM) and trophectoderm, which are grades A to C and A to B respectively. ICM: Grade A–tightly packed, many cells; Grade B–Loosely grouped; several cells; Grade C–Very few cells. Trophectoderm A–many cells forming a cohesive epithelium; B–few cells forming a loose epithelium. The highest score possible is AA. Blastocysts are eligible for transfer if they have a score of at least 4 AA on Day 5 of development. The protocol for blastocyst culture is given in Appendix 1.

Although blastocyst transfer appears to be ideal for choosing the right embryo, there are certain disadvantages. To date all reported studies (Bungum *et al,* 2003[7], Rienzi *et al,* 2002)[8] including a randomized controlled trial (Coskun *et al,* 2000[9)] show no evidence to prove that transfer of embryos at the blastocyst stage is superior to Day 2 or day 3 embryo transfers,. Studies on transfer of a single blastocyst versus transfer of a single early cleaving embryo have not been carried out. Additionally, cryopreservation of blastocysts is far less successful than cryopreservation of early stage embryos.

The extended period of culture involved in blastocyst culture means additional expense as well as increased workload and responsibility for the embryology laboratory. Extreme care is required to see that embryos are not exposed to suboptimal conditions that would compromise their viability. In certain countries such as Germany, very strict embryo protection laws are in force and such selection of embryos by prolonged culture is not permitted. Hence blastocyst culture is not feasible as a routine procedure in every IVF laboratory.

However blastocyst culture is essential for patients needing preimplantation diagnosis for genetic diseases or chromosomal defects and for those having defects in oocyte quality who require their embryos to be assessed for an extended period. It may also be useful for patients having a large cohort of embryos and for those undergoing ICSI with testicular sperm (Virant-Klun *et al,* 2003).[10]

EARLY APPROACHES TO EMBRYO GRADING

The alternative to blastocyst culture is to characterise features in oocytes, zygotes and early embryos which correlate with a high rate of blastocyst development and implantation. If embryo viability could be ascertained at an early stage, then extended culture could be avoided. Thus various systems of grading or scoring embryos have been developed. As a prelude to discussing these systems,it is necessary to survey the various characteristics of oocytes, zygotes and early embryos which aid in 'guesstimating' the 'right' embryo.

FOLLICULAR OXYGENATION

Doppler analysis of several hundred follicles has demonstrated that the degree of perifollicular vascularization is highly individual, such that adjacent follicles with virtually identical appearance on B mode ultrasound examination, exhibit very different blood flow rates. Follicular blood flow correlates with the percentage of dissolved oxygen in the corresponding follicular fluid. For most IVF patients with the same protocol of follicular stimulation and comparable number of follicles aspirated, 30 to 40 percent of the follicles had perifollicular blood flow patterns consistent with a level or follicular oxygenation greater than 3 percent. Other follicles displayed little or no detectable blood flow, and dissolved oxygen in follicular fluid was at or less than 2 percent. An association between follicular oxygen content, embryo development competence and subsequent ongoing pregnancy has been suggested with the use of Doppler (Van Blerkom, 1997).[11]

Similar results have been reported by Nargund et al,1996[12] and Chui et al, 1997[13] who observed that human embryos derived from follicles with high degree of perifollicular vascularization showed superior implantation potential.

OOCYTE MORPHOLOGY

Oocyte Dysmorphisms

Oocyte morphology as a predictor of outcome is applicable mainly to intracytoplasmic sperm injection (ICSI), since the cumulus oophorus is denuded prior to injection allowing direct inspection of the oocyte. Serhal et al, 1997[14] performed ICSI on 538 oocytes with normal cytoplasm, 142 oocytes with excessive granularity and 112 with cytoplasmic inclusions (vacuoles, refractile bodies and smooth endoplasmic reticulum (SER). Although fertilization rates and the percentage of grade 1 (good quality) embryos were similar in all 3 groups, pregnancy rate was 24 percent per patient in the group with embryos derived solely from normal oocytes while the pregnancy rate was only 3 percent in the group where oocytes had cytoplasmic abnormalities. Thus outcome of ICSI depends on the quality of the oocytes retrieved, as suggested by the findings of this study and the fact that oocytes with abnormal cytoplasmic morphology have been reported to have high frequency of aneuploidy (Van Blerkom and Henry, 1992).[15]

In a review by Van Blerkom, 1994[16] the association of ooplasmic abnormalities and aneuploidy was discussed. It seems clear that organelle clustering, appearing as dark clusters, SER aggregation, or a dark and granular cytoplasm, is associated with a high frequency ($> = 40\%$) of aneuploidy. Other ooplasmic abnormalities, such as vacuoles, were associated with a lower aneuploidy rate ($< 10\%$). However, the developmental potential of oocytes with such cytoplasmic abnormalities was still significantly reduced, obviously for reasons other than aneuploidy.

Kahraman et al, 2000[17] found overall fertilization rates and early embryo development to be normal in oocytes with centrally located granular cytoplasm. However in those couples undergoing PGD, 52.3 percent of the blastomeres biopsied were chromosomally abnormal. Although the pregnancy rate was 28.2 percent, 54.5 percent of these resulted in abortion,which is likely to be due to the high aneuploidy rate. Implantation rate was only 4.2 percent.

Tracking of oocyte dysmorphisms for ICSI patients has been reported by Meriano et al, 2001.[18] In all three groups in their study, embryos derived from normal looking oocytes were transferred. Significantly low pregnancy and implantation rates (3.1 and 1.7%) were observed ($p = 0.005$) where the cohort contained >50 percent phenotypically dysmorphic oocytes with repetition of the same dysmorphisms from the previous cycle. Dysmorphic features included central dark cytoplasm, SER, vacuoles, necrotic inclusions and perivitelline debris. In comparison, clinical pregnancy and implantation rate were 28 and 15 percent respectively in the group with > 50 percent dysmorphic oocytes but no repetition from the previous cycle. The control group with < 30 percent dysmorphic oocytes had a 45.5 percent pregnancy rate and a 26.5 percent implantation rate.

Cytoplasmic Texture

Quantitative assessment of cytoplasmic texture of oocytes has been studied to find out if it could predict oocyte and embryo quality (Ryan et al,

2002).[19] Texture analysis was done on grey scale images taken on a digital camera at the time of ICSI and fertilization check. These images were quantitatively analysed using MRI analysis software and different numerical parameters were generated that described various aspects of texture. Analysis of Day 0 images of oocytes and day 1 images of zygotes identified subsets of parameters that were indicative of blastocyst development and implantation. One parameter termed teta 3 was observed to vary significantly between oocytes of varying maturity. Oocytes with teta 3 values close to the mean had higher rates of implantation from the resulting embryos.

First Polar Body Morphology

Xia et al,1997[20] graded oocytes on the basis of first polar body size and texture, size of perivitelline space and cytoplasmic inclusions. These three parameters correlated significantly with fertilization rate and embryo quality after ICSI. Oocytes with intact first polar body, normal perivitelline space and without inclusions had significantly higher fertilization rates and embryo quality after ICSI.

Ebner et al,1999[21] graded oocytes based on first polar body morphology. Embryo transfers were performed on day 2. In the study group, selection of embryos for transfer was based on first polar body morphology, first preference being given to embryos derived from grade 1 first polar body (ovoid with smooth surface), as compared to grade 2 (ovoid with rough surface), grade 3 (fragmented) and grade 4 (large). In the control cohort, selection of embryos for trans-fer was based exclusively on degree of fragmentation. The pregnancy and implantation rates in the study group (35.7 and 20.4%) was significantly higher than the control group (23.3 and 10.5%) respectively. Multiple pregnancy rate was also significantly higher in the study group.

Giant Oocytes

Cohorts of oocytes may contain oocytes which are at least 30 percent larger in diameter than normal oocytes (mean diameters 200.4 µm and 154.7 µm respectively) (Balakier et al, 2002).[22] The incidence of these oocytes is about 0.3 percent. These giant oocytes may fertilise normally or abnormally following IVF or ICSI. Normally fertilised giant oocytes are also capable of development to blastocysts. However cytogenetic and fluorescence in situ hybridization (FISH) analysis have revealed that these giant oocytes are diploid or chromosomally abnormal. They may play an important but underestimated role in causing digynic triploidy (Rosenbusch et al, 2002).[23]

The sequence of events during fertilization are:
- Sperm head decondenzation
- Second polar body extrusion
- Central appearance of male pronucleus (PN)
- Female PN accompanies male PN or appears shortly thereafter (female PN forms near second polar body)
- Both PN initially have small nucleoli
- Female PN is drawn centrally towards male PN until the two abut
- Growth of PN occurs
- Coalescence of nucleoli within PN
- Withdrawal of cytoplasmic organelles from the cortex towards centre of the oocyte, giving rise to a halo at the periphery of the oocyte (Payne et al,1997).[24]

POLAR BODY PLACEMENT

Orientation of the polar bodies relative to the pronuclear axis is also believed to relate to embryo morphology. The ooplasm and/or pronuclei may rotate to orient the axis through the abutted pronuclei towards the second polar body. This might correct anomalies in polarity which may arise from fertilization and prepare the zygote for subsequent cleavage. The sperm centrosome controls the plane of the first mitotic cleavage. Therefore the orientation and polarity of the male pronucleus may be more critical than that of the female. Garello et al,1999[25] observed that with increasing magnitude of the angle between the PN axis and the distal polar body (probably the first polar body), the quality of ICSI embryos decreased significantly.

ZYGOTE MORPHOLOGY

A novel approach is the noninvasive assessment of the oocyte at the zygote or bipronuclear stage (2 PN stage).

- Oocytes are generally checked for fertilization about 16 to 18 hours postinsemination or post ICSI. This time (at least for ICSI) includes the maximum time required for abuttal of PN. Failure of abuttal is due to abnormal function of the sperm-derived centriole and its associated microtubule organizing region.

- Failure of pronuclear growth is related to incomplete nuclear protein transition in the male gamete. This leads to developmental failure of the zygote. The occurrence of this phenomenon is low when mature sperms are used for IVF and ICSI as compared to immature sperm (e.g. testicular sperm).

As the pronuclei assemble, their chromosomes reorganise and nucleolar precursors are synthesized. This process known as nucleologenesis, comprises the assembly, growth and fusion of nucleolar precursor bodies. Formation of these nucleoli indicates early pronuclear transcriptional activity (synthesis of ribosomal RNA). It also depends on factors in the ooplasm that appear during maturation (Tesarik and Kopecny, 1990).[26]

Polarization of the nucleoli of both pronuclei represents an important step in the establishment of embryonic axes. This is an absolute requisite for subsequent cell determination in the pre-implantation embryo. Polarization of nucleoli occurs progressively with time, with smaller nucleoli gradually coalescing to form larger ones. Zygotes at an earlier stage of development may show approximately equal distribution of nonpolarized nucleoli in each pronucleus while those which are advanced may show complete polarization. Interpronuclear synchrony is more important than actual polarity.

Scott and Smith,1998[27] were the first to perform scoring at the 2 PN stage. At 16 to 18 hours postinsemination, zygotes were scored for alignment of pronuclei, nucleoli and appearance of the cytoplasm, generating an embryo score (Table 44.1).

TABLE 44.1: Embryo scoring

Parameter	Score
PN Close or aligned	5
PN well separated or very unequal in size	1
Nucleoli aligned	5
At pronuclear junction beginning to align	4
Scattered	3
Cytoplasm heterogenous with clear halo	5
Clear homogenous cytoplasm, pitted or dark cytoplasm	3
Nuclear membrane breakdown or cleavage to two cell	10

The minimum score of an embryo was 7 and the maximum was 25. There was strong correlation between corrected score, CS (average score of the embryos transferred), implantation and delivery rates. CS of more than 15 resulted in 71 percent pregnancies/OPU (34/48), 28 percent implantation and 65 percent delivery rate. CS less than 14 resulted in 8 percent pregnancy rate and 2 percent implantation rate. Thus oocyte quality and pronuclear embryo morphology are related to implantation.

Ludwig et al, 2000[28] used the scoring system of Scott and Smith (1998) for assessment of zygotes. The criteria for assessment after pronuclear membrane breakdown or first cleavage division were omitted. A mean PN score of less than 13 resulted in a pregnancy of 4 percent while a mean score of 13 or greater, resulted in a pregnancy rate of 22 percent.

Tesarik and Greco,1999[29] suggested new evaluation criteria to predict the developmental fate of human embryos at the pronuclear stage. Zygotes were designated as pattern 0 if they possessed the following characteristics: (i) the difference in the number of nucleolar precursor bodies (NPB) between both pronuclei did not exceed three, (ii) the distribution of NPB (random versus polarized) was the same in both pronuclei, and (iii) there were at least three NPB in each pronucleus. If NPBs were less than seven in each PN they were polarized, i.e. accumulating near the poles at which the pronuclei were associated. Alternatively if NPBs exceeded seven in each PN, they were never polarized. This pattern 0 was defined on the basis of nucleoli patterns seen in zygotes in 100 percent implantation cycles. Other

TABLE 44.2: Development of pattern 0 and pattern non 0 zygotes				
Nucleoli pattern	*Zygote No.*	*No. early cleaving embryos (%)*	*Early arrested embryos (%)*	*Grade 1 Embryos (%)*
Pattern 0	124	88 (70.9)	3/124 (2.4)	80 (64.5)
Non 0	164	83 (50.6)	15/164 (9.1)	85 (51.8)

patterns of nucleoli distribution were earlier designated as patterns 1 to 5, but subsequently all these patterns were defined as nonpattern 0.

In a retrospective cohort analysis of 380 fresh embryo transfers according to conventional criteria (equal-sized blastomeres, less than 10 percent fragments and clear nongranulated cytoplasm), Tesarik et al, 2000[30] reported that those embryos developed from pattern 0 zygotes gave significantly higher pregnancy (44.8%) and implantation rates (30.2%) compared with pregnancy (22.1%) and implantation rates (11.2%) for the transfer of nonpattern 0 zygotes.

Menezes et al 2000[31] conducted a prospective pilot study where embryo selection was done on the basis of nucleoli patterns in zygotes (2 PN stage) and subsequent early cleavage at 26 to 27 hours postinsemination or ICSI. The zygotes were cultured individually in microdroplets of EBSS (Universal IVF medium, Medicult) so that their further development could be monitored. Zygotes were assessed at 16 to 18 hours post IVF or ICSI under an inverted microscope at a magnification of 200x. All observations were videotaped to enable accurate assessment. Embryo transfers were performed on day 2. A maximum of 3 embryos were transferred. The observations on nucleoli patterns in zygotes and early cleavage were taken into account in the selection of embryos.

A total of 288 zygotes were analysed according to their nucleolar pattern and subsequent development. Comparisons between pattern 0 and non 0 zygotes were made using the Chi-squared test. Pattern 0 zygotes produced a higher percentage of early cleaving and grade 1 embryos and fewer arrested embryos than pattern non 0 zygotes (Table 44.2). Edwards and Beard[32] emphasized the need to determine whether pronucleate embryos with high scores as per the criteria used by Scott and Smith, 1998[27] are the embryos which grow to blastocysts in vitro. Hence some sibling embryos were cultured further in vitro using G1/G2 media (Scandinavian IVF Science) and their development monitored until blastocyst formation or hatching. Both clinical pregnancy rate as well as blastocyst development were significantly higher in embryos with nucleoli pattern 0 (Table 44.3). Thus observations on pronuclear morphology provide valuable information for assessment of embryo quality and selection for transfer.

Scott et al, 2000[33] scored zygotes according to distribution and size of nucleoli within each nucleus. They showed that zygotes showing equality between nuclei resulted in 49.5 percent blastocysts whereas zygotes with unequal size, numbers or distribution of nucleoli had only 28 percent blastocyst formation. Cleaving embryos selected primarily by zygote and secondarily by

TABLE 44.3: Outcome of embryo transfer and culture with embryos derived from pattern 0 and non 0 zygotes				
Nucleoli pattern	*No. ET's*	*No. of clinical pregnancies (%)*	*No. sibling embryos cultured*	*No. blastocysts (%)*
Pattern 0	45*	13 (28.9) [a]	30	11/30 (36.7) [b]
Non 0	10**	nil (0) [a]	56	8/56 (14) [b]

* ET's done with at least one pattern 0 embryo
** ET's done with only pattern non 0 embryo (s)
[a] $p < 0.005$
[b] $p < 0.01$

day 3 morphology, had increased implantation and pregnancy rates (31 and 57%) compared with those selected by morphology alone (19 and 33%) respectively.

EARLY CLEAVAGE

When several embryos with similar characteristics are present in the same cohort, the selection of the best embryos is left to chance. In order to ascertain which embryos are superior, the time of the first cleavage division is noted. Those which cleave early, that is around 27 hours post-ICSI or IVF are selected. Clinical pregnancies and implantation rates have been significantly more in the early cleavage group (25.9 and 14% compared with 5.9 percent in the "no early cleavage" group (Sakkas et al,1998).[34]

Bos-Mikich et al, 2001[35] reported a 55 percent clinical pregnancy rate in the early cleavage group compared to 25 percent in the group that did not display early cleavage between 25 and 29 hours post insemination/ICSI. Compelling evidence of higher developmental competence of early cleaving embryos in elective single embryo transfer procedures has also been given by Salumets et al,2003[36], who reported a 50 percent clinical pregnancy rate after transfer of early cleaving embryos compared to 26.4 percent for ones that did not cleave early.

DAY 2 CLEAVAGE RATE

There is substantial clinical evidence for an optimal cleavage rate for embryos as reported by Cummins et al, 1986.[37] Analysis of 1539 embryo transfers resulting in 232 clinical pregnancies, showed that embryo development rate and embryo quality scores (based on blastomere size, fragmentation and quality of cytoplasm) were of value in predicting success. Clinical pregnancies resulted from embryos with a moderate to good quality score coupled with average or above average growth rates. Poor quality and very slow or very rapidly growing embryos were under-represented in cycles leading to pregnancy. Ziebe et al, 1997[38] did a retrospective study of 1001 IVF cycles which included a consecutive series of single transfers (341), dual transfers

(410) and triple transfers (215) where all the transferred embryos in each cycle were of identical quality score and cleavage stage. Embryo transfers were performed on day 2. Transfer of 4-celled embryos resulted in a significantly higher pregnancy rate compared with 2-celled, 3-celled or greater than 4-celled embryos.

Giorgetti et al, 1995[39] described the implantation potential of a well-defined type of embryo. They reported significantly higher pregnancy rates after transfer of 4-celled embryos. These embryos implanted two fold more than embryos at other cell stages, thus implying an optimal cleavage rate of embryos.

These results indicate the policy to be used when weighing the two main morphological criteria namely quality and cleavage stage. A 4-cell embryo, even in presence of minor amount of fragments, should be preferred to a 2-cell embryo without fragments.

FRAGMENTATION

Fragments are small membrane enclosed, usually anucleate bits of cytoplasm which are seen budding off from intact blastomeres. These are visible under low magnification under a stereomicroscope but a better vision is obtained if observed at high magnification (200-400x) under an inverted microscope. Fragments may be scattered or localized. Alikani and Cohen, 1995[40] found that implantation potential was highest in embryos having less than 5 percent fragments or localised fragments, than in those having scattered, large or extensive fragments. Embryos of certain patients show fragmentation in repeated IVF cycles, irrespective of the stimulation protocol given.

Fragmentation may be related to oocyte aging or the process of IVF itself. Reactive oxygen species released from dying sperm, genetic abnormality resulting from polyspermy, changes in culture conditions, follicular stimulation, as well as changes in genetic control of apoptosis during cleavage can all predispose to fragmentation (Braude, 1999).[41] Some forms of spontaneous fragmentation are not lethal. They appear as transient structures which disappear by resorption. The occurrence and fate of fragments may be related to transient and focal ATP deficiencies in blastomeres as well as mitochondrial deficiencies or absence (Van Blerkom et al, 2001).[42] Excessive fragmentation however, is generally believed to reflect poor quality of an embryo as Magli et al, 2001[43] have reported an increase in chromosome abnormalities proportional to the percentage of fragmentation; 90 percent chromosome abnormalities were found in embryos with greater than 40 percent fragmentation.

MULTINUCLEATION

Multinucleation may be observed in one or more blastomeres of an embryo. This can arise due to karyokinesis in the absence of cytokinesis with subsequent arrest of the blastomere or the entire embryo. Multinucleation may also be caused by partial fragmentation of nuclei or by defective migration at mitotic anaphase. The presence of multinucleation is not necessarily related to gross morphology of the embryos viewed under the stereomicroscope. Pelinck et al, 1998[44] reported a clinical pregnancy rate of 16.9 percent in a study group where embryos with multinucleated blastomeres (MNBs) were transferred as compared to a pregnancy rate of 23.2 percent in the control group. Similarly implantation rate was 6 percent in the MNB group versus 11.3 percent in the control group.

In another study, Jackson et al,1998[45] observed that the live birth rate dropped from 28 percent in cycles with no multinucleate embryos to 8 percent in cycles having 50 percent or more of embryos with MNBs and to 4 percent in cycles with 100 percent multinucleation. When greater than 50 percent of transferred embryos contained MNBs there was a significant reduction in implantation (3.4 vs 14.7%) and clinical pregnancy (9.1 vs 29.1%), when compared with transfer of control embryos. When embryos with MNBs were cultured, the majority got arrested at the 2 cell to 16 cell stage and there was significantly lower blastocyst formation. This is probably the consequence of cytokinetic and chromosomal anomalies (Balakier and Cadesky,

1997.[46] Kligman et al, 1996[47] found that 74.5 percent of MNB embryos were chromosomally abnormal compared to 32.3 percent of embryos with mononucleated blastomeres.

More recently Hardarson et al, 2001[48] reported that embryos with uneven sized blastomeres displayed a much higher multinucleation rate and aneuploidy, which eventually resulted in a lower implantation rate.

In a large retrospective analysis of 10,388 cleaved embryos from 1395 IVF/ICSI cycles, multinucleation was observed in 33.6 percent of embryos in 79.4 percent of cycles, more frequently on day 2 than on day 3 (27.4 vs 15.1% (Van Royen et al, 2003)[49] Multinucleated embryos had a decreased implantation rate: 4.3 percent for single and 5.7 percent in double embryo transfers. These figures are comparable to those reported by Jackson et al,1998.[45] On day 2, four cell embryos showed minimal multinucleation (16.8%) while 8 cell embryos on day 3 showed minimal multinucleation (15.5%).

MNB cycles had higher estradiol levels, more follicles on the day of hCG injection, higher number of oocytes retrieved, higher fertilization rate and embryos per patient. Some patients with high incidence of multinucleated embryos show a repetitive pattern in consecutive cycles, suggesting a patient linked predisposition.

Biochemical pregnancies, spontaneous abortions and termination of pregnancy due to chromosomally abnormal fetus have all been reported following the transfer of MNB embryos (Pelinck et al,1998,[44] Balakier et al,1997).[46] The ongoing implantation rate, though low, can be explained by the fact that blastomeres are believed to be totipotent till around the 8 cell stage. Hence sibling blastomeres can develop further if chromosomally normal. Live births originating from MNB embryos have been reported (Jackson et al,1998,[45] Balakier and Cadensky, 1997,[46] Van Royen et al, 2003).[49]

Since multinucleation is a factor which highly discriminates between embryos with high and low implantation rate, the evidence given above is a strong argument in favour of thorough and systematic screening of the nuclear status of the embryos at high magnification (200-400x), as the presence of MNBs could often be missed when observations are done only under the stereo-microscope. MNB embryos should not be transferred unless they are the only ones available. In such cases patients should be adequately counseled about the consequences.

ZONA PELLUCIDA THICKNESS VARIATION

The variation in thickness of the zona pellucida has been positively correlated to good embryo scores (Host et al, 2002).[50] The degree of zona thickness variation of transferred embryos in pregnancy cycles has also been reported to be significantly higher (p < 0.005) than that of embryos in nonpregnant cycles (Zhou et al, 2002).[51]

EMBRYO SCORING

Several scoring systems have been used to define embryo quality. Scoring based on early cleavage and cleavage rate have already been described. The cumulative embryo scoring (CES) system proposed by Steer et al,1992[52] is a simple system to enable selection of an optimal number of embryos for transfer on day 2, while reducing the incidence of multiple pregnancies. This CES system combines embryo morphology, cleavage rate and number of embryos transferred into a single figure, representing their collective quality. CES is defined as the sum of the products of number of blastomeres and morphological gradings of transferred embryos (Table 44.4).

TABLE 44.4: Morphological gradings of transferred embryo

Grade	Description
4	More than 2 cell; equal blastomeres, smooth membrane; translucent cytoplasm; nil fragments
3	Similar to 4 but one morphological characteristic not ideal or less than 3 blastomeres
2	Moderate fragmentation and/or more than one characteristic less than ideal
1	Extensive fragmentation or aberrations in most morphological characteristics

Visser et al,1993[53] calculated and analysed the scores of 602 IVF embryos transferred to determine the CES system's relationship to pregnancy rate, pregnancy outcome and incidence of twin and triplet pregnancies. Pregnancy rate was found to increase from 4 percent with scores between 1 and 10, to 35 percent in the 41 to 50 group. The score of 20 was the criterion for separating patients into poor and good pregnancy prognosis groups. Birth rates below and above a score of 20 (2.8 and 19.2% respectively) differed significantly (p = 0.0005).

Van Royen et al,1999[54] characterized top quality embryos on the basis of 23 transfers where 2 embryos had been transferred and resulted in ongoing twin pregnancies. A top quality embryo was defined as one having 4 to 5 blastomeres on day 2, at least 7 blastomeres on day 3, less than 20 percent fragmentation on day 3 and no MNBs. Using this definition, 221 transfers of 2 embryos each, in patients less than 38 years of age were analysed. Ongoing pregnancy rate was 63 percent when there were 2 top embryos, 58 percent with one top embryo and 23 percent with nil top embryos. The corresponding implantation rates were 49, 35 and 12 percent respectively. The twin pregnancy rate was significantly higher when two top embryos were transferred (57%) compared to 21 percent when only one top embryo was transferred.

Hu et al,1998[55] retrospectively analysed the effect of the mean cumulative embryo morphology score on implantation, pregnancy and multiple conception rates in 2,686 embryos from 754 patients. All embryo transfers were done on Day 3. Embryos which were at least 5 cells with equal sized blastomeres and nil fragments were given a score of 4. Five or greater celled embryos with less than 30 percent fragments scored 3. Embryos with at least 5 cells with unequal sized blastomeres and nil fragments scored 2. Embryos with at least 5 cells with blastomeres of equal size and 30-50 percent fragments as well as similar celled embryos with unequal sized blastomeres and 1-50 percent fragments scored 1. Embryos having less than 5 cells of any size and any embryo with greater than 50 percent fragments scored 0. The cumulative score was the embryo score multiplied by the number of blastomeres and the mean cumulative score (MCES) was the average cumulative score of embryos transferred. Embryos with MCES of >19 were termed good, those with scores from 10-19 were termed fair and those with scores below 10 were termed poor.

For women < 36 years of age, as MCES increased, implantation rates increased significantly from 13 percent to 20 percent to 29 percent (p < 0.01) and pregnancy rates changed significantly from 29 percent to 46 percent to 59 percent in the three groups respectively (p < 0.001). For women between 36 and 39, implantation rates increased significantly from 11 percent to 17 percent to 22 percent (p < 0.05) and pregnancy rates changed significantly from 26 percent to 42 percent to 43 percent respectively (p < 0.04). For women above 39 years of age, none of the effects was significant. Implantation rates were 4, 8 and 13 percent while pregnancy rates were 9, 23 and 27 percent respectively.. The drawback of this study is that up to 5 embryos were transferred per patient resulting in an overall high multiple pregnancy rate of 12.8 percent.

The Graduated Embryo Score (GES) for predicting blastocyst formation and pregnancy rates has been described by Fisch et al, 2001.[56] This system awards a total possible score of 100 points, based on evaluation at 16-18 hours, 25-27 hours and 64-67 hours post insemination and weighting for nucleoli arrangement, regular cleavage, degree of fragmentation and day 3 morphology. Nucleoli that were aligned on the pronuclear axis scored 20 points. Zygotes that had cleaved symmetrically to 2 cell scored 30 points. At this stage embryos with 0, < 20 percent and > 20 percent fragmentation received 30, 25 and 0 points respectively. On day 3, embryos with 7 cells, nil fragments, 8 cells with equal or slightly unequal blastomeres and 9 cells with nil fragments scored 20 points, embryos from 7 to 11 cells as well as compacting embryos scored 10 points. Maximum cumulative score for an embryo was 100 points. The blastocyst formation, pregnancy and implantation rates were 44 percent, 59 percent and 79 percent respectively with embryos scoring 70 to 100 points. For embryos scoring 0-65 points, the corresponding figures were 34 percent, 34 percent and 24 percent.

Recently, De Placido et al, 2002[57] reported a new scoring system to predict preimplantation embryo quality., which included a combination of in vitro growth rate and morphology of both zygotes and embryos. The design for zygote scoring was equally distributed into three factors: (1) position, size and apposition of pronuclei, (2) position and type of nucleoli and (3) presence of cytoplasmic halo. The maximum score for each factor was 5, which meant that the maximum score for a perfect zygote would be 15. For cleavage embryos on day 2 and day 3, the scoring factors were: (1) size of blastomeres (2) level of multi-nucleation and (3) degree of fragmentation. Here too the maximum score for each factor was 5, with a maximum score of 15. The scoring system was weighted with the equation: (embryo score X number of blastomeres)x zygote score, the rationale being to balance embryo quality and zygote quality, since poor quality embryos can develop from good quality zygotes and vice versa. Thus top quality embryos could maximally score 900 and 1800 points on day 2 and day 3 respectively. Cohorts of embryos were divided into 3 groups depending on the mean quality of the cohort. Top quality embryos (Group 1) had a zygote score and embryo scores of at least 14 each with at least 4 or 8 blastomeres on days 2 and 3 respectively. Medium scoring embryos (Group 2) were zygotes and embryos scoring between 10 and 13.9 and were 2-3 cells on day 2 and/or 4-7 cells on day 3. Low scoring embryos (Group 3) had zygote and embryo scores of less than 10 and were less than 2 and 4 cells on days 2 and 3 respectively. Day 2 weighted scores were > = 600, 400-599 and < 400 for the three groups while day 3 weighted scores were >1000, 500-999 and < 500 respectively.

The correlation coefficient between zygote score, day 2, day 3 and cumulative scores was low where as the weighted scores which took into account both zygote and embryo characteristics resulted in a high correlation between scores and pregnancy as well as implantation. It was also observed that when no top quality embryos were present in the transferred cohort, a pregnancy rate of 33.3 percent was obtained but the implantation rate was low (9.4%). The pregnancy and implantation rates increased progressively as the number of top quality embryos increased from 1 to 4 (38, 50, 47, 75; 12, 13, 17, 28). This demonstrates that embryos scored as top quality using the weighted score are characterized by a significantly higher potential for implantation than lower scoring embryos. These authors also observed that maternal age heavily reduced both pregnancy and implantation rates but this was not due to any effect on the embryo score.

At our clinic, Sjoblom *et al*, 2001[58] described an embryo scoring system that was a cumulative score of scores from day 0 to 2/3. The original scoring system was modified as follows. Day 0 observations were made only on oocytes that were meant for ICSI, as they could be carefully assessed for morphology after the cumulus cells had been denuded. No score was assigned to the oocytes on day 0 but presence of bull's eye (Figure 44.1), aggregation of smooth endoplasmic reticulum (Figure 44.2),nature of the polar body (Figure 44.3) and zona pellucida (Figure 44.4) were noted. The elasticity of the membrane during injection was also noted.

Embryos resulting from bull's eye and/or SER oocytes were generally not transferred. Occasionally a cohort contained a giant oocyte. Such giant oocytes (Figure 44.5) were not

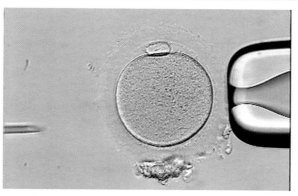

FIGURE 44.3: Normal Metaphase II oocyte with grade 1 (smooth, ovoid) polar body

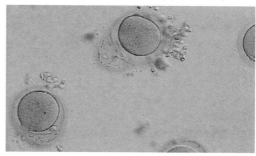

FIGURE 44.4: Abnormal zona pellucida in two oocytes

injected as they are known to be chromosomally abnormal. In IVF if giant oocytes were observed to be normally fertilized they were not transferred for the same reason.

On day 1 at fertilization check (16-18 hours post insemination or ICSI), the oocytes were scored for the orientation of polar bodies, presence of halo, texture of cytoplasm, condition of the oocyte membrane, features of the pronuclei and nucleoli (Figures 44.6 to 44.8), as

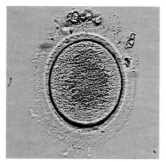

FIGURE 44.1: Oocyte with central dark cytoplasm (bull's eye)

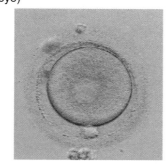

FIGURE 44.2: Oocyte with aggregation of smooth endoplasmic reticulum (SER) (clear fluid filled space)

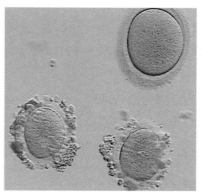

FIGURE 44.5: Giant oocyte(top) with 2 normal sized immature oocytes

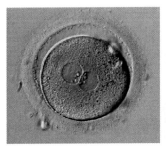

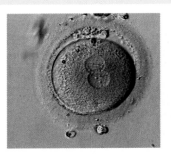

FIGURE 44.6: Zygote showing cytoplasmic halo and polarized nucleoli

FIGURE 44.8: Zygote with nonpolarised nucleoli

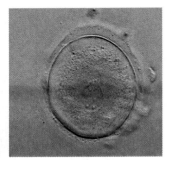

FIGURE 44.7: Zygote with unequal sized pronuclei

given in Table 44.5. At 25 to 27 hours the zygotes were checked for early cleavage. The maximum score for a perfect zygote on day 1 would be 15.

On day 2 and day 3, about 41-44 hours and 64-68 hours post insemination or ICSI respectively, the cleaved embryos were scored for texture and thickness variation of zona pellucida (Figure 44.9), number, size and shape of blastomeres, volume occupied by blastomeres, membrane texture, cytoplasmic texture, fragmentation and presence of MNBs (Figures 44.10 to 44.15) (Table 44.6). Again the total score for a perfect embryo on day 2 or day 3 would be 15. The maximum cumulative score for a perfect embryo would be 30 on day 2 and 45 on day 3. If MNBs were present, the percentage of blastomeres containing MNBs was deducted from the total score. For example, if a 4 cell embryo scoring 12 on day 2, had one blastomere containing MNBs, then the percentage of MNB blastomeres would be $1/4 \times 100 = 25$. Therefore 25 percent of the score, $(25/100 \times 12 = 3)$ would be deducted, giving a final corrected score of 9 (12 minus 3).

TABLE 44.5: Day 1 score		
		Score
Polar Body orientation	< 45° between PN axis & distal pb	1
	> 45° angle	0
Halo	Present	1
	Faint or Absent	0
Cytoplasmic Texture	Normal	2
	Slightly granular	1
	Vacuoles, Bull's eye, very granular, SER etc	0
Membrane	Smooth	1
	Jagged	0
PN Size	Equal	1
	Unequal	0
PN Apposition	Apposed	1
	Apart	0
PN Position	Central	1
	Eccentric	0
Nucleoli Pattern	Equal numbers (< 8) and aligned	5
	Equal numbers and scattered	2
	All other patterns	0
25 hrs post insem/ICSI check	2 cell	2
	Syngamy (disappearance of PNs)	1
	PNs intact	0
Total score		**15**

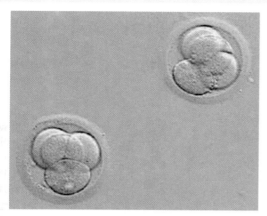

FIGURE 44.9: Embryos with thickness variation of their zonae

Generally 1 or 2 embryos with the highest scores were transferred per patient irrespective of age (average 1.9). Due to the high incidence of twin pregnancies (21% of clinical pregnancies)

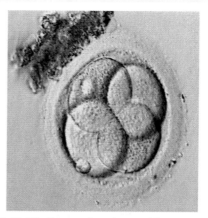

FIGURE 44.10: Four cell embryo with equal sized and regular shaped blastomeres

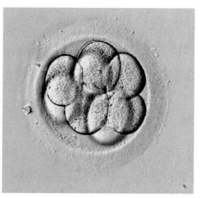

FIGURE 44.11: Eight cell embryo with equal sized and regular shaped blastomeres

TABLE 44.6: Day 2/3 score		
		Score
Zona Pellucida thickness/variation	Variable	1
	Uniform	0
Zona Pellucida texture	Normal thickness and texture	1
	Very thick/abnormal shape	0
Blastomere size	Equal	1
	Unequal	0
Blastomere shape	Regular	1
	Irregular	0
Volume occupied by blastomeres	Blastomeres fill zona	1
	Large space between cells and zona	0
Membrane	Smooth	1
	Jagged	0
Cytoplasm	Clear	1
	Granular, vacuoles etc.	0
Fragmentation	< 10%	2
	10-30%	1
	> 30%	0
Development rate	Day 2 4 cell	6
	2, 3, 5, > 5 cell	3
	uncleaved	0
	Day 3 8 cell	6
	6, 7, > 8 cell	3
	< 6 cell	0
Presence of MNBs	If present deduct percentage of score dependent on number of cells displaying multinucleation	
	Total score	**15**

Day 2 Cumulative Score/30
Day 3 Cumulative Score/45

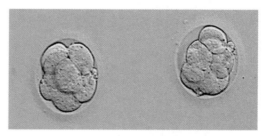

FIGURE 44.12: Compacting eight cell embryos

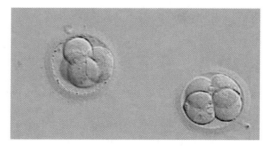

FIGURE 44.13: Two 4 cell embryos with left embryo showing wide space between blastomeres and zona

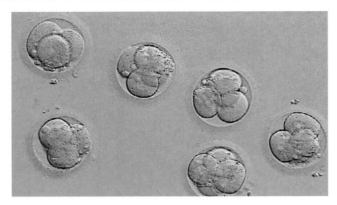

FIGURE 44.14: Embryos with 10% fragments

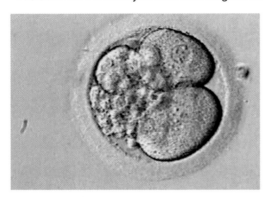

FIGURE 44.15A: Embryo with unequal size and shape of blastomeres, MNBs and > 30% fragments

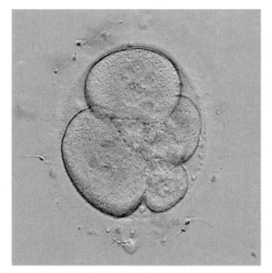

FIGURE 44.15B: Embryo with MNBs in 2 blastomeres

at our clinic following transfer of two embryos, good prognosis patients who were under 35 years opted for single embryo transfer. Three embryos were transferred only in women who

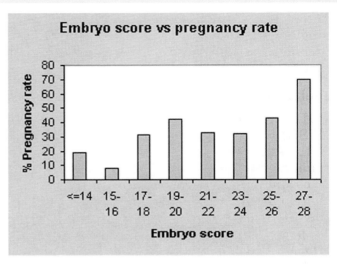

FIGURE 44.16: Day 2 Embryo score versus pregnancy rate

were 40 and above and additionally had repeated failures with poor oocyte/embryo quality. The average score of the transferred embryos was strongly correlated to the pregnancy rate (Spearman rank order correlation, $r = 0.881$, $p < 0.005$). As seen from Figure 44.16, transfer of high scoring day 2 embryos resulted in excellent pregnancy rate.

OTHER METHODS OF SELECTING EMBRYOS

Amino Acid Profiles

The depletion or appearance of amino acids brought about by single human embryos conceived by IVF has been studied by Hughton et al,2002.[59] Amino acid profiles have been obtained for human embryos from day 2 or 3 of development, during the compacting 8 cell to morula stage and the morula to blastocyst transition. Profiles of alanine, arginine, glutamine, methionine and asparagine predicted the potential for blastocyst development at > 95 percent. Leucine was the most consistently depleted amino acid throughout development by embryos which formed blastocysts. Alanine was the most conspicuous amino acid produced. There were marked differences in amino acid turnover between embryos that developed to blastocyst and those which arrested. On the basis of these results, it has been suggested that noninvasive amino acid profiling has the potential to select developmentally competent single embryos for transfer which will not only increase the success rate but eliminate multiple births as well.

Preimplantation Genetic Diagnosis (PGD)

PGD using fluorescence *in situ* hybridization (FISH) technique has been of great advantage in the study of the chromosomal complement of human preimplantation embryos. The incidence of chromosomal abnormalities in preimplantation embryos is high, ranging from approximately 25 percent in young patients to more than 85 percent in older patients (Gianaroli *et al*, 1997).[60] The frequency of chromosomal abnormalities is related to advanced maternal age, multiple IVF failures, altered karyotype, repeated miscarriages and use of epididymal or testicular sperm. Assessment of embryos for common aneuploidies found in spontaneous abortions and live births, with transfer of euploid embryos has resulted in high pregnancy and implantation rates for this group of patients (Magli *et al*, 1998).[61] This technology is presently expensive, is not widely available and has drawbacks as only one or two blastomeres of each embryo are analysed. Other techniques such as Complete Genomic Hybridization (CGH) (Vouillaire *et al*, 2002)[62] hold promise, but this technique is not commonly available.

CRYOPRESERVATION

A good cryopreservation programme is absolutely essential to improve the overall preg-

nancy rate when the transfer of fewer embryos especially single embryo is being advocated. This means that freezing and thawing techniques must be robust. Commercial media providers have modified the original freeze thaw protocols of Lasalle *et al*,1985.[63] In Quinn's Advantage freeze thaw kits supplied by Sage, phosphate buffered saline (PBS) has been replaced by HEPES buffered human tubal fluid (HTF) medium. HTF is the medium in which the embryos are cultured and HEPES buffer aids in pH control when freezing and thawing is done outside the CO_2 incubator. Another modification is that freezing and thawing procedures are done at 37°C, preferably under oil and not at room temperature.

Following thawing, a high percentage of embryos should survive with at least 50 percent of their blastomeres and zona pellucida intact. Survival of embryos with 100 percent of their blastomeres intact along with additional mitosis during overnight culture after thawing is indicative of embryos with the highest implantation potential (Van der Eldst,1997[64], Ziebe *et al*,1998[65] Guerif *et al*, 2000,[66] Edgar *et al*, 2000).[67] Another important factor that contributes to success is the accurate detection of the LH surge during natural cycles for frozen thawed embryo replacement or adequate preparation of the endometrium in hormone replacement therapy (HRT) cycles.

With frozen thawed embryo transfers included, a cumulative delivery rate per pick up of 52.8 percent has been reported (Tiitinen *et al*,

TABLE 44.7: Elective SET vs double ET					
	Singleton clinical pregnancies / ET			*Twin clinical pregnancies / ET*		
	e SET	*SET*	*2ET*	*e SET*	*SET*	*2ET*
Vilska *et al* (1999)[69]	22/74 (29.7)	19/94 (20.2)	218/742 (29.4)	0/74 (0)	0/94 (0)	52/742 (7)
Van Royen *et al* (1999)[54]	6/28 (21)	—	70/221 (31.7)	0/28 —	— (20.4)	45/221 (20.4)
Tiitinen *et al* (2001)[68]	49/127 (38.6)	17/94 (18.1)	203/517 (40)	1/127 (0.8)	1/94 (1)	42/517 (8)
Martikainen *et al* (2001)[70]	21/74 (28.3)	—	17/70 (24.3)	1/74 (1.35)	—	11/70 (15.7)
Gerris *et al* (2002)[71]	105/299 (35.1)	—	309/853 (36.2)	1/299 (0.3)	— (12.2)	104/853 (12.2)
De Neubourg *et al* (2002)[72]	54/127 (43)	—	36/116 (31)	0/127 (0)	—	11/116 (0.5)

2001).[68] Thus efficient cryopreservation will be highly effective for pursuing single embryo transfers.

Current Reports on Elective SET (eSET) Versus SET and 2 Embryo Transfers

Some European countries, Scandinavian countries in particular, have pioneered work on single embryo transfers. Their results shown in Table 44.7 show that pregnancy rates are not compromised by transferring a single embryo and offers the additional advantage of twin pregnancies being almost completely eliminated. Pregnancy rates following SET have been lower than eSET for the obvious reason that only one embryo was available.

Recently in Australia, a multicentre, double blind randomized controlled trial called the Australian Study of Single Embryo Transfer (ASSET), has been launched, to compare pregnancy outcomes following either single or double embryo transfer in an optimal group of patients undergoing IVF/ICSI.

CONCLUSION

In the new millennium the high incidence of iatrogenic twins following IVF, is no longer considered an unavoidable price to be paid in order to achieve a satisfactory ongoing pregnancy rate. The huge expense incurred in countries due to multiple pregnancies should be diverted towards preventing such catastrophes. Though this goal could ideally be achieved by employing elective single embryo transfer (eSET) as a routine, it is hampered by several factors. The major hurdle is the accuracy of identifying embryos with very high implantation potential and hence the fear of reducing existing pregnancy rates. However once eSET becomes the gold standard of IVF practice, centres will have to focus on implantation rates instead of pregnancy rates and further this to livebirth per embryo transferred,as a criterion of excellence of any ART centre. Live birth per embryo is a statistical criterion which is negatively influenced by the incidence of multiple pregnancies (Hazenkamp et al, 2000).[73]

Several different embryo scoring techniques have been used to identify embryos with high implantation potential. At present it is not known clearly whether identification of embryos on day 1 at the 2PN stage, day 2, day 3 or blastocyst stage have independent or overlapping value. Although all these techniques have their merits, the one which is most efficacious, simple, quick and cheap is likely to be universally adopted. For the present it would seem prudent to adopt an individualized embryo transfer policy depending on the patient's age, cause of infertility and other related factors. With the rapid progress that is being made in this area, the day is probably not far off when every clinician will confidently advise their IVF patients " Have as many embryos put back as you like-one at a time" (Templeton, 2000).[74]

ACKNOWLEDGEMENT

The authors gratefully acknowledge Dr Stephen Steigrad, Dr Graeme Hughes and Dr John Tyler, Directors of IVFAustralia, for their support.

REFERENCES

1. Quinn P. Where have the high pregnancy rates come from?–Culture media. Proceedings of the 21st Annual Scientific Meeting of the FSA: 2002;22.
2. De Sutter P, Gerris J, Dhont M. A health economic decision-analytic model comparing double with single embryo transfer in IVF/ICSI. Hum Reprod 2002;17 (11):2891-96.
3. Lambert R. Safety issues in assisted reproductive technology. The children of assisted reproduction confront the responsible conduct of assisted reproductive technologies. Hum Reprod 200217 (12):3011-15.
4. Gardner DK, Lane M. Culture of viable human blastocysts in defined sequential serum free media. Hum Reprod 1998;13 (Suppl 3):48-59.
5. Coates A, Rutherford AJ, Hunter H et al. Glucose free medium in human in vitro fertilization and embryo transfer: A large scale, prospective randomized clinical trial 1999;72:229-32.
6. Gardner DK, Lane M, Stevens J et al. Blastocyst score affects implantation and pregnancy outcome towards a single blastocyst transfer. Fertil Steril 2000;73: 1155-58.
7. Bungum M, Bungum L, Hamaidan P. Day 3 versus Day 5 embryo transfer: a prospective randomized study. Reprod Biomed Online 2003;7 (1):98-104.
8. Rienzi L, Ubaldi F, Iacobelli M et al. Day 3 embryo transfer with combined evaluation at the pronuclear

and cleavage stages compares favourably with day 5 blastocyst transfer. Hum Reprod 2002;17 (7):1852-55.

9. Coskun S, Hollanders J, Al-Hassan S et al. Day 5 versus day 3 embryo transfer: a controlled randomized trial. Hum Reprod 2000;15 (9):1947-52.

10. Virant-Klun I, Tamazevic T, Zorn B et al. Blastocyst formation-good indicator of clinical results after ICSI with testicular spermatozoa. Hum Reprod 2003;18 (5):1070-76.

11. Van Blerkom J. Can the developmental competence of early human embryos be predicted effectively in the clinical laboratory? Hum Reprod 1997;12 (8):1610-14.

12. Nargund G, Bourne R, Doyle P et al. Association between ultrasound indices of follicular blood flow, oocyte recovery and preimplantation embryo quality. Hum Reprod 1996;11:109-113.

13. Chui D, Pugh N, Walker S et al. Follicular vascularity: The predictive value of transvaginal Doppler ultrasonography is an in vitro fertilization programme: a preliminary study. Hum Reprod 1997;12:191-06.

14. Serhal RF, Ranieri DM, Kinis A et al. Oocyte morphology predicts outcome of intracytoplasmic sperm injection. Hum Reprod 1997;12 (6):1267-70.

15. Van Blerkom J, Henry G. Oocyte dysmorphism and aneuploidy in meiotically mature oocytes after ovarian stimulation. Hum Reprod 1992;7:379-90.

16. Van Blerkom J. Developmental failure in human reproduction associated with chromosomal abnormalities and cytoplasmic pathologies in meiotically mature oocytes. In: The Biological Basis of Early Human Reproductive Failure. Applications to medically assisted conception. Ed: J van Blerkom, Oxford University Press, New York, 1994;283.

17. Kahraman S, Yakin K, Donmez et al. Relationship between granular cytoplasm of oocytes and pregnancy outcome following intracytoplasmic sperm injection. Hum Reprod 2000;15 (11):2390-93.

18. Meriano J, Alexis J, Visram-Zaver S. Tracking of oocyte dysmorphisms for ICSI patients may prove relevant to the outcome in subsequent patient cycles. Hum Reprod 2001;16 (10):2118-23.

19. Ryan J, Lemcke S, Pike I. Cytoplasmic texture of human embryos as a predictor of development. Proceedings of the Fertility Society of Australia, 21st Annual Scientific Meeting 2002;38.

20. Xia P. Intracytoplasmic sperm injection: Correlation of oocyte grade based on polar body, perivitelline space and cytoplasmic inclusions with fertilization rate and embryo quality. Hum Reprod 1997;12 (8):1750-55.

21. Ebner T, Yaman C, Moser M et al. Elective transfer of embryos selected on basis of first polar body morphology is associated with increased rates of implantation and pregnancy. Fertil Steril 1999;72 (4):599-603.

22. Balakier H, Bouman D, Sojecki A et al. Morphological and cytogenetic analysis of human giant oocytes and giant embryos. Hum Reprod 2002;17 (9):2388-93.

23. Rosenbusch B, Schneider M, Glaser B et al. Cytogenetic analysis of giant oocytes and zygotes to assess their

relevance for the development of digynic triploidy. Hum Reprod 2002;17 (9):2388-93.

24. Payne D, Flaherty SP, Barry MF et al. Preliminary observations on polar body extrusion and pronuclear formation in human oocytes using time–lapse video cinematography. Hum Reprod 1997;12:532-41.

25. Garello C, Baker H, Rai J et al. Polar body placement and embryo quality after intracytoplasmic sperm injection and in vitro fertilization: further evidence for polarity in human oocytes? Hum Reprod 1999;14 (10):2588-95.

26. Tesarik J, Kopecny V. Assembly of the nucleolar precursor bodies in human male pronuclei is correlated with an early RNA synthetic activity. Exp Cell Res 1990;191:153-56.

27. Scott LA, Smith S. The successful use of pronuclear embryo transfers the day following oocyte retrieval. Hum Reprod 1998;13:182-87.

28. Ludwig M, Schopper B, Al-Hasani S et al. Clinical use of a pronuclear stage score following intracytoplasmic sperm injection: Impact on pregnancy rates under the conditions of the German embryo protection law. Hum Reprod 2000;15:325-29.

29. Tesarik J, Greco E. The probability of abnormal preimplantation development can be predicted by a single static observation on pronuclear stage morphology. Hum Reprod 1999;14:1318-23.

30. Tesarik J, Junca AM, Hazout A et al. Embryos with high implantation potential offer intracytoplasmic sperm injection can be recognized by a simple, non invasive examination of pronuclear morphology. Hum Reprod 2000;15:1396-99.

31. Menezes J, Gunasheela S, Sathananthan H. Assessment of embryo quality as a predictor of IVF outcome. In Rao KR, Brinsden PR (Eds), The Infertility Manual, FOGSI India, 2001;428-37.

32. Edwards RG, Beard HK. Blastocyst stage transfer: Pitfalls and benefits. Is the success of human IVF more a matter of genetics and evolution than growing blastocysts? Hum Reprod 1999;14:1-6.

33. Scott L, Alvero R, Leondires M et al. The morphology of human pronuclear embryos is positively related to blastocyst development and implantation. Hum Reprod 2000;15 (11):2394-2403.

34. Sakkas D, Shoukier Y, Chardonner D et al. Early cleavage of human embryos to the 2 cell stage after intracytoplasmic sperm injection as an indicator of embryo viability. Hum Reprod 1998;13 (1):182-87.

35. Bos-Mikich, Mattos A, Ferrari A. Early cleavage of human embryos: an effective method for predicting successful IVF/ICSI outcome. Hum Reprod 2001;16 (12):2658-61.

36. Salumets A, Hyden-Granskog C, Makinen S et al. Early cleavage predicts the viability of human embryos in elective single embryo transfer procedures. Hum Reprod 2003;18 (4):821-25.

37. Cummins JM, Breen JM, Harrison KL et al. A formula for scoring human embryo growth rates in in vitro

fertilization-its value in predicting pregnancy and in comparison with visual estimates of embryo quality. In Vitro Fertil Embryo Transfer 1986;3 (5):284-95.

38. Ziebe S, Peterson K, Lendenberg S et al. Embryo morphology or cleavage stage: How to select the best embryo for transfer after in vitro fertilization. Hum Reprod 1997;12 (7):1545-49.

39. Giorgetti C Terriou P, Auquier P et al. Embryo score to predict implantation after in vitro fertilization based on 957 single embryo transfers. Hum Reprod 1995;10: 2427-31.

40. Alikani M, Cohen J. Patterns of cell fragmentation in the human embryo in vitro. J Assist Reprod Genet 1995;12 (Suppl):28s.

41. Braude PR. Embryo quality and implantation In: Templeton A, Cooke I, Shaughn, O'Brien PM (Eds): Evidence Based Fertility Treatment: In vitro Fertilization 1999;5:283-94.

42. Van Blerkom J, Davis P, Alexander S: A microscopic and biochemical study of fragmentation phenotypes in stage-appropriate human embryos. Hum Reprod 2001;16 (4):719-29.

43. Magli M, Gianaroli L, Ferraretti A. Chromosomal abnormalities in embryos: Molecular and Cellular Endocrinol 2001;183:S29-34.

44. Pelinck MJ, De Vos M, Van Der Elst J et al. Embryos cultured in vitro with multinucleated blastomeres have poor implantation potential in human in vitro fertilization and intracytoplasm sperm injection. Hum Reprod 1998;13 (4):960-63.

45. Jackson KV, Ginsburg ES, Horntstein MD et al. Multinculeation is normally fertilized embryos is associated with an accelerated induction response and lower implantation and pregnancy rate in "in vitro" fertilization and embryo transfer cycles. Fertil Steril 1998;70 (1):60-66.

46. Balakier H, Cadesky K. The frequency and developmental capability of human embryos containing multinucleated blastomeres. Hum Reprod 1997;12:800-04.

47. Kligman I, Benadiva C, Alikani M et al. The presence of multinucleated blastomeres in human is correlated with chromosomal abnormalities. Hum Reprod 1996;11:1492-98.

48. Hardarson T, Hanson C, Sjogren A. Human embryos with unevenly sized blastomeres have lower pregnancy and implantation rates: indications for aneuploidy and multinucleation. Hum Reprod 2001;16 (2):313-18.

49. Van Royen E, Mangelschots K, Vercruyssen M et al. Multinucleation in cleavage stage embryos. Hum Reprod 2003;18 (5):1062-69.

50. Host E, Gabrielsen A, Lindenberg S et al. Apoptosis in human cumulus cells in relation to zona pellucida thickness variation, maturation stage and cleavage of the corresponding oocyte after intracytoplasmic sperm injection. Fertil Steril 2002;77 (3):511-15.

51. Zhou Y, Huang X, Bilu Y et al. Relationship between the degree of zona pellcida thickness variation of

transferred embryos and clinical outcomes in IVF-ET cycles. Fertil Steril 2002;78:S227.

52. Steer CV, Mills CL, Tan SL et al. The cumulative embryo score: A predictive embryo scoring technique programme. Hum Reprod 1992;7:117-19.

53. Visser D, Fourie F le R. The applicability of the cumulative embryo score system for embryo selection and quality control in an in vitro fertilization embryo transfer programme. Hum Reprod 1993;8 (10):1719-22.

54. Van Royen E, Mangelshots K, De Neubourg D et al. Characterization of a top quality embryo, a step towards single embryo transfer. Hum Reprod 1999;9:2345-49.

55. Hu Y, Maxson W, Hoffman D et al. Maximizing pregnancy rates and limiting higher order multiple conceptions by determining the optimal number of embryos to transfer based on quality. Fertil Steril 1998;69 (4):650-57.

56. Fisch J, Rodriguez H, Ross R et al. The Graduated Embryo Score (GES) predicts blastocyst formation and pregnancy rate from cleavage stage embryos. Hum Reprod 2001;16 (9):1970-75.

57. De Placido G, Wilding M, Strina I et al. High outcome predictability after IVF using a combined score for zygote and embryo morphology and growth rate. Hum Reprod 2002;17 (9):2402-09.

58. Sjoblom P, Cummins L, Menezes J et al. A cumulative embryo score for pregnancy detection. Proceedings of the 17th World Congress on Fertility and Sterility, PB 2001;29:134.

59. Houghton F, Hawkhead J, Humpherson P et al. Non-invasive amino acid turnover predicts human embryo developmental capacity. Hum Reprod 2002;17 (4):999-1005.

60. Gianaroli L, Magli M, Munne S et al. Preimplantation genetic diagnosis increases the preimplantation rate in human IVF by avoiding the transfer of chromosomally abnormal embryos. Fertil Steril 1997;68: 1128-31.

61. Magli M, Gianaroli L, Munne S et al. Incidence of chromosomal abnormalities from a morphologically normal cohort of embryos in poor prognosis patients. J Assist Reprod Genet 1998;15:297-301.

62. Voullaire L, Wilton L, McBain J et al. Chromosome abnormalities identified by comparative genomic hybridisation. Mol Hum Reprod 2002;8 (11):1035-41.

63. Lasalle B, Testart J, Renard J. Human embryo features that influence the success of cryopreservation with the use of 1, 2 propanediol. Fertil Steril 1985;44:645-51.

64. Van der Elst J, Van den Abbeel E, Vitrier S et al. Selective transfer of embryos with further cleavage after thawing increases delivery and implantation rates. Hum Reprod 1997;12:1513-21.

65. Ziebe S, Bech B, Petersen K et al. Resumption of mitotis during post thaw culture: a key parameter in selecting the right embryos for transfer. Hum Reprod 1998;13: 178-81.

66. Guerif F, Bidault R, Cadoret V et al. Parameters guiding selection of best embryos for transfer after

cryopreservation: a reappraisal. Hum Reprod 2002;17 (5):1321-26.

67. Edgar D, Bourne H, Speirs A et al. A quantitative analysis of the impact of cryopreservation on the implantation potential of human early cleavage stage embryos. Hum Reprod 2000;15 (1):175-79.

68. Tiitinen A, Halttunen M, Harkki P et al. Elective single embryo transfer: the value of cryopreservation. Hum Reprod 2001;16 (6):1140-44.

69. Vilska S, Tiitinen A, Hyden-Granskog C et al. Elective transfer of one embryo results in an acceptable pregnancy rate and eliminates the risk of multiple birth. Hum Reprod 1999;14 (9):2392-95.

70. Martikainen H, Tiitinen A, Tomas C et al. One versus two embryo transfer after IVF and ICSI: a randomised study. Hum Reprod 2001;16 (9):1900-03.

71. Gerris J, De Neubourg D, Mangelschots K et al. Elective single day 3 embryo transfer halves the twinning rate without decrease in the ongoing pregnancy rate of an IVF/ICSI programme. Hum Reprod 2002;17 (10): 2626-31.

72. De Neubourg D, Mangelschots K, Van Royen E et al. Impact of patients choice for single embryo transfer of a top quality embryo versus double embryo transfer in the first IVF/ICSI cycle. Hum Reprod 2002;17 (10): 2621-25.

73. Hazenkamp J, Bergh C, Wennerholm U et al. Avoiding multiple pregnancies in ART. Consideration of new strategies. Hum Reprod 2000;15 (6):1217-19.

74. Templeton A. Avoiding multiple pregnancies in ART. Hum Reprod 2000;15 (8):1662.

APPENDIX 1
PROTOCOL FOR BLASTOCYST CULTURE

CONSUMABLES REQUIRED

BD Falcon 60 mm petri dishes(Catalogue No. 3002) or 35 mm dishes(Catalogue No. 3001).

Culture Media

- Day 0-Quinn's Advantage Fertilization Medium(HTF), Sage, USA–Catalogue No. 1020.
- Day 1 to Day 3-Quinn's Advantage Cleavage Medium– Catalogue No. 1026
- Day 3 to Day 5-Quinn's Advantage Blastocyst Medium- Catalogue No. 1029

All the above media were supplemented with 10 percent (v/v) of Human Serum Albumin(100 mg/ml), Sage-Catalogue No. 3003

All embryos were cultured individually in 10 microlitre droplets under oil (Sage,Catalogue No. 4008), Sage. Two extra drops were accommodated in each dish to serve as wash drops.

Prepared dishes were equilibrated overnight at 37°C in an atmosphere of 5% CO_2/5% O_2/90% N2.

Embryo checks-All embryo assessments were done under an inverted microscope (at 200 to 400 × magnification) provided with a heated stage. All media changes were conducted on heated stages of stereomicroscopes. The dishes containing embryos were not left out of the CO_2 incubator for more than 2 minutes.

Day 1 Check

Oocytes were checked for fertilization at 16 to 17.5 hours post insemination or ICSI. Normally fertilized oocytes with 2 pronuclei were transferred to dishes containing cleavage medium. Care was taken to wash each oocyte in the cleavage medium wash drops prior to transfer, to avoid carry over of fertilization medium.

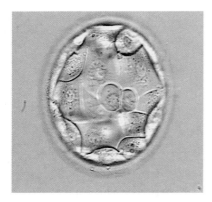

FIGURE 44.17: Day 5 blastocyst (3 BB)

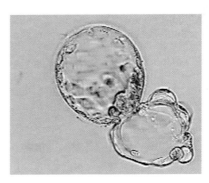

FIGURE 44.18: Hatching blastocyst

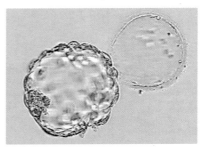

FIGURE 44.19: Hatched blastocyst

Day 2 Checks

These were done on the morning of Day 2 (41 to 44 hours post insemination or ICSI). Embryos were scored as described earlier. MNB embryos were not used for subsequent transfer unless they were the only ones available and provided the MNBs were not present in 100 percent of the blastomeres. No media change occurred on day 2.

Day 3 Checks

These were done on the morning of Day 3 (64 to 68 hours post insemination or ICSI). Embryos were scored and degree of compaction if any was recorded for each embryo. All embryos that were 6 cell or beyond were transferred to BCM, after thorough washing in BCM wash drops.

No Checks Were Done on Day 4

Day 5 Checks

On the morning of Day 5 (112 to 116 hours post insemination or ICSI), embryos were checked for blastocyst development (Figures 44.17 to 44.19). Assessment of blastocysts was done according to Gardner's classification for both ICM and trophectoderm.

• Indira Hinduja • Firuza Kharas • Kusum Zaveri

45

Intracytoplasmic Sperm Injection (ICSI)

The birth of Louise Brown following fertilization of an oocyte *in vitro* and transfer of the resulting embryo in the uterus was a historical event in medical science. Initially, the technique of *in vitro* fertilization and embryo transfer (IVF-ET) was advocated for irreparably damaged fallopian tubes.[1] Subsequently other forms of infertility, such as unexplained infertility,[2] endometriosis,[3] cervical factor,[4] immunological infertility[5] and male factor[6] were treated successfully utilizing this technique. The pregnancy rates in male infertility were disappointing because fertilization rates were low,[7-10] which in turn are directly proportional to abnormal semen parameters. Since medical and surgical line of treatment did not improve semen quality, efforts were directed to improve the fertilization rate with the existing sperm parameters. The technique of micromanipulation of human gametes was a breakthrough, bypassing the major blocks for sperm penetration namely the zona pellucida and sperm cell membrane.

Direct injection of spermatozoa into the cytoplasm of the oocytes of various animal species has resulted in the birth of live young ones.[11] Initially, in humans this technique did not have much success.[12] The zonal procedures such as zona drilling,[13] zona-cracking[14] and zona dissection[15] followed by macroinsemination methods of assisted fertilization resulted in occasional pregnancies. In 1988, Ng[16] and his associates were the first to report the birth of a baby by injecting spermatozoa into the subzonal

space (SUZI), formerly called microinsemination of sperm transfer (MIST). These authors, however, expressed caution as direct ooplasmic sperm injection was an invasive technique with a high incidence of oocyte degeneration.[17]

In 1992, Palermo *et al*[18] announced the first live human birth by intracytoplasmic sperm injection (ICSI), followed by a series of publications documenting significantly higher successes in fertilization, implantation and live birth.[19, 20] When compared for severe male factor infertility and success rates, ICSI performed better than SUZI.[19, 21]

Today, the technique of ICSI has replaced a number of treatment modalities for male factor infertility and has achieved fertilization and pregnancies with microinjection of spermatozoa or precursor cells from the ejaculate, epididymis or testes, regardless of the underlying pathophysiology.

INDICATIONS FOR INTRACYTOPLASMIC SPERM INJECTION (ICSI)

ICSI can be applied in the following:
  i. Male factor infertility
 ii. Female factor infertility
iii. Preimplantation genetic diagnosis (whenever indicated).

Male Factor Infertility

Ejaculated Sperm

a. Normal sperm parameters:
   i. Presence of antisperm antibodies

ii. Repeated fertilization failure
iii. Cryopreserved sperm
b. Abnormal sperm parameters:
    i. Oligoasthenoteratozoospermia (OAT)
    ii. Globozoospermia
    iii. Necrozoospermia
    iv. Immotile cilia syndrome.

Epididymal Sperm

i. Congenital absence of vas deferens
ii. Acquired vasal block
iii. Failed vasoepididymal anastomosis
iv. Ejaculatory duct obstruction.

Testicular Sperm

i. Failure to retreive sperm from epididymis
ii. Testicular failure: Maturation arrest, Germ cell aplasia.

Ejaculatory Disorders

i. Anejaculation
ii. Retrograde ejaculation.

Female Factor Infertility

a. Low number of oocytes
b. Oocyte abnormality (like thick zona)
c. Repeated failure of fertilization following IVF.

Preimplantation Genetic Diagnosis

Normal sperm parameters and deviation from these criteria have been reported by the World Health Organization (WHO).[22] Conventional IVF-ET has shown poor prognosis in cases having sperm parameters below the value reported by WHO.[23] The practice of ICSI has proved that there is no difference in the fertilization rate in men with demonstrable or suspected male factor infertility. Nagy et al, in 1995,[24] have shown, the count and motility of sperm are least important for fertilization with ICSI. Abnormal sperm head characteristics are attributed to small or large head size, amorphous head and globozoospermia. There is no significant difference in fertilization with small or large head, where as chromosomal aberrations in spermatozoa with amorphous

head and sperm with rounded head has shown very low fertilization rates.[25, 26]

The success of ICSI diminished considerably with low sperm motility, especially of ejaculated sperm. Immotile spermatozoa are differentiated from dead sperm by hyperosmotic swelling test (HOS) for selection of sperm for ICSI.[27] There is no significant difference in fertilization rates between spermatozoa from the ejaculate in OAT, epididymal and testicular spermatozoa in obstructive and testicular spermatozoa in non-obstructive azoospermia[28] as also sperm retrieved from the urinary bladder in cases of retrograde ejaculation. The comparison of fresh and cryopreserved spermatozoa has no difference in fertilization and pregnancy rates.[29]

The incidence of testicular cancer has increased two to four fold over the last 40 years. Cryo-preservation of spermatozoa, even of poor quality for future use in ICSI has become part of the treatment modality. The treatment of autoimmune infertility in the male is very disappointing. ICSI in such cases is very effective and the results are not affected by the type of immunoglobulin bound to spermatozoa.

When preimplantation genetic diagnosis is indicated, ICSI has an advantage over IVF, since during blastomere biopsy, contamination with genetic material of additional spermatozoa present on the zona or in the perivitelline space is precluded.

Failure of fertilization in conventional IVF, with normal or abnormal semen parameters could be due to inability of spermatozoa to penetrate the zona pellucida, because of gamete abnormalities or failure of oocyte activation or decondensation of sperm head nucleus. Currently, ICSI is the most effective technique to overcome failure of fertilization. Among the female factors, less number of oocytes, thick zona and oocyte defects are common causes of infertility. Traditional IVF yielded poor results and ICSI comparatively has shown better results.

Procedural Details

The success of ICSI, besides quality of gametes depends upon skill and experience of the operator, microtools and the actual sperm injection procedure.

In order to obtain a large number and uniformly matured oocytes, the ovarian stimulation protocol is very important. The combination of gonadotrophin releasing hormone agonist starting from 23rd day of the previous cycle, with human menopausal gonadotrophin for development of the follicles, is commonly used. Ovulation is induced by human chorionic gonadotrophin (10,000 IU) when at least three follicles are equal to or more than 18 mm and serum estradiol level is1000 pg/ml. The USG guided transvaginal oocyte retrieval is carried out 36 hours after hCG administration.

Oocyte Preparation

To assess the maturity and to allow precise sperm injection, denudation of corona cumulus complex is an essential step before ICSI. The enzyme hyaluronidase is used for decoronising the oocyte, followed by repeated mechanical aspiration of oocyte in and out of the pipette. The high concentration of hyaluronidase or prolonged exposure to it raises the problem of premature activation and degeneration of oocyte. Different concentrations of hyaluronidase were used by Vander Velde et al.[30] who showed that 10 IU/ml in combination with a pipette size of at least 1000 μm can be used successfully. Denuded oocytes are observed under an inverted microscope for presence or absence of germinal vesicle, and presence or absence of polar body. All oocytes with first polar body are selected for ICSI (Figure 45.1).

Preparation of Sperm

The sperm preparation technique for the selection of morphologically normal and motile sperm from ejaculate, epididymal aspirate, testicular biopsy, frozen and thawed semen sample or from urinary bladder is a critical aspect of ICSI.

Sperm Preparation for Assisted Fertilization

Accurate assessment of semen samples prior to the procedure, gives the information to choose

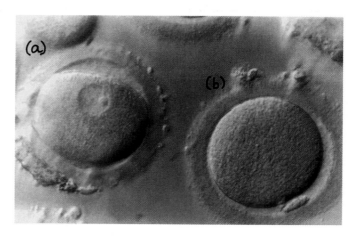

FIGURE 45.1: Oocyte maturing is checked after cumulus-corona cell removal: (a) An immature oocyte showing presence of germinal vesicle. (b) A typical mature metaphase II oocyte showing the presence of polar body 1

the appropriate sperm preparation technique for ICSI. The sperm sample showing good count and a good forward progressive motility can be prepared using standard swim-up technique. Discontinuous Percoll or buoyant density gradient centrifugation is used for samples having low count and poor forward motility, and a high concentration of debris.

Standard Swim-up Method

The entire ejaculate is divided into a number of tubes each containing 1 ml of semen sample over which is layered 2 ml of the sperm preparation medium. These tubes are tightly capped and are allowed to stand in a dark environment at room temperature for 1 hour. The middle cloudy layer is aspirated and centrifuged at 200 g for 5 minutes. Supernatant is removed and the pellet is mixed with 2 ml medium and centrifuged again for 5 minutes. Supernatant is discarded and the pellet is layered with 1 ml medium and incubated in 5 percent CO_2 environment for a period of 30 minutes before insemination. The count and motility is assessed before use. Sometimes when the semen volume is low, the entire semen sample is mixed with one and a half times volume of medium and centrifuged and pellet is washed twice as described above.

Discontinuous Density Gradient Centrifugation

Since percoll is no more used in ART, buoyant-density gradient is commonly used for poor quality semen sample and the kits are commercially available. Two or three discontinuous gradients are used to isolate the motile sperm fraction. Buoyant density gradients apparently protect the sperm from the trauma of centrifugation and better quality of sperm can be recovered. Two step gradient i.e., 80 percent followed by 40 percent is done and the semen sample is layered on top of the 40 percent buoyant in a conical centrifuge tube. The tube is centrifuged for 20 min at 600 g, the pellet or lower most 80 percent layer is washed twice with sperm preparation medium and final pellet is layered by 0.4 ml of medium and incubated for 30 minutes. Similarly a mini gradient (95/70/50) technique is used for a very poor sample. The semen sample is diluted 1:1 with the culture medium and layered over 0.3 ml each of 95, 70 and 50 percent, centrifuged at 600 g for 5 min. The pellet is resuspended in 0.5 ml of medium and centrifuged for 5 minutes at 200 g. The supernatant is discarded. The pellet is layered by 0.2-0.4 ml of medium.

High Speed Centrifugation and Washing

The sample having occasional spermatozoa or cryptozoospermia are directly centrifuged at 1800 g for 5 min. The pellet is washed with a small volume of medium and centrifuged at 200 g for 5 min. This pellet with minimal quantity of medium is incubated in the form of a droplet which is overlayered with mineral oil.

The Hypo-osmotic Swelling (HOS) Test

The HOS test determines viability and functional integrity of the sperm membrane. The live spermatozoa withstand the hypo-osmotic environment and their tails swell and get coiled. The dead spermatozoa whose plasma membrane is broken do not show swelling of the tail. The sperm with coiled tail is selected for microinjection.

Collection of Sperm

In case of azoospermia, sample can be obtained from the epididymis by open microsurgical technique or by microepididymal sperm aspiration (MESA). This requires general anesthesia. However, a much simpler procedure like percutaneous epididymal sperm aspiration (PESA) can be performed under local anesthesia. In case of failure of retrieving sperm from the epididymis, needle aspiration of sperm from the testis Testicular sperm aspiration (TESA) or Testicular sperm fine needle aspiration (TEFNA) is often successful in harvesting sufficient sperm for ICSI. Occasionally open testicular biopsy becomes necessary when all other techniques fail to obtain spermatozoa.

In cases having retrograde ejaculatory dysfunction, before ejaculation the bladder is emptied via a catheter and approximately 20 ml of the culture medium is instilled. After ejaculation, the bladder is again emptied and the entire sample is collected and centrifuged. The resulting pellet is washed twice, the supernatant is discarded and the pellet is re-suspended in the medium.

Epididymal sperm can be prepared by buoyant density gradient centrifugation or swim-up technique. The sample with fewer spermatozoa is washed twice in micro-drops and the final pellet is deposited in petri-dishes covered with mineral oil for motile spermatozoa to swim out to the periphery of the droplets.

The testicular biopsy tissue is either crushed between two microslides or is dissected by two needles or microscissors under the microscope. The other methods are either to milk out the contents of the tubules or slit open the tubules for release of the cells. Incubation at 32°C for a short time may further help to release cells. It is important to cryopreserve the remaining sperm or tissue for future use.

In cases with severe testicular dysfunction only sperm precursor cells, round and elongating or elongated spermatids can be identified. The fertilization and pregnancy rates are extremely low following use of spermatid injection for ICSI. Round spermatids must be distinguished from other round cells such as spermatogonia, spermatocytes, leukocytes, lymphocytes and erythrocytes. The identification is according to size, shape, amount of cytoplasm and size of tail. The round spermatid is round with smooth nucleus and three-dimensional appearance. The acrosomal structure may be observed as a bright spot or small protrusion on one side of the nucleus. Elongated spermatid has an elongated nucleus at one side of the cell and a large cytoplasm on the other side surrounding the developing tail.

Microtools

The success of ICSI also depends upon the microtools. The preparation of microtools is time consuming and painstaking and requires an expertise on the job. Sterile and ready-to-use microtools are also commercially available. The holding pipette is used to hold the oocyte at the blunt end. The outer diameter of the holding pipette is of 0.080 to 0.150 mm and the inner diameter is of 0.018 to 0.025 mm. The outer diameter of the injection pipette is 0.0060 to 0.007 mm and the inner diameters of 0.005 to 0.006 mm. Both these microtools are bent to an angle of ~30° to 35° at the distal end. This angle facilitates horizontal positioning within culture dishes.

The smooth and gentle injection of spermatozoon in ooplasm is the key to success of ICSI. Good quality microtools and appropriate optical system having Hoffman modulation for better depth and differentiation, equipped with two manipulators in order to allow microinjection are available. In order to prevent oocyte damage, microscopes are mounted with heating stage to maintain the temperature at 37°C. Two identical micromanipulators are mounted on the microscope to allow holding pipette on the left side to hold an oocyte and injection pipette on the right side to inject a spermatozoon. The manipulators are either mechanical or electrical for coarse movements having hanging or vertical joysticks for fine movements. Both the injectors and micropipette holders are connected to air tight 0.8 ml glass syringe via Teflon tubing,

which is filled with mineral oil. The equipment is installed on vibration free table-top in the dust free laboratory. The instrumentation and methodology is also discussed in the next chapter.

PREPARATION FOR ICSI

Micropipettes

Thin walled glass capillary tubes (1 mm OD, 0.6 mm ID) are used for the preparation of micropipettes and oocyte-denuding pipettes.

The micropipettes are fabricated using the puller, and polished and angled at 35° using the microforge.

The sharp and beveled tips for microinjection needles are created using the Grinder/beveler.

These micropipettes are washed in sterile water and stored in large clean sterile petri-dishes using moulding clay or tape which holds them in place.

The inner and outer diameters of the micropipettes are as follows:

Holding pipette   : ID 20-30 μ OD 80-100 μ
Microinjection needle : ID 5-8 μ   OD 10-15 μ

Readymade micropipettes are also available commercially.

For denudation of oocytes, three types of pipettes are used:
1. Fire-polished pasteur pipettes.
2. 170 μ denuding pipettes.
3. 140 μ denuding pipettes.

Media and Chemicals

1. EBSS supplemented with 21 mM HEPES, 4 mM sodium bicarbonate, 0.16 mM pyruvate, 100 U/ml penicillin, and 50 ug /ml streptomycin.

                    or

   Commercially available ready-to-use sequential media.
2. Polyvinylpyrrolidone (PVP)
   Ten percent PVP prepared in IVF culture media.

   Preparation Add 2 ml IVF culture media to 0.2 gm PVP (i.e. 10%). Vortex in cyclo-mixer till PVP dissolves totally. Centrifuge for 10 minutes to remove all air bubbles. Filter with 0.45 μ filter into small aliquots. Store in deep freeze till further use.

3. Hyaluronidase
   800 IU/ml hyaluronidase prepared as stock solution in EBSS, filtered and kept in small aliquots in the deep freeze. Used as a final concentration of 20 IU/ml in IVF culture media.
   (Add 10 μl of stock to 400 μl of IVF culture media during preparation of denudation dish)

4. Mineral oil
   Sterile mineral oil equilibrated in 5 percent CO_2 overnight.

ICSI PROCEDURE

Prepare hyaluronidase denuding dish overnight. Overlay with sterile, washed, equilibrated mineral oil.

1. Transfer 3-4 oocytes into hyaluronidase drop with firepolished pipette. Aspirate few times till cumuli is removed and only corona radiata remains.
2. Transfer to drop (1) of IVF culture media with 170 μ pipette. Aspirate till oocyte passes easily.
3. Transfer to drop (2) of IVF culture media with 140 μ pipette. Aspirate till most of corona is removed.
4. Transfer to drop (3) of IVF culture media with 140 μ pipette. Aspirate till oocyte is complete denuded.
5. Transfer to wash-dish. Wash thoroughly in 3 drops of IVF media. Incubate in IVF culture media drop for 2-3 hrs. before doing ICSI.

Prepare ICSI dishes (as shown in the diagram). Culture drops are prepared using oocyte wash buffer. Incubate these dishes for at least 1/2 hour before loading the sperm and oocytes.

After ICSI procedure, wash oocytes in wash dish and culture them in IVF culture media at 37°C and 5 percent CO_2.

The procedure is carried out in specially prepared injection dishes as described above. The dish is prepared by pipetting small droplets of HEPES buffered cultured medium for individual oocyte. Two large drops in the center, one of the sperm sample and the second of 10 percent polyvinylpyrrolidone (PVP) used to impair sperm motility prior to immobilization and aspiration into the injection pipette. In case the sperm count is around 5 million, 3.0–5.0 μl of sperm suspension is added to PVP. In case the sperm count is very low, morphologically normal sperm is selected from the sperm droplet and brought to the PVP droplet to immobilize it by touching the tail with the injection needle before injection. The viscous solution of PVP facilitates sperm handling and prevents the sperm cells from sticking to the injection pipette during the procedure. Selected immobilized sperm is aspirated in the injection pipette, tail first, and positioned ~10-15 μm from the tip. The oocyte droplet is brought in the position. Using the two microtools, i.e. the holding and the injecting pipette, the oocyte is rotated to position it so that the polar body is at 6 or 12 O'clock to minimize the possibility of damaging the meiotic spindle. The injection pipette is brought closer to the oocyte and the sperm is brought near the beveled tip. The pipette is advanced through the zona and ooplasm until the needle tip almost reaches a 9 O'clock position. The membrane may rupture spontaneously or may be ruptured by gentle negative pressure. When it breaks, a sudden flux of cytoplasm is seen in the injection pipette. The sperm is injected slowly into the oocyte with a minimum amount of the fluid after which the needle is gently removed. This procedure is repeated for all the other oocytes to be injected.

Once the injection procedure is complete, the oocytes are washed four times in the culture medium and incubated overnight in the CO_2 incubation. Sixteen to eighteen hours after injection, the oocytes are assessed for the presence of pronuclei under an inverted microscope (Figure 45.2). Further evaluation for cleavage is done 24 hours later.

The failure of fertilization could be due to faulty technique, expulsion of spermatozoon, non-motility of the spermatozoon or the injection of round headed spermatozoon. In some cases, the failure may be due to injecting a morphologically abnormal or fragile oocyte or

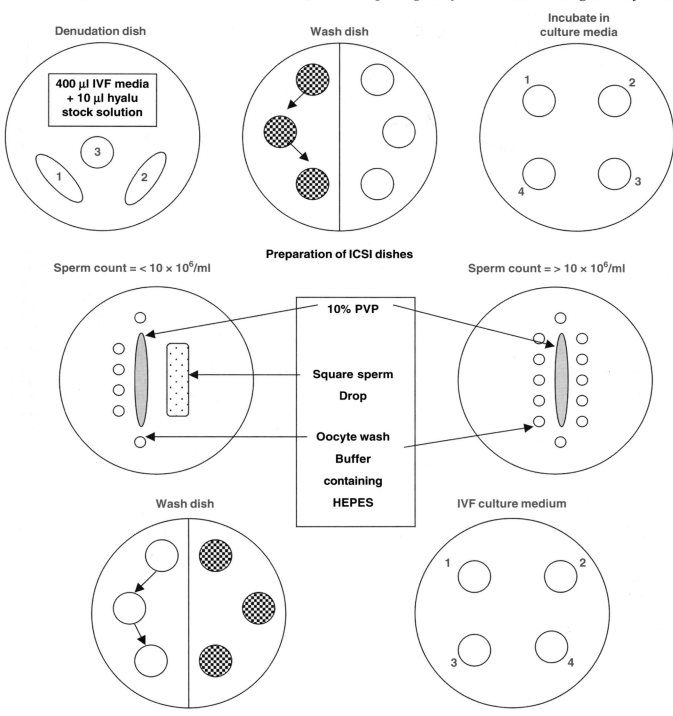

Preparation of ICSI dishes

Flow chart for ICSI procedure

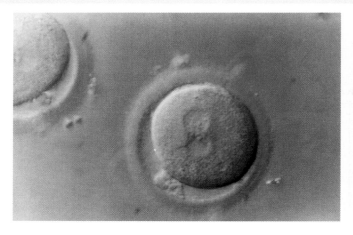

FIGURE 45.2: A normally fertilized oocyte showing presence of two clearly visible pronuclei

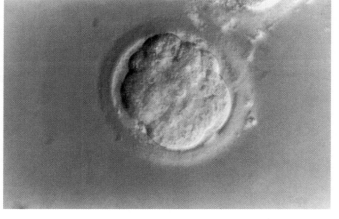

FIGURE 45.4: Day 5 embryo showing good compaction

some occult gamete abnormality, which may be responsible for unexplained infertility.

Observation for fertilization is very important because the oocyte having one or more than two pronuclei also have a potential to cleave similar to the two pronuclei zygotes. Such zygotes are not selected for transfer. On the third day, the quality of the embryo is evaluated for the number and size of blastomeres and presence of fragments[31] (Figure 45.3). Every clinic has its own criteria according to their success rate for the transfer of embryos. Some prefer to transfer at the 2-8 cell stage on day two or three of the ovum pick-up (OPU) or culture further in

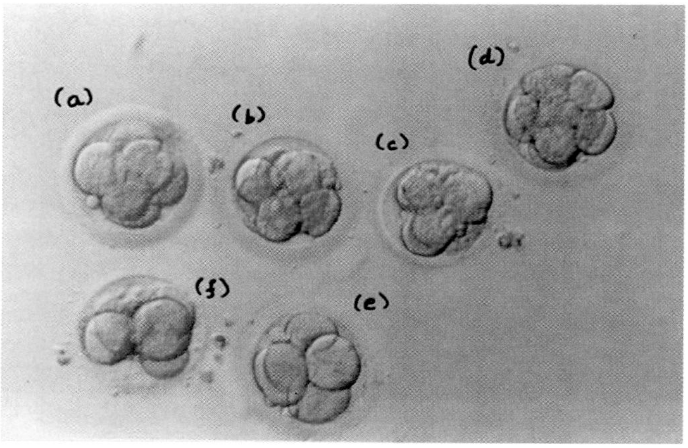

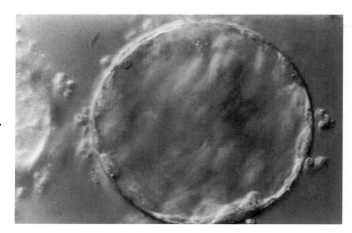

FIGURE 45.5: A well-expanded blastocyst

sequential media until blastocysts form on day five or six of OPU (Figures 45.4 to 45.6). A maximum of three embryos or blastocysts are transferred, however; in older women transfer of more than three embryos have given better results. Recently, assisted hatching on day 3 of retrieval either by laser or acid Tyrode, especially in women over 35 years of age and those with repeated failure of implantation is routinely done.

Our experience of 740 ICSI cycles from January 1997 to December 1999 includes 8.9 percent using ejaculatory spermatozoa, 7.9 percent epidydimal, 2.8 percent testicular spermatozoa and 0.3 percent spermatid injec-

FIGURE 45.3: Grading of cleaved embryos (clockwise) (a), (b), (d) and (e)—Grade I embryos, 6-8 cell, (c) and (f)—Grade II embryos, with 10 percent fragmentation

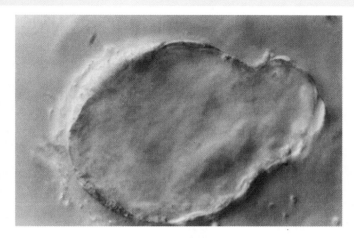

FIGURE 45.6: Blastocyst showing early hatching

tions. ICSI procedure was not performed in 20 cases. The procedure could not be performed either because there were no metaphase II (M II) oocytes or spermatozoa were not available for microinjection. The total number of oocytes retrieved were 6734 (9.1%) per treatment cycle. 87 percent of the oocytes were at M II, 4 percent at M I and 9 percent at the germinal vesicle (GV) stage. Successful micro-injections were performed in 97 percent of the cases, including those oocytes that matured later (M I and GV). 71 percent fertilization was attained with 2 PN, 2 percent with single PN and 2.9 percent with 3 PN.

The clinical pregnancy rate is 43 percent in cases where the transfer was done on the second or third day of retrieval, whereas it is 49 percent when at least one blastocyst is transferred along with other embryos of either morula or compaction stage on day 5 or 6 after retrieval. 17 percent of these pregnancies have ended in first trimester abortions and 3.2 percent in ectopic pregnancies.

The complete information up to six months after birth is available in 200 babies born with ICSI. Low birth weight was seen in five sets of twins and one triplet gestation. Ninety-three were males and one hundred and seven were females. Major malformation requiring surgery was found in three children. Meningocele in one, harelip cleft palate in the second and inguinal hernia in the third.

Future Directions

Male infertility is the reason for infertility in almost 50 percent of all infertile patients. In about 30 percent of these cases, genetic disorder is suspected. Severe oligoasthenoteratozoospermia or azoospermia is the presenting finding. The major breakthrough in the treatment of such males was the introduction of ICSI, which requires the presence of only very few vital spermatozoa for injection. According to Engel and Schmidt,[32] assisted reproduction does not significantly influence the human genetic pool; but the potential risk factors involving genetically transmitted diseases and conceiving a malformed child still exists. Therefore the evaluations of chromosomal status of the couple and their inheritance is of utmost importance prior to selection for ICSI.

Men who are affected by congenital absence of bilateral vas deferens have 60 percent heterozygous mutations in the cystic fibrosis transmembrane conductance regulator (CFTR) gene including compound heterozygotes. i.e. different mutations in each gene copy.[33] Patients with obstructive azoospermia should be investigated for mutations in CFTR gene. The deletions of the Y chromosome and the androgene receptors are future additional investigations. Age-related aneuploidy is also an important factor that may lead to chromosomally abnormal off spring.

Preimplantation genetic diagnosis (PGD) is an important step to prevent the transmission of genetic disorders. Prospective PGD facilities have become the vital component of the laboratories that cater to assisted fertilization techniques. In other words, PGD facilities are a part of an ICSI laboratory. The delivery rate per cycle of PGD is similar to that of IVF or ICSI. The long-term follow up of children born with ICSI and applications of PGD will show the possible risks, and outcome of both the procedures.

REFERENCES

1. Steptoe PC, Edwards RG. Birth after the re-implantation of a human embryo (letter). Lancet 1978;2:366.
2. Lopata A, Johnson WIH, Leeton JF, et al. Use of in vitro fertilization in the infertile couple. In: Pepperell RJ, Hudson B, Wood C (Eds.): "The infertile couple". Edinburgh, Churchill Livingstone 1980;209-28.

3. Mahadevan MM, Trounson AO, Leeton JF. The relationship of tubal blockage, infertility of unknown cause, suspected male infertility and endometriosis to succes of in-vitro fertilization and embryo transfer. Fertil Steril 1983;40:755-62.

4. Hewett J, Cohen J, Krishnaswamy V, et al. Treatment of idiopathic infertility, cervical mucus hostility and male infertility. Artificial insemination with husband's semen or in-vitro fertilization? Fertil Steril 1985;44:350-55.

5. Aitken RJ. A free-radical theory of male-infertility. Reprod Fertil Devp 1994;6:19-24.

6. Yovich JL, Stanger JD, Yovich JM, et al. Treatment of male infertility by in vitro fertilization. Lancet 1984;2:169-70.

7. de Kretser DM, Kerr JB. The cytology of the testis. In: Knobil E, Neill JD(Eds.): Physiology and Reproduction. Raven Press, New York, 1994;1177-1290.

8. Kruger TF, Acosta AA, Simmons KF, et al. Predicting value of abnormal sperm morphology factor in in vitro fertilization. Fertil Steril 1988;49:112-17.

9. Oehninger S, Acosta AA, Kruger T et al. Failure of fertilization in in vitro fertilization: the "occult" male factor. J IVF ET 1988;5:181-87.

10. Yates CA, Trounson AO, deKretser DM. Male factor infertility and in vitro fertilization. 4th. International congress in Andrology, Florence, Italy 1989;14-18:Abstract, 263.

11. Markert CL. Fertilization of mammalian eggs by sperm injection. J Exp Zool, 1983;228:195-201.

12. Lazendorf SE, Malomey MK, Veek LL, et al. A preclinical evaluation of pronuclear formation by microinjection of human spermatozoa into human oocytes. Fertil Steril 1988:49:835-42.

13. Gordon JM, Grunfeld L, Garrisi GJ, et al. Fertilization of human oocytes by sperm from infertile males after zona pellucida drilling. Fertil Steril 1988;50:68-73.

14. Odawara Y, Lopata A. A zona opening procedure for improving in vitro fertilization at low sperm concentration: A mouse model. Fertil Steril 1989;51:699-704.

15. Cohen J, Maltev H, Fchilly C, et al. Implantation of embryo after partial opening of oocyte zona pellucida to facilitate sperm penetration. Lancet 1988;2:162.

16. Ng S-C, Bongso TA, Ratnam SS, et al. Pregnancy after transfer of multiple sperm under the zona. Lancet ii, 1988;790.

17. Ng S-C, Bongso TA, Ratnam SS. Microinjection of human oocytes: A technique for severe oligoastheno-teratozoospermia. Fertil Steril 1991;56:1117-23.

18. Palermo G, Joris H, Devroey P, et al. Pregnancies after intracytoplasmic injection of a single spermatozoon into an oocyte. Lancet, 1992;340:17-18.

19. Palermo G, Joris H, Derbe M-P, et al. Sperm characteristics and outcome of human assisted fertilization by subzonal insemination and intracytoplasmic sperm injection. Fertil Steril 1993;59:826-35.

20. Van Steirteghem AC, Liu J, Joris H, et al. Higher success rate by intracytoplasmic sperm injection than by subzonal insemination. Report of a second series of 300 consecutive treatment cycles. Hum Reprod 1993a;8:1055-60.

21. Abdalla IH, Leonard T, Pryor J, et al. Comparison of SUZI and ICSI for severe male factor. Hum Reprod 1995;10:2941-44.

22. World Health Organization. Laboratory manual for Examination of human semen and sperm-cervical mucus interaction. 3rd edition. Cambridge University Press, New York 1992.

23. Ryder T, Mobberley M, Hughes L, et al. A survey of the ultrastructural defects associated with absent of impaired human sperm motility. Fertil Steril 1990;53:556-60.

24. Nagy ZP, Liu J, Joris H, et al. The result of intra-cytoplasmic sperm injection is not related to any of the three basic sperm parameters. Hum Reprod 1995;10:1123-29.

25. Lee JD, Kamiguchi Y, Yanagimachi R. Analysis of chromosome constitution of human spermatozoa with normal and aberrant head morphology after injection into mouse oocytes. Hum Reprod 1996;11:1942-46.

26. Rybouchkin A, Dozortsev D, De Sutter P, et al. Analysis of the oocyte activating capacity and chromosomol complement of round-headed human spermatozoa by injection into mouse oocyte. Hum Reprod 1996;11:2170-75.

27. Casper RF, Meriano JS, Jarvi KA et al. The hypo-osmotic swelling test for selection; of viable sperm for intracytoplasmic sperm injection in men with complete asthenozoospermia. Fertil Steril 1996;65:972-76.

28. Ghazzawi IM, Sarraf MG, Taher MR et al. Comparison of the fertilizing capability of spermatozoa from ejaculates, epididymal aspirates and testicular biopsis using intracytoplasmic sperm injection. Hum Reprod 1998;13:348-52.

29. Friedler S, Raziel A, SofferY et al. Intracytoplasmic injection of fresh and cryopreserved testicular spermatozoa in patients with non-obstructive azoospermia—a comparative study. Fertil Steril 1997;68:892-97.

30. Van de Velde H, Nagy ZP, Joris H et al. Effect of different hyaluronidase concentrations and mechanical procedures for cumulus cell removal on the outcome of intracytoplasmic sperm injection. Hum Reprod 1997;12:2246-50.

31. Staessen C, Camus M, Khan I et al. An 18-month survey of infertility treatment by in vitro fertilization, gamete and zygote intrafallopian transfer, and replacement of frozen-thawed embryos. J IVF ET 1989;6:22-29.

32. Engel W, Schmidt M. Gibt es genetische Risiken der mikroassistierten Reproduction? Fertilitat 1995;11:214-28.

33. Patrizio P, Asch RH. The relationship of the congenital absence of the vas deferens (CBAVD), cystic fibrosis (CF) mutations, and epididymal sperm. Assist Reprod Rev 1994;4:95-100.

• Swee-Lian Liow, Soon-Chye Ng

46

Intracytoplasmic Sperm Injection: Instrumentation and Methodology

INTRODUCTION

For the last one-and-a-half decade of the 20th century, many micromanipulation techniques such as partial zona dissection (PZD; Cohen *et al*, 1988), subzonal sperm injection (SUZI; Ng *et al*, 1988) and intracytoplasmic sperm injection (ICSI; Palermo *et al*, 1992) have been developed and refined to overcome some of the problems of human infertility. However, direct injection of a single sperm into an oocyte provided a major breakthrough in the field of assisted fertilization in human when Palermo *et al* (1992) reported the first human pregnancies following ICSI. Since then ICSI has evolved over the last few years as the most effective treatment for severe oligo-asthenoteratospermia with many IVF centers reporting a significant improvement in pregnancy rate and take-home baby rate. With modifications from the ICSI procedure, it is also now possible to inject testicular spermatozoa and spermatids directly into the oocyte to assist conception and delivery of live babies.

As in all micromanipulation techniques, ICSI involves intricate and precise maneuvers of microtools on the oocytes and sperm under an inverted microscope. Although the skill and experience of the embryologist in performing ICSI is important, the outcome of the procedure depends largely on the quality of the microtools such as the microinjection needles. Other factors such as equipment and environment within the IVF laboratory can also affect the success of the

ICSI programme. The instrumentation and methodology of ICSI have also been reviewed by Mansour (1998) and discussed by Joris *et al* (1998).

The Micromanipulation System

Requirements of a microscope for ICSI and other micromanipulation techniques:

1. An inverted microscope with × 10, × 20 and × 40 objectives.
2. A magnification of × 400 is required for ICSI.
3. A long working distance condenser
4. A heating stage set at 38°C.

The Hoffman Modulation Contrast system is preferred to the Normarski system [also known as differential interference contrast (DIC)] as the former is designed to compensate for the effect of plastic; in Normarski system clear images can be obtained from glass dishes.

Micromanipulation system (Figure 46.1a) is comprised of:

1. A set of left and right arms of the micromanipulators that are either electronically or mechanically controlled by their respective joysticks (Figure 46.1b).
2. A set of joysticks that allow control of coarse and fine three-dimensional (x-y-z) positioning and also precise linear displacement simultaneously. The joysticks are either hydraulically driven based on de Fonbrune's system or electronically driven. A combination of both types of joystick is also possible (Figure 46.1c).

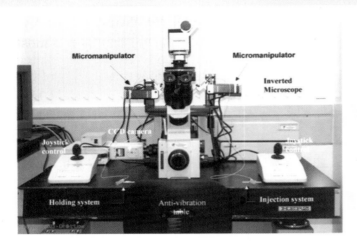

FIGURE 46.1A: The micromanipulation system

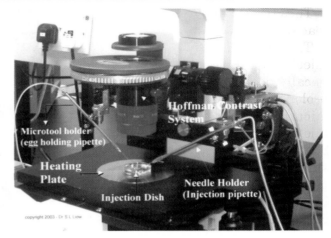

FIGURE 46.1B: Micromanipulation stage

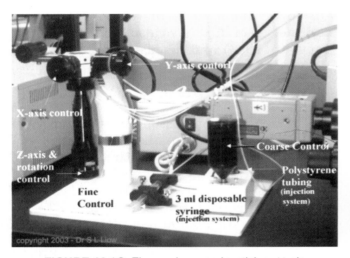

FIGURE 46.1C: Fine and coarse joystick controls
(Narishige, Japan)

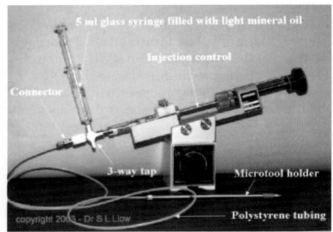

FIGURE 46.1D: Lubricant-filled injection and holding units

3. A holding unit that is similar to the injection unit. Both of these units are either filled entirely with lubricant or air (Figure 46.1d)
4. An injection unit that is comprised of a completely air-tight syringe connected to the micropipette holder by a Teflon plastic tubing with air-tight fittings (Figure 46.1e)

The microscope and the micromanipulation system are mounted on an anti-vibration table to prevent vibrations from interfering with the injection procedure.

Accessories to the micromanipulation system:
1. A high quality camera
2. A television monitor
3. A video tape recorder/player

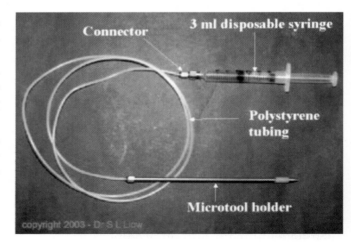

FIGURE 46.1E: Air-filled injection and holding units

These accessories are useful for documentation, teaching and demonstration purposes.

The micromanipulators that control the injection and holding systems should be ergonomically positioned to prevent back pains due to prolonged work (an occupational hazard) on the micromanipulation system. For instance, the injection is done from the right micromanipulator but the joystick controller is placed on the left side of the microscope. Likewise, the holding pipette is placed on the left micromanipulator but its movements are controlled by the joystick controller on the right side of the microscope.

Preparation of Capillary Tubes

Capillary tubes made from borosilicate glass with inner diameter (ID) of 0.75 mm and outer diameter (OD) of 1.0 mm and a length of 10 cm are used for the preparation of holding pipettes and microinjection needles (Figure 46.2). Prior to use, the capillary tubes are soaked in 10 percent HCl for 24 hours in a glass cylinder and rinsed with Milli-Q water twenty times to remove all traces of the acid. They are then dried in an oven at 150°C for 4 hours. Alternatively, the capillary tubes are washed by sonication for 30 min in Milli-Q water containing 2 percent detergent and rinsing in Milli-Q water for at least 30 min. These steps are repeated but sonication is done without detergent. The capillary tubes are then dried in hot air and sterilized at 120°C for 6 hours (Joris *et al*, 1998).

Preparation of Microinjection Pipettes

Injection of sperm into the ooplasm is the most invasive micromanipulation technique in assisted conception. Hence, the design and quality of the microtools, especially the injection pipettes is of utmost importance as the size and shape of these needles will determine the success or failure of a micromanipulation procedure.

The instruments that are necessary to make microinjection needles are:
1. Micropipette puller
2. Microforge
3. Microbeveller or micropipette grinder.

Micropipette Puller

A horizontal micropipette puller is preferred to the vertical one as the former produces needles of uniform shapes (Figure 46.3). An example of a good pipette puller is the one produced by Sutter Instruments, USA (Model P-87 or P-97). The quantity of heat, pull speed and strength can be stored in the programs. The desired shape of the needle should be one that has a long and uniform tapering end with a length of about 10 mm. The variation in the diameter of the taper end of the needle is approximately 1 µm per 100 µm. The internal diameter (ID) of the needle should be between 5 and 8 µm. This is essential as the amount of ooplasm and fluid aspirated into the injection pipette before re-injection is directly related to the inner diameter of the injection pipette.

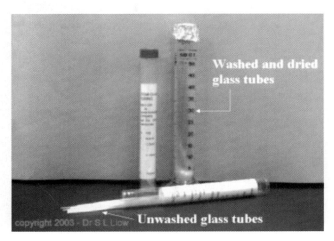

FIGURE 46.2: Preparation of capillary tubes

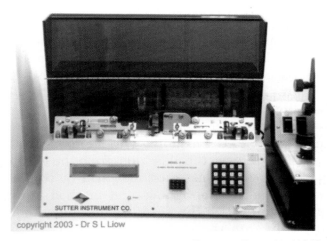

FIGURE 46.3: Micropipette puller (Sutter puller p-87, USA)

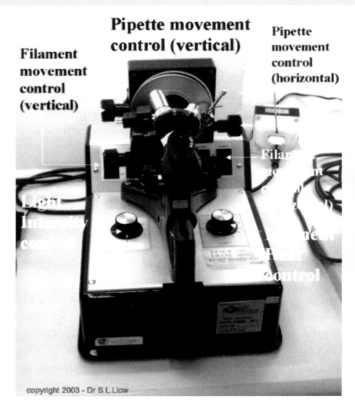

FIGURE 46.4: Microforge (Technical Product Instruments, USA)

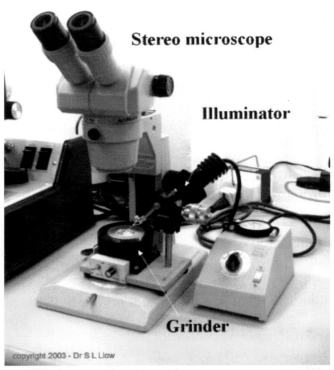

FIGURE 46.5A: Micropipette grinder (Narishige, Japan)

Microforge

A microforge is an instrument that allows the operator to make microinjection needles and holding pipettes of a specific size (Figure 46.4). The microforge works by squaring and breaking the micropipettes with its filament.

Micropipette Grinder

A microbeveller or micropipette grinder makes needles by bevelling and polishing the micro-pipette at a desired angle preferably at 45° (Figures 46.5a and b). There are two methods of bevelling the micropipettes. The first method is wet grinding in which saline is dropped at intervals onto the grinding surface to lubricate as well as remove the glass dust from the needle. However, some glass dust may still be trapped within the needle. The second method is dry grinding in which the needle is ground without any saline on the grinding surface. The dust accumulated in the needle is washed away with

10 percent hydrofluoric acid and Milli-Q water (Figure 46.5c). The latter method produces cleaner needles.

Spiking the Needle

Making a spike at the tip of the needle facilitates easy penetration of the needle into the egg thus

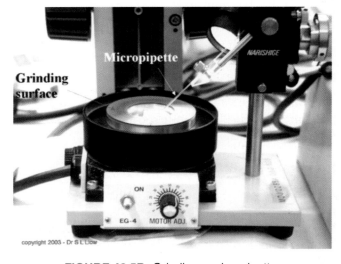

FIGURE 46.5B: Grinding a micropipette

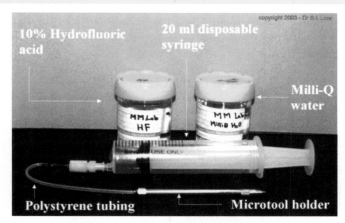

FIGURE 46.5C: Needle washing apparatus

minimizing trauma. The length of the spike should be as short as possible since a long spike tends to pierce through the egg thus killing it (Figure 46.6). 'Spiking' the needle is done with the microforge.

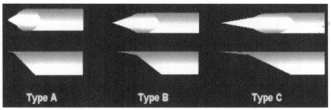

FIGURE 46.6: Front and side views of microinjection pipettes (A) a microinjection pipettes have normal bevel opening and a short spike. Most suitable for ICSI procedure, (B) Microinjection pipettes have slightly elongated bevel opening and a longer spike. They can be used for ICSI but damage to oocytes can occur more frequently, and (C) microinjection pipettes have elongated bevel opening and a long spike. They are not recommended for ICSI as damage to oocytes is certain *(Copyright 2003—Dr SL Liow)*

Bending of Microinjection Needle and Holding Pipette

The microinjection needle and holding pipette are bent at 30-35° with a microforge to allow a horizontal displacement on the microscope stage.

Preparation of a Holding Pipette

A holding pipette is a tool that holds an egg firmly for a micromanipulation procedure. Basically, a holding pipette is a micropipette with a blunt end that has been squared and broken and then fire-polished by a microforge. The outer diameter (OD)

of the holding pipette is preferably the same as that of an egg. The ID of the holding pipette is about 15 µm. This is to ensure that the oocyte is held firmly but gently during the ICSI procedure to prevent unnecessary movements that could traumatize the oocyte.

Storage of Holding Pipettes and Microinjection Needles

In an ICSI program, it is advisable to prepare sufficient microinjection needles and holding pipettes for a week. It is recommended that for every ICSI procedure, there will be 2 microinjection needles or at least 10 needles per week. This is to ensure that the program is not affected by a sudden depletion of needles. Sterilizing the needles at 150°C for 2 hours before a procedure is essential.

Keeping the holding pipettes and the micro-injection needles away from dust is important. This is because dust that gathers over time will not only contaminate the microenvironment in which the micromanipulation procedure is performed but also interfere with the procedure. To avoid this problem, the holding pipettes and the needles are stored in a stainless steel container that is wrapped up with a layer of aluminium foil (Figure 46.7).

Commercial Microinjection Needles and Holding Pipettes

Microinjection needles and holding pipettes for the ICSI procedure are now easily available

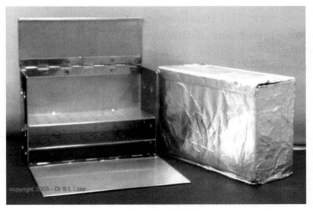

FIGURE 46.7: Storage of holding pipettes and microinjection needles

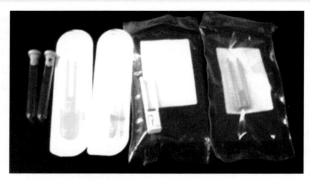

Figure 46.8: Commercial microinjection needles and holding pipettes *(Copyright 2003—Dr SL Liow)*

commercially (Figure 46.8). Their availability has eliminated the needs of investing a substantial amount of capital and time in acquiring equipment for microtool making and skill in making microinjection needles and holders respectively. However, the quality of the microinjection needles and holding pipettes differ among the makers. Therefore, one has to choose a reliable maker that can produce these microtools with high quality consistently.

Lubricant-filled Injection and Holding Units

Both the injection and holding units are comprised of a tool-holder that holds the needle in place, Teflon plastic tubing and a graduated syringe supported by a body. These units are filled with endotoxin-free light mineral oil (Sigma M8410). Tiny air bubbles are sometimes trapped within the syringe or silicon tubing or the tool-holder. These air bubbles if they are not removed will cause havoc to the entire micromanipulation procedure. For instance, instead of a smooth and slow deposition of the sperm into the cytoplasm of the egg, a sudden uncontrollable force pushes the sperm and some medium into the egg. This sudden expulsion may disrupt the integrity of the oocyte and consequently it may degenerate because of differential rates of expansion and contraction between the air bubbles and the mineral oil. Flushing the injection unit for at least 3 times or until all the air bubbles are expelled can prevent the occurrence of this problem. It is also important to push out all the air bubbles from the tool-holder before loading the needle into it. The disadvantage of this procedure is that it is

an unpleasant and tedious task that soils the embryologist's hand and the needle holder with mineral oil.

Air-filled Injection and Holding Units

Air-filled injection and holding units are developed in our laboratory to overcome this problem. Each of the air-filled systems consists of a microtool holder connected to a 3 ml disposable syringe by a Teflon plastic tubing. Loading of the microinjection pipette or holding pipette into the unit is simple and neat. The equilibrium within the injection pipette is established by placing the needle into a droplet of 10 percent polyvinylpyrrolidone (PVP) for a few minutes. As the needle is being lowered into the droplet, mineral oil followed by the PVP are passively sucked into the needle by capillary action until equilibrium is established.

Preparation of Oocytes for ICSI

The oocytes are recovered by vaginal ultrasound-guided puncture 34-36 hours after hCG. Longer pre-incubation time might be necessary for some oocytes to reach full cytoplasmic maturity, leading to a higher activation rate upon microinjection (Rienzi *et al*, 1998). Usually 4-6 hours after oocyte recovery, the cumulus-oocyte-corona complex (COC) are exposed to hyaluronidase (80 units/ml) in HEPES-buffered medium to remove the cumulus cells. Higher concentration of hyaluronidase would increase degeneration rate of the oocytes and formation rate of single pronuclear oocytes (Joris *et al*, 1998).

The removal of the cumulus cells to assess the maturity and clear image of the oocyte is an essential step in ICSI. The speed of removing the cumulus cells is hastened when the COC is first manually aspirated in and out of a Pasteure pipette (Van de Velde *et al*, 1997). When most of the cumulus have been removed, the oocyte is further aspirated with drawn-out Pasteur pipettes with an opening of about 200 µm and 180 µm in diameter respectively. Oocytes with tight corona can be further removed with a 150 µm drawn-out Pasteur pipette. These denuded oocytes are then washed through 3 microdroplets of HEPES-

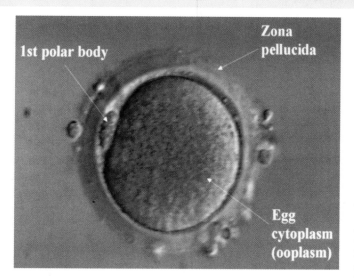

FIGURE 46.9: A denuded metaphase II oocyte
(Copyright 2003—Dr SL Liow)

buffered medium and assessed for their maturity, i.e. germinal vesicle stage or metaphase I or metaphase II stage (Figure 46.9). The oocytes are then transferred to another dish and washed through three 50 µl microdroplets of HEPES-free medium. These oocytes are then left in the final microdroplet and incubated at 37°C in 5 percent CO_2 until needed. Usually 4-6 OCC are denuded at one time. The exposure of the oocytes to hyaluronidase should be minimized to avoid parthenogenetic activation (Pickering *et al*, 1988). Although a stage warmer is generally used during oocyte and embryo manipulation under the microscope, prolonged period of exposure of the oocytes outside the incubator environment could result in irreversible disruption of the meiotic spindle (Pickering *et al*, 1990).

Preparation of Ejaculated Sperm for ICSI

Discontinuous gradients (90-70-40) separation method is used for preparation of ejaculated sperm. The gradients are layered from bottom to top, i.e. 90-70-40 percent (2 ml per layer) in a 14 ml tube. The semen is then layered on the top of the gradients. After centrifugation at 300 g for 20 minutes, the whole column of semen and gradients are discarded leaving behind the pellet that remains at the bottom of the tube. The pellet is washed with 2 ml fresh medium at 300 g for 10

minutes. The washing procedure is repeated three times. After the last washing, about 200 ml of the supernatant and the pellet remains. The pellet is re-suspended in this supernatant and incubated at 37°C and 5 percent CO_2 in a humidified atmosphere until needed. Sperms with good morphology and motility are generally obtained from this method.

Preparation of Testicular Sperm for ICSI

A sample of testicular biopsy is teased with a pair of 21G hypodermic needles in a dish containing HEPES-buffered medium. The clumps of seminiferous tubules are separated and cut into very fine pieces by the needles. The cells in the suspension are then processed by discontinuous 90-70-40 gradient separation procedure. After the separation and washing procedure, the pellet is re-suspended in about 100 µl of supernatant. The final cell suspension contains mainly testicular sperm and immature sperm cells with minimal erythrocytes.

Preparation of Microinjection Dish

The microinjection dish is prepared on the cover of a 35 × 10 mm Petri dish. Four to six 5 µl droplets of HEPES buffered medium are placed on the left, close to the centre of the dish. These droplets are numbered to avoid confusion during ICSI. A 5 µl droplet of 10 percent PVP is placed on the right, close to the centre of the dish. The PVP droplet is spread longitudinally to flatten it. The whole dish is then over-laid with mineral oil as soon as possible. The oil should just cover the droplet completely. One µl of sperm is placed on the right side of PVP droplet. This is to allow sperm to swim towards the left side of the droplet in a few minutes. A metaphase II oocyte is placed into each of the droplet of HEPES-buffered medium. The ICSI procedure is carried out on the 38°C heated stage of the microscope with magnifications of × 50, × 100 and × 200.

Alignment of Injection and Holding Pipettes

Aligning the injection and the holding pipettes over the microinjection dish so that they look 'straight' under the microscope would ensure a smooth and easy performance of the ICSI procedure.

Before loading the needle and holding pipette into the respective microtool holders, it would be advisable to loosen the plunger of the 3 ml syringe and then leave it at 1.5 ml mark. Alignment of the needle and holding pipette is done over a 35 mm × 10 mm petri dish cover. At the centre of the petri dish cover is a "flatten" droplet made up of 1 μl HEPES-buffered medium and 5 μl 10 percent PVP, over-laid with light mineral oil. This dish is used to align and stabilize the pressure within the needle. The dish cover is put on the stage of the microscope and the needle placed above the droplet. The needle is then adjusted so that a "straight" pipette is seen at low magnification (× 5 objective). The outline of the droplet is then focused before the needle is lowered into the droplet. The pipette is then checked for smooth x-y movement along the bottom of the dish. Smooth and gentle aspiration and expulsion of the PVP is also checked. The needle is left in the PVP for a few minutes to allow equilibrium to establish. The control within the needle could be enhanced if a short column of mineral oil is first aspirated into the needle. The holding pipette, that is mounted on the left micromanipulator and controlled by the right joystick, is also placed above the droplet and adjusted to be 'straight'. It is important that the holding pipette should not be placed into the PVP droplet or contain traces of the PVP. This is because shrinkage of the oocyte can occur if the oocyte has intimate contact with PVP.

Intracytoplasmic Sperm Injection

Although the timing of sperm injection does not significantly affect the survival and fertilization rates of the oocytes and embryo quality (Van de Velde, 1998) higher number of good quality embryos can be obtained when ICSI is performed between 1 and 9 hours after oocyte recovery (Yanagida *et al*, 1998). The ICSI technique performed by most centres requires that the oolemma is broken at the point of injection before the sperm is delivered into the ooplasm (Dozortsev

et al, 1995; Palermo *et al*, 1996; Vanderzwalmen *et al*, 1996; Joris *et al*, 1998; Carrillo *et al*, 1998). The aspiration of the ooplasm into the needle to induce breakage is a delicate part of the technique. Gentle ooplasmic aspiration within the needle would result in higher survival rate of the oocytes and embryo quality (Vanderzwalmen *et al*, 1996; Carrillo *et al*, 1998). The amount of ooplasm aspirated is dependent upon the size of the needle and the speed in which it is performed. Minimal amount of ooplasm aspirated with a slow and gentle aspiration ensures that the oocyte is not unduly traumatised. On the other hand, large amount of ooplasm aspirated with or without a sudden aspiration will alter the integrity of the oocyte resulting in degeneration, failure to fertilise or poor embryo quality. Likewise, gentle re-injection of sperm with minimal amount of polyvinylpyrrolidone (PVP) is preferred. This can be achieved by placing the spermatozoon at the tip of the pipette that has already been positioned close to the zona pellucida prior to injection.

Role of Polyvinlpyrrolidone (PVP) in ICSI

Polyvinylpyrrolidone (PVP; molecular weight 360,000) when dissolved in a solution becomes very viscous. Palermo *et al* (1992) used 10 percent (w/v) PVP to slow down the sperm for manipulation and injection of a single sperm that resulted in the first ICSI pregnancy. Since then many IVF centres are using PVP for the ICSI procedure even though there is the potential risk of PVP as a carcinogen (Ashwood-Smith, 1971; Feichtinger *et al*, 1995) and may interfere with sperm nuclear decondensation (Dozortsev *et al*, 1995). A few centers that have avoided using PVP in the ICSI procedure have reported better fertilization rates in PVP-free medium even though embryo quality and implantation rates remain the same (Hlinka *et al*, 1998; Tsai *et al*, 2000). The advantage of PVP over culture medium is that the viscosity of the PVP allows better control of the ooplasmic aspiration and sperm injection procedures. PVP will still be the substance of choice in ICSI unless its potential harmful effects are proven to be true or a safer and better alternative is found.

Storage and Thawing of Polyvinylpyrrolidone (PVP)

A small volume of PVP (30-50 µl) is usually stored in a sterile 0.5 ml centrifuge tube at -20°C. Prior to its use, the PVP is allowed to thaw at room temperature and then centrifuged at 3000 rpm for 5 minutes. This procedure allows water droplets that were evaporated passively and frozen on the inner surface of the tube to return to the PVP so that its concentration of 10 percent is maintained.

Technique of ICSI

The needle with the immobilized sperm is brought to the droplet containing the oocyte. The 6 O'clock polar body orientation is achieved by rotating the oocyte at the tip of the holding pipette with the needle or by gentle motion suction and releasing of the oocyte by the holding pipette. While the oocyte is held firmly by the holding pipette, the needle is brought close to the oocyte. The needle is then focused to the same focal plane as the oolemma by moving the joystick control along the z-axis (vertical plane). The sperm is then gently pushed towards the tip of the needle. When the sperm is sufficiently close to the tip, the needle is then slowly advanced through the zona pellucida and into the ooplasm at 3 O'clock position. After puncturing and breaking the oolemma by gently aspirating minute amount of cytoplasm (1-2 pl), a single sperm is gently deposited into the ooplasm with minimal volume of PVP (about 1-2 pl).

Ooplasmic aspiration has been considered as an integral part of the ICSI procedure as it ensures that the sperm is in the oocyte and in intimate contact with the ooplasm. Factors that are present in the ooplasm promote the formation of the male pronucleus (Tesarik and Kopecny, 1989; Montag et al, 1992). Cytoplasmic aspiration is also proposed to trigger the initial steps in inducing activation of the oocyte by an artificial calcium influx generated by ICSI (Tesarik et al, 1994; Tesarik, 1998). Vigorous aspiration of the ooplasm as advocated by Tesarik and Sousa (1995) as a crucial step to the success of ICSI would instead increase the rate of oocyte damage and did not improve fertilization rate. The average time taken to inject an oocyte is about one minute. Occasionally, it is difficult for the needle to pierce the oolemma even to the extent of piercing through the oocyte at the 9 O'clock position. Joris et al (1998) described different patterns of membrane breakage to overcome this problem. After all the oocytes have been injected, they are rinsed 4 times in medium before incubation at 37°C and 5 percent CO_2 in air.

Positioning of the Oocyte for ICSI

A metaphase II oocyte is held under minimal suction by the holding pipette with orientation of the polar body at either 6 or 12 O'clock. This position has been used in the first ICSI pregnancy and subsequently thereafter (Palermo et al, 1992) as damage to the metaphase spindle can be avoided. Although there was no significant difference in the survival or normal fertilization rates when the injections of oocytes were compared between 6 and 12 O'clock polar body orientation, injections of the oocytes at 6 O'clock polar body orientation resulted in higher number of good quality embryos (Nagy et al, 1995) and possibly pregnancy rates (Van Der Westerlaken et al, 1999). Except for the injection of the oocyte at 9 O'clock polar body, normal fertilization can occur irrespective of the other polar body orientations. However, the polar body orientation that could result in the sperm deposited near the metaphase spindle could result in better development of the embryo. Recently, in a retrospective analysis of oocyte fertilization and embryo development with respect to sperm deposition during ICSI, Blake et al (2000) demonstrated that injections of human oocytes with the polar body oriented at 7 or 11 O'clock position resulted in higher number of high quality embryos, significantly more than the conventional 6 or 12 O'clock polar body orientation.

Immobilization of Sperm

Immobilization of motile sperm prior to ICSI, by touching the tail with the needle is mandatory even with totally non-motile spermatozoa (Fishel et al, 1995; Van den Bergh et al, 1995; Vanderzwalmen et al, 1996). Immobilization of a spermatozoon induces permeabilization of the sperm membrane that may result in the release of a cytosolic factor that diffuses into the ooplasm with subsequent intracellular calcium oscillations and hyperpolarization of the oocyte (Homa and Swann, 1994; Dale *et al*, 1999). This phenomenon is known as activation. The activation of the oocyte triggers a series of biochemical processes in the ooplasm that would eventually lead to sperm nuclear decondensation (Tesarik and Kopecny, 1989; Montag *et al*, 1992), second polar body emission, pronuclear formation and exocytosis (Stice and Robl, 1990; Swann, 1990). Injection of this sperm cytosolic factor could also lead to embryonic development up to at least the blasto-cyst stage in the mouse (Swann and Lawrence, 1996). The components of the sperm cytosolic factor have been shown to be heat-sensitive proteins and only effective when injected into the ooplasm (Stice and Robl, 1990; Swann, 1990; Dozortsev *et al*, 1995; Palermo *et al,* 1997; Tesarik, 1998; Perry *et al*, 1999). Full mammalian oocyte activation is initiated by the coordinated action of one or more heat-sensitive protein constituents of the peri-nuclear matrix and at least one heat-stable sub-membrane component of sperm-borne oocyte-activating factors (SOAFs) (Perry *et al*, 1999; 2000).

At the edge of the sperm-PVP droplet, a morphologically normal motile sperm is immobi-lised by touching its tail with the needle. The sperm flagellum is then crushed by sliding the needle on the mid-portion of the flagellum until a kink on the flagellum is seen. It is then aspirated tail first into the needle. Care should be taken not to damage the mid-piece because it contains the male centrosome that contributes a major role in fertilization in humans. Proper immobilisation technique is necessary to ensure leakage of SOAFs into the ooplasm. These heat-sensitive proteins have significant functions in the fertilization process.

ICSI with Very Few Sperm

In cases of very few spermatozoa found in the final sperm sample, one or two 5 µl micro-droplets of sperm sample are placed beside the PVP droplet.

Using the needle, catch and aspirate the required number of motile sperm and transfer them into the PVP droplet. Place a small droplet of oil in the PVP as a reference for the location of these sperm. Replace the 5µl droplets of HEPES-buffered medium with the same fresh medium before placing the oocytes into them. Proceed with ICSI.

ICSI with Testicular Sperm

The approach to this procedure differs from intracytoplasmic injection of ejaculated sperm into an oocyte. As in preparation of microinjection dish, place one or two 5µl micro-droplets of testicular sperm sample beside the PVP droplet. Using the needle, select and aspirate the required number of 'twitching' or occasionally motile sperm and transfer them into the PVP droplet. Place a small droplet of oil in the PVP as a reference for the location of these sperm. Then place the oocytes into the 5µl droplets of HEPES-buffered medium. Aggressive immobilization of testicular sper-matozoa, by permanently crimping the sperm tail between the mid-piece and the rest of the tail, prior to ICSI can improve fertilization and preg-nancy rates (Palermo *et al*, 1996). This procedure is necessary because the molecular structure of the plasma membrane between testicular sperm and ejaculated sperm are different. There is a considerable reorganization of the molecular structure of the plasma membrane of sperm during maturation in the epididymis and that some of the changes are brought about by a direct interaction with epididymal secretory proteins (Brown *et al*, 1983).

ICSI with Immotile Spermatozoa

Sperm that are immotile are not necessarily dead. As long as the sperm is viable fertilization can occur when the ICSI procedure is done properly and pregnancies have been reported (Liu *et al*, 1997; Ved *et al*, 1997). It is difficult to differentiate between a viable and a dead sperm per se. To overcome this problem a test has been devised by exposing the sperm in a hypo-osmotic solution. In this hypo-osmotic swelling (HOS) test the tail of a dead sperm remains rigid as it is exposed to the hypo-osmotic solution. On the other hand, the tail of a viable sperm curls almost instantly. This phenomenon is known as sperm curling. Once the sperm has been determined to be viable it is quickly washed in PVP; its tail crimped with the needle prior to injection into the oocyte. The morphologically normal, immotile but viable spermatozoa have an aneuploidy rate similar to that of normal motile spermatozoa (Zeyneloglu, 2000). A solution composed of 50 percent culture medium and 50 percent water is to be preferred for the selection of viable immotile spermatozoa for ICSI (Verheyen *et al*, 1997).

REFERENCES

1. Ashwood-Smith MJ. Polyvinylpyrrolidone solutions used in plasma expanders: potential carcinogens? Lancet. 1971;1(7712):1304.
2. Blake M, Garrisi J, Tomkin G, Cohen J. Sperm deposition site during ICSI affects fertilization and development. Fertil Steril 2000;73(1):31-37.
3. Brown CR, von Glos KI, Jones R. Changes in plasma membrane glycoproteins of rat spermatozoa during maturation in the epididymis. J Cell Bio 1983;96: 256-64.
4. Carrillo AJ, Atiee SH, Lane B, Pridham DD, Risch P, Silverman IH, et al. Oolemma rupture inside the intracytoplasmic sperm injection needle significantly improves the fertilization rate and reduces oocyte damage. Fertil Steril 1998;70:676-79.
5. Cohen J, Malter H, Fehilly C, Wright G, Elsner C, Kort H, et al. Implantation of embryos after partial opening of oocytezona pellucida to facilitate sperm penetration [Letter]. Lancet 1988;16(2):162.
6. Dale B, Marino M, Wilding M. Sperm-induced calcium oscillations. Soluble factor, factors or receptors? Mol Hum Reprod 1999;5(1):1-4.
7. Dozortsev D, Rybouchkin A, De Sutter P, Dhont M. Sperm plasma membrane damage prior to intracytoplasmic sperm injection: a necessary condition for sperm nucleus decondensation. Hum Reprod 1995;10: 2960-64.
8. Feichtinger W, Obruca A, Brunner M. Sex chromosomal abnormalities and intracytoplasmic sperm injection. Lancet 1995;346(8989):566.
9. Fishel S, Lisi F, Rinaldi L, Green S, Hunter A., Dowell K, et al. Systematic examination of immobilizing spermatozoa before intracytoplasmic sperm injection in the human. Hum Reprod 1995;10:497-500.
10. Hlinka D, Herman M, Vesela J, Hredzak R, Horvath S, Pacin J. A modified method of intracytoplasmic sperm injection without the use of polyvinylpyrrolidone. Hum Reprod 1998;13:1922-27.
11. Homa ST, Swann K. A cytosolic sperm factor triggers calcium oscillations and membrane hyperpolarizations in human oocytes. Hum Reprod 1994;9:2356-61.
12. Joris H., Nagy Z, Van de Velde H. et al. Intracytoplasmic sperm injection: Laboratory set-up and injection procedure. Hum Reprod 1998;13 (Suppl 1):76-86.
13. Liu J, Tsai YL, Katz E, Compton G, Garcia JE, Baramki TA. High fertilization rate obtained after intracytoplasmic sperm injection with 100% nonmotile spermatozoa selected by using a simple modified hypo-osmotic swelling test. Fertil Steril 1997;68:373-75.
14. Mansour R. Intracytoplasmic sperm injection: a state of the art technique. Hum Reprod Update 1998;4: 43-56.
15. Montag M, Tok V, Liow SL, Bongso A, Ng SC. *In vitro* decondensation of mammalian sperm and subsequent formation of pronuclei-like structures for micromanipulation. Mol Reprod Dev 1992;33:338-46.
16. Nagy Z, Liu J, Joris H, Bocken G et al. The influence of the site of sperm deposition and mode of oolemma breakage at intracytoplasmic sperm injection on fertilization and embryo development rates. Hum Reprod 1995;10:3171-77.
17. Ng SC, Bongso A, Ratnam SS, Sathananthan H, Chan CL, Wong PC, et al. Pregnancy after transfer of sperm under zona. Lancet 1988;2:790.
18. Palermo G, Joris H, Devroey P, Van Steirteghem AC. Pregnancies after intracytoplasmic injection of single spermatozoon into an oocyte. Lancet 1992;340:17-18.
19. Palermo GD, Alikani M, Bertoli M, Colombero LT, Moy F, Cohen J, et al. Oolemma characteristics in relation to survival and fertilization patterns of oocytes treated by intracytoplasmic sperm injection. Hum Reprod 1996;11:172-76.
20. Palermo GD, Avrech OM, Colombero LT, Wu H, Wolny YM, Fissore RA, et al. Human sperm cytosolic factor triggers Ca_2^+ oscillations and overcomes activation failure of mammalian oocytes. Mol Hum Reprod 1997;3(4):367-74.
21. Perry AC, Wakayama T, Yanagimachi R. A novel trans-complementation assay suggests full mammalian oocyte activation is coordinately initiated by multiple, submembrane sperm components. Biol Reprod 1999; 60:747-55.
22. Perry AC, Wakayama T, Cooke IM, Yanagimachi R. Mammalian oocyte activation by the synergistic action of discrete sperm head components: induction of calcium transients and involvement of proteolysis. Dev Biol 2000;217(2):386-93.
23. Pickering SJ, Johnson MH, Braude PR, Houliston E. Cytoskeletal organization in fresh, aged and spontaneously activated human oocytes. Hum Reprod 1988;3:978-89.
24. Pickering SJ, Braude PR, Johnson MH, Cant A, Currie J. Transient cooling to room temperature can cause irreversible disruption of the meiotic spindle in the human oocyte. Fertil Steril 1990;54:102-08.

25. Rienzi L, Ubaldi F, Anniballo R, Cerulo G, Greco E. Preincubation of human oocytes may improve fertilization and embryo quality after intracytoplasmic sperm injection. Hum Reprod 1998;13:1014-19.

26. Stice SL, Robl JM. Activation of mammalian oocytes by a factor obtained from rabbit sperm. Mol Reprod Dev 1990;25:272-80.

27. Swann K. A cytosolic sperm factor stimulates repetitive calcium increases and mimics fertilization in hamster oocytes. Development 1990;110:1295-1302.

28. Swann K, Lawrence Y. How and why spermatozoa cause calcium oscillations in mammalian oocytes. Mol Hum Reprod 1996;2:388-90.

29. Tesarik J, Kopecny V. Developmental control of the human male pronucleus by ooplasmic factors. Hum Reprod 1989;4:962-68.

30. Tesarik J. Oocyte activation after intracytoplasmic injection of mature and immature sperm cells. Hum Reprod 1998;13(Suppl 1):117-27.

31. Tesarik J, Sousa M. Mechanism of calcium oscillations in human oocytes: a two-store model. Mol Hum Reprod 1996;2:383-86.

32. Tesarik J, Sousa M, Testart J. Human oocyte activation after intracytoplasmic sperm injection. Hum Reprod 1994;9:511-18.

33. Tsai MY, Huang FJ, Kung FT, Lin YC, Chang SY, Wu JF, et al. Influence of polyvinylpyrrolidone on the outcome of intracytoplasmic sperm injection. J Reprod Med 2000;45:115-20.

34. Van de Velde H, Nagy ZP, Joris H, De Vos A, Van Steirteghem AC. Effects of different hyaluronidase concentrations and mechanical procedures for cumulus cell removal on the outcome of intracytoplasmic sperm injection. Hum Reprod. 1997;12:2246-50.

35. Van de Velde H, De Vos A, Joris H, Nagy ZP, Van Steirteghem AC. Effect of timing of oocyte denudation and micro-injection on survival, fertilization and embryo quality after intracytoplasmic sperm injection. Hum Reprod 1998;13:3160-64.

36. Van den Bergh A, Bertrand E, Biramane J, Englert Y. Importance of breaking a spermatozoon's tail before intracytoplasmic injection: A prospective randomized trial. Hum. Reprod 1995;10:2819-20.

37. Van Der Westerlaken LA, Helmerhorst FM, Hermans J, Naaktgeboren N. Intracytoplasmic sperm injection: position of the polar body affects pregnancy rate. Hum Reprod 1999;14:2565-69.

38. Vanderzwalmen P, Bertin G, Lejeune B, Nijs M, Vandamme B, Schoysman R. Two essential steps for a successful intracytoplasmic sperm injection: injection of immobilized spermatozoa after rupture of the oolema. Hum Reprod 1996;11:540-47.

39. Ved S, Montag M, Schmutzler A, Prietl G, Haidl G, van der Ven H. Pregnancy following intracytoplasmic sperm injection of immotile spermatozoa selected by the hypo-osmotic swelling-test: A case report. Andrologia 1997; 29:241-42.

40. Verheyen G, Joris H, Crits K, Nagy Z, Tournaye H, Van Steirteghem A. Comparison of different hypo-osmotic swelling solutions to select viable immotile spermatozoa for potential use in intracytoplasmic sperm injection. Hum Reprod Update 1997;3:195-203.

41. Yanagida K, Yazawa H, Katayose H, Suzuki K, Hoshi K, Sato A. Influence of oocyte preincubation time on fertilization after intracytoplasmic sperm injection. Hum Reprod 1998;13:2223-26.

42. Zeyneloglu HB, Baltaci V, Ege S, Haberal A, Batioglu S. Detection of chromosomal abnormalities by fluorescent in-situ hybridization in immotile viable spermatozoa determined by hypo-osmotic sperm swelling test. Hum Reprod 2000;15:853-56.

• Peter R Brinsden

47

Cryopreservation in an ART Program

INTRODUCTION

Human embryo freezing plays a vital part in most Assisted Conception Units. Ovarian follicular stimulation is almost universally practised in *in vitro* fertilisation and other assisted conception treatments, in order to maximise the chance of achieving a pregnancy. Following stimulation, the average number of oocytes produced is around 10-12. In the United Kingdom, the maximum number of embryos that may be transferred to the uterus is three and the strong recommendation of most authorities and practitioners in the UK is that this should be reduced to two. In about 50 percent of women therefore, surplus embryos will be available to freeze. The advantage of freezing supernumerary embryos is that no viable normal embryos are wasted and the chance of achieving a pregnancy in subsequent replacement cycles is enhanced, without the need for further ovarian stimulation. There are, however, a number of ethical and moral dilemmas that have been thrown up by the relatively new technology of embryo freezing and a number of these are only just becoming evident. In particular, the fate of stored embryos on the death or divorce of couples, the "ownership" of embryos and the accumulation in freezers around the world of large numbers of unclaimed embryos.

In addition to embryo freezing, most assisted reproductive technology (ART) programmes will use frozen semen samples for donor insemination and other indications. Other aspects of cryo-preservation involve the freezing of human oocytes, and the freezing of ovarian tissue samples, either in young women who are about to undergo cancer chemotherapy or radiotherapy and possibly for certain social indications.

HISTORY OF CRYOPRESERVATION IN ART

Donor insemination programmes have used frozen semen since 1953, when the first pregnancies were achieved.[1] Although the freezing process degrades the quality of semen, normal semen generally freezes and thaws well. The same cannot be said for oocytes however, and attempts have been made to freeze oocytes for many years,[2] but in general they have met with little success, although pregnancies and births have been reported as a result of these techniques.[3-5]

Edwards and Steptoe, in the earliest days of *in vitro* fertilisation (IVF) pointed out the potential benefits of freezing surplus human embryos, although the earliest attempts were not successful.[6] It was not until 1983 that the first pregnancy[7] was reported following the transfer of frozen/thawed human embryos. Since then, embryo freezing has become an integral part of the majority of programmes practising ART, both in the United Kingdom and worldwide. More than 1100 babies have been following transfer of frozen/thawed embryos at Bourn Hall since the first pregnancy was reported[8] by our program.

More recently, considerable advances have been made in oocyte freezing and Bourn Hall started a clinical oocyte freezing programme in the year 2000. The possibility of freezing ovarian tissue and possibly obtaining mature oocytes, either by *in vivo* maturation at a later time or by *in vitro* maturation, have been extensively discussed.[9-11] Bourn Hall have frozen ovarian tissue since 1992 for young women who are about to embark on chemotherapy or radiotherapy and whose ovarian function is therefore likely to be severely compromised. It is not possible yet to guarantee these young women that the ovarian tissue will be able to be used, either by *in vitro* or *in vivo* development of oocytes, but many, after proper counselling, do feel it is worth freezing tissue nevertheless.

CLINICAL APPLICATIONS FOR EMBRYO FREEZING

The principle indications to freeze human embryos in ART programmes are:
- Storage of surplus embryos following super-ovulation for IVF
- When there is a high risk of the development of ovarian hyperstimulation syndrome (OHSS) after superovulation for IVF
- When problems develop during an IVF cycle: i.e. endometrial polyps, poor endometrial development, illness or domestic reasons
- Before cancer chemotherapy or radiotherapy
- Storage of donated embryos for future embryo research.

  Many assisted conception units, both in the United Kingdom and elsewhere, have active embryo donation and IVF surrogacy programs. Embryos are usually donated by couples who have some frozen but who have achieved all the children they want for themselves or by couples who may have decided to discontinue their treatment. Because of the requirement in the United Kingdom to "quarantine" embryos to guard against the possibility of transmission of HIV, clinics freeze all embryos for at least 6 months, confirm negative HIV status and then proceed to embryo transfer.

  Frozen embryos may also act as a source of research embryos. Many couples with embryos remaining in storage after completing their families offer to donate their embryos to research projects approved by local Ethics Committees and,

in the UK, by the Human Fertilisation and Embryology Authority (HFEA).

CLINICAL MANAGEMENT OF FROZEN EMBRYO TRANSFER CYCLES

Frozen/thawed embryos may be transferred to the uterus either in a natural monitored cycle or in a hormone controlled cycle. The chance of achieving a pregnancy have been reported to be the same as for fresh embryo transfer.[12, 13]

Replacement in a Natural Cycle

Natural cycle replacement is generally recommended when the woman is young and has normal regular menstrual cycles. Women in this group attend the clinic from day 10 in the menstrual cycle to monitor follicular growth and ovulation by serial ultrasound scanning, with measurement of serial levels of serum oestradiol, luteinising hormone (LH) and progesterone. When the spontaneous LH surge has been detected, the day of embryo replacement is timed for three days later. No luteal phase support is given in these cycles.

Replacement in a Hormone Controlled Cycle

Older women and those with irregular cycles will usually be treated in cycles brought under control by the use of gonadotrophin releasing hormone agonists, such as buserelin or nafarelin. Daily doses of the agonist are usually started on or about preceding cycle day 21. Pituitary down regulation is confirmed on the second day of menstruation. If "baseline levels" have been reached and the ovaries are quiescent on ultrasound scanning, the dose of agonist is reduced and hormone replacement therapy with oestradiol valerate tablets are given in doses of 2 mg orally daily, increasing to 4 mg on day 6 and 6 mg on day 10, reducing again to 4 mg from day 14 onwards. Progesterone in the form of Cyclogest® or, more recently, Crinone® 8 percent are given from cycle day 15 onwards.[12]

ADVANTAGES AND DISADVANTAGES OF HUMAN EMBRYO FREEZING

The advantages of an active and successful freezing program in an ART unit have already been outlined in the introduction. The major benefit is that not a single good, potentially viable embryo from a stimulation cycle is wasted. This maximises the chance of achieving a pregnancy for each couple and reduces the stress, trauma and cost to couples.

The major disadvantage to ART clinics of freezing embryos is that large numbers of embryos belonging to couples who have lost contact with the clinics are tending to accumulate in freezers. In the United Kingdom, the Human Fertilization and Embryology Act (1990) makes it mandatory that all such "orphaned" embryos should be disposed of after 5 years of storage. A revision of the regulation in the UK extended the allowed storage period to 10 years. Other ethical dilemmas have arisen following the death of one or both of the partners of couples with embryos in store, and custody battles for embryos have followed divorce or separation of couples. Another major disadvantage of freezing embryos is the cost. The equipment required for freezing is expensive, the freezing procedure is labor intensive and many clinics report poor pregnancy rates following the transfer of frozen/thawed embryos of only 5-10 percent. In general, however, experienced units with active embryo freezing programmes should be able to achieve success rates equivalent to or just less than the results of fresh embryo transfer.[16]

RESULTS OF
FROZEN EMBRYO TRANSFER

A number of different factors might be considered to affect the outcome of the replacement of frozen/thawed embryos. However, in a recent review of 1009 cycles of frozen embryo replacement carried out at Bourn Hall, the only factors that appeared to have a significant effect were: patient age, the number of embryos replaced, and whether or not the embryos originated from a cycle in which all embryos had been frozen to avoid the effects of ovarian hyperstimulation.

The effect of age on the outcome of frozen embryo replacement is shown in Table 47.1. Pregnancy rates are significantly lower in patients over 40, although there was no significant difference in the number of embryos replaced, and no difference in success between the other age groups.

TABLE 47.1: The effect of patient age on the outcome of frozen embryo replacement

Age	No. transfers	Mean No. Embryos replaced	No. pregnant (%)
< 30	165	2.6	43 (26%)
30-34	426	2.5	113 (27%)
35-39	331	2.5	88 (27%)
40+	87	2.5	15 (17%)

Table 47.2 shows the relationship between the number of embryos replaced, and pregnancy rates, clearly demonstrating the increase in potential for pregnancy with increased numbers of embryos.

TABLE 47.2: Pregnancy rate in relation to the number of embryos replaced

No. of embryos replaced	No. transfers	No. pregnant (%)
1	120	8 (7%)
2	259	54 (21%)
3	630	187 (29.7%)

The outcome of frozen embryo replacement in relation to the type of replacement cycle, whether natural or hormone controlled, is shown in Table 47.3. Although it appears that these two treatment methods are equally successful, it should be remembered that patients are assigned to these two groups using different criteria, and it is therefore not surprising that the one method does not demonstrate a significant advantage over the other.

TABLE 47.3: Pregnancy rate in relation to the type of replacement cycle

	No. Transfers	Mean age	Mean No. Embryos replaced	No. pregnant (%)
Natural Cycles	410	33.1	2.54	117 (28%)*
HRT Cycles	599	34.1	2.61	142 (24%)*
* Not significant				

In Table 47.4, the relationship between the stimulation regim in the originating IVF cycle and the pregnancy rate from the subsequent frozen embryo replacement is shown. These data suggest that the ovarian stimulation regimen used in the originating cycle does not influence the outcome of frozen embryo replacement.

TABLE 47.4: Pregnancy rates in relation to the ovarian stimulation regimen in the originating cycle

Stimulation protocol	No. transfers	No. pregnant (%)
Long GnRH Agonist/HMG/FSH	798	206 (26%)
Short GnRH Agonist/HMG/FSH	146	37 (25%)
Clomiphene/HMG/FSH	65	16 (25%)

Table 47.5 shows that the cause of infertility does not appear to affect pregnancy rates; neither, in this series, did pregnancy in the originating cycle increase the chance of pregnancy from frozen embryo replacement (Table 47.6). However, those cases in which the embryos originated from cycles in which all the embryos were frozen to avoid the potential danger of hyperstimulation, had a significantly higher pregnancy rate.

TABLE 47.5: The effect of the cause of infertility on the outcome of frozen embryo replacement

Diagnosis	No. transfers	No. pregnant (%)
Tubal Damage	300	78 (26%)
Unexplained Infertility	162	41 (25%)
Male Factor	172	44 (26%)
Mixed (Male and Female)	202	50 (25%)
Others	173	46 (27%)

It appears therefore that pregnancy rates following frozen embryo replacement are influenced by the same factors as fresh embryo replacement, i.e. age and number of embryos replaced. The fact that the cause of infertility has no influence may be due to the fact that having sufficient embryos to freeze indicates that these patients are the better responders in each group,

TABLE 47.6: Pregnancy rates in relation to the outcome of originating cycle

Outcome of originating cycle	No. transfers	No. pregnant (%)
Pregnant	96	22 (23%)
Non-pregnant	623	137 (22%)
Freeze-all Embryos	290	110 (38%)

having produced sufficient oocytes to have enough to transfer fresh and still freeze some. It also excludes all patients with problems related to fertilization, those with limited response to stimulation, and those who have poor quality oocytes or embryos.

There has been concern that the length of time embryos have been kept in storage might have a detrimental effect on the outcome of frozen embryo transfer and might also cause an increase in fetal abnormalities. Table 47.7 shows that there is no apparent effect, although it will be seen that the numbers in some of the groups are small. However this is the biggest series examined to date, and so far there is no indication that extended storage is detrimental.

REGULATION OF HUMAN EMBRYO FREEZING

The Human Fertilization and Embryology Authority (HFEA) regulate all infertility treatment involving the use of donor gametes or treatments in which human embryos are created *in vitro* and all storage of gametes and embryos in the United Kingdom.

There has been considerable debate about the fate of embryos, the genetic parents of which have not been able to be traced. It has been suggested that these so called "orphaned" embryos should be donated to other infertile couples or used for ethically approved research projects. Neither of these options is possible, since the genetic "parents" of these embryos will not have given their specific consent.

Presently, all couples in this Clinic are contacted annually and asked whether they would like their embryos to:
• Remain in storage for a further year
• Be allowed to perish
• Be donated to a research project
• Donated to infertile couples
In spite of our best efforts at tracing the genetic "parents" of many embryos, contact has been lost. Many couples have not been in contact at all with the Clinic since their embryos were frozen.

At Bourn Hall Clinic the embryo freezing program started in 1984. An internal audit of the first 10 years of our program showed that 3,700 couples had embryos frozen and there were 8,500 remaining in store. During this same 10 year period, 590 of the 3,700 couples made decisions on the disposal of their embryos: 160 couples donated their embryos to research programs and 80 donated their embryos to other couples in the embryo donation program: 350 couples asked to have their remaining embryos destroyed. For those couples who have kept in contact, there has not been a problem, but there has been a real problem for those who have lost contact with the clinic. In excess of 800 embryos were destroyed on 1 August 1996 and thereafter small numbers are required to be destroyed each month in compliance with the instructions of the Human Fertilization and Embryology Authority.

CONCLUSIONS ON HUMAN EMBRYO FREEZING

The ability to freeze human embryos surplus to IVF treatment cycles is of great benefit to couples who are fortunate enough to have embryos left over from their IVF stimulation cycles. It allows many couples to have second or third attempts at embryo transfer with, in many Clinics, an equal chance of achieving a pregnancy; freezing maximises the use of these embryos and minimises their waste.

The Ethics Committee of the American Society for Reproductive Medicine, in a discussion document on the ethics of human embryo cryo-preservation,[17] states "the advantages are so compelling that the Committee believes that cryopreservation capacity is an essential component of all programs offering IVF". They cite the most important reasons for this strong statement as: decreasing cost, decreasing the risk of multiple pregnancies, decreasing the need for controlled ovarian hyperstimulation and decreasing the number of oocyte recovery cycles required for a pregnancy to occur with IVF. They go on to conclude that the long term risks and benefits of the procedure, although not as yet fully assessed, "appears to be safe". Similarly, the HFEA have encouraged the setting up of cryopreservation programs in IVF units in the United Kingdom in order to maximise the effectiveness of stimulated

IVF cycles and minimise the wastage of human embryos.

However, although there are very real benefits to freezing embryos, a previously unforeseen consequence of this technique is that large numbers of embryos are accumulating in freezers around the World, as many Clinics have lost contact with the genetic "parents". The fate of these embryos is causing concern to clinicians and scientists in Assisted Conception Units everywhere, and has also provoked considerable discussion among the public and in the media about the ethical aspects of this treatment.

CRYOPRESERVATION AND PATIENTS UNDERGOING CANCER THERAPY

A small group of patients who will benefit from cryopreservation technology are those young men and women who are about to undergo cancer chemotherapy or radiotherapy for a number of different conditions, usually one of the leukemias or lymphomas. Testicular tumors are increasingly common among young men and even young women suffer from breast or gynaecological cancers. The problem arises because increasing numbers of these young people are now surviving because of improvements in treatment and they are, and should very reasonably be, concerned about their fertility prospects after they have recovered from treatment. Very often the effect of the cancer chemotherapy or radiotherapy on the gonads is unpredictable and will vary according to the dosage and duration of therapy.[18] It should be remembered that spermatogenesis is often impaired before the treatment is started. Young men should be reassured that there is no evidence of increased genetic abnormalities occurring in any children that may be born as a result of this treatment.

Other indications to freeze semen are in ART cycles when difficulties in producing a semen sample due the stresses of treatment are anticipated and also when sperm has to be "quarantined" before certain treatments, such as IVF surrogacy. An increasing number of men are also freezing semen before having vasectomy procedures, as a back up in case they re-marry in the future.

Oocyte Freezing

Oocyte freezing is now possible and Bourn Hall have just introduced a clinical program. Oocyte cryopreservation may be indicated prior to cancer chemotherapy, prior to oophorectomy, in oocyte donation programs and there may be social or personal reasons why a woman may wish to freeze her eggs while she is young for possible future use when she is older. In general, the success of oocyte cryopreservation programs is governed by the successful thaw rate of the oocytes—approximately 50-60 percent survive and ICSI is required to assist fertilization, since the zona pellucida tends to harden with freezing. However, clinical pregnancy rates of 30-40 percent can be achieved with single embryo implantation rates of 15-20 percent.

Ovarian Tissue Freezing

Ovarian tissue freezing is another option which has been used in this clinic for 8 years, with the hope that the technology will become available to develop mature oocytes from the tissue by *in vitro* maturation techniques or possibly by *in vivo* maturation. The freezing technology is straightforward, but requires small samples of ovarian tissue, which are usually obtained by laparoscopic punch biopsies or, if a laparotomy is being carried out, by direct ovarian biopsy. The major problem is that the technology for *in vitro* maturation is not yet available and, when young women are being counselled before undertaking this option, they must be very carefully advised of this. It is possible that the technology may never develop but it is likely to be available within the next 10 years.

It is our belief that all young men and women should be fully counselled on their future fertility prospects before proceeding to any treatment which may jeopardise their fertility prospects. All their concerns about their future health and their fitness to carry any children should be addressed and the chances of a successful outcome should be realistically discussed with them.

THE SAFETY OF HUMAN EMBRYO FREEZING

There has been no indication that the babies born following transfer of frozen embryos have any increased incidence of abnormality.[19, 20] The oldest children born as a result of frozen embryo transfer are only in their early teens and it is important that they be followed up in the future, as with all assisted conception treatments. Frozen embryo technology has been used in the animal livestock industry for many years, but so far the only indication of any problems with the long term safety of the use of frozen embryos has been as a result of research on mice.[21] To date, no developmental defects had been observed in humans. A review of the world literature on the safety of cryopreservation by Wood[22] was reassuring.

CONCLUSIONS

Embryo and oocyte cryopreservation facilities should be an integral part of all ART programs. The benefits to infertile couples of cryopreservation are evident and proven. Recent developments indicate that oocyte and ovarian tissue cryopreservation will be successful in the future in helping some young women who need to delay having a family.

REFERENCES

1. Bunge RG, Sherman JK. Fertilizing capacity of frozen human spermatozoa. Nature 1953;172:767-68.
2. Whittingham DG. Fertilization in vitro and development to term of unfertilized mouse oocytes previously stored at-196°C. J Reprod Fertil 1977;49:89-94.
3. Chen C. Pregnancy after human oocyte cryopreservation. Lancet 1986;1: 884-86.
4. Van Uem JF. Birth after cryopreservation of unfertilised oocytes. Lancet 1987;1:752-53.
5. Porcu E, Fabbri R, Seracchioli R, Ciotti P, Magrina IO, Flamigni C. Birth of a healthy female after intracytoplasmic sperm injection to cryopreserved human oocytes. Fertil Steril 1997;68:724-26.
6. Edwards RG, Steptoe PC. A Matter of Life. London. Hutchinson. 1980;135-37.
7. Trounson AO, Mohr L. Human pregnancy following cryopreservation, thawing and transfer of an eight-cell embryo. Nature 1983;305:707-09.
8. Cohen J, Simons RS, Fehilly CB, Fishel SB, Edwards RG, Hewitt J, Rowland GF, Steptoe PC, Webster JM. Birth after replacement of hatching blastocyst cryopreserved at expanded blastocyst stage. Lancet 1985;1:647.
9. Newton H, Aubard Y, Rutherford A, Sharma V, Gosden R. Low temperature storage and grafting of human ovarian tissue. Hum Reprod 1996;11:1487-91.

10. Shaw J, Bowles J, Koopman P, Wood EC, Trounson AO. Fresh and cryopreserved ovarian tissue samples from donors with lymphoma transmit the cancer to graft recipients. Hum Reprod 1996;11:1668-73.

11. Donnez J, Bassil S. Indications for cryopreservation of ovarian tissue. Hum Reprod Update 1998;4:248-59.

12. Sathanandan M, Macnamee MC, Rainsbury P, Wick K, Brinsden P, Edwards RG. Replacement of frozen–thawed embryos in artificial and natural cycles: A prospective semi-randomised study. Hum Reprod 1991;6:6 85-87.

13. Queenan JT, Veek LL, Seltman HJ, Muasher SJ. Transfer of cryopreserved-thawed pre-embryos in a natural cycle or a programmed cycle with exogenous hormonal replacement yields similar pregnancy results. Fertil Steril 1994;62:545-50.

14. Brinsden PR, Avery SM, Marcus SF, Macnamee MC. Frozen embryos: Decision time in the UK. Hum Reprod 1995;10:3083-84.

15. Saunders DM, Bowman MC, Grierson A, Garner F. Frozen embryos: The dilemma ten years on. Hum Reprod 1995;10:3081-82.

16. Avery SM. Embryo cryopreservation. A Textbook of In Vitro Fertilization and Assisted Reproduction (2nd edn). Brinsden PR (Ed.): Parthenon Pubs. 211-17.

17. The Ethics Committee of the American Fertility Society. Ethical Considerations of Assisted Reproductive Technologies. The cryopreservation of pre-embryos. Fertil Steril 1994;62 (Suppl 1):56S-59S.

18. Lass A, Akagbuso F, Abusheikha N, Hassouneh M, Blayney M, Avery SM, Brinsden P. A programme of semen cryopreservation for patients with malignancies in a tertiary infertility centre: lessons from eight years experience. Hum Reprod 1998;13:3256-61.

19. Olivennes F, Schneider Z, Remy V, Blanchet V, Kerbrat V, Fanchin R, Hazout A, Glissant M, Fernandez H, Dehan M, Frydman R. Perinatal outcome and follow-up of 82 children aged 1-9 years old conceived from cryopreserved embryos. Hum Reprod 1996;11:1565-68.

20. Sutcliffe AG, D'Souza SW, Cadman J, et al. Outcome in children from cryopreserved embryos. Arch Dis Child 1995;72:290-93.

21. Dulioust E, Toyama K, Busnel MC, et al. Long term effects of embryo freezing in mice. Proc Natl Acad Sci USA 1995;92:589-93.

22. Wood MJ. Embryo freezing: is it safe? Hum Reprod 1997;12(Natl Suppl: J Brit Fert Soc):32-37.

• Luca Gianaroli • Marco Toschi
• M Cristina Magli • Anna Pia Ferraretti

48

Vitrification of the Human Oocyte: A Practical Guide

Human oocyte cryopreservation represents an attractive option to the range of infertility treatments available at present. It could provide indeed an alternative to embryo preservation with consequent avoidance of the associated ethical problems. However, while embryo cryopreservation is a successful procedure, oocyte cryopreservation has poorer results (Bernard and Fuller, 1996) and only a few successful pregnancies have arisen (Chen, 1988; Van Uem et al, 1988; Serafini et al, 1995; Tucker et al, 1996; Porcu et al, 1997; Antinori et al, 1998; Borini et al, 1998; Polak de Fried et al, 1998; Yang et al, 1998; Young et al, 1998). The lack of success has been primarily attributed to the poor survival, fertilization, and development of cryopreserved human oocyte (Trounson and Kirby, 1989; Van Blerkom and Davis, 1994).

The difficulties encountered with the freezing of human mature oocytes (metaphase II) were postulated to arise mainly from inherent problems associated with the susceptibility of the mammalian spindle to freeze-thaw damage. Several forms of cryo-injury could be responsible for the relative lack of success in preserving human oocytes. These include damage to the meiotic spindle (Magistrini and Szollosi, 1980; Sathananthan et al, 1988 a; 1988 b; Pickering et al, 1990; Van der Elst et al, 1992; Gook et al, 1993), to the microfilaments essential for polar body extrusion, pronuclear migration and cytokinesis (Vincent et al, 1990), to the zona pellucida forming breaches and hardenings (Johnson et al, 1988; Johnson, 1989; Todorow et al, 1989), and to the cortical granules causing a premature cortical reaction (Schalkoff et al, 1989; Vincent et al, 1990; Gook et al, 1993; Al-Hasani and Diedrich, 1995).

Studies using metaphase II oocytes showed that morphological and biophysical factors affect the survival rate after cryopreservation. Among the morphological factors, the maturative stage, the quality and the dimensions of the cell seem to play an important role. Regarding the maturative stage, cryopreservation procedures and the concomitant use of cryoprotectants can damage the organization of the cell spindle resulting in an elevated rate of chromosomal dislocation, aberration and aneuploidy. In addition, the notable heterogeneity in the distribution and organization of the cytoplasmic organelles and the great variability in the membrane's permeability make oocytes very sensitive to the entire cryopreservation process. Regarding dimensions, the big volume, characteristic of human oocytes, affects negatively the survival rate after thawing as the cell needs a long time to equilibrate with the cryoprotectant solution.

The intracellular ice formation is the main biophysical factor conditioning cell survival and this is due to piercing of the membrane caused by ice crystals. As the human oocyte is a big cell containing a large quantity of water, it requires a long time to reach adequate dehydration before lowering the temperature, making it more difficult to avoid ice crystals formation.

Intracellular ice formation depends on the presence of the cryoprotectant in the freezing solution, and on the freezing and thawing rates. Furthermore, it is extremely important to establish what the optimal exposure time of the oocyte to cryoprotectant solutions is: it has to be long enough to permit sufficient dehydration of the cell, but not so long as to damage the cell by altering the intracellular pH.

The majority of pregnancies from cryopreserved oocytes in humans were achieved by the slow freezing technique (Chen, 1986; Porcu et al, 1998; Tucker et al, 1998). The vitrification method seemed to be promising according to results from mammalian experiments (Nakagata, 1989; Hotamisligil et al, 1996; Martino et al, 1996; Vajta et al, 1998) and based on the observations that it is a potentially less damaging procedure than freezing because it avoids the formation of intracellular ice. This should minimize the consequent damaging osmotic effects that occur as a result of ice formation during equilibrium cooling and warming. Nevertheless, although successful case reports have been documented (Hong et al, 1999; Kuleshova et al, 1999), the value of this technique for human oocytes remains elusive (Hunter et al, 1995).

THE TECHNIQUE

Vitrification may be defined as a physical process by which a highly concentrated solution of cryoprotectant solidifies during cooling without formation of ice crystals. The solid, called a glass, retains the normal molecular and ionic distribution of the liquid state and can be considered to be an extremely viscous supercooled liquid (Mazur, 1990; Rall and Fahy, 1985; Rall, 1987; Fahy et al, 1984; Fahy, 1989). Theoretically, it is advantageous with respect to freezing because it avoids the damage caused by intracellular ice formation and the osmotic effects related to extracellular ice formation.

Three factors affects the process (or probability) of vitrification:
1. Cooling rate
2. Viscosity

3. Volume

as expressed by the formula:

$$\text{Vitrification probability} = \frac{(\text{cooling rate})(\text{viscosity})}{(\text{volume})}$$

The probability of vitrification increases proportionally to viscosity or cooling rate, or by decreasing the volume (Arav et al, 2002). When optimizing vitrification conditions, it has to be considered that a high viscosity causes an increase of tossicity due to the concentration of cryoprotectants.

Normally, vitrification is achieved simply by plunging the sample directly into liquid nitrogen at -196°C (Rall and Fahy, 1985). In this way, the heat transferred from the sample to the liquid nitrogen leads to the evaporation of liquid nitrogen around the sample, resulting in the formation of a nitrogen gas layer, which acts as an insulator. This phase, defined as insulation, reduces the heat transfer and makes it impossible to achieve uniform and rapid cooling rates. To reduce this phenomenon, a machine has been proposed by Arav and colleagues (Arav et al, 2002), that is able to reduce the liquid nitrogen temperature from -196 to -210°C by applying a negative pressure. The aim is to enhance the temperature interval at which nitrogen turns from liquid to fumes, resulting in a dramatically increased cooling rate (@ 30.000°C/min). Using the machine, the cooling rate is especially enhanced in the first stage of cooling (from 20°C to -10°C) being six times higher when using 0.25 ml straws, four times with open pulled straws (OPS) or two times with electron microscope grids. Between -10°C and -150°C, the cooling rate is only doubled but that was found to be enough to reduce the chances of devitrification and recrystallization during warming.

All the authors agree that the volume reduction enhances the vitrification success and the cooling rate and volume, but not viscosity, as the paths to optimize the process (Martino et al, 1996; Arav and Zeron, 1997; Vajta, 2000). Several attempts were made in the past to develop solutions with increased viscosity by using high concentrations of permeating (glycerol, DMSO, propylene glycol, ethylene glycol) or not permeating (Ficoll, sucrose, trehalose, PVP) cryoprotectants. However, the cryoprotectant solutions obtained were often damaging because of their toxicity or osmotic effects.

Moreover, a decrease in the volume of the solution reduces the probability of ice crystal formation and allows successful vitrification in the presence of lower and non toxic concentrations of cryoprotectant.

Following this path, Arav and colleagues proposed a new technique known as minimum drop size in which very small volumes (0:1-0:5 µl) of vitrification solution (VS) are cooled and warmed. In this way, working on the volume and not on the concentration of cryoprotectant, the probability of ice crystals formation is reduced (Arav, 1992; Arav *et al* 1993 a; 1993 b; Arav and Zeron, 1997).

Another problem associated with vitrification is the fracture of the glassy solution that occurs only when the volume is above 1 µl. For volumes of 1 µl, fractures have been observed when the concentration of the VS was high (100% VS = 38% ethylene glycol, 0.5 M trehalose and 4 percent Bovine Serum Albumin in TCM medium). At half-concentration of VS (50%), fractionations were observed only at a high cooling rate. The explanation of this phenomenon resides in the following equation:

$$\text{Probability of fractionation} = CR\,(\Delta T/V)$$

Where:
  CR = cooling rate.
  ΔT = temperature difference between glass transition and
        liquid nitrogen temperature.
  V = volume.

The reason for the increasing probability of fractionation in high concentrations of VS is thought to be related to the glass transition temperature. Fractions can form only at temperatures below that at which the liquid turns into glass and above the temperature of liquid nitrogen (-196°C). It is known that a solution with a higher concentration will have a higher glass transition temperature. Consequently, if the temperature gradient increases, as in the case of higher glass transition temperature, the probability of fractionation will increase accordingly.

Some protocols for human oocyte cryopreservation include the exposure to a vitrification solution made of ethylene glycol (40%) and sucrose (0.6 mol/l). This concentration assures a stable solution during the vitrification processes but can result in toxicity when the cells are exposed for more than two minutes at a temperature higher than 25°C (Kasai *et al*, 1992).

In a different approach, some protocols are based on fast passages through increasing solutions of cryoprotectant to achieve, at the same time, both the entrance of the cryoprotectant into the cell and the volume reduction. Arav and colleagues (Arav *et al*, 2002) proposed a vitrification protocol which provides the short exposure at increasing concentration of VS (10%, 50% and 75%) mainly composed by ethylene glycol (38%) and trehalose (0.5 mol/l). These phases are fundamental and their length is species-specific.

The oocyte in 10 percent VS starts to shrink in volume. This partial dehydration is due to a water flow from the intra to the extra-cellular area caused by the difference in the osmotic pressure across the cell membrane. At the same time, an inflow starts due to the entrance of the cryoprotectant from the extracellular area (where it is at higher concentration) to the intracellular compartment, this flow being slightly delayed with respect to the water flow towards the extracellular compartment. The net result is the return to the previous volumetric dimensions of the oocyte due to a restored balance with the external environment. During this process of water balancing, the cell loses a portion of the intracellular fluids soaking up, at the same time, the cryoprotectant which results to be at the same external concentration of 10 percent. This phase must be long enough to leave the cell the time to reach a balance with the solution. The time requirement can change depending on permeability properties of the plasmalemma which is also related to the composition of the membrane and changes from species to species. Conversely, the following steps into the 50 and 75 percent solutions have to occur very rapidly for two main reasons: (1) a high concentration of cryoprotectants causes an important toxic effect and (2) the overall result of these passages is the reduction in volume of the cell; therefore, no time must be given for an inflow to occur.

The whole process can be graphically represented:

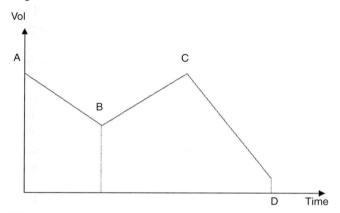

Where:
A = 100 percent initial volume
B = maximal dehydration in the 10 percent solution
C = acquisition of the initial volume (10% solution)
D = dehydration of the cell in the 50-75 percent solutions.

The phases A to C occur in the 10 percent VS, whereas phases C to D occur in the 50 and 75 percent VS.

Laboratory tests on mouse metaphase II oocytes had registered positive effects arising from the addition to the VS (6 M DMSO) of polyethylene glycol (PEG 1mg/ml). Vitrified oocytes with no PEG showed a fertilization rate of 60 percent a blastocyst development of 55 percent. These results increased significantly in the presence of PEG to values of 91 percent and 73 percent respectively (O'Neil *et al,* 1997).

Devitrification

For the devitrification process, a sequence of steps has been proposed in solutions at a decreasing molarity of sucrose or trehalose (1M; 0.5M; 0.25M; 0.125M) at 37°C.

The aim of these steps is removing gradually the cryoprotectant from the oocytes in order to avoid osmotic shock. Afterwards, the oocytes are transferred to the culture medium according to the used techniques (Kuleshova *et al,* 1999).

Hong *et al,* (1999) pointed out that the devitrification conditions affect in a significant way the pre-implantation phases of the embryos deriving from vitrified oocytes. One of the most important variables is the period of time at which the oocyte is kept in the different concentrations of sucrose. The authors proposed two protocols, both of them made of four steps: in the first one (short protocol) the intervals were of 2.5 minutes vs. 5 minutes in the second one (long protocol). The results of this study demonstrated that even if the survival, maturation and fertilization rates were not different, embryos coming from oocytes in the short protocol developed to two cells, four cells, eight cells and blastocysts at a higher percentage compared to the long protocol.

Clinical Application

The scientific literature reports only a few cases of pregnancy obtained from human vitrified oocytes. Kuleshova *et al,* (1999) published the birth of a healthy baby girl from a 47 year old woman entering the oocyte donor program. Mature oocytes were vitrified following a protocol with solutions of rising concentration of cryoprotectant. In this study the survival rate was 65 percent the fertilization rate 67 percent (Figures 48.1 and 48.2). One embryo with regular morphology was biopsied for chromosomal analysis and was identified as disomic for chromosomes X, 13, 14, 15, 16, 18, 21 and 22. It was transferred at 93 h after insemination into the uterine cavity yielding a clinical, regularly on term pregnancy.

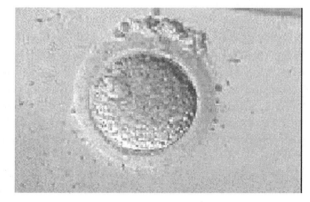

FIGURE 48.1: Metaphase II human oocyte after thawing. The aspect of the cytoplasm is very granular

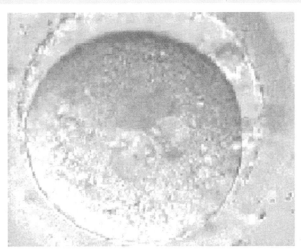

FIGURE 48.2: Regularly fertilized oocyte with two pronuclei and two polar bodies. Nucleoli are aligned within pronuclei and the aspect of the cytoplasm is still granular

The Protocol for Human Oocytes Vitrification

According to Kuleshova *et al*, (1999), cumulus denuded mature metaphase II oocytes are transferred to 10 percent ethylene glycol solution in phosphate buffered saline (PBS) containing 10 mg/ml human serum albumin (HSA) for 40 seconds. Oocytes are then transferred to 20 percent ethylene glycol in PBS+ 10mg/ml HSA for 30 seconds and finally to 40 percent ethylene glycol and 20.54 percent (0.6 mol/l) sucrose in PBS+10 mg/ml HSA for a further 60 seconds. All the procedures are carried out on a warm stage at 37°C.

The oocytes are then drawn into the OPS, a finely drawn plastic straw, by capillary action and rapidly cooled to –196°C by direct plunging to liquid nitrogen.

Oocytes are warmed by transfer of the vitrified OPS content into pre-warmed sucrose solutions maintained on a warm stage at 37°C. The oocytes are expelled into 13.69 percent sucrose (0.4 mol/l) in PBS + 10 mg/ml HSA for 2-3 min, then to 8.56 percent sucrose (0.25 mol/l) in PBS + 10 percent mg/ml HSA for 2-3 min and finally 4.28 percent sucrose (0.125 mol/l) in PBS + 10 mg/ml HSA for 3-6 min. Oocytes were washed in IVF 50 medium (Vitrolife), incubated for 4 h before, inseminated by intracytoplasmic sperm microinjection and returned to culture in fresh IVF 50 medium.

Preimplantation Genetic Diagnosis (PGD) of Vitrified Oocytes

At the S.I.S.Me.R. Reproductive Medicine Unit, the chromosomal analysis in preimplantation embryos is routinely proposed when experimental programs have a clinical application, such as for oocyte vitrification. The numerical analysis of interphase chromosomes is based on the use of specific fluorescence-labelled DNA probes in the fluorescence *in situ* hybridisation technique (FISH). Working on single cells imposes obvious limits on the number of chromosomes that can be screened during PGD. The use of multiple probes permits the simultaneous analysis of different chromosomes and can be completed by successive rounds of FISH using additional probes. In this way, diagnosis on up to nine chromosomes is currently available, including those whose aneuploidies are more frequently detected in spontaneous abortions and on term pregnancies: XY, 13, 14, 15, 16, 18, 21, 22.

Embryo Biopsy

Embryo biopsy is generally carried out at 62-64 hours after insemination. At this time, compaction starts to take place and cellular damage is very likely to occur if the biopsy is performed when cell-cell interactions and junctions begin to assemble. The biopsy procedure entails an opening in the zona pellucida of approximately 20-25 mm diameter, which is performed chemically by using acid Tyrode's solution. The position of the embryo is selected in order to have a nucleated blastomere at the 3 O'clock position that is removed by using a polished glass needle and gently released in the medium (Figure 48.3). Extreme attention is taken to avoid rupture of the cell membrane and damage to the surrounding blastomeres. The biopsied embryo is removed from the biopsy disk, washed and incubated in fresh medium, whereas the blastomere undergo genetic analysis.

FISH

The biopsied blastomere is transferred to hypotonic solution (1% sodium citrate) fixed in

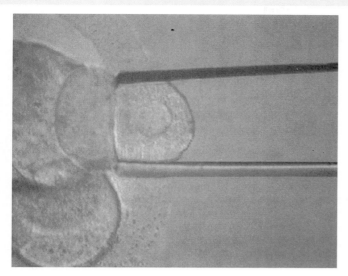

FIGURE 48.3: A blastomere is biopsied from an eight-cell embryo using a polished glass needle

methanol: acetic acid (3:1) on a glass slide, and dehydrated in ethanol series (70%, 85% and 100%, 2 minutes each solution) (Figure 48.4). The fluorescent probes are then added and let to hybridize at 37°C after DNA denaturation (Figure 48.5). After washing off the unbound probe in 0.7 percent SSC-0.3 percent NP 40, the diagnosis is made at the fluorescent microscope. For a second round hybridization, the whole procedure is repeated starting from dehydration in ethanol.

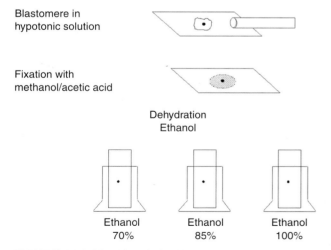

FIGURE 48.4: The biopsied cell is lysed in hypotonic solution and the nucleus fixed on a glass slide using a methanol:acetic acid solution. Then, it is dehydrated in increasing ethanol series

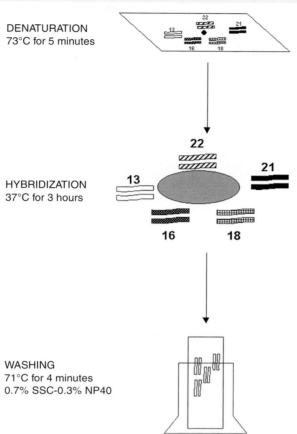

DENATURATION
73°C for 5 minutes

HYBRIDIZATION
37°C for 3 hours

WASHING
71°C for 4 minutes
0.7% SSC-0.3% NP40

FIGURE 48.5: The hybridizing solution is put on the nucleus; denaturation follows and hybridization takes place for 3 hours at 37°C. A washing step is then performed to eliminate the excess of unbound probe

Results

The following table shows the results of FISH analysis on a group of embryos generated by vitrified oocytes.

No. cycles 10	
No. generated embryos	27
No. FISH analysed embryos	17
• FISH normal	9
• FISH abnormal	8
No. transferred cycles	6
No. transferred embryos	8
No. clinical pregnancies	1

The detected chromosomal abnormalities were: one monosomy, one trisomy, one haploidy and 5 complex abnormalities (Figures 48.6 to 48.9).

The FISH screening of embryos generated by thawed oocytes revealed that a normal

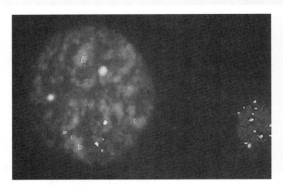
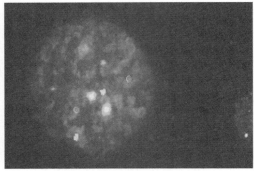

FIGURE 48.6: A blastomere is analyzed for the chromosomes 13, 16, 18 21 and 22 in the first round FISH (a) and for the chromosomes XY, 14 and 15 (b). The blastomere was diagnosed as normal for the tested chromosomes. The signals were (a): Red = LSI 13, Aqua = CEP 16, Purple = CEP 18, Green = LSI 21, Yellow = LSI 22; (b) Aqua = CEP X, Red = Tel 14, Green = CEP 15. LSI refers to locus specific probes, CEP to centromeric probes and Tel to telomeric probes

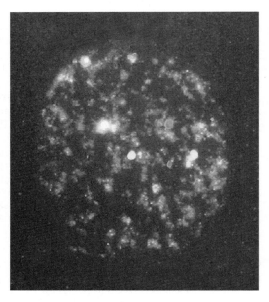

FIGURE 48.7: A blastomere analyzed for the chromosomes 13, 16, 18 21 and 22 in the first round FISH was diagnosed as monosomic for the chromosome 18. The signals were (a): Red = LSI 13, Aqua = CEP 16, Purple = CEP 18, Green = LSI 21, Yellow = LSI 22. LSI refers to locus specific probes and CEP to centromeric probes

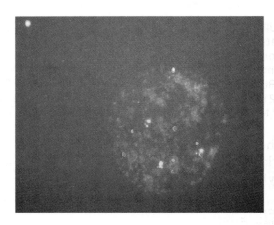

FIGURE 48.8: A blastomere analyzed for the chromosomes 13, 16, 18 21 and 22 in the first round FISH was diagnosed as trisomic for the chromosome 22. The signals were (a): Red = LSI 13, Aqua = CEP 16, Purple = CEP 18, Green = LSI 21, Yellow = LSI 22. LSI refers to locus specific probes and CEP to centromeric probes

chromosomal status is associated with a regular embryo development (Kuleshova *et al*, 1999). These data were confirmed by another study, in which the chromosomal constitution of oocytes cryopreserved with the slow freezing technique was comparable to that observed in the controls (Cobo *et al*, 2001). As expected, the most frequent abnormalities is represented by complex abnormalities that are mainly related to slow cleavage or blockage, suggesting that oocyte freezing may affect the cytoskeleton and consequently the mitotic process.

CONCLUSIONS

The positive results with animal oocytes, greatly encouraged the use of vitrification in the human. Despite the report of several pregnancies, the technique still seems to be far from being optimal. After a series 66 thawed cycles where only 20 underwent embryo transfer yielding 3 clinical pregnancies, the implantation rate per oocyte resulted to be 1 percent. Therefore, reconsideration

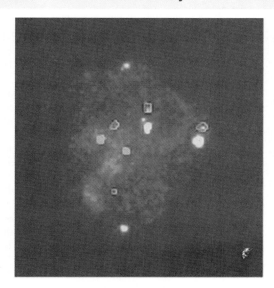

FIGURE 48.9: A blastomere analyzed for the chromosomes 13, 16, 18 21 and 22 in the first round FISH carried complex abnormalities: 1 copy of chromosome 13, 3 copies of chromosome 21 and 3 of chromosome 22. The signals were (a): Red = LSI 13, Aqua = CEP 16, Purple = CEP 18, Green = LSI 21, Yellow = LSI 22. LSI refers to locus specific probes and CEP to centromeric probes

of the whole protocol is recommended as further work is needed to improve the conditions for human oocyte cryopreservation.

REFERENCES

1. Al-Hasani S, Diedrich K. Oocyte storage. In Grudzinskas JG, Yovich JL (Eds): Gamete/ The Oocyte. Cambridge University Press, Cambridge 1995.
2. Antinori S, Dani G, Selman HA, et al. Pregnancy after sperm injection into cryopreserved human oocytes. Hum. Reprod 1998;13(Abstract Bk 1):157-58.
3. Arav A. Vitrification of oocytes and embryos. In: Lauria A., Gandolfi F (Eds.): New Trends in Embryo Transfer. Portland Press, Cambridge, UK, 1992;255-264.
4. Arav A, Yavin S, Zeron Y, et al. New trends in gamete's cryopreservation, Mol. Cell. Endocrinol 2002;187:77-81.
5. Arav A, Rubinsky B, Fletcher G, et al. Cryogenic protection of oocytes with antifreeze proteins. Mol. Reprod. Dev 1993b;36:488-93.
6. Arav A, Shehu D, Mattioli M. Osmotic and cytotoxic study of vitrification of immature bovine oocyte. J. Reprod. Fert 1993a;99:353-58.
7. Arav A, Zeron Y. Vitrification of bovine oocytes using modified minimum drop size technique (MDS) is effected by the composition and the concentration of the vitrification solution and by the cooling conditions. Theriogenology 1997;47:341-42.
8. Bernard A, Fuller BJ. Cryopreservation of human oocytes: a review of current problems and perspectives. Hum. Reprod Update 1996;2:193-207.
9. Borini A, Baffaro MG, Bonu MA, et al. Pregnancies after freezing and thawing. Preliminary data. Hum. Reprod. 1998;13(Abstract Bk1):124-25.
10. Chen C. Pregnancy after human oocyte cryopreservation. Lancet i, 1986;884-86.
11. Chen C. Pregnancies after human oocyte cryopreservation. Ann. NY Acad. Sci 1988;541:541-49.
12. Fahy GM, MacFarlane DR, Angell CA et al. Vitrification as an approach to cryopreservation, Cryobiology 1984;21:407-26.
13. Fahy GM. Vitrification, in Low Temperature Biotechnology: Emerging Applications and Engineering Contributions, McGrath, JJ, Diller KR, (Eds.): BED 1989;Vol. 10/HTD Vol. 98.
14. Gook D, Osborn S, Johnston W. Cryopreservation of mouse and human oocytes using 1, 2 propanediol and the configuration of the meiotic spindle. Hum. Reprod 1993;8:1101-09.
15. Hong SW, Chung HM, Lim JM, et al. Improved human oocyte development after vitrification : a comparison of thawing methods. Fertil. Steril 1999;72:142-46.
16. Hotamisligil S, Toner M, Powers RD. Changes in membrane integrity, cytoskeletal structure, and developmental potential of murine oocytes after vitrification in ethylene glycol. Biol. Reprod 1996;55:161-68.
17. Hunter JE, Fuller BJ, Bernard A, et al. Vitrification of human oocytes following minimal exposure to cryoprotectants; initial studies on fertilization and embryonic development. Hum. Reprod 1995;10:1184-88.
18. Johnson MH. The effect of fertilization of exposure of mouse oocytes to dimethyl sulfoxide: an optimal protoco. J. In Vitro Fertil. Embryo Transfer 1989;6:168-175.
19. Johnson MH, Pickering SJ, Gorge MA. The influence of cooling on the properties of the zona pellucida of the mouse oocyte. Hum Reprod 1988;3:383-87.
20. Kasai M, Nishimori M, Zhu SE. Survival of mouse morulae vitrified in an ethylene glycol-based solution after exposure to the solution at various temperature. Biol Reprod 1992;47:1134-39.
21. Kuleshova L, Gianaroli L, Magli MC, et al. Birth following vitrification of a small number of human oocytes: case report. Hum Reprod 1999;14:3077-79.
22. Magistrini M, Szollosi D. Effects of cold and of isopropyl N-phenylcarbamate on the second meiotic spindle of mouse oocytes. Eur J Cell Biol 1980;22:699-707.
23. Martino A, Ansen N, Leibo SP. Development into blastocysts of bovine oocytes cryopreserved by ultrarapid cooling. Biol Reprod 1996;54:1059-69.
24. Mazur P. Equilbrium, quasi-equilibrium, and non-equilibrium freezing of mammalian embryos, Cell Biophys 1990;17:53-92.
25. Nakagata N. High survival rate of unfertilized mouse oocytes after vitrification. J Reprod Fertil 1989;87:479-83.

26. O'Neil L, Paynter SJ, Fuller BJ. Vitrification of mature oocytes: improved results following addition of polythylene glycol to dimethyl sulfoxide solution. Cryobiology 1997;31(3):295-310.

27. Pickering S, Braude P, Johnson M, et al. Transient cooling to room temperature can cause irreversible disruption of the meiotic spindle in the human oocyte. Fertil Steril 1990;54:102-08.

28. Polak de Fried E, Notrica J, Rubinstein M et al. Pregnancy after human donor oocyte cryopreservation and thawing in association with intracytoplasmic sperm injection in a patient with ovarian failure. Fertil Steril 1998;69:555-57.

29. Porcu E, Fabbri R, Seracchioli R, et al. Birth of a healthy female after intracytoplasmatic sperm injection of cryopreserved human oocytes. Fertil Steril 1997;68:724-30.

30. Porcu E, Fabbri R, Seracchioli R et al. Birth of six healthy children after intracytoplasmatic sperm injection of cryopreserved human oocytes. Hum Reprod 1998;13:724-26.

31. Rall WF, Fahy GM. Ice-free cryopreservation of mouse embryos at −196°C vitrification. Nature 1985;313:573-75.

32. Rall WF. Factors affecting the survival of mouse embryos cryopreserved by vitrification, Cryobiology 1987;24:387-402.

33. Sathananthan AH, Ng SC, Trounson A, et al. The effects of ultrarapid screening on meiotic and mitotic spindles of mouse oocytes and embryos. Gamete Res 1988a; 21:385-401.

34. Sathananthan AH, Trounson A, Freeman L, et al. The effects of cooling human oocytes. Hum Reprod 1988b;8:968-77.

35. Schalkoff ME, Oskowitz SP, Powers RD. Ultrastructural observations of human and mouse oocytes treated with cryopreservatives. Biol Reprod 1989;40:379-93.

36. Serafini P, Tran C, Tan T. Cryopreservation of human oocytes. A clinical trial. J Assist Reprod Genet 1995;12:1S-220S.

37. Todorow SJ, Siebzehnrubl ER, Spitzer M, et al. Comparative results on survival of human and animal eggs using different cryoprotectants and freeze-thawing regimens. II. Human Hum Reprod 1989;4:812-16.

38. Trounson A, Kirby C. Problems in the cryopreservation of unfertilized eggs by slow cooling in dimethyl sulfoxide. Fertil Steril 1989;52:778-86.

39. Tucker M, Wright G, Morton P, et al. Preliminary experience with human oocyte cryopreservation using 1, 2 propanediol and sucrose. Hum Reprod 1996; 11:1513-15.

40. Tucker MJ, Morton PC, Wright G, et al. Clinical application of human egg cryopreservation. Hum. Reprod 1998;13:3156-59.

41. Vajta G. Vitrification of the oocytes and embryos of domestic animals. Anim Reprod Sci 2000;60-61:357-64.

42. Vajta G, Holm P, Kuwayama M, et al. Open pulled straw (OPS) vitrification: a new way to reduce cryoinjuries of bovine ova and embryos. Mol Reprod Dev 1998;51:53-58.

43. Van Blerkom J, Davis PW. Cytogenetic, cellular, and developmental consequences of cryopreservation of immature and mature mouse and human oocytes. Microsc Res Tech 1994;27:165-93.

44. Van der Elst J, Van der Abbeel E, Nerinckx S, et al. Parthenogenetic activation of pattern and microtubular organization of the mouse oocytes after exposure to 1-2 propanediol. Cryobiology 1992;29:549-62.

45. Van Uem JFHM, Siebzehnrubl ER, Schuh B, et al. Birth after cryopreservation of unfertilized oocytes. Lancet, ii, 1988;752-53.

46. Vincent C, Pickering SJ, Johnson MH. The zona hardening effect of dimethyl sulfoxide requires the presence of an oocyte and is associated with reduction in the number of cortical granules present. J Reprod Fertil 1990;89:253-59.

47. Yang DS, Blohm PL, Winslow L, et al. A twin pregnancy after microinjection of human cryopreserved oocyte with a specially developed oocyte cryopreservation regime. Fertil Steril 1998;S239, P-357.

48. Young E, Kenny A, Piugdomenech E, et al. Triplet pregnancy after intracytoplasmatic sperm injection of cryopreserved oocytes: case report. Fertil. Steril 1998;70:360-61.

• **Meheranghiz B Minbattiwalla**

49

Preimplantation Genetic Diagnosis

"Genes" are the genetic codes within the 23 sets of chromosomes in a human body. Approximately, there are about 100,000 genes in the 22 pairs of autosomes and the sex chromosomes X and Y, each coding for a particular protein or a trait. Any change in the genic pattern will alter the function of the relevant protein. Each cell in the human body contains two copies of every gene. The back-up copy usually recognizes any gene mistake and repairs it before passing it on to its offspring. Sometimes, the cell's DNA repair mechanisms fail or the cell surveillance becomes less efficient, e.g. due to age. The accumulation of gene mistakes results in "mutations" serious enough to cause genetic disease. About 5000 human genes are known to have mutations. Mutated genes are either inherited from parents or acquired spontaneously.

An estimated 60 percent of all *in vitro* fertilization (IVF) pregnancy losses are associated with chromosomal abnormalities in the embryo.[1] Performing preimplantation genetic diagnosis (PGD) prior to embryo transfer could prevent the initiation of abnormal pregnancies in IVF patients, especially in women over 35 years or older where aneuploidies and other genetic abnormalities of the embryo are more frequent, increasing the risk of spontaneous miscarriage or the development of an abnormal fetus. It is also favourable for couples who have a family history of a specific genetic disease and for those with moral objections to termination of pregnancy.

PGD was developed in the late 1980s as an alternative to prenatal diagnosis. The first successful cases of PGD were performed in 1988, but since then this technique has progressed slowly, mainly due to the time taken to develop single-cell diagnostic techniques with polymerase chain reaction (PCR) in order to obtain a representative sample for analysis.

PGD takes an advantage of IVF techniques, so that embryos are generated *in vitro*. When the embryo is at the 6-8 cell stage (day 3) embryo biopsy is performed and 1-2 blastomeres are excised for genetic diagnosis. Traditionally embryo biopsy is performed using Acid Tyrode's solution, but more recently a non-contact laser is also used. Two blastomeres are mostly removed so that two independent genetic diagnoses can be obtained. This is of advantage when chromosomal mosaicism and dominant chromosomal disorders exist. For cases where aneuploidy screening is required in order to improve IVF pregnancy rate, one blastomere is generally removed. The first and the second polar bodies can also be used for aneuploidy screening but only for maternally inherited diseases.

The genetic material–deoxyribonucleic acid (DNA) in a blastomere is analyzed either by Fluorescent *in situ* Hybridization (FISH) or PCR. FISH utilizes different fluorescent colored probes, which are specific for a given chromosome. Up to 11 chromosomes can be examined in a single cell using this method. However, all the 11 probes cannot be used in one attempt, as it is not possible to examine more than five chromosomes in an interphase nucleus at one time, therefore the biopsied cells are re-probed with additional probes.

Sexing by FISH is probably the simplest PGD test to perform, using three probes, for each sex chromosomes and an autosome. The sex chromosome FISH probes bind rapidly to the nuclei and results can be made available in a few hours. FISH is most convenient for sexing the embryos in case of X-linked diseases like, haemophilia and Duchenne Muscular Dystrophy. It is also an easy technique for aneuploidy screening for infertile couples going through IVF with advanced maternal age, recurrent IVF failure or recurrent miscarriage provided the couple has a normal karyotype.

The various color combinations of the FISH probes help in distinguishing normal cells from cells with aneuploidy and therefore, common mutations viz. an extra number 21 chromosome (trisomy 21—Down's syndrome), missing X chromosome (Turner's syndrome), an extra X chromosome (XXY–Klinefelter's syndrome), an extra number 13 chromosome (trisomy 13–Patau's syndrome) and an extra number 18 chromosome (trisomy 18–Edward's syndrome) can be easily detected. For Robertsonian translocations, probes are available for the acrocentric chromosomes (13, 14, 15, 21 and 22). Few commercial FISH probes are available for specific chromosomal sites. For reciprocal translocations, three color FISH probes are used on either side of the break points, but often a high level of abnormal chromosomes are observed, which makes it difficult to develop a PGD program for this group. PGD for chromosome abnormalities could be possible in future when more commercial probes are available or with the development of techniques like "Comparative Genomic Hybridization (CGH)."

The *PCR* technique is best suited for single cell genetic diagnosis, particularly for the detection of single gene disorders. Single cell PCR helps in establishing molecular analysis with rapid amplification and analysis of the concerned gene. It is particularly important when the amount of genetic material available is considerably limited. Diagnosis of single copies of genes within a single cell is an attractive possibility for PGD, since prevention of the disease through carrier identification and genetic counseling cannot diminish the impact of the genetically transmitted diseases. Single cell PCR besides being a technically challenging procedure has risks of contamination and allele dropout (ADO). Since only one cell is amplified, if another cell or another piece of DNA enters the reaction tube, it will also be amplified. Therefore, ICSI is performed for the embryos to be biopsied, to ensure that there are no more than one sperm present to avoid paternal contamination and cumulus is removed entirely to avoid maternal contamination. Stringent conditions are employed to ensure that no other contamination occurs; therefore, unlinked polymorphic markers are incorporated to be sure that the DNA is of embryonic origin. Parents and other family members should also be tested to find an informative marker and used in a multiplex fluorescent PCR protocol.

ADO in the PCR technique is the preferential amplification of one allele over another. It poses a problem for PGD of dominant disorders or where two different mutations are carried for a recessive disorder, if only one mutation is being analyzed.[2] Modifications of PCR protocols or pretreatment of the cell before PCR decreases the ADO rate or may even eliminate it entirely depending upon the number of primers within the multiplex. Multiplex cells provide multiplex copies to amplify, with the result, effects of ADO become either insignificant or are balanced by ADO of other alleles.[3] ADOs do occur more frequently in multiplex PCR, when cell numbers are decreased;[4, 5] however, low rates of ADOs are reported with preferential amplification.[6] Reduced quantity of dNTP and *Taq* in a PCR reaction balances the rate of amplification of alleles, avoiding the phenomenon of ADO.[7]

Microsatellites in multiplex PCR enhances reliability and accuracy of single cell diagnosis. Microsatellites, which are a category of short tandem repeat (STR) sequences show variability and stability and are ideal genetic markers. They help in tracing the contamination source by matching to all sources of potential contamination. Thus, contamination can be identified and controlled especially when single cell reactions are to be performed for PGD.

With conventional PCR if the product yield is low, it will indicate a faint signal on the gel and the migration rate across the gel may also differ; thus the standard values produced will be inaccurate. But, sensitivity can be improved many-fold by labeling the primers with fluorescent markers and using an ultrasensitive system fluorescent DNA sequencer like the "gene-scanner" that separates, detects and analyzes the fluorescent labeled PCR products. Its other advantage is that several primers can be multiplexed together even if the product range overlap each other as different dyes can be simultaneously determined.[8] Fluorescent PCR also reduces misdiagnosis caused by contamination. This technique is most feasible for PGD so that embryos are neither wrongly replaced nor discarded; however, it is an expensive investment. Nevertheless, there are conventional PCR protocols that can function under stringent resources,[7] so that PGD in IVF centers can be regarded more critically and within an open scope for preferential preimplantation screening.

Patients opting for PGD should be given proper counseling and be made aware of the limitations, advantages and risks of the technique. They should know:

i. that, they would have to undergo IVF procedure(s) including ovarian stimulation even if they are fertile.

ii. that, the procedure entails moral, legal, technical and financial issues.

iii. that, there could be misdiagnosis, inconclusive diagnosis and possible long-term negative effects, which at present are unknown.

The data from European Society of Human Reproduction and Embryology (ESHRE) PGD consortium[9] shows that the pregnancy rates from PGD are around 20 percent. This is low, as many good quality embryos having implantation potential are rejected, because they are genetically or chromosomally abnormal. Till date PGD babies

have not been exposed to risks of neonatal problems or malformations.[10]

Potential Advantages of PGD

- Few malformed babies and pregnancy terminations.
- Less genetic testing during pregnancy (amniocentesis and chorionic villus sampling).
- Increase in implantation rate after IVF.
- Reducing spontaneous abortions by transferring normal embryos.
- Eliminating the step of cryopreservation, which often results in loss of embryos.
- Avoiding the transmission of genetic diseases.

Risks Involved in PGD

- There could be accidental damage to an embryo during biopsy.
- Removal of 1-2 blastomeres could delay embryo development but will not affect the embryo's ability to grow and result in normal pregnancy.
- Misuse of the technique for sex selection.
- Abortion could kill one baby at a time, but PGD may eliminate more than one embryo, depending on the number of embryos analyzed.
- Misdiagnosis could occur due to contamination from foreign DNA if strict sterility is not observed during the procedure.

PGD is being globally used for an increasing number of genetic and chromosomal abnormalities

PGD for Fragile X

Fragile X syndrome is a common single-gene disorder of neuro-developmental disability that leads to varying degrees of mental retardation and physical disorder. Individuals with this syndrome inherit it from their mother who carries a "premutation" or a "full mutation allele". This syndrome occurs due to an unstable region of DNA within the FMR-1 gene on the X-chromosome. Affected individuals carry the full mutation (>200 CGG repeats), which originates from the premutation allele (52-200 CGG repeats) on the maternal X chromosome. The FMR-1 gene contains a set of CGG repeat sequences that are polymorphic within the population. Normal alleles have 6-54 repeat sequences. "Premutation" alleles have the capacity to expand and cause disease in the next generation.[11]

PGD for Sickle Cell Anemia

Sickle cell anemia is the most common autosomal recessive disorder in humans. Indications for diagnosis include a homozygous (one β^s gene on each chromosome) or compound heterozygous states with the β^s gene on one chromosome and β-globin chain defects viz. HbC, HbD and severe β-thalassemias (β^0CD39 and IVSl-ntl mutations) on the other, the latter completely destroying β-globin chain synthesis and the β^+IVS-nt 110 genotype, which curtails β-globin production.[12]

The first DNA diagnostic procedure for prenatal purpose was reported 23 years ago,[13] which recognized that the mutation of this disease itself affected the cleavage site of a restriction enzyme, *DdeI* that recognizes the DNA sequence of CTNAG (N = A, T, C or G). DNA from a normal allele (CTGAG) is digested by the enzyme, but DNA from an affected allele, in which A is substituted by T, (CTGTG) is not digested.[14,15] The resulting differences between DNA fragment sizes are recognized by electrophoresis. *HpaI* restriction fragment length polymorphism (RFLP) was used earlier to distinguish β^A-globin and β^S-globin genes.[13,16,17] With the advent of PCR, mutated region (CCT **G**AG GAG to CCT **G**TG GAG, codons 5-7) is amplified for diagnosis using: (i) Oligonucleotide hybridization technique, which is a synthetic labeled oligonucleotide (~20 kilobases) binding specifically to the CCT GTG GAG sequence under stringent conditions, but not to CCT GAG GAG. The reaction is carried out on a membrane using a drop of PCR product and the binding site is seen using probes tagged with radioactive isotopes or enzymatic chromogenes. There are several variations of this technique;[18,19] therefore, cross-checks with control probes, e.g. β^A sequence are essential. (ii) Analysis of restriction endonuclease site identifies the mutation by the absence of a restriction endonuclease site with the Southern blot technique on extracted DNA; the lost cleavage site produces a larger RFLP fragment.[14,15] Using

enzyme *MstII*, the normal CCT-GAG-GAG sequence is cut into two DNA fragment, 228 and 202 bp sizes. The enzyme cannot cleave the mutant sequence, CCT-GTG-GAG and yields a single 430 bp DNA fragment[20] Other enzymes that recognize the CCTGTGGAAG mutation are *DdeI* and *Bsu361* (an isoschizomer of *MstII*).[21, 22]

The first PGD for sickle cell anemia was performed in mouse model[23] and the first unaffected pregnancy resulting from PGD for this disease in humans was reported by Xu and co-workers.[24]

PGD for Spinal Muscular Atrophy (SMA)

SMA is a neuromuscular autosomal recessive disorder, affecting 1 in 6,000 babies. The disease is divided in three clinical subtypes (I, II, III), characterized by decreasing severity of symptoms. More than 95 percent of the patients are homozygous for a deletion of exon 7 of the survival motor neuron (SMN) gene. Most of the patients with SMA lack both copies of SMN1 exon 7 and most carriers have only one copy of SMN1 exon 7.[25] Detection of the deletion could be hampered by the presence of a highly homologous SMN2. With multiplex quantitative PCR assay, using restriction enzyme digestion *DraI*, differentiation between SMN2 from SMN1 is possible;[25] both the genes differ by only one nucleotide. In the absence of the SMN1 gene, patients carry one or more copies of the highly homologous SMN2 gene. But in the absence of the SMN2 gene, a mutant SMN2 A2G transgene is unable to rescue the embryonic lethality. In the presence of SMN2, the A2G transgene delays the onset of motor neuron loss, resulting in mild SMA.[26]

DNA molecular studies[27] of the SMN gene on the long arm of chromosome 5(5q11.2q13.3) revealed homozygous deletion of exon 7 along with a homologous deletion of exon 8. There may therefore be 5q-unlinked SMA or SMA due to other mutations. With quantitative Southern blot analysis, a severe and homogeneous decrease in the content of muscle mtDNA in relation to nuclear DNA in SMA patients is possible along with a two-to-three fold reduction of the nuclear-encoded complex II (succinate dehydrogenase) activity in SMA muscle tissue.[28] With western blot analysis reduction of both mitochondrial-and nuclear-encoded cytochrome C oxidase subunits is possible.

PGD for Fanconi Anemia (FA)

FA is an inherited anemia initiating bone marrow failure (aplastic anemia), that eventually develops acute myelogenous leukemia (AML). It is a recessive disorder. If both the parents carry a mutation in the same FA gene, then each of their children has a 25 percent chance of inheriting the defective gene from both parents to acquire FA. There are at least seven FA genes: A, C, D2, E, F, G and BRCA2 and six of these genes, which account for > 85 percent of the cases of FA have been cloned. Mutations in FA-A and FA-C, account for FA in 76 percent of patients worldwide.

Cytogenetic studies have shown that since particular mutation predisposes to multiple chromosome breaks, spontaneous chromosome breakage is a feature of FA with interchanges usually between non-homologous chromosomes. A high frequency of monosomy 7 and duplications involving 1q are found[29] with no occurrences of t(8; 21), t(15; 17) or abnormalities of 11q, which are associated with M2, M3 and M5 leukemias, respectively. Several markers of telomeric integrity and function with high frequency of extra chromosomal TTAGGG signals, and of chromosomes ends with undetectable TTAGGG repeats suggests an intensive breakage at telomeric sequences. Quantitative FISH analysis showes an accelerated telomere shortening of 0.68 kb in both arms of FA chromosomes and a 10-fold increase in chromosome end fusions despite normal binding of TRF2, a telomere binding factor that protects human telomeres from end fusions.[30]

Complementation studies on molecular basis[31-38] have postulated that FA mutations are allelic. Heterogeneous responses suggest genetic heterogenecity.[39, 40] With transfection experiments,[41] two DNA sequences, that are the hallmarks of FA, can be corrected: spontaneous chromosome breakage and hypersensitivity to the cell killing, and clastogenic effects of the difunctional alkylating agent diepoxybutane.

These experiments have opened a way for cloning the 'FA gene', mapping it and determining its gene product and precise function.[42]

PGD for FA Combining with HLA Matching

DNA analysis of single blastomeres for the IVS4 + 4A→T (adenine to thymine) mutation in the FA complement C (FANCC) gene has identified the genetic status and HLA markers of each embryo before implantation for an affected sibling requiring stem cell transplant.[43]

PGD for Alpha 1-antitrypsin Deficiency

Alpha 1-antitrypsin deficiency is a very common autosomal recessive disorder in the white population. This 52-kDa glycoprotein, accounts for 90 percent of the total alpha 1-globulin in plasma. Despite its name, its major function is to inhibit the activity of elastase generated by neutrophils in the lungs. Activated neutrophils elaborate elastase and release oxygen radicals and chlorinated oxidants that oxidize methionine at the active site of alpha 1-antitrypsin. Such oxidation introduces a 2000-fold decrease in the rate of association of the specific serine protease inhibitor with the neutrophil elastase, reducing the ability to inhibit elastase activity. This unopposed elastase activity can cause severe destruction of lung tissue. The major phenotype of alpha 1-antitrypsin deficiency is destruction of pulmonary alveoli resulting in chronic obstructive pulmonary disease or emphysema.

The gene for alpha 1-antitrypsin is highly polymorphic with more than 70 percent different alleles found in the European population. The different forms of alpha 1-antitrypsin, frequently designated as Pi for proteinase inhibitor, can be distinguished by the differences in electrophoretic mobility. The most common allele is the PiM with an allele frequency of 0.95. Two mutant alleles S and Z, account for most of the disease associated with alpha 1-antitrypsin deficiency. Homozygous PiSS reduces alpha 1-antitrypsin activity by 50-60 percent but does not cause the disease, while PiZZ is associated with 10-15 percent of normal activity and accounts for most of the illness associated with alpha 1-antitrypsin deficiency. PiZZ also accounts for the accumulation of the abnormal protein secondary to failure of the hepatocyte to secrete it causing liver disease, with the result approximately 20 percent of children with this genotype develop juvenile cirrhosis and ~20 percent of adults develop cirrhosis of the liver with an increased risk of primary carcinoma of the liver. Heterozygous PiSZ individuals have 30-35 percent normal activity and may develop emphysema. Many rare alleles can also cause severe deficiency or absence (null alleles) of detectable alpha 1-antitrypsin.

The gene of alpha 1-antitrypsin is cloned and mapped on the long arm of chromosome 14. The PiS variant results from a GAA to GTA mutation in exon 3 causing the substitution of valine for glutamic acid at position 264, resulting in the production of an inhibitor with decreased stability. The PiZ variant results from a mutation in exon 5 changing GAG to AAG, encoding Glutamic acid at position 342. Although alpha 1-antitrypsin gene is highly polymorphic, only two mutations, Z and S cause the majority of disease associated with a deficiency of this protein inhibitor. Therefore, relevant regions of DNA are amplified with PCR using allele-specific oligonucleotide probes specific for the normal or mutant sequence. Highly accurate diagnosis is accomplished using a combination of allele-specific oligonucleotide probes and RFLPs.[44]

PGD for Tay-Sachs Disease

Tay-Sachs is yet another autosomal recessive hereditary disorder affecting the central nervous system (CNS). The classic infantile type is the most common. Babies with Tay-Sachs lack hexosaminidase A (hexA), an enzyme necessary for breaking down certain fatty substance in the brain and nerve cells. These substances build up and gradually destroy brain and nerve cells, until the entire CNS stops working. Death occurs by age 5. In cases where hexA levels are low symptoms begin later in life and death generally occurs by age 15.

A Tay-Sachs carrier has one normal gene for hexA and one Tay-Sachs gene. High-risks couples,

have a 25 percent chance with each pregnancy of conceiving a child with the same condition, a 50 percent chance of producing a carrier child and a 25 percent chance that a child will be neither be a carrier nor affected with the disease. If only one parent is a carrier, none of their children will have the disease, but each child will have a 50-50 chance of inheriting the Tay-Sachs gene and being a carrier. DNA-based genetic testing can determine whether the embryo has infantile Tay-Sachs or another hexA deficiency and its severity. The test can also look for known mutations in the hexA gene that cause the disease.

PGD for Canavan Disease

Canavan disease is also an autosomal recessive trait that belongs to a group of conditions known as leukodystrophies, which result from defects in myelin—a substance made up of proteins and lipids, which forms an integral component of the nervous system. The function of myelin or 'white matter' in the brain is to protect nerves and allow messages to be sent to and from the brain. One of the earliest signs of the disease is overall low muscle tone and lack of head control beginning during infancy. In the affected child, the white matter begins to deteriorate due to a deficiency of enzyme aspartoacylase, which leads to the accumulation of a chemical, N-acelyl-aspartic acid (NAA), in the brain that causes destruction of myelin. Both the parents of an affected child are carriers of an altered gene on chromosome 17, which is responsible for synthesizing aspartoacylase. A carrier parent is healthy because he/she has one functional copy of the gene, which produces a sufficient amount of the enzyme. A child who receives two altered copies of the gene, one from each parent is unable to produce any aspartoacylase and will develop the Canavan disease.

PGD for Achondroplasia (ACH)

ACH is the most common genetic form of short-limbed dwarfism, inherited as an autosomal dominant trait with 100 percent penetrance. 90 percent of the cases are sporadic with an increased risk correlated with paternal age at the time of conception suggesting a *de novo* and paternal origin of the mutation.[45] Homozygosity of the ACH alleles leads to a more severe phenotype with embryonal lethality.[46] ACH is due to a unique amino acid substitution of a glycine to an arginine at position 380 (G380R) in the transmembrane domain of the fibroblast growth factor receptor 3 (FGFR3).[47] This missense mutation at position 1138 is due to a G to A transition in 97 percent of the cases and a G to C transversion in the rest of the cases.[48] The first attempt at PGD testing two mutations for ACH[49] involved a substitution at G380R position of FGFR3 for *SfcI* or *MspI* restriction sites.

PGD for Cystic Fibrosis (CF)

The initiated disorder CF is characterized by mucous membrane abnormalities in the lungs. The disease occurs frequently in patients with asthama and in those with allergic rhinitis. CF disorder is diagnosed by the presence of alterations in a gene known as Cystic Fibrosis Transmembrane Conductance Regulator (CFTR). People with CF carry two copies of an altered CFTR gene, which affects the membranes in the lungs and leads to accumulation of thick, sticky mucous. CF mutation analysis have characterized 80 different mutations, accounting for ~91 percent of CF genes and generating 103 different genotypes. The most frequently occurring mutation, Δ-508, is the single amino acid deletion in exon 10 of chromosome 7, which codes for a portion of the first nucleotide binding function (NBF-1) domain of the CFTR gene. The other common mutations are, M470V, L997E, E528E, 621 + IG > T, G542X, N1303K, 2789 + 5G > A, 2183AA > G, E822X and R1158X.[50,51] Approximately, 48 mutations can be tested. Findlay *et al*[6] first reported ADO and preferential amplification in single cell PCR analysis for CF along with sex determination in the same reaction.

PGD for Down's Syndrome and Sex Determination

PGD can be performed simultaneously for chromosome 21 and sex determination using 3-color FISH technique. An accurate, rapid and cost-effective diagnostic system can be offered by using quantitative multiplex fluorescent PCR for simultaneous diagnosis and conformation of sex and trisomy using two markers for chromosome 21 in single cells.[52]

PGD for Susceptibility and Late on-set Conditions

There are susceptibility genes that trigger late in life and are inherited from the parents. A healthy child at birth may develop Li-Fraumeni syndrome, breast cancer or schizophrenia later in life. PGD can be carried out to avoid the birth of a child with P53 mutations for Li-Fraumeni syndrome[53,54] and early on-set Alzheimer's disease.[55] PGD may be sought for BRCA1 and 2, susceptibility for breast cancer or for potential linkage on chromosome 22q12-q13.1 susceptibility for schizophrenia or schizoaffective disorders.[56]

PGD for HLA Matching for an Existing Child

Parents opting for a child to produce stem cells for an affected child, would prefer to have PGD as it will enable them to transfer only those embryos free of the disease and HLA matched to the existing child. PGD was sought for conceiving a child who would serve as a source for providing haematopoitic stem cells from the umbilical cord blood, for a child suffering from Fanconi anemia.[43] Without the stem cell transplant, chances for survival of the first child were remote and non-sibling matches are normally not safe and effective as sibling donations. Parents could have conceived coitally for the same purpose, but if the new fetus was not the HLA-match for the suffering child, it could be a burden and even put up for adoption.[57] Instead, IVF-PGD helped in choosing the embryos that served as HLA-matched donor(s) for the suffering child.

PGD for Gender Selection

The controversial use of PGD for sex selection, i.e. to have preference for a particular gender rather than the health of the child is abusive. When families with 'culturally-founded sexist notions' want the first born to be a male child and

PGD is attempted to select the Y-bearing embryo, then the technique is misused and unfair to the female gender.

On the other hand if PGD is done for the purpose of 'gender variety' in a family, whereby the sex of the second or subsequent children is sought, the application becomes less controversial and defensive. It gives the legitimacy of wanting to raise children of both genders. Another acceptable use of PGD for gender variety is to select male off-spring as the second child for couples who already have a daughter.[58] For this purpose of 'balancing' a family, PGD appears to be justified with fewer disparities in the sex ratio. These choices do not express a hierarchy or inequality between sexes and hence are not "sexist".

PGD for Non-medical Traits

PGD for selection for inheritable phenotypic traits such as hearing ability, sexual orientation, intelligence, height, beauty etc., although not feasible, its use in future may be possible. PGD can be applied to test for GJB2 mutations for deafness, which is the most common phenotypic trait.[59] It would be appropriate to offer PGD for people with a family history of deafness, to screen embryos with this mutation.

Partial list of other Genetic disorders available through PGD:
1. Aneuploidies of chromosomes 13, 16, 18, 21, 22, X and Y
2. Adrenal Leukodystrophy + HLA
3. Alloimmune Thrombocytopenia
4. Alzheimer's Disease (early on-set)
5. Becher Muscular Dystrophy
6. Beta Thalassemia
7. Beta Thalassemia + HLA
8. BRCA 1 and 2
9. Charcot Marie Disease
10. Connexin 26 (mutations E47X and 30delG)
11. Cri du Chat
12. Chronic Granulomatosis Disease
13. Duschenne Muscular Dystrophy
14. Epidermolysis Bulosa
15. Familial Dysautonomia–IKAP
16. Gaucher's disease
17. Hemophilia Factor VII
18. Hemophilia Factor X
19. HLA alone (leukemias)
20. Hunter's Syndrome
21. Huntington's Disease
22. Hurler Syndrome
23. Hyper IGM + HLA
24. Kleinfelter's Syndrome
25. Lesch-Nylan Syndrome
26. Li-Fraumeni Syndrome (to detect p53 mutations)
27. Lymphoproliferative Dx (X-linked)
28. Marfans
29. Mendelian Disorders
30. Metachromatic Leukodystrophy (some mutations)
31. Myotonic Dystrophy
32. Pachyonychia Congenita
33. Pelizaens–Merzbacher Syndrome
34. Polycystic Kidney Disease
35. Prader—Willi Syndrome or Angelman Syndrome
36. Retinitis Pigmentosa
37. Rh(D) Genotype
38. Spinocerebellar Ataxia
39. Wiscott—Aldrich

Sixty-five more genetically inheritable single gene defect diseases can be detected.

The Ethical Implications of PGD

PGD was hindered by misdiagnosis; therefore in 1997, a PGD consortium was established as part of the ESHRE and ever since annual reports of the world data on PGD are produced. As with most technological advances, there is always the potential for abuse; thus ethical issues in PGD are important to consider as this technique is already been used for HLA matching[43] and sexing for social reasons.[58]

This ingenious technology has not only ushered a conception for the end of genetic disorders but has also triggered a debate regarding fetal rights versus parental rights. In principle, it is the diagnosis for a specific disease mutation or chromosomal aberration. It spares the off-spring the burden of having to make similar decisions for their own reproduction. Two groups of "pro-lifers" view PGD with different perspectives making the issue controversial.

For the "orthodox" pro-lifers, PGD is unthinkable and an abuse, as abortion kills one baby at a time, PGD eliminates several embryos at a time if they are tested genetically unfit for transfer. Secondly, the selection of embryos itself is objectionable. There are fears that genetic screening of prospective children will move us towards a eugenic world in which children would be valued for their genotype than for their inherent characteristics. This would eventually start a vogue of "designer" children produced with the help of genetic engineering and the essence of procreating naturally will be lost.

For the "moderate" pro-lifers, PGD is far less emotionally traumatic than the traditional abortion. Preventing implantation and pregnancy is reasonably acceptable than getting pregnant and aborting the fetus later. This "infanticide" is crueler than selective implantation. Although the preimplantation embryos can be considered as living entities, it is not appropriate to bestow "rights" for them as they are yet in a rudimentary stage of development;[60] nevertheless, they are to be respected as the first stage towards a new person.[61] With this perspective, PGD should be made ethically acceptable, to be used for preventing offsprings with serious genetic disease, i.e. progressing towards establishing a 'clean gene pool'.

It is likely for scientific technology to be misused as scientists unravel the mysteries of life; but if careful ethical analysis is brought about with legitimate and legal concerns, open public debates and appropriate policy issues, any misuse of technology can be averted. It is important that all countries establish strict criteria for the use of PGD to avoid eugenics. Development of newer scientific technologies is in the interest of mankind, for improving the quality of life, towards the process of eradicating the real enemy of life— "the suffering", it should therefore be used cautiously as Aldous Huxley[62] suggests in the foreword of Brave New World: "as though, like the Sabbath, they had been made for man, not (as at present and still more so in the Brave New World) as though man were to be adapted and enslaved to them."

PGD at the moment seems the only realistic approach and allows better use of the available resources for the existing patient populations until gene therapy or other approaches can cure or significantly improve the clinical impact of the conditions. In situations where an affected individual has a family history of the genetic disease it may be possible to identify the mutation in that family and use the information for PGD-DNA testing rather than identifying individual mutations, which could be costly and time consuming. Another method would be "linkage analysis", which is a form of DNA testing that compares the DNA of the embryo to that of affected and unaffected relatives, to determine if the embryo is affected.

The goal of gene therapy, where scientists transfer a normal gene into cells to replace an abnormal or missing gene,[63] is to cure or alleviate the symptoms of certain genetic diseases. This revolutionary new form of treatment is being tested in patients with several genetic diseases. This approach holds promise in completely nullifying inheritable disorders.

REFERENCES

1. Minbattiwalla MB. Chromosomal status of failed fertilized oocytes. In: "Predicting Reasons For In-Vitro Fertilization Failure: Understanding ultrastructural, cytogenetics and immunological disorders." Ph.D thesis, University of Bombay 2001.
2. Rechitsky S, Freidine M, Verlinsky Y, et al. Allele dropout in sequential PCR and FISH analysis of single cells (cell recycling). J Ass Reprod Gen 1996;13:115-24.
3. Findlay I, Matthews P, Quirke P. Multiple genetic diagnosis from single cells using multiplex PCR: reliability and allele dropout. Prenat Diagn 1998;18: 1413-21.
4. Lygo JE, Johnson PE, Holdaway DJ, et al. The validation of short tandem repeat (STR) loci for use in forensic casework. Int J Legal Med 1994;107:77-89.
5. Ray P, Handyside A. Single cell analysis for diagnosis of cystic fibrosis and Lesh-Nyham syndrome in human embryos before implantation. Miami Bio-Technology Short Reports: Proceedings of the Miami Bio-Technology European Symposium. Advances in Gene Technology: Molecular Biology and Human Genetic Disease; IRL, Oxford Univ Press. 1994;5-46.

6. Findlay I, Ray P, Quirke P et al. Allelic dropout and preferential amplication in single cells and human blastomeres: implication for preimplantation diagnosis of sex and cystic fibrosis. Hum Reprod 1995;10:1609-18.

7. Minbattiwalla MB, Mukhopadhyaya R, Hinduja I, et al. Modified 2-step method for single and duplex PCR on single cells and its applications. Ind J Hum Genet (in press).

8. Findlay I, Quirke P. Fluorescent polymerase chain reaction: Part I. A new method allowing genetic diagnosis and DNA fingerprinting of single cells. Hum Reprod Update 1996;2:137-52.

9. ESHRE PGD Consortium Steering Committee ESHRE Preimplantation Genetic Diagnosis (PGD) Consortium: data collection II. Hum Reprod 2000;15:2673-83.

10. The ESHRE Ethics Taskforce. Taskforce 5: Preimplantation Genetic Diagnosis. Hum Reprod 2003;18:649-51.

11. Sermon K, Seneca S, VanderFaeillie A, et al. Preimplantation diagnosis for Fragile X syndrome based on the detection of the non-expanded paternal and maternal CGG. Prenat Diagn 1999;19:1223-30.

12. Voskaridou E, Kollia P, Loukopoulos D. Sickle Cell Thalassemia in Greece. Identification and contribution of the interacting β-thalassemia genes. Ann NY Acad Sci 1990;612:508-09.

13. Kan YW, Dozy AM. Antenatal diagnosis of sickle-cell anaemia by DNA analysis of amniotic fluid cells. Lancet 1978;2:910-12.

14. Chang JC, Kan YW. A sensitive new prenatal test for sickle-cell anemia. N Engl J Med 1982;307:30-32.

15. Orkin SH, Little PFR, Kazazian HH Jr, et al. Improved detection of the sickle mutation by DNA analysis. N Engl J Med 1982;307:32-36.

16. Kan YW, Dozy AM. Polymorphism of DNA sequences adjacent to the human β-globin structural gene: relationship to sickle mutation. Proc Natl Acad Sci 1978;75:5631-35.

17. Kazazian HH jr, Phillips JA, Boehm CD, et al. Prenatal diagnosis of β-thalassemia by amniocentises; linkage analysis of multiple polymorphic restriction endonuclease sites. Blood 1980;56:926-30.

18. Saiki RK, Walsh PS, Levenseon CH, et al. Genetic analysis of amplified DNA with immobilized sequence specific oligonucleotide probes. Proc Natl Acad Sci USA 1989;17:2503-16.

19. Greever RF, Wilson LB, Nallaseth HH Jr, et al. Improved detection of the sickle cell mutation by DNA analysis: application to prenatal diagnosis. N Engl J Med 1982;307:32-36.

20. Embury SH, Sharf SJ, Saiki RK, et al. Rapid prenatal diagnosis of sickle cell anemia by a new method of DNA analysis. N Engl J Med 1987;316:656-61.

21. Gurgey A, Becsac S, Mesci L, et al. Prenatal diagnosis of sickle cell anemia using PCR and restriction enzyme DdeI. Turkish J Pediatr 1993;35:159-62.

22. Husian SM, Kalavathi P, Anandaraj MP. Analysis of sickle cell gene using the polymerase chain reaction and restriction enzyme Bsu 361. Ind J Med Res 1995;101:273-76.

23. Sheardown SA, Findlay I, Turner A, et al. Preimplantation diagnosis of a human β-globin transgene in biopsied trophectoderm cells and blastomeres of the mouse embryo. Hum Reprod 1992;7:1297-1303.

24. Xu K, Shi Z, Veeck L, et al. First unaffected pregnancy using preimplantation genetic diagnosis for sickle cell anemia. JAMA 1999;281:1701-06.

25. Ogino S, Wilson RB. Quantification of PCR bias caused by a single nucleotide polymorphism in SMN gene dosage analysis. J Mol Diag 2002;4:185-90.

26. Monani U, Pastore MT, Gavrilina TO, et al. A transgene carrying an A2G missense mutation in the SMN gene modulates phenotypic severity in mice with severe (type I) spinal muscular atrophy. J Cell Biol 2003;160:41-52.

27. Shawky RM, Abdel-Aleem K, Rifaat MM, et al. Molecular diagnosis of spinal muscular atrophy in Egyptians. East Mediterr Health J 2001;7:229-37.

28. Berger A, Mayr JA, Meierhofer D, et al. Severe depletion of mitochondrial DNA in spinal muscular atrophy. Acta Neuropathol (Berl) 2003;105:245-51.

29. Auerbach AD, Allen RG. Leukemia and preleukemia in Fanconi anemia patients: a review of the literature and report of the International Fanconi Anemia Registry. Cancer Genet Cytogenet 1991;51:1-12.

30. Callen E, Samper E, Ramirez MJ, et al. Breaks at telomeres and TRF2-independent end fusions in Fanconi anemia. Hum Mol Genet 2002;11:439-44.

31. Poon PK, O'Brien RL, Parker JW. Defective DNA repair in Fanconi anaemia. Nature 1974;250:223-25.

32. Hirsch-Kauffmann M, Schweiger M, Wagner EF, et al. Deficiency of DNA ligase activity in Fanconi's anemia. Hum Genet 1978;45:25-32.

33. Fujiwara Y, Tatsumi M, Sasaki M. Cross-link repair in human cells and its possible defect in Fanconi's anemia cells. J Mol Biol 1977;113:635-49.

34. Wunder E. Further studies on compartmentalization of DNA-topoisomerase I in Fanconi anemia tissue. Hum Genet 1984;68:276-81.

35. Duckworth-Rysiecki G, Cornish K, Clarke CA. Identification of two complementation groups in Fanconi anemia. Somat Cell Mol Genet 1985;11:35-41.

36. Schweiger M, Auer B, Burtscher HJ, et al. DNA repair in human cells: biochemistry of the hereditary diseases Fanconi's anemia and Cockayne syndrome. Europ J Biochem 1987;165:235-42.

37. Auerbach AD: Fanconi anemia and leukemia: tracking the genes. Leukemia 1992;6(Suppl 1):1-4.

38. Strathdee CA, Gavish H, Shannon WR, et al. Cloning of cDNAs for Fanconi's anaemia by functional complementation. Nature 1992;356:763-67.

39. Moustacchi E, Diatloff-Zito C. DNA semi-conservative synthesis in normal and Fanconi anemia fibroblasts following treatment with 8-methoxypsoralen and near

ultraviolet light or with X-rays. Hum Genet 1985;70: 236-42.

40. Diatloff-Zito C, Papadopoulo D, Averbeck D, et al. Abnormal response to DNA cross-linking agents of Fanconi anemia fibroblasts can be corrected by transfection with normal human DNA. Proc Nat Acad Sci 1986;83:7034-38.

41. Shaham M, Adler B, Ganguly S, et al. Transfection of normal human and Chinese hamster DNA corrects diepoxybutane-induced chromosomal hypersensitivity of Fanconi anemia fibroblasts. Proc Nat Acad Sci 1987;84:5853-57.

42. Chaganti RSK, Houldsworth J. Fanconi anemia: a pleotropic (sic) mutation with multiple cellular and developmental abnormalities. Ann Genet 1991;34:206-11.

43. Verlinsky Y, Rechitsky S, Schoolcraft W, et al. Preimplantation diagnosis for Fanconi anemia combined with HLA matching. JAMA 2001;285:3130-33.

44. Gelehrter, Collins. Principles of Medical Genetics, Williams & Wilkins, 1990.

45. Wilkin DJ, Szabo JK, Cameron R, et al. Mutations in fibroblast growth-factor receptor 3 in sporadic cases of achondroplasia occur exclusively on the paternally derived chromosome. Am J Hum Genet 1998;63: 711-16.

46. Pauli RM, Conroy MM, Langer LO Jr, et al. Homozygous achondroplasia with survival beyond infancy. Am J Med Gen 1983;16:459-73.

47. Rousseau F, Bonaventure J, Legeai-Mallet L, et al. Mutations in the gene encoding fibroblast growth factor receptor-3 in achondroplasia. Nature 1994;371:252-54.

48. Bellus GA, Hefferon TW, Ortiz De Luna RJ, et al. Achondroplasia is defined by recurrent G380R mutations of FGFR3. Am J Hum Genet 1995;56: 368-73.

49. Moutou C, Rongieres C, Bettahar-Lebugle K, et al. Preimplantation genetic diagnosis for achondroplasia: genetics and gynaecological limits and difficulties. Hum Reprod 2003;18:509-14.

50. Maire F, Brenvenu T, Ngukam A et al. Frequency of CFTR gene mutations in idiopathic pancreatitis. Gastroenterol Clin Biol 2003;27:398-402.

51. Kanavakis E, Efthymiadou A, Strofalis S, et al. Cystic fibrosis in Greece: molecular diagnosis, haplotypes, prenatal diagnosis and carrier identification amongst high-risk individuals. Clin Genet 2003;63:400-09.

52. Findlay I, Matthews P, Toth T, et al. Same day diagnosis of Down's syndrome and sex in single cells using multiplex fluorescent PCR. Mol Pathol 1998;51:164-67.

53. Simpson JL. Celebrating preimplantation genetic diagnosis of p53 mutations in Li-Fraumeni syndrome. Reprod Biomed Online 2001;3:2-3.

54. Verlinsky Y, Rechitsky S, Verlinsky O, et al. Preimplantation diagnosis of P53 tumor suppressor gene mutations. Reprod Biomed Online 2001;2:102-05.

55. Verlinsky Y, Rechitsky S, Verlinsky O, et al. Preimplantation diagnosis for early-onset Alzheimer's disease caused by V717L mutation JAMA 2002;283:1018-21.

56. Pulver AE, Karayiorgou M, Wolyniec PS, et al. Sequential strategy to identify a susceptibility gene for schizophrenia: report of potential linkage on chromosome 22q12-q13.1: Part 1. Am J Med Genet 1994;54: 36-43.

57. Auerbach AD. Umbilical cord blood transplants for genetic disease: diagnostic and ethical issues in fetal studies. Blood Cells 1994;20:303-09.

58. Malpani A, Malpani A, Mody D. Preimplantation sex selection for family balancing in India. Hum Reprod 2002;17:11-12.

59. Nance WE, Pandya A. Genetic epidemiology of deafness. In: Keats BJB, Popper AN, Fay RR (Eds.): Genetic & Auditory Disorders. Springer-Verlag, New York, USA, 2002;67-91.

60. Robertson JA. Extending preimplantation genetic diagnosis: the ethical debate. Hum Reprod 2003;18: 465-71.

61. American Society of Reproductive Medicine: Ethics Commette, Ethical considerations of assisted reproductive technologies. Fertil Steril 1994;62(Suppl): 32S-37S.

62. Huxley A. "Brave New World", Harper and Brothers, England, p.ix, 1932.

63. Castaldo G, Nardiello P, Bellitti F, et al. Haemophilia B: from molecular diagnosis to gene therapy. Clin Chem Lab Med 2003;41:445-51.

• Orly Lacham-Kaplan

50

Haploidization of Somatic Cells Following Nuclear Transfer into MII Mouse Oocytes

INTRODUCTION

Embryos and offspring from injections of nuclei isolated mechanically from haploid and diploid germ cells such as elongating and round spermatids, and secondary spermatocytes were reported in animals with varied success rates (Lacham-Kaplan and Trounson 1997; Sofikitis *et al* 1998). Mice (Kimura and Yanagimachi 1995) and human (Sofikitis *et al* 1997) secondary spermatocytes, which are diploid germ cells, are able to enter metaphase and undergo meiosis following insertion into MII oocytes and artificial activation. Two-second polar bodies were extruded from the activated oocyte; one contained half of the oocyte chromosomes and the other contained half of the spermatocyte chromosomes. Following embryo transfer, live healthy offspring were born in mice (Kimura and Yanagimachi 1995) and a birth has also been claimed in the human (Sofikitis *et al* 1997).

Injection of germ cells into mature oocytes has also been attempted in humans to overcome male infertility related to obstructive and non-obstructive azoospermia (Tesarik 1996; Aslam *et al* 1998; Vanderzwalmen *et al* 1998). However, the small number of cells obtained and the failure to distinguish between the different stages of germ cell development and other cell types resulted in a limited number of oocytes injected, fertilization failure and reduced embryo development (Vanderzwalmen *et al* 1998; Verheyen *et al* 1998).

Nuclear transfer of adult somatic cells into human oocytes resulted in the formation of haploid pronuclei following artificial activation or insemination with sperm (Takeuchi *et al* 2001; Tesarik *et al* 2001). Replacement of an oocyte's chromosomes with those of a somatic cell, creating a new "healthy" oocyte, has also been suggested as a treatment for female patients with ovarian failure (Sauer *et al* 1991) or defective oocytes (Rosenwaks, 1987).

It has been demonstrated in mouse cloning studies that somatic cells undergo haploidization within metaphase II (MII) oocytes (Wakayama *et al* 1998). The cell chromosomes divide into two poles in 64 percent of reconstituted oocytes and progress to the formation of 2-pronuclei following artificial activation in the presence of cytochalasin B (Wakayama *et al* 1998). Recently we have been able to demonstrate that mouse embryos can be produced from diploid somatic cells (Lacham-Kaplan *et al* 2001) as a replacement for sperm (Figure 50.1).

Embryo Normality Following Haploidization

In comparison to the high fertilization rate (75%) following nuclear transfer of diploid spermatocytes in mice the efficiency in producing diploid zygotes following haploidization of somatic cells within MII oocytes is very low (10-29%). Moreover, although two second polar bodies are produced and two pronuclei are formed, the capacity of the reconstituted oocytes to develop *in vitro* is limited

Fertilization with somatic cells:

Oocyte - MII
Donor cell - diploid in G_0 or G_1

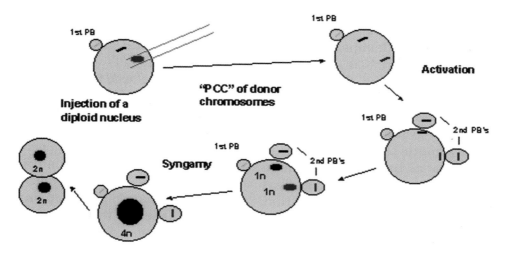

FIGURE 50.1: Haploidization of somatic cells following nuclear transfer into mature MII oocytes

(0-17%) and no offspring have been reported following the transfer of somatic cell derived embryos to recipient females. Kimura and Yanagimachi (1995) reported 65 percent of oocytes injected with secondary spermatocytes develop to blastocysts and 24 percent developed to live offspring. Sofikitis *et al* (1997) reported that from a total of 30 human oocytes injected with secondary spermatocytes isolated from testicular biopsies, 12 (40%) formed two pronuclei and developed normally in culture before being transferred to three patients resulting in one (8%) pregnancy.

Haploidization of cumulus cells within enucleated human oocytes was confirmed by Fluorescent *In situ* Hybridisation (FISH) analyses on the second polar bodies separated from the ooplasm of reconstituted oocytes after fertilization by sperm (Tesarik *et al* 2001). A single signal for the chromosomes 13, 18, 21 and X were identified in the polar bodies of two of the three oocytes analyzed, indicating that they were haploid sets. In another study (Takeuchi *et al* 2001), insertion of cumulus cells into enucleated human oocytes resulted in the formation of one or two pronuclei within the oocytes with no extrusion of a polar

body. Nonetheless, when two pronuclei were formed each contained a haploid set of chromosomes as identified by FISH using specific probes for chromosomes 16, 18 and X. Unlike nuclear transfer into human oocytes, which results in either one or two pronuclei or one pronucleus and one polar body (Takeuchi *et al* 1999; Tsai *et al* 2000; Takeuchi *et al* 2001; Tesarik *et al* 2001), somatic cells inserted into enucleated mouse oocytes were reported to produce two or more pronuclei (Wakayama *et al* 1998). Although two pronuclei appeared in the majority of oocytes (64%) the rest (36%) had three or more pronuclei suggesting that the separation of the chromosomes is random and that not all cells are capable of normal haploidization in MII oocytes in these species. In contrast all oocytes that extruded two-second polar bodies in the study by Lacham-Kaplan *et al* (2001) formed two pronuclei. One originated from the oocyte and the other from the cell inserted.

DNA was identified in both second polar bodies extruded from the oocytes and two distinct groups of DNA were identified within the cytoplasm (Lacham-Kaplan *et al* 2001). Although the somatic cell derived pronuclei were assumed to be haploid and therefore, the resultant embryos diploid, their abnormal development may be related to structural aberrations of the chromosomes. This will need to be examined in further studies. Normal chromosome structure is important for gene expression during preimplantation development of the mammalian embryo (Thompson 1996). A recent study by Tateno *et al* (2003a) found that the number of chromosomes in the majority (91.1%) of mouse oocytes following haploidization is either greater or lesser than the expected number (n=20) in the group of chromosomes originated from the somatic cell.

It is also of importance to identify the more optimal cytoplasm to induce haploidization. Tsai *et al* 2000; Takeuchi *et al* 2001, have shown that immature GV oocytes are more likely to induce haploidization of somatic cells. Their suggestion was contradicted by Fulka *et al* (2002) who demonstrated that somatic cell nuclei are unable to proceed through the reduction division when introduced into an immature oocytes meiotic cytoplasm.

Haploidization and Imprinting

It has been suggested that the correct imprint of genes is required for normal development but this may be overemphasized because of epigenetic modifications that occur following fertilization and embryo development are more likely to effect embryo development (Reik *et al* 1993). Following fertilization a widespread demethylation of the zygotic DNA occurs, with the exception of imprinted genes, as the DNA is reprogrammed to enable the correct pattern of embryonic gene expression to be established (Monk *et al* 1987). The high level of DNA methylation present in somatic cells is likely to affect this process. The maternally and paternally inherited alleles of imprinted genes are distinguished by epigenetic modifications, notably methylation, which allow the developing embryo to express either allele as and when required for normal development (Surani 1998). In secondary spermatocytes both alleles are imprinted similarly to sperm, hence, inheritance of either allele would have no adverse

effect on the expression of imprinted genes in the resulting embryo. In somatic cells, however, only one allele is imprinted, either maternally or paternally. In this case, inheritance of the maternal set of chromosomes or a random separation of chromosomes could result in the abnormal inheritance and ultimately expression of imprinted genes (Trounson 2001). When three blastocysts developed from male fibroblast zygotes produced by haploidization (Lacham-Kaplan *et al* 2001), the inheritance of the maternally imprinted *snrp* gene appeared to be random. Two of the embryos did not express the gene, which indicated that they inherited a maternally imprinted allele and, one expressed the gene indicating that in this embryo the paternally imprinted allele was inherited. It is yet to be established if chromosomal separation during the expulsion of the second polar body of the somatic nucleus is random in all cases. Following artificial activation the reconstituted oocytes would be expected to extrude a second polar body from both somatic cells and form two pronuclei, resulting in diploid zygotes. However, it is necessary to determine if epigenetic regulation of imprinted genes will allow normal development because the alleles derived from the somatic cells will probably retain the signature of their origins rather than the balanced set derived from male and female gametes. Unlike cloning where the complete set of alleles are derived from the somatic cell imprints, only half the genomic complement needs reprogramming because the oocytes chromosomes are retained for making artificial germ cell procedures. It would be interesting if this produces better outcome for the normality of development than does cloning (Trounson 2001).

Regardless of whether the chromosomes are separated according to their origin or not, it is not known how this event occurs as the information obtained from human and mouse studies is very limited. In mice, the nucleus of the somatic cell is transformed into disarrayed chromosomes 3 hours after injection (Wakayama *et al* 1998). Single condensed chromatids are each attached to a single spindle and are therefore not aligned on a metaphase plate. At about 1 hour after activation the chromosomes are segregated into two groups and about 5 hours later two pronuclei appear. In the human, induction of premature chromosome condensation (PCC) in Hela cells, which are in a different stage of the cell cycle following fusion to metaphase cells, was not accompanied by the appearance of a mitotic spindle although the chromosomes migrated to two poles in the next cell division cycle (Johnson and Rao 1970). Some evidence from Tateno *et al* (2003a) indicate that the single chromatids of the somatic nucleus are randomly arranged on the spindle before pseudo polar body extrusion.

The Procedure

Media

All media (Appendix A-E) components to be prepared under sterile conditions in a laminar flow hood and the pH and osmolarity of the medium should be determined. Media can be prepared fortnightly and stored at 4°C.

Media that can be used:

1. KSOMaa-culture media (Summers *et al* 2000) (Appendix A)
2. Hepes KSOMaa-handling media–modification of KSOMaa (Appendix A)
3. M16-culture media (Whittingham 1971) (Appendix B)
4. M2-handling media (Quinn *et al* 1982) (Appendix C)

M2 and Hepes KSOMaa media are to be used for oocyte collection. M16 and KSOMaa are to be used for oocyte and embryo culture. Media should be prepared by weighing separate constituents and adding sterile deionized water (CSL, Parkville, Vic, Australia). All media should be supplemented with 4-mg/ml bovine serum albumin (BSA; Cat# 11020-021, Gibco, BRL, Auckland, New Zealand), and sterilized by filtration through 0.22 µm filters (Flowpore D26 filters: Flow Laboratories, North Ryde, Australia) into 10 ml sterile plastic test tubes (Falcon, Becton Dickinson Lab ware, NY, USA). Media can be stored up to 2 weeks.

Media used for oocyte, and embryo culture should be incubated overnight in an atmosphere of 5 percent CO_2 in air at 37°C before use.

Mice

Mice used in these studies should be of the hybrid F1 strains (C57BL female X CBA male or C57BL female X DBA male). These strains are likely to induce haploidization in greater rates than inbred mice. Somatic cells [cumulus cells, fibroblasts, embryonic stem (ES) cells) may be originated from any strain. ES cells] from a 129 background are more likely to undergo haploidization.

Preparation of Oocytes and Cumulus Cells

Induce superovulation of 4 to 6 week of age female mice by the injection of 10 IU of Pregnant Mare's Serum Gonadotropin (PMSG; Folligon; Intervet, Lane Cove, Australia) and 10 IU human Chorionic Gonadotropin (hCG; Choralon; Intervet) 48 hour later. Oocytes can be recovered from the oviducts of superovulated females 13 to 14 hour after hCG injection. Oocyte-cumulus cell complexes should be liberated into warm handling medium containing 40 IU hyaluronidase (Fraction IV-S; Sigma Chemicals Co. St. Louis, MO). Incubate oocyte cumulus cell complexes in the hyaluronidase solution for 5 min to separate cumulus cells from the oocytes. Cumulus-free oocytes should be collected and washed in fresh warm handling medium before being cultured in culture medium previously equilibrated at 37°C in a 5 percent CO_2 in air atmosphere for 15 hour. The remainder, hyaluronidase solution containing cumulus cells is to be collected into a 5 ml plastic tube (Falcon, Becton Dickenson, NSW, Australia). Add an additional 2 ml of fresh warm culture medium to the tube before centrifugation at 300 *g* for 5 min. Remove the supernatant and transfer the cells located at the bottom of the tube into a drop of 5 percent CO_2 in air equilibrated culture medium. Both oocytes and cumulus cells should be cultured under mineral oil (Sigma) at 37°C in 5 percent CO_2 in air until used 1 hour later for injection.

Preparation of Embryonic Stem (ES) Cells

Cultured somatic cells and ES cells to be prepared according to established protocols for cell lifting. Medium is removed of cultured cells and flasks are washed with PBS (5 ml/25 ml flasks). PBS is removed and Trypsin/EDTA (0.05% Trypsin + 0.4% EDTA, Sigma) is added for about 3 minute. The flasks are shaken to improve lifting of cells. After 1 minute cell suspensions are mixed by pipetting them up and down using a glass pipette for at least 6 times. An equal amount of medium containing FCS is then added to flask to neutralise the Trypsin. About 10 ml of cell suspension is collected into 15 ml tubes. Tubes are centrifuged for 2 minute at 300 g. The supernatant is removed and cells are resuspended in handling medium used for injection and centrifuged again for 5 minute at 300 g. Cumulus cells are collected from the hyaluronidase drops into 5 ml plastic tube. About 1ml of handling medium is added to the tube. The tube is centrifuged for 5 min at 300 g. The supernatant is removed and the cells are diluted to a concentration of 10,000 cells/ml. Cells are then diluted (at 1:4 ratio) in 10 percent (polyvinylpyrrolidone) (ICN Biomedical Inc, Ohio, USA) w/v in M2 or in Hepes KSOMaa medium. Polyvinylpyrrolidone is prepared by weighing 0.1 g into a 5 ml sterile plastic tube (Falcon, Becton Dickinson Lab ware, NY, USA) containing 1 ml of M2 or Hepes KSOMaa media. The falcon tube containing PVP in M2 or Hepes KSOMaa is left at 4°C to dissolve overnight (optional). The next morning the solution should be filtered through 0.8 µm filters (Millipore Corporation, Bedford, MA01730, USA).

Preparation of Adult Fibroblasts

Adult male fibroblasts were prepared as previously described by Lacham *et al* (2000). The muscle and skin tissues from adult male mice were removed and chopped finely using surgical blades. The tissue fragments were treated with 0.25 percent Trypsin (Sigma) and 0.4 percent EDTA (Bochiringer Mennheim, Mennheim, Germany) in Ca Mg-free PBS (Oxid, Hampshire, England) for 30 min at 37°C. Disaggregated cells were washed and cultured in Dulbecco's modified Eagles medium (DMEM, Trace Biociences, NSW, Australia) supplemented with 2 mM L-glutamine (Gipco, Life Technology, NY, USA), 26 mM sodium bicarbonate (BDH, Dorset, England, 100 IU/ml penicillin (Life Technologies) and 100 µg/ml Streptomycin (Life Technologies) and 10 percent

Fetal Calf Serum (FCS) (Life Technologies) in 10 cm Petri dishes (Falcon) at 37°C under 5 percent CO_2 in air. The primary culture was allowed to reach 100 percent confluence before being passaged into 75 cm culture flasks (Falcon). Cells were stored at passage 2, frozen in 90 percent FCS and 10 percent DMSO (Sigma) at–80°C. For nuclear transfer, cells were thawed at 37°C in a water bath then washed and cultured in DMEM containing 10 percent FCS up to passage 4. The cell monolayer was trypsinized to detach cells from the tissue culture flasks and centrifuged at 1000 rpm for 5 min. The cell pellet was re-suspended in M2 medium containing 4 mg/ml BSA (Fraction IV, Sigma).

Microinjection (Figure 50.2)

A thin walled (0.78 mm inner diameter) glass capillary (Clark Electro Medical Instruments, Pangbourne, Reading, UK) with outer diameter of 1.00 mm is used to prepare the injection and holding pipettes. The capillaries are pulled on a Sutter instrument (Model P-87, Sutter instrument Co., USA). The injection takes place on an inverted microscope with the aid of a Piezo drill manipulator (optional) (Piezodrill, Burleigh Instruments Inc, Burleigh Pork, Fishers NY).

Prepare 3 drops (50 µl) on the cover of 150 mm plastic dish (Nunclon, Denmark), the first is the cell suspension, the second is M2 or Hepes KSOMaa wash drop and the third an M2 or Hepes KSOMaa drop for the oocytes. Cover the drops with oil.

Cells are pulled in and out of the injection pipette for 2-3 times before the microinjection

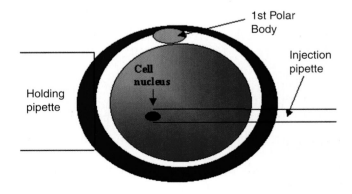

FIGURE 50.2: Nuclear transfer

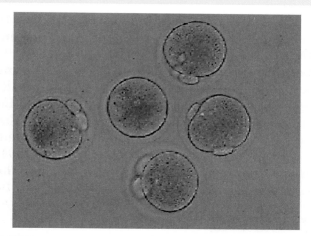

FIGURE 50.3: Mouse zygotes following the injection of cumulus cells and artificial activation by 8 percent ethanol 9 hour after injection. A clear 2-2nd polar bodies and 2 pronuclei are evident

pipette is passed through the rinse M2 or Hepes KSOMaa drop to the injection drop. When using Piezo, the injection pipette is cut at about 3-5 µm (for cumulus cells) or 7-8 µm (for fibroblasts). With the aid of the holding pipette one mature oocyte is held by suction. A single Peizo pulse is used to core the zona pellucida, and a second Peizo pulse is used to break the oolemma of the oocyte. A single nucleus is expelled from the injection pipette into each oocyte. The expected survival rate using this procedure is 50 to 70 percent.

For manual injection the pipette is broken on the micro-forge before mounting onto the micromanipulation system. The break should be at 3-5 µm (for cumulus cells) or 7-8 µm (for fibroblasts). Pipette can also be broken after mounting on the system using the holding pipette to break its' tip. Cells are also pulled in and out of the pipette 2-3 times. The pipette is pushed through the zona pellucida into the perivitelline space. The nucleus is brought closer to the opening of the pipette. The pipette is pushed towards the oolemma. The oolemma is sucked into the pipette until its break. The oocyte content and the nucleus are expelled slowly into the oocyte. The survival rate using this procedure is 30 to 40 percent.

Oocyte Activation

Leave injected oocytes in culture for 3 hour before they are subjected to artificial activation. Activation can be done by the exposure of oocytes to 8 percent ethanol, by electricity or by chemicals such as strontium. When ethanol is used, dilute 100 percent ethanol in M2 or Hepes-KSOMaa to a concentration of 8 percent (0.8 ml of 100% ethanol in 92 ml handling medium). Oocytes are added to a 100 µl drop of 8 percent ethanol mixture covered with mineral oil for 5 minute in room temperature. After 5 minute oocytes are washed in fresh handling medium and transferred to culture medium for up to 6 hours.

For strontium activation, oocytes are cultured in calcium free culture medium supplemented with 5 mM strontium (Sigma) for 4-6 hours. At the end of the incubation time, remove, wash and culture the oocytes further in calcium containing culture medium.

Embryo Development

Separate reconstituted zygotes exhibiting 2-second polar bodies and 2-pronuclei and culture them up to 5 days to examine their development to blastocysts (Table 50.1). It is expected that about 70 percent of the oocytes injected with somatic cells will survive the procedure. From these about 30 to 40 percent should produce 2nd polar bodies as demonstrated in Figure 50.2 and in Figure 50.3. The development to blastocyst is impaired though and only about 15 percent of those will reach this stage *in vitro*.

TABLE 50.1: The time sequence of mouse preimplan–tation embryo development after haploidization

Day	In vitro development
0 (6 hr after NT)	Survived and fertilization
1 (24 hr after NT)	2-cell
2 (48 hr after NT)	4-cell
3 (72 hr after NT)	8 cell/Morula
4 (96 hr NT)	Blastocysts

CONCLUSIONS

A few studies examined the possibility of producing embryos and offspring from somatic cells in mice (Lacham-Kaplan *et al* 2001; Tesarik *et al* 2001; Tekeuchi, 2001). These studies confirm that mouse somatic cells are able to enter metaphase within the cytoplasm of metaphase II (MII). In all studies, somatic cells were able to continue as metaphase cells resulting in their chromosomes separating into two poles. Following artificial activation (Tsai *et al* 2000; Takeuchi, 2001, Lacham-Kaplan *et al* 2001) or insemination with sperm (Tesarik *et al* 2001), the oocytes extrude two-second polar bodies and two pronuclei or, two pronuclei were produced within the oocyte with no polar body extrusion. While Tesarik (2001) and Takeuchi (2001) used somatic cells to replace the oocyte chromosomes and artificially activated or inseminated the reconstituted oocytes with sperm to produce embryos, Lacham-Kaplan (2001) used somatic cells to reconstitute diploidy in the oocyte. Mouse female or male somatic cells were injected into non-enucleated MII oocytes, which were activated 2-3 hour later, resulting in the formation of 2-second polar bodies and 2-pronuclei.

The subject of producing embryos and more so live offspring from somatic cells used as germ cells, is controversial and as such raises negative views. Tateno *et al* (2003a,b) have concluded that the proposal of using haploidization for assisted reproduction is biologically unsound, given the fundamental limitations of chromosomes segregation and genomic imprinting. The calculations demonstrated in those studies should not discourage researchers but support further examination into the topic. It took over a 100 embryos to produce 2 pups in the initial cloning studies in mice (Wakayama*et al* 1998; Wakayama, Yanagimachi 1999). The proportion of live offspring from mice cloning increased only slightly with time. The more recent mouse cloning studies reported 3–7 percent live offspring (Ogura *et al* 2000; Wakayama *et al* 2000). This minor improvement was related to the cell type used and the identification of the most receptive cytoplasm. For a more efficient production of somatic cell zygotes with higher capability to develop to blastocysts and to term, other artificial activation procedures should be investigated (Sasagawa, Yanagimachi 1996) using different cell types (Wakayama *et al* 1998; Wakayama, Yanagimachi, 1999; Ogura *et al* 2000; Ono *et al* 2000).

The success of the present technique will be measured by the ability to produce progeny and if the progeny is genetically, physiologically and morphologically normal. If successful, the method will allow the production of embryos for couples where the male partner is sterile. Established cell lines from skin or muscle cells of men with spermatogenesis arrest or sterile men following chemotherapy or X-irradiation can be stored for many repeated treatment cycles. It would be also possible in the future to combine the artificial oocyte (Tesarik *et al* 2001; Takeuchi *et al* 2001) and artificial germ cell procedures, by injecting two somatic cells into enucleated oocytes.

BIBLIOGRAPHY

1. Aslam I, Fishel S, Green S, et al. Can we justify spermatid microinjection for severe male factor infertility? Human Reproduction Update 1998;4:213-22.
2. Humphreys D, Eggan K, Akutsu H, et al. Epigenetic instability in ES cells and cloned mice. Science 2001;293:95-97.
3. Fulka J Jr, Martinez F, Tepla O, Mrazek M, Tesarik J. Somatic and embryonic cell nucleus transfer into intact and enucleated immature mouse oocytes. Hum Reprod 2002;17:2160-64.
4. Johnson RT, Rao PN. Mammalian cell fusion: Induction of premature chromosome condensation in interphase nuclei. Nature 1970;226:717-22.
5. Kimura Y, Yanagimachi R. Development of normal mice from oocytes injected with secondary spermatocyte nuclei. Biology of Reproduction 1995;53:855-62.
6. Lacham-Kaplan O, Trounson A. Fertilization and embryonic developmental capacity of epididymal and testicular sperm and immature spermatids and spermatocytes. Reproductive Medicine Review 1997; 6:55-68.
7. Lacham-Kaplan O, Diamente M, Pushett D, Hall H, Lewis I, Trounson A. Developmental competence of nuclear transfer cow oocytes following direct injection of fetal fibroblast nuclei. Cloning 2000;2:2-9.
8. Lacham-Kaplan O, Daniels R, Trounson A. Fertilization of mouse oocytes using somatic cells as male germ cells. Reproductive Biomed Online 2001;3:205-11.
9. Monk M, Boubelik M, Lehnert S. Temporal and regional changes in DNA methylation in the embryonic, extraembryonic and germ cell lineages during mouse embryo development. Development 1987;99:371-82.
10. Ogura A, Inoue K, Ogonuki N, et al. Production of male cloned mice from fresh, cultured and cryopreserved immature Sertoli cells. Biology of Reproduction 2000; 62:1579-84.
11. Ono Y, Shimozawa N, Ito M, Kono T. Cloned mice from cells arrested at metaphase by a serial nuclear transfer. Biology of Reproduction 2001;64:44-50.
12. Quinn P, Barros C, Whittingham DG. Preservation of hamster oocytes to assay the fertilizing capacity of

human spermatozoa. Journal of Reproduction and Fertility 1982;66:161-68.

13. Reik W, Romer I, Barton SC, et al. Adult phenotype in the mouse can be affected by epigenetic events in the early embryo. Development 1993;119:933-42.

14. Rosenwaks Z. Donor eggs: Their application in modern reproductive technologies. Fertility and Sterility 1987;47:895-909.

15. Sasagawa I, Yanagimachi R. Comparison of methods for activating mouse oocytes for spermatid nucleus transfer. Zygote 1996;4:269-74.

16. Sauer M, Paulson R, Macoso T, et al. Oocyte and pre-embryo donation to women with ovarian failure: An extended clinical trail. Fertility and Sterility 1991;55:39-43.

17. Sofikitis N, Mantzavinos T, Loutradis D, et al. Delivery of a healthy male after ooplasmic injection of secondary spermatocytes. Proceedings of the 23rd Annual Meeting of the American Society of Andrology, 1997;57 (Abs 129).

18. Sofikitis N, Miyagawa I, Yamamoto Y, et al. Micro and macro-consequences of ooplasmic injections of early haploid male gametes. Human Reproduction 1998;4:197-212.

19. Summers MC, McGinnis LK, Lawitts JA, Raffin M, Biggers JD. IVF of mouse ova in a simplex optimized medium supplemented with amino acids. Human Reproduction 2000;15:1791-801.

20. Surani MA. Imprinting and the initiation of gene silencing in the germ line. Cell 1998;93:309-12.

21. Takeuchi T, Ergun B, Hua T, et al. A reliable technique of nuclear transplantation for immature mammalian oocytes. Human Reproduction 1999;14:1321-17.

22. Takeuchi T, Kaneko M, Veeck LL, et al. Creation of viable human oocytes using diploid somatic nuclei. Are we there yet? Human Reproduction 2001;16:5(Abs 0-011).

23. Tateno H, Akutsu H, Latham KE, Yanagimachi R. Inability of mature oocytes to create functional haploid genomes from somatic cell nuclei. Fertility and Sterility 2003a;79:216-17.

24. Tateno H, Latham KE, Yanagimachi R. Reproductive semi-cloning respecting biparental origin. Human Reproduction 2003b;18:472-75.

25. Tesarik J. Fertilization of oocytes by injecting spermatozoa, spermatids and spermatocytes. Review of Reproduction 1996;1:149-52.

26. Tesarik J, Nagy ZP, Sousa M, et al. Fertilizable oocytes reconstructed from patient's somatic cell nuclei and donor ooplasts. Reproductive Biomedicine Online 2001:2;160-64.

27. Thompson EM. Chromatin structure and gene expression in the preimplantation mammalian embryo. Reproductive Nutr Development 1996;36:619-35.

28. Trounson A. Nuclear transfer in human medicine and animal breeding. Reproduction Fertility and Development 2001;13;31-39.

29. Tsai MC, Takeuchi T, Bedford JM, et al. Alternative source of gametes: Reality or science fiction? Human Reproduction 2000;15;988-98.

30. Vanderzwalmen P, Nijs M, Schoysman R, et al. The problems of spermatid microinjection in the human: The need for an accurate morphological approach and selective methods for viable and normal cells. Human Reproduction 1988;13:515-19.

31. Verheyen G, Crrabe E, Joris H, et al. Simple and reliable identification of the human round spermatid by inverted phase-contrast microscopy. Human Reproduction 1998;13:1570-77.

32. Wakayama T, Perry ACF, Zuccotti M, et al. Full-term development of mice from enucleated oocytes injected with cumulus cell nuclei. Nature 1998;394:369-73.

33. Wakayama T, Yanagimachi R. Cloning of male mice from adult tail-tip cells. Nature Genetics 1999;22:127-28.

34. Wakayama T, Tateno H, Mombaerts P, et al. Nuclear transfer into mouse zygotes. Nature Genetics 2000; 24:108-09

35. Wittingham DG. Culture of mouse ova. Journal of Reproduction and Fertility 1971;14(Suppl):7-21.

APPENDICES

APPENDIX A
KSOMaa CULTURE AND HANDLING MEDIUM
(ADAPTED FROM SUMMERS ET AL 2000)

Components	Culture KSOMaa		Hepes KSOMaa (Handling)	
	g / 100 ml	mM	g / 100 ml	mM
NaCl	5.552	95	5.552	95
KCl	0.186	2.5	0.186	2.5
KH_2PO_4	0.048	0.35	0.048	0.35
$MgSO_4.7H_2O$	0.049	0.2	0.049	0.2
Sodium Lactate	1.868	10.0	1.868	10.0
D-Glucose	0.991	5.5	0.991	5.5
$NaHCO_3$	2.10	25	2.10	25
Sodium-pyruvate	0.22	0.2	0.22	0.2
*$CaCl_2.2H_2O$	2.5	1.71	2.5	1.71
EDTA	0.038		0.038	
NaOH	0.01		0.01	
Hepes	8		8	
Phenol red	1.46		1.46	
Glutamine	1.0 mg/ml		4.0 mg/ml	
BSA				

EAA (Eagle's essential amino acids)
NEAA (Eagle's non-essential amino acids)
*For activation medium, omit calcium and replace with $SrCl_2$.

APPENDIX B
M16 CULTURE MEDIA (WHITTINGHAM 1971)

Components	mM	g / 100 ml
NaCl	94.66	5.533
KCl	4.78	0.352
$MgSO4 \times 7H_2O$	1.19	0.293
KH_2PO_4	1.19	0.162
Sodium Lactate	23.28	2.610 or 4.349 of 60% syrup
Glucose	5.56	1.000
Penicillin	100 U/ml	0.06
Streptomycin sulphate	50 µg/ml	0.05
$NaHCO_3$	25.00	2.102
Phenol Red	0.001	0.01
Sodium pyruvate	0.33	0.036
*$CaCl_2. 2H_2O$	1.71	0.252

Osmolarity 290-300
*For activation medium, omit calcium and replace with $SrCl_2$.

APPENDIX C
M2 HANDLING MEDIA (QUINN ET AL 1982)

Components	g / 100 ml	mM
NaCl	5.533	94.66
KCl	0.352	4.78
$MgSO_4 \times 7H_2O$	0.293	1.19
KH_2PO_4	0.162	1.19
Sodium Lactate	2.610 or 4.349 of 60% syrup	23.28
Glucose	1.000	5.56
Penicillin	0.06	100 U/ml
Streptomycin sulphate	0.05	50 μg/ml
HEPES	4.969	20.85
$NaHCO_3$	2.102	25.00
Phenol Red	0.01	0.001
Sodium pyruvate	0.036	0.33
$CaCl_2. 2H_2O$	0.252	1.71
Osmolarity 290-300		

• **Nalini Krishnan**

51

Histopathology and its Role in Infertility

PATHOLOGY OF FEMALE INFERTILITY

Female infertility is a complex problem for which a simple answer is rarely available. A detailed investigation of the infertile status entails a gynecological, endocrinological, immunological and cytogenetic assessment, and it is a known fact that histopathology has only a minor role to play. But it must be emphasized that in certain situations the histopathologists opinion plays a crucial role in the diagnosis, line of treatment and ultimately the outcome.

This chapter will highlight only those areas where histopathology could play a role in diagnosing or confirming the cause of infertility.

Classification of Infertility[1]

Infertility is basically divided into two categories: anovulatory and ovulatory which in turn may be due to different factors.

Anovulatory Infertility

Hypothalamic-pituitary factors
• Gonadotrophin deficiency
• Hyperprolactinemia.

Ovarian factors
• Gonadal dysgenesis, e.g. Turner's syndrome with pure XO or a variety of XO mosaics.
  1. Streak ovaries

2. Indefinite demarcation between cortex and medulla
3. Whorled foci of ovarian-like stroma
4. Presence of germ cells in early embryonic life which totally disappears by puberty
5. XO mosaics may retain ova, menstruate and become pregnant.

• *Gonadotrophin-resistant ovary syndrome.* This is also known as Savage syndrome. Features are:
  1. Congenital or aquired.
  2. Increased estrogen levels.
  3. Decreased gonadotrophin levels.
  4. Anovulation.
  5. Ovarian biopsy shows numerous primordial follicles but which do not progress to maturation.
  6. Said to be due to lack of FSH receptors resulting in no response of ovary to exogenous gonadotrophins.

• Premature ovarian failure
  1. High gonadotrophin levels.
  2. Absence of primordial follicles.

• Autoimmune ovarian failure
  Antibodies are directed against steroid-producing cells of the ovary.

Histologically the ovary is atrophic/fibrotic or a lymphocytic infiltration is seen around the developing follicles.

- Luteinized unruptured follicle syndrome

  This syndrome is characterized by
  1. Luteinization of granulosa and theca cell layers
  2. Normal development of an ovum-containing corpus luteum,
  3. But no release of the ovum.

- Polycystic ovarian syndrome

  Characterized by:
  1. Bilateral ovarian enlargement,
  2. Fibrous thickening of tunica albuginea.
  3. Multiple subcapsular follicular cysts.
  4. No corpora lutea or corpora albicantes so no evidence of ovulation.

- 17-hydroxylase deficiency
  1. Rare enzyme deficiency.
  2. Decreased adrenal and gonadal synthesis of steroid hormones.
  3. Defective ovarian synthesis of estrogens.
  4. Failure of follicular maturation.
  5. Ovary contains multiple small follicular cysts.

- Ovarian neoplasms

  Thecomas and granulosa cell tumors which secrete estrogen and androblastomas which secrete androgens cause anovulation mainly because of their effect on the feedback mechanism.

Ovulatory Infertility

The hypothalamic-pituitary-ovarian axis is intact in ovulatory infertility. The infertility is mainly due to abnormality or pathology of the reproductive tract.

Tubal Factors

The fallopian tube has a very important role to play in fertility since fertilization takes place in the tube. Salpingitis or inflammation of the fallopian tube may be acute or chronic.

Granulomatous salpingitis is mainly due to tuberculosis and is one of the important causes for infertility. Histopathologically typical tubercle granulomas are seen in the wall of the tube.

Endometrial factors

- *Endometrial biopsy*: It plays an important role in the investigation of female infertility. The abnormality may be intrinsic as in inflammation or extrinsic as a result of abnormal gonadal function.

Timing of the biopsy	
Anovulatory cycle Luteal phase defect	Later stages of the cycle
Nonspecific endo-metritis	Preovulatory phase, because if it is done in the later stages the premenstrual inflammatory infiltrate could confuse the picture
Tuberculous endo-metritis	Premenstrual biopsy since the tubercles would be well developed

An important point to be noted is that when a women who is being investigated for infertility gives a history of irregular periods a β-hCG level check should be done prior to an endometrial biopsy. Otherwise we may inadvertently disrupt a conceptus! and the histopathologist would find the following picture under the microscope (Figure 51.1).

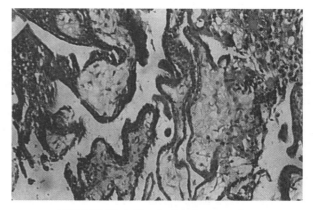

FIGURE 51.1: Products of conception

ENDOMETRITIS

The diagnosis of endometritis is difficult due to the fact that the usual indicators of an inflammatory process in other tissues are actually found in the normal endometrium, (i.e. lymphocytes, lymphoid aggregates, lymphoid follicles) and polymorphonuclear leukocyte infiltrate interstitial hemorrhage and tissue necrosis are seen in normal menstruation.

Endometritis may be infective or noninfective and this can be identified histologically based on the type of inflammatory cell infiltration and changes in the endometrial development and maturation.

Acute Endometritis

It is not a very significant factor in infertility for this condition is of short duration and usually resolves completely. It is only when the basal layers are involved that there will be a re-emergence of the inflammatory process again.

Causes could be due to retained products, microorganisms, physical, thermal and chemical agents. Histologically there is a heavy focal or diffuse infiltration of polymorphonuclear leukocytes which surround and penetrate the glandular lumina and which can also lead to the destruction of the tissue.

Chronic Nonspecific Endometritis

Chronic nonspecific endometritis occurs when the inflammation persists in the basalis or other parts which are not shed. The causative agents are similar to those causing acute endometritis.

Histologically there is focal or diffuse infiltration of lymphocytes and plasma cells. They may even infiltrate and destroy the glandular epithelium, though destruction is less common (Figure 51.2).

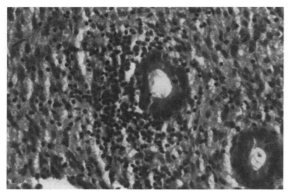

FIGURE 51.2: Nonspecific endometritis

Tuberculous Endometritis

Tuberculous endometritis is generally associated with a tuberculous salpingitis. Very rarely it could

be due to a hematogenous spread of a pulmonary focus.

Histologically, the extent of the inflammation may vary profoundly. The findings may be diffuse or focal stromal infiltration of lymphocytes and plasma cells with involvement and destruction of the glands, or classical tubercular granulomas characterized by focal collections of epithelioid cells, a few Langhans type of giant cells surrounded by a cuff of lymphocytes (Figure 51.3).

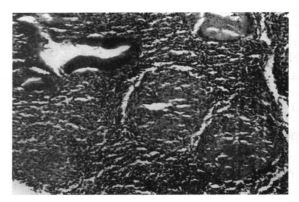

FIGURE 51.3: Tuberculous endometritis

Specific Endometritis Caused by Rare Microorganisms

- Sarcoidosis
- *Cryptococcus glabratus*
- *Blastomyces dermatitidis*
- *Mycoplasma*
- Actinomycosis
- Candidiasis
- Herpes virus endometritis
- Cytomegalovirus (CMV) endometritis
- Chlamydial endometritis
- Toxoplasmosis
- Schistosomiasis
- Gonorrheal endometritis.

FOREIGN BODY GRANULOMA

Talc Granuloma

Histologically, there is a histiocytic infiltrate surrounding the talc particles with or without multinucleate foreign body type of giant cells. Lymphocytes and plasma cells may also be seen.

IUCD Endometritis

An intrauterine contraceptive device (IUCD) acts like a foreign body inducing endometritis in some women. Histologically there is seen an infiltration of polymorphonuclear leukocytes, lymphocytes and plasma cells.

ANOVULATION

Complete absence of ovulation is known as anovulation. Disorders of ovulation account for approximately 30 to 40 percent of all cases of female infertility. Normally anovulatory cycles occur at the beginning and the end of the reproductive period.

Hammerstein (1965) distinguished three types of anovulatory cycles based on how the estrogen levels are high and how long the secretion of estrogen persists.

Type A

The follicle continues to secrete for 7 to 10 days (persistent follicle resulting in irregular proliferation). Histologically the glands vary in their size and distribution with pseudostratification or multilayering.

Type B

There is an additional secretion of gonadotrophin (LH) taking place with little luteinization of the follicle (abortive secretion).

Histologically there is focal abortive secretion among the proliferative glands.

Type C

The follicle becomes insufficient early and the estrogen levels remain low (insufficient follicle resulting in deficient proliferation).

Histologically the growth of the glands and stroma are retarded when compared with those of the normal proliferative phase. The glands are usually straight and slender.

Thus with the waxing and waning of the hormonal levels, the histological picture of the endometrium varies from atrophy to hyperplasia.

Histologically the most important criteria for making a diagnosis from endometrial curettings is the absence of secretory changes in the second half of the cycle. Ideally if a proliferative endometrium is seen just prior to or at the onset of the period, it would be highly suggestive of an anovulatory cycle.

LUTEAL PHASE DEFECT

Luteal phase defect occurs when two endometrial biopsies show a delay of more than 2 days beyond the actual day of cycle in the histologic development of the endometrium (Table 51.1)—as assessed by the criteria of Noyes et al.

TABLE 51.1: Functional disturbances of the endometrium in infertility[2]	
Morphology	*Possible causes*

Atrophy	• Non-functioning ovaries
	  Gonadal dysgenesis
	  Deficient follicular development
	  Gonadotrophin-resistant ovary syndrome
	• Hormone-refractive endometrium

Deficient proliferation	• Deficient follicular maturation or stimulation with deficient (and after prolonged) anovulatory cycle • Endometrium partially refractive to estrogen
Irregular proliferation or hyperplasia	• Central defect Polycystic ovary syndrome (repeated anovulatory cycles or persistent follicle) • Endometrium refractive to progesterone
Deficient secretory phase • With coordinated apparent delay • With coordinated true delay • With dissociated delay Abortive secretion	Central defect • Persistent follicle and delayed ovulation (relative corpus luteum deficiency) • Inadequate FSH stimulation (absolute corpus luteum insufficiency) • Inadequate LH stimulation with or without hyperprolactinemia Non-ovulating, insufficient follicle with sporadic luteinization
Arrested secretion	Gestagen stimulation without ovulation, mostly exogenic
Asynchronous cycle	Disturbance of central regulation (direct or indirect by negative feedback mechanism)

ENDOMETRIAL HYPERPLASIA

Endometrial hyperplasia represents biologic and morphologic changes ranging from an exaggerated physiologic state to a carcinoma-*in situ.*

Basically they evolve in a proliferative endometrium resulting from an unopposed, prolonged estrogen stimulation.

The most recent classification scheme endorsed by the International Society of Gynecological Pathologists is based on both architectural and cytologic features.

Classification of Endometrial Hyperplasia

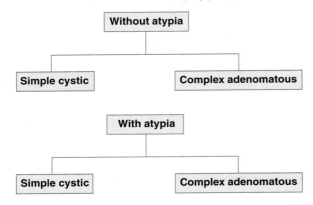

Histologically in simple cystic (without atypia) there are enlarged cystically dilated glands with variable size and shape and an increased gland:stroma ratio.

In complex adenomatous (without atypia) there is papillary infolding and budding and crowding of glands.

In simple cystic and complex adenomatous with atypia there is cytological atypia represented by enlarged nuclei of variable size and shape and loss of polarity with an increase in nucleocytoplasmic ratio, prominent nucleoli, irregular clumping of chromatin and parachromatin clearing.

Progression to cancer increases with the degree of atypia (Figures 51.4 and 51.5).

DATING OF THE ENDOMETRIUM

No discussion on endometrium is complete without dating of the endometrium.

It is impossible to precisely date the endometrium in the proliferative phase since the

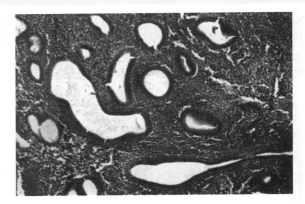

FIGURE 51.4: Simple cystic hyperplasia

duration may vary between 10 and 20 days even under physiological conditions. Therefore, the proliferative phase is divided into three stages: early, mid and late proliferative phase.

In contrast, the secretory phase can be fairly precisely related to the day of the cycle.

Proliferative Phase[4]

Early Proliferative Phase [Day 5 to day 7]

The endometrial glands are straight and narrow with the cut surface being round. The lining epithelium is cubocolumnar and basophilic and with occasional mitosis. The stromal cells are oval to elongated to spindly with scant cytoplasm and ill-defined cytoplasmic borders. Mitotic activity can be seen. Thin walled blood vessels are also seen (Figure 51.6).

Midproliferative Phase (Day 8 to day 10)

The glandular epithelium is taller with more obvious stratification and increased mitotic

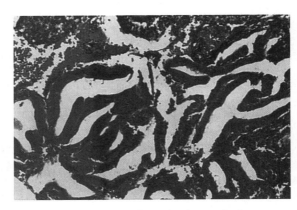

FIGURE 51.5: Complex hyperplasia

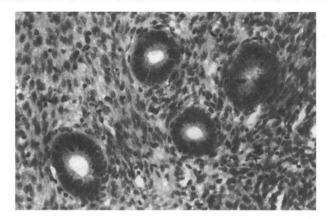

FIGURE 51.6: Early proliferative phase

activity. The stroma shows mitotic activity and transient stromal edema. Numerous capillaries are also seen.

Late Proliferative Phase [Day 11 to day 14]

Here the glandular growth exceeds stromal growth. Therefore the glands are variable in size and tortuous. The epithelium is still stratified, but the mitotic activity has decreased. The stroma shows minimal edema and reduced mitosis (Figure 51.7).

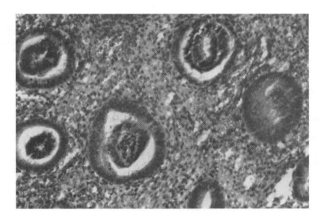

FIGURE 51.7: Late proliferative phase

Secretory Phase[5-7]

The normal corpus luteum after ovulation develops and involutes at a definite rhythm and in a precise sequential manner causing changes in the endometrium to occur at the same rate.

In the first 24 to 36 hours postovulation there is no apparent change in the histological appea-

rance of the endometrium. Endometrial dating from 16th to 28th day is according to Noye's criteria.

Day 16

- Subnuclear vacuoles
- Pseudostratification
- Mitoses, glands and stroma.

Day 17

- More or less orderly row of nuclei
- Cytoplasm above nuclei and subnuclear vacuoles below gland and stromal mitosis (Figure 51.8).
- Very, minimal secretion.

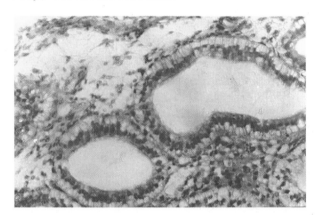

FIGURE 51.8: Secretory phase-day 17

Day 18

- Vacuoles above and below nuclei
- Improved linear arrangement of nuclei
- Gland mitosis rare
- Stromal mitosis rare
- Bubbles of secretion seen at luminal border.

Day 19

- A few vacuoles remain in cell, but mainly active evaluation with intraluminal secretion
- No gland or stromal mitosis
- May look like day 16 but no pseudostratification.

Day 20

- Peak secretion with "ragged" luminal border
- Vacuoles are rare.

Day 21

- Abrupt onset of stromal edema
- Gland secretion prominent
- "Naked" stromal nuclei begin to appear.

Day 22

- Peak edema
- Marked appearance of "naked" stromal nuclei
- Active secretion, but subsiding
- Rare stromal mitosis.

Day 23

- Prominent spiral arterioles
- Periarteriolar cuffing with enlargement of stromal cell nuclei and cytoplasm (earliest predecidual change)
- Stromal mitoses.

Day 24

Definite predecidual cells around arterioles with early subepithelial changes
- Greater stromal mitoses
- Ragged cell borders, i.e. secretory exhaustion (Figure 51.9).

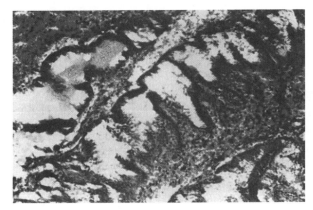

FIGURE 51.9: Secretory phase-day 24

Day 25

- Definite subcapsular predecidua

- Inspissated secretion noted to begin
- Early stromal infiltration with lymphocytes and occasional polymorphonuclear leukocytes.

Day 26

- Generalized decidual reaction
- Polymorphonuclear leukocytic invasion
- Inspissated secretion.

Day 27

- Solid sheet of decidua
- Marked leukocytic infiltrate
- Inspissated secretion with variable intracellular secretory activity.

Day 28

- Focal necrosis and hemorrhage
- Peak leukocytic infiltration
- Cells may show secretory exhaustion or active secretion (variable).

Menstruating

- Stromal clumping
- Glandular break-up and hemorrhage
- Variable leukocytic infiltration
- Edema
- After 24 hours, metaplastic alterations on surface.

RECENT ADVANCES IN ENDOMETRIAL RECEPTIVITY AND IMPLANTATION

Detection of pinopode formation on the surface epithelium by surface electron microscopy (SEM) appears to be one of the accurate markers for endometrial receptivity,[8] and hence a very important tool in ARTs.

Another set of workers have identified three markers: pinopodes from day 20 onwards and β_3 and α_4 integrins on day 22 to 23.[9]

PATHOLOGY OF MALE INFERTILITY

Histopathological examination of the male genital system with respect to infertility is largely confined to the testes. Hence, a brief account of what is normal is given and then what is pathological or abnormal.

Normal Testis

- Mean volume—20 mL
- Tubule volume—14 to 15 mL
- Leydig cell volume—0.5 to 1.2 mL. Occupies 1/5th of the intertubular space
- Mean tubular diameter—180 µm
- Mean tubular length—500 m.

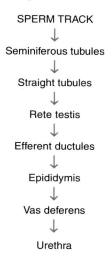

SPERM TRACK
↓
Seminiferous tubules
↓
Straight tubules
↓
Rete testis
↓
Efferent ductules
↓
Epididymis
↓
Vas deferens
↓
Urethra

Normal Biopsy

Tubules should be uniform in size. Tubular cross-section should show active spermatogenesis and, in about half of them, sperm heads should be seen in the lumen or at the luminal border.

The basement membrane should be thin throughout. Leydig cells should be seen occupying one-fifth of the intertubular space (Figure 51.10).

Abnormal or Pathological Testis[10]

Lesions which are commonly encountered in biopsies taken for investigating the cause of infertility are described below.

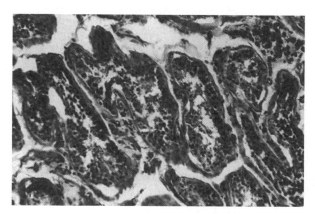

FIGURE 51.10: Normal testes

Destructive Lesions

Tuberculous Orchitis

Tuberculous orchitis is not a very uncommon lesion and it almost invariably begins in the epididymis and spreads to the testis.

Histopathological findings are classical with focal collections of epithelioid cells, and Langhans type of giant cell, surrounded by a cuff of lymphocytes.

Testis with No Spermatogenic Activity

The tubules are not totally destroyed despite no spermatogenic activity.

Major tubular atrophy with no germ cells
- Typically seen in XXY-type Klinefelter's syndrome
- Majority of the tubules are narrow solid and hyalinized (ghost tubules)
- Few tubules are larger and lined by Sertoli cells
- An occasional instance of an odd tubule containing germ cells may be seen
- More than half of the testis is occupied by nodular masses of Leydig cells
- Leydig cell atrophy in case of older men (Figure 51.11).

Minor tubular atrophy with no germ cells
Also known as del Castillo's syndrome/No germ cell syndrome/Chromatin negative Klinefelter's syndrome and Sertoli cell only syndrome.

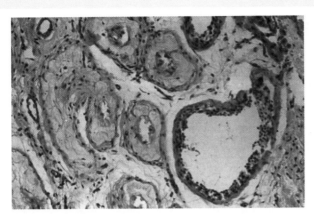

FIGURE 51.11: Tubular atrophy

The histopathological findings are:
- Tubules well preserved but lined by Sertoli cells
- The tall columnar Sertoli cells line the tubule with no intervening spermatogonia
- Tubules are smaller than normal (less than half)
- Pseudohyperplasia of the Leydig cells are seen (Figure 51.12).
- *Inactive germ cells present*

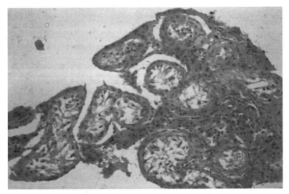

FIGURE 51.12: Sertoli cell only

Usually occurs due to suppression of LH and FSH by exogenous estrogens as part of the therapy for cancer of the prostate or as the result of endogenous secretion seen in cirrhosis of the liver going into failure

Testis with subnormal or below normal spermatogenic activity. This could be generalized as in maturation arrest or could be patchy.

Maturation arrest: Tubules appear to show spermatogenic activity but stop short of producing sperms, sometimes spermatids and even spermatocytes. Hormonal treatment may be of help.

Patchy spermatogenesis: In this situation, the entire spectrum is seen from apparently normal to Sertoli cell only (Figure 51.13).

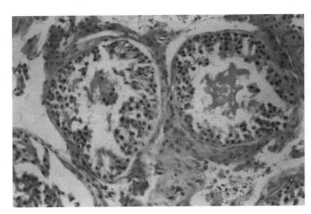

FIGURE 51.13: Maturation arrest

Obstructive Lesions of the Epididymis

The epididymis which is a single 5 m long coiled tubule is just not a passive conveyer of sperms. The epididymis conveys the non-motile non-fertilizing sperm with the testicular fluid. During their 12-day transit through the epididymis they undergo maturation, increasing motility as a result of microscopic and biochemical changes and are stored in the tail of the epididymis for about 2 months.

Testicular biopsies nowadays have been to a large extent replaced by other less invasive procedures to evaluate the spermatogenic activity and to extract sperm for ART procedures.

Microscopic Epididymal Sperm Aspiration (MESA)

This technique was first described in 1985 and initially used in the treatment of patients with secondary obstructive azoospermia.[11] Results showed that epididymal sperms were capable of fertilization *in vitro*[11-13] and also result in pregnancy.

REFERENCES

1. Fox H, Buckley CH: Pathology of female infertility. In Anthony PP, Macsween RNM (Eds): Recent Advances in Histopathology 11. Churchill Linvingstone, 1981; 119-34.

2. Dallenbach-Hellweg Q. Histopathology of the endometrium. Pub. Springer-Verlag, 1987.

3. Lurain JR. Uterine cancer. In Berek JS, Adashi EY, Hillard PA (Eds): Novak's Gynaecology Williman and Wilkins, 1996;1059-61.

4. Buckley CK, Fox H. Biopsy Pathology of the Endometrium. Published by Chapman and Hall Ltd., 1989;38-47.

5. Noyes RW, Hertig AT, Rock J. Dating the endometrial biopsy. Fertil Steril 1950;1:3-25.

6. Noyes RW, Haman JO. Accuracy of endometrial dating: Correction of endometrial dating with basal body temperature and menses. Fertil Steril 1953;4:504-17.

7. Novak ER, Woodruff JD (Eds): Novak's Gynaecologic and Obstetric Pathology with Clinical Relations. WB Saunder Company, 1974;161.

8. Nikas G, Makrigiannakis A, Hovatta O et al. Surface morphology of the human endometrium. Annals NY Academy of Sciences, 316-24.

9. Acosta AA, Elberger L, Barghi M et al. Endometrial dating and determination of the window of implantation in healthy fertile women. Fertil Steril 2000;73(4): 788-98.

10. Lennox B. The infertile testis. In Anthony PP, Macsween RNM (Eds): Recent Advances in Histopathology 11. Churchill Livingstone, 1981;135-48.

11. Temple-Smith PD, Southwick GJ, Yates CA et al. Human pregnancy by in vitro fertilisation (IVF) using sperm aspiration from the epididymis. J in Vitro Fertil Embryo Transfer 1985;2:119.

12. Silber SJ, Balmaceda J, Borrero C et al. Pregnancy with sperm aspiration from the proximal head of the epididymis—a new treatment for congenital absence of the vas deference. Fertil Steril 1988;50:525.

13. Silber SJ, Ord T, Balmaceda J et al. Congenital absence of the vas deference: The fertilisation capacity of human epididymal sperm. N Engl J Med 1990;323:1788.

Section 8

Ethical and Legal Issues

• Peter R Brinsden

52 The Regulation of Assisted Reproductive Technology: The United Kingdom Experience

INTRODUCTION

Treatment of the more severe causes of subfertility by assisted reproduction technology (ART) has, since the very earliest days of Robert Edwards and Patrick Steptoe, produced a number of ethical, legal and political problems and dilemmas. In the late 1960's and 1970's, research by Steptoe and Edwards, which led to the birth of Louise Brown,[1] provoked considerable comment and indeed criticism, not only in the United Kingdom (UK), but Worldwide. In the very early days of their research, these two pioneers advocated the setting up of ethics committees and guidelines to help to resolve some of the contentious issues.

In 1982, four years after the birth of Louise Brown, the government of the United Kingdom decided to set up a committee to make recommendations on the regulation of ART in the UK. In 1984, the 'Warnock Report'[2] was published. This recommended that all practitioners and premises should be licensed when human embryos were created, that all treatments using donor eggs and sperm, the freezing and storage of gametes and embryos and all research on human embryos should be licensed. This report formed the basis upon which, after a period with Voluntary and Interim Licensing Authorities, legislation was drafted. Following a vigorous and free vote in the House of Commons, the Human Fertilisation and Embryology Act (1990)[3] was passed. Following passage of this Act, the Government created the

Human Fertilisation and Embryology Authority (HFEA), which became effective on 1st August 1991. The HFEA subsequently developed a Code of Practice,[4] which is now the "rulebook" by which all Clinics providing licensed treatment must abide. The HFEA regulate and licence all treatment involving embryos, as recommended in the Warnock report, storage of gametes and embryos and all human embryo research. At the same time as this regulatory process was being developed in the UK, a number of other countries were developing their own regulations and guidelines. Some countries, such as Germany, have developed much more strict regulation covering the use and storage of embryos; other countries have more liberal regulation, mainly in the form of guidelines. Many countries at this time still have no formal regulation, such as the United States, Italy and Japan.

Following passage of the HFE Act in 1990, a few problems arose when it was found that the Act was in fact too restrictive. The very strict 'confidentiality clause', which allows all infertile couples to insist on total confidentiality in their treatment, such that even their own doctors cannot be informed of the treatment if the couple do not wish it, did cause considerable disquiet amongst ART clinicians.[5] The Act also recommended that charges be levied for treatment, and larger licensed clinics are now paying upwards of £ 50,000 per annum in a levy, which has to be paid ultimately by infertile couples. There has been some disquiet also amongst clinics on the publication of the results of individual clinics, which has inevitably led to 'league tables' being published by newspapers. The annual "Patients' Guide"[6] generally is an excellent document, but concern has been expressed that those clinics which have done worst may be put out of business; while others believe that if they are performing so badly, perhaps that is what should occur.

No other group of clinicians and scientists in the World is regulated as strictly as ART practitioners in the UK. In spite of this, the large majority of clinicians and scientists feel comfortable with the legislation that has come out, although there are some reservations about possible restriction of clinical freedom and freedom to carry out research. The benefits to infertile couples are very considerable and it has also helped to promote quality in laboratory and clinical practice.

The stated aim of the Code of Practice is: "to support the best clinical and scientific practices, while guarding against the undoubted risk to exploitation of people at a time when they may be particularly vulnerable and to ensure the safety and efficacy of treatment and research and to be concerned about certain fundamental ethical and social questions such as:

1. The respect which is due to human life at all stages of its development;
2. The right of people who are or may be infertile to the proper consideration of their request for treatment;
3. A concern for the welfare of the children, which cannot always be adequately protected by concern for the interests of the adults involved;
4. A recognition of the benefits, both to individuals and to society which can flow from the responsible pursuit of medical and scientific knowledge".[7]

By July 1992, the end of the 'transitional period' allowed by the Act, 121 centres in the UK had been visited and inspected and 65 licenses issued for IVF, 37 for donor insemination only, 32 for research and 8 for gamete storage only. In 2003, 75 clinics hold licenses from the HFEA to practise IVF and related licensed techniques.

THE EFFECTS OF LEGISLATION UPON CLINICAL AND SCIENTIFIC PRACTICE IN THE UK

The HFEA's Code of Practice has radically affected the practice of assisted conception in the UK. No other medical speciality or other area of research has ever been brought under such strict control. The need for some degree of control has never been questioned by clinicians and scientists in the field, but there are many who have voiced their concerns at being so strictly regulated. In general, however, even the critics have come around to appreciate that such a strict system can work and is of benefit, both to patients and to the public, by ensuring that clinical and scientific standards are maintained.

The Code of Practice is comprehensive and deals with all aspects of treatment and research provided at licensed clinics. It distinguishes between guidelines which 'should' be followed and rules laid down in the Act that 'must' be observed. Those areas which most affect the doctors, scientists and patients are briefly summarised below, under their separate sections within the Code:

Part 1: Staff

Provides that a 'person responsible' shall take full responsibility for ensuring that the staff of licensed units are sufficiently qualified, that proper equipment is used, that genetic material is kept and disposed of properly and that the centre complies with the conditions of its license. Guidelines for minimum standards and qualifications of clinical, nursing, scientific and counseling staff are laid down. Failure of the 'person responsible' to comply with the Code of Practice can lead to his/her removal or prosecution, or to suspension of the clinic's license.

Part 2: Facilities

Covers the standards expected in the provision of clinical, laboratory and counseling care. Proper systems for monitoring and assessing practices and procedures are required in order to optimise and improve procedures and outcome.

Part 3: Assessing Clients, Donors and Welfare of the Child

This part deals in detail with the need to ensure that all clients' needs are fully assessed and their specific treatment requirements are met. Certain subjects within this part are dealt with in detail:

1. *Confidentiality* Any information about clients and donors must be kept confidential. No information about the treatment of couples provided under a treatment license may be disclosed to anybody other than the Authority or persons covered by a license, except with the consent of the persons to whom the information relates or in an emergency. It is the person's right to decide what information will be passed on and to whom.

2. *Welfare of the child* The future welfare of any child born as a result of treatment is considered of paramount importance. 'A woman shall not be provided with treatment services unless account has been taken of the welfare of any child born as a result of treatment, (including the need of that child for a father) and of any other child who may be affected by the birth'.

3. *Assessment of potential gamete donors* This section sets out guidelines for the screening of prospective donors with regard to their history, suitability, screening for inherited conditions and HIV and other testing. The guideline on age states that 'genetic gametes should not be taken from female donors over the age of 35, and from male donors over the age of 55, unless there are exceptional reasons for doing so. Gametes should not be taken for the treatment of others from anyone under the age of 18.[7]

Part 4: Information

There are a number of regulations covering the proper provision of information before licensed treatment is given. 'Such relevant information as is proper' must be given.[7] In particular, information should be given on the limitations and results of treatment, possible side-effects, the techniques involved, comparison with other available treatments, the availability of counseling, the cost of treatment, as well as a number of provisions about the rights of the child and the need for a center to keep a register of outcomes of treatment.

Part 5: Consent

No licensed treatment should be given without the written consent of the couple to all the possible stages of that treatment, including the possible freezing of supernumerary embryos. A standard consent form recommended by the HFEA is to be used by all centers. Specific consent must be obtained from couples who have gametes or embryos frozen and for what is to be done with them if he/she dies, or becomes incapable of varying or revoking his or her consent.

Part 6: Counseling

People seeking licensed treatment must be given a suitable opportunity to receive proper counseling about the implications of treatment and proposed steps before they consent to treatment. No one is obliged to accept counseling but it is generally recognised as being beneficial and couples should be encouraged to take it up. The provision of implications counseling is mandatory and couples should be referred for support and therapeutic counseling as appropriate.

Part 7: Use of Gametes and Embryos

This section covers the transport of embryos within the UK and the import and export of embryos to the UK. The main clauses cover the safety and handling of gametes and embryos for clinical use. Clause 7.9 states that 'no more than three eggs or embryos should be placed in a woman in any one cycle, regardless of the procedure used'. In the next revised Code of Practise to be published in 2003, the HFEA are very likely to limit the number of embryos that may be transferred to two. Neither should women be treated with 'gametes nor with embryos derived from gametes of more than one man or woman during any one treatment cycle'. A number of clauses in this section apply to the provision of donor insemination. A limit has been imposed of ten live children to any one gamete donor, be it of sperm or oocytes. Clauses 7.19-7.21 give guidance on the disposal of human embryos no longer required for treatment or those to be used for research and recognise that the 'special status' of the human embryo is fundamental to the provision of the Act.

Part 8: Storage and Handling of Gametes and Embryos

Clauses in this part provide for the 'highest possible standards' in the storage and handling of gametes and embryos, their security and the recording and identification of fresh and stored gametes and embryos.

Part 9: Research

All research that involves the creation, keeping or use of human embryos outside the body must be licensed by the Authority. A center must apply to the Authority for a separate license for each research project.

    Research licenses may only be granted:

1. To promote advances in the treatment of infertility;
2. To increase knowledge about the cause of congenital disease;
3. To increase knowledge about the causes of miscarriage;
4. To develop more effective techniques of contraception;
5. To develop methods for detecting the presence of gene or chromosomal abnormalities in embryos before implantation.

    The Authority will not give licenses unless it is satisfied that the use of human embryos is essential for the purposes of that research.

Additionally

1. No embryos may be kept or used after the appearance of the primitive streak or after 14 days:
2. No human embryos may be placed in a non-human animal;

3. The genetic structure of a cell may not be altered while it forms part of an embryo.

    All research projects must be approved by local Ethics Committees before submission to the Authority.

Part 10: Records

All paper and computer records are confidential and no information about patients may be given to any person other than a member of the Authority, a person covered by the license or under the following circumstances:

1. To the person himself or herself receiving treatment;
2. With the specific consent of the patient to specified people or to unspecified people who need to know in connection with medical or financial audit;
3. In a medical emergency to avert imminent danger to the health of the person concerned;
4. In connection with legal proceedings or formal complaints procedures.

Part 11: Complaints

All licensed centers are required to have procedures for acknowledging and investigating complaints and to have a nominated person to deal properly with such complaints. The Authority must be informed of the number of complaints made in any year and those that are outstanding.

ADVANTAGES AND DISADVANTAGES OF A STRICT REGULATORY SYSTEM

To Clinicians and Scientists

A strict national regulatory system generally promotes good clinical and laboratory practices in this special area. In particular, it reassures patients that they are receiving treatment that is of a certain standard and it reassures the public that unreasonable practices cannot occur in licensed clinics in the United Kingdom. A regulatory body such as the HFEA can also act as a source of advice and support for clinicians and scientists, and the annual inspection process of clinics ensures a form of 'peer review'.

The major disadvantages of a strict regulatory system are not so much due to the rules and regulations, but more to the increased bureaucracy caused by the process and the considerable costs involved, with larger clinics paying as much as £ 50,000-£ 60,000 per year in license fees. Another problem that has been experienced with legislating on treatment is that there is a loss of flexibility, since it is difficult to change laws to allow the speciality to 'move with the times'.

To Infertile Couples

There is little doubt that small groups of infertile couples have their chances of achieving a pregnancy reduced by the imposition of strict regulation. The guideline that treatment should not be initiated for women over the age of 50 prevents a very few women from receiving treatment. The large majority of people are happy that a limit be placed on age, since the idea of women in their 60's having families is not one that it is acceptable to most in society. Some women in their 40's, and others who have had multiple failed attempts at treatment, may be disadvantaged by only allowing three, or soon only two embryos to be transferred. The number of couples affected by this restriction are, in fact, very few and most practitioners accept that the move to only allowing a maximum of three embryos was reasonable, and most are in favor of moving to limit the number to two embryos.

In a recent legal case, the restrictions placed on the use of a woman's deceased husband's sperm, seemed harsh. However, the HFEA had no choice, in that the law is quite clear that treatment could not be allowed to proceed in the United Kingdom, as the husband had not given his informed consent to the procedure. After much legal debate, the problem was settled by allowing the woman to transfer the sperm and to undertake treatment in another country. This was generally felt to be an unsatisfactory compromise, but the reasons for it were understood.

In 1996, at the end of the first-five years of regulation covering the storage of embryos, it was found that there were large numbers of embryos being held in storage for couples with whom contact had been lost.[8, 9, 10] The law required these embryos to be destroyed if consent could not be obtained to extend the storage for another five years. The mass destruction of several thousand embryos in the United Kingdom caused an outpouring of criticism and debate in the World Press. That hurdle has now been overcome and there is now no reason why such problems should occur again, as the regulations are made absolutely clear to couples at the time of signing their consents for storage.

With the huge increase in access to the 'Internet', concerns have been expressed about the potential for traffic of patients between countries seeking gamete donors and surrogate hosts. Donor sperm and oocytes can be purchased over the Internet and couples can see pictures and details of the donors to help them choose. Permission to import donor sperm, eggs or embryos must be sought from the HFEA and a license obtained. It is possible for couples who cannot obtain treatment in the UK to travel to countries where they can. A recent example is of a gay couple who travelled to the United States and had twins by a surrogate host.[11]

ETHICAL ISSUES

A number of interesting social and ethical issues have been addressed by the HFEA since it came into power. They have developed a process of 'discussion documents', which have provided a healthy forum for the debate of contentious issues before they have made a final decision. This process has ensured that the opinions of all interested groups are obtained. The process is rather cumbersome and the collection of data and the decision-making process arrived at from analysis of that data must be difficult; it is also possible for certain pressure groups to respond to a discussion document in strength and thereby influence the balance of opinion. The HFEA does not need to go through this discussion process, but it is generally perceived that it shows their desire to listen to and be influenced by people's opinions before making their final decision. A number of interesting issues have been dealt with by the HFEA during the last eight years which have affected clinical practice; these include:

1. The process of sex selection was reviewed and a discussion document issued. This was not strictly within the remit of the HFEA, as it did not cover licensed treatment, unless IVF or donor gametes were involved. Nevertheless, following discussion, the HFEA allowed sex selection by the process of sperm selection for inherited conditions, but not for social reasons.

2. The use of foetal ovarian tissue was another issue that the HFEA addressed. Many felt very uncomfortable with the concept of oocytes being cultured from foetal ovarian tissue for donor egg programs. Following a full review using the discussion document process, the HFEA decided that research with foetal ovarian tissue should be allowed to continue, but that it should not be used as a source of donor gametes or for any other clinical use.[12]

3. Payment of egg and sperm donors has been discussed at some length and has recently been the subject of a discussion document. Most interested groups in the United Kingdom agree that payment of large sums of money to gamete donors should not be allowed, but most clinicians and scientists believe that a modest payment to donors should be acceptable. The HFEA have decided that the previous maximum payment of £ 15 to sperm and egg donors should continue, but that some "benefits in kind", such as having a concurrent sterilisation procedure for ovum donors, should be allowed.

4. The issue of 'egg sharing', to improve the availability of donor oocytes, has caused considerable controversy. Most practitioners have felt uncomfortable with the concept of infertile women giving eggs to infertile couples for free treatment. Nevertheless, there are many advantages to such an idea and it has been pursued successfully by one particular group in the United Kingdom.[13] The HFEA have, somewhat unexpectedly, said that this idea would not be banned and they have recently drawn up guidelines.

5. Together with the Human Genetics Advisory Commission, the HFEA have recently reported to the Government on human cloning. Their recommendation was that cloning of humans should not be allowed, but the cloning of human tissues for medical treatment and the associated research should be allowed. The Government have not accepted this recommendation in full and are seeking further consultation before making a decision.

6. There are other treatments that are acceptable in the United Kingdom that are not accepted in many other countries. The donation of embryos surplus to a couple's requirement to another couple is accepted in the UK and the treatment is successful. It is certainly preferable to many couples than the adoption of babies or children, which is becoming increasingly difficult in the UK.

7. The practice of IVF surrogacy or gestational surrogacy in the United Kingdom is accepted, but only for exceptional and specific indications. Most countries in Europe do not allow surrogacy.

CONCLUSION

The Human Fertilisation and Embryology Authority were appointed by the UK Government following the passing of the Human Fertilisation and Embryology Act 1990 to regulate the provision of infertility treatment by IVF, donor gametes, the storage of gametes and embryos and all research involving human embryos. They took on full statutory responsibility for this regulation on 1 August 1991. Since then, the Authority and those it licenses have dealt with the very complex provisions of the Act in a spirit of mutual help and co-operation. We have all felt our way through the complex legal minefield. Intense debate has been achieved on many of the most contentious issues through discussion documents put out by the HFEA. The Code of Practice, which is the 'bible' by which all licensed clinics must abide, clearly explained what 'should' and what 'must' be complied with. The HFEA is able to, and does, respond to changes, and a revised Code of Practice is published every 2 or 3 years.

In general, patients are reassured by the 'authority of the Authority'. Practitioners are generally content that the best possible job of regulation is being effected by an Authority which is set a seemingly impossible task–the regulation of the socially and ethically very difficult area of assisted human reproduction. The lay public should, and I believe generally does, feel reassured that there is a watchdog body to oversee this often contentious area and that it will act, along with local independent Ethics Committees, as the conscience of the public and to assure good clinical and scientific practice.

There are a number of areas into which the Authority is now being drawn and over which the original Act did not grant them regulatory powers. Sex selection and the possible use of foetal ovarian tissue are examples of this. Some consider that they should not become involved with these contentious areas, as they are outside their currently specified area of authority. Some clinicians and scientists are concerned that more and yet more regulation of their practices will occur; and yet there is at present no more qualified body to consider these matters. Surely it is better that this Authority, with its greater depth of knowledge and experience than any other, should be tasked with debating these problems, rather than some other new imposed authority of lesser experience.

From the earliest days of assisted conception, it was clinicians and scientists pioneering the work who felt the need for guidance and some regulation.[14] It was they who asked for Ethics Committees to be set up and who encouraged proper Government legislation in this difficult area. We in the UK now have a statutory Authority controlling our practice–the only medical speciality to have one. It is not perfect, but no Authority could have been set up with much more forethought, with 8 years of deliberation–through the Warnock Report, the Voluntary and Interim Licensing Authorities and two Acts of Parliament. The end result–the Human Fertilisation and Embryology Authority– is reassuring to our patients and to the general public. It is to be hoped that all the experience on regulating assisted reproduction treatment gained during the past 13 years might help other countries, which have yet to legislate, to do so more easily.

REFERENCES

1. Steptoe PC, Edwards RG. Birth after the reimplantation of human embryo. Lancet 1978;2:366.
2. Report of the Committee of Enquiry into Human Fertilisation and Embryology Her Majesty's Stationery Office, London 1984.
3. Human Fertilisation and Embryology Act Her Majesty's Stationery Office, London 1990.
4. Human Fertilisation and Embryology Authority. Code of Practice: et seq to 2001. Her Majesty's Stationery Office, London 1991.
5. Brinsden PR. Confidentiality taken to the extreme. Lancet 1991;2:851-52.
6. The Patient's Guide to Donor Insemination and In Vitro Fertilization Clinics. Human Fertilisation and Embryology Authority 1995 and annually.
7. Human Fertilisation and Embryology Authority. Code of Practice: Her Majesty's Stationery Office, London 1993.
8. Brinsden PR, Avery SM, Marcus SF, Macnamee MC. Frozen embryos: decision time in the UK. Hum Reprod 1995;10:3083-84.
9. Edwards RG, Beard H, Bradshaw J. UK Law dictated the destruction of 3000 cryopreserved human embryos. Hum Reprod 1997;12:3-5.
10. Deech R. Destruction of cryopreserved embryos: a reply from the Chairman. Hum Reprod 1997;12:5-6.
11. The Independent. Gay couple to be fathers of test-tube twins. Thursday 2nd September 1999;7.
12. Review of the Guidance on the Research use of Fetuses and Fetal Material (CM762) Her Majesty's Stationery Office, London 1989.
13. Ahuja KK, Mostyn BJ, Simons EG. Egg sharing and egg donation: attitudes of British donors and recipients. Hum Reprod 1997;12:2845-52.
14. Edwards RG, Sharpe DJ. Social values and research in human embryology. Nature (London) 1972;231:87-91.

• Pushpa M Bhargava

53

The Infertility Treatment Scene in India: Strengths, Problems and Solutions

INTRODUCTION

Indian civilization is one of the most ancient. During the entire history of our sub-continent, the emphasis on the family has been paramount, and family means children. Thus, having a child has been of the greatest importance not only to the couple but also to their larger family. Socially, a stigma is attached to a couple (traditionally, to the woman partner) if the couple does not have a child. Economically, children have been a couple's best insurance for old-age, and continue to be so even today, as there is no adequate social security system operative in the country. For those belonging to the lower strata of the society, including many farming families in our villages, children provide help in augmenting the family's income by sharing the family's work.

But some 15 percent of couples in India, as elsewhere are infertile. With the population of India at one billion, the number of infertile couples could be well over 20 million-much more than the entire population of Australia and New Zealand.

The new medical techniques that attempt to obtain a pregnancy by manipulating the sperm or/and the oocyte outside the body, and transferring the gamete or the embryo into the uterus, have opened up new avenues for treatment of infertility, specially in the last two and a half decades, so much so that, today, it is possible to take care of some 85 percent of the cases of infertility. There is, therefore, a huge market for the new techniques such as assisted reproductive technologies (ART), to treat infertility in India.

India is widely regarded as one of the scientifically and technologically most advanced country of the world! The last decade has seen a virtual mushrooming of infertility clinics all over the country as we have no law that would require compulsory registration of such clinics. We do not know the exact number of infertility clinics in any city or in the country. Various estimates give the number as between 200 and 300, not counting those that may not be advertising themselves, as they may have a niche market in their geographical area.

THE INFERTILITY CLINICS

While India has no doubt, many infertility clinics the facilities and quality of which would match with similar clinics anywhere else in the world, the unfortunate element in the story is that there are also many which have inadequate facilities and staff.

It is also widely known that many clinics, including some of those that have excellent facilities and staff, engage in a number of unethical practices. Further, lack of a system of accreditation and supervision of clinics that handle gametes *in vitro* and practice ART, has the potential of leading to several undesirable situations. Let us look at some examples.

Many instances are known where a patient has only been given intra-uterine insemination (IUI) but charged for *in vitro* fertilization (IVF). Such malpractices become possible in India because 70 percent of the country is rural and about half the women of the country (a much larger proportion in the villages) are illiterate. The situation is made worse by the fact that the average per capita income in the country is about the lowest in the world, if one takes away the upper creamy layer of the society which, say, pays tax and represents a very small proportion (less than 5 percent) of the population. Therefore paying for IVF when only IUI has been done on an infertile couple, must cause an immense financial strain on the couple. Often, people in the villages sell their land and/or other assets to come to an infertility clinic. It would, therefore, be not only unethical but even criminal from the social point of view for such a couple to be charged for IVF if only IUI has been done.

There have also been advertisements in Indian newspapers by ART clinics saying that their success rate in IVF has been more than three times the average success rate around the world. Such clinics have been clearly misleading the people through such an advertisement to gain advantage over other infertility clinics.

There have also been advertisements in the recent past in our newspapers by infertility clinics saying that they can give a couple a child of the desired sex by pre-natal sex selection-that is separation of the X and Y spermatozoa, when the fact is that no established technique yet exists which would separate X and Y sperm with one hundred percent efficiency.

In many infertility clinics in the country today, there is no professional counseling available. There is no codified system to decide as to when the couple must be asked to give up the treatment on ethical grounds, and advised to adopt a child; instead, the treatments are prolonged unnecessarily over a large number of cycles in spite of the fact that the gynecologist knows that the expense that the couple would be incurring would be infructuous. There is no way in the country to prevent such a malpractice. Some gynecologists engage in artificial insemination by the husband's semen (AJH) or by donor semen

(AID), when no adequate facilities exist with the gynecologist for processing of semen, or for doing appropriate checks in case the semen has been obtained from outside, or for documentation of what is being done.

In my estimate, unethical practices such as those mentioned above, today, perhaps, result in an infructuous expenditure of several hundred million rupees by the people of the country, most of whom would have sacrificed a great deal to be able to pay the expenses of treatment at an infertility clinic.

THE ETHICAL ISSUES

i. An important issue in the practice of ART in India is, who should be the donor of semen for AID? In this regard, we ought to remember that a vast majority of the population in India today stills lives as a part of the larger joint family.

If a couple is infertile in India, the family lays the blame on the woman even though, in about half the diagnosable cases, a male factor is the cause of infertility. The mother-in-law would, however, rarely acknowledge in public that her son, and not the daughter-in-law, is at fault. Therefore, even if she is convinced of the biological fact that the daughter in-law is fine but her son has a problem, she would want to make sure that her son's infertile status is kept as close a secret as possible. Therefore, she takes the daughter-in-law to an infertility clinic and, following the advise of the clinic that the daughter-in-law needs to be inseminated by donor semen, the mother-in-law asks the clinic to inseminate the daughter-in-law by the semen of the husband's brother or of a close family friend. The daughter-in-law would normally have no say in this regard, no matter how opposed she might be to the idea of being inseminated by the semen of someone whom she has been and would continue to see all the time. The psychological stress that the daughter-in-law will go through for the rest of her life, including during pregnancy, on account of the knowledge that the biological father of the child she is carrying is someone whom she knows and has social intercourse all the time, would not be a matter of concern to the rest of the family.

In such a scenario, quarrels between a mother-in-law and her daughter-in-law are not yet a thing of the past in India. Against this background, imagine the following scenario. At the instance of the mother-in-law, a woman is inseminated with the semen of her husband's brother or friend. A few years later, the mother-in-law and the daughter-in-law quarrel. The mother-in-law then says publicly that her daughter-in-law has committed adultery and names the person with whom the adultery has been committed. DNA fingerprinting-a technology which has been widely used in India since 1986 and in the development of which in the country I had a small role-will establish that the basis of mother-in-law's allegation that the child is not her son's child but of another man, is correct. As the infertility clinics are, as of today, not required to keep appropriate records, there will be no way that the daughter-in-law can establish that she never slept with the man who is the biological father of the child, and that she was artificially inseminated with that man's semen with the express approval-even suggestion-of the mother-in-law.

When we asked the National Commission for Women, a statutory organization set up by the Government of India, as to their opinion in regard to the anonymity or otherwise of donors of semen in cases such as the ones mentioned above, the Commission was strongly of the opinion that all sperm and egg donation must be anonymous. The situation I have outlined above would seem to support this view.

ii. The second major question that the ART clinics in India are facing today, pertains to donation of the oocyte. Who should be an oocyte donor? As of today, in India, it is almost always a close relative from the side of the man or the woman. The idea of having a close relative or friend of the family as

donor of the sperm or the egg, is that the entire story is kept within the family-friend boundary. The other implications-including the genetic and the social implications-of such donation are not understood for reasons mentioned in the preceding section in respect of sperm donation.

Do we need to have sperm banks that would also keep track (for example, through appropriate advertisement) of possible oocyte donors against monetary compensation? Do we also need to encourage the system of egg sharing in which an indigent infertile couple that needs financial resources for ART agrees to donate oocytes to an affluent infertile couple wherein the wife can carry the pregnancy through but cannot produce her own oocyte, for *in vitro* fertilization with the sperm of the male partner of the affluent couple, for a monetary compensation that would take care of the expenses of an ART procedure on the indigent couple? These questions need to be answered.

iii. The third question being raised in the country in regard to the practice of ART pertains to surrogacy. Who may act as the surrogate mother? As of now it, again, is a close relative-for example, the mother of the male partner or the sister of the female partner. Thus, in many cases in the country, a woman has given birth to her own grandchild without incest. On the other hand, there are also regular advertisements, for example in the magazine, Woman's Era, for surrogate motherhood. I believe that it is unethical to have a close relative act as a surrogate mother especially in the Indian environment where family ties are very close. In a closely-knit family, the fact that the child was delivered by so-and-so will always be known to the members of the family and, eventually, to the child when it grows older. Carrying a child in one's own womb is, in the Indian society, the epitome of a close relationship. Therefore, it would be difficult for a child and the surrogate mother, if they see each other everyday, for such a relationship not to come in the way of the child establishing the expected relationship with the biological mother, without confusion in the child's mind. Will the best solution under our circumstances be what is already being practiced by some in the country, that is, to advertise for a surrogate, and strike an appropriate financial arrangement that will adequately compensate the woman who agrees to act as a surrogate mother?

Another relevant issue that is exercising the minds of people in regard to surrogacy is whether or not surrogacy in India should be considered ethical if the reason is only convenience of the couple. There is a view that surrogacy by assisted conception should be considered only for those for whom it would be physically or medically impossible or undesirable to carry a baby to term, and not for those who are perfectly capable of producing a child in the normal way but desire a surrogate mother because the woman does not want to go through the pregnancy for the sake of convenience, or for reasons such as a break in professional service, or simply the risk of having one's vital statistics affected.

iv. Then there is the question of the right of the child born through donation of a germ cell, to know who its biological father or mother is, when the child attains adulthood, assuming that the sperm or the egg donation has been anonymous. In the Indian environment, it has been argued, it may be both impractical and unethical to give the right to the child. Given the closeness of relationships in India, such a right would be psychologically unfair to the child, to the donor and to the couple who have brought up the child; the child, of course, must continue to have the right to know everything else (except the name and address) about the person who donated the oocyte or the sperm.

Let us look at this issue in a little greater detail. We have the technique of DNA fingerprinting available today which establishes the biological parenthood without any doubt. If a need arises for DNA fingerprinting to be done on the child, it would become obvious that the couple who brought up the child does not comprise both the biological parents of the child. Such a discovery for the child, all of a sudden, could alienate him from his parents whom he could accuse of deliberately hiding the truth from him. Therefore, there may be no harm in the couple's telling the child at an appropriate time that he/she was born following anonymous sperm or egg donation.

v. There are also several other issues that have needed to be resolved in respect of practice of ART in India. For example, what should be the age limits-upper and lower-for germ cell donation or surrogacy, and the number of times one can act as a surrogate mother.

vi. There is also the question of what the infertility clinics should do with spare embryos which would be the main source of totipotent embryonic stem cells. As of today, there is no regulation in the country prescribing what should be done with such embryos.

The silver lining is that the Indian Council of Medical Research (ICMR) released, on 4th September 2002, a draft national guidelines for accreditation, supervision and regulation of ART clinics in India following the recommendations of a high-power committee set up by the ICMR. These guidelines have since been publicly debated in the country at Chennai, Bangalore, Kolkata, Jodhpur, Hyderabad and Mumbai. They are now in the process of being finalized and eventually sent to the Parliament for passing an appropriate Act.

THE RECOMMENDATIONS

I now give several important recommendations that are before the Expert Group appointed by the ICMR for formulating the national guidelines on accreditation, supervision and regulation of infertility clinics in India, for finalisation, as of 15th April 2003:

1. **Classification of infertility clinics.** The infertility clinics will be categorized in four groups:

- *Level-1A (L-l A)* infertility clinics would be those that do not engage in IUI (intra-uterine insemination) and thus do not handle gametes that have been donated, collected or processed *in vitro*. They would not require accreditation.
- *Level-IB, Level-2 and Level-3 (L-1B, L-2 and L-3, respectively)* infertility clinics that would handle gametes that have been donated, collected or processed *in vitro*, would require accreditation. They would differ only in respect of the infrastructure and the type of facilities and expertise that they would offer to the patients. The guidelines state these facilities in detail. Level-IB, Level-2, and
- *Level-3* infertility clinics would encourage appropriately qualified gynaecologists of Level-1A clinics to use their facility.

2. **Infrastructural requirements for Level-B, Level-2 and Level-3 clinics**. The requirements in terms of space have been divided into the non-sterile area and the sterile area. The non-sterile area would include a reception and meeting room for patients, a room with privacy, a general purpose clinical laboratory, a store room, a record room, an autoclaving room, a semen collection room, a semen processing laboratory and a clean room for IUI. The sterile area would include the operation theatre, a room for intrauterine transfer of embryos, and the embryology laboratory. Some of the spaces mentioned above can be combined (that is, the same space can be used for more than one purpose) as long as such a step does not compromise the quality of service. However, space provisions for the sterile area cannot be combined with those for the non-sterile area, and vice-versa.

All instruments would be required to be calibrated periodically-at least once every year.

The infertility clinics need not have in-house facilities to perform all the procedures necessary to diagnose infertility. They can be farmed out to speciality laboratories specia-lizing in delivering such services. (It would clearly be of advantage for the infertility clinic to use a laboratory that has been duly accredited, for example, by the National Accreditation Board for Calibration and Testing Laboratories.)

3. **Requirement of staff.** The guidelines state the requirements for staff for L-1B, L-2, L-3 infertility clinics. The minimal qualifications for the staff are also stated. The need for appropriately qualified gynecologist, andro-logist, clinical embryologist and counselor, in addition to the Director (or the Program Coordinator) of an infertility clinic at any of the above levels, is emphasized. The mini-mum qualifications and experience that an individual in the above categories of staff, should have, is also stated. Provision has been made for sharing the services of an andro-logist, a clinical embryologist and a coun-selor by more than one infertility clinic, as long as the quality of the service is not compromised. The responsibility for ensuring that such sharing does not lead to such a compromise would lie with the clinic. The minimal qualification for a gynecologist in a Ll-B, L-2 orL-3 clinic would be a post-graduate degree, with adequate experience the details of which are provided in the guidelines. A person with a BSc or BVSc degree with at least five years of first-hand, hands-on experience of the appropriate techniques that are mentioned in the guidelines, would be acceptable for function-ing as a clinical embryologist. A person who has at least a degree in social sciences, life sciences or medicine, and who has a good knowledge of the various causes of inferti-lity, its social and general implications, and the possibilities offered by various treat-ment modalities, could be considered as qualified to serve as a counselor.

4. **Procedures for treatment of infertility.** The guidelines list the procedures that are currently employed for treatment of inferti-lity. If a new procedure is discovered and comes in vogue, it could be used by an

infertility clinic of L-1B, L-2 or L-3, but the clinic using it first must inform, within six months of the first use, the appropriate accreditation committee about this usage; the committee would be obliged to give its decision on whether the procedure should be continued or not continued, within eight weeks of its receiving the information from the clinic. Once the procedure has been approved the other clinics would be free to use it without asking for permission.

5. **Protocol for screening of patients.** Basic details of a protocol for such a screening are provided in the guidelines to help the infertility clinics to decide as to which procedure might be best suited for the particular patient, taking into account the cost factor and the socio-economic status of the patient.

6. **Responsibilities of the clinic and information and counseling to be given to patients.** Two separate sections in the guidelines, give the details of the responsibilities of the clinic, and the information and counseling to be given to patients.

7. **Requirements for sperm donor, for surrogate mothers, and for semen banks.** These requirements are given in detail in the guidelines.

8. **Method of sourcing semen and oocyte donors and surrogate mothers.**

   The guidelines permit the sourcing of the above through appropriate advertisement; the protocol for such sourcing has been laid down. Payment to gamete donors or to surrogate mothers is not prohibited but guidelines laid down.

9. **Spare embryos.** Directions for preservation, utilization or destruction of spare embryos are given in the guidelines. The use of spare embryos for research, for example, for work on stem cells, with permission from the owners of the embryos, is recommended to be encouraged.

10. **Rights of the patients.** The guidelines lay emphasis on the information that must be provided to the patients to enable him/her to exercise a well-reasoned choice that would be in the best interests, taking all factors into consideration. The guidelines also require appropriate record keeping and transparency in all dealings. The document emphasises the requirement of a high level of professionalism in respect of the techniques used and in counseling. It also lays emphasis on honesty and integrity that must be exhibited by the clinic in respect of having the consent forms filled. Model consent forms are also provided.

11. **Recommendations on some other important issues.** The gamete donors must be anonymous but all possible information about the donor (except the name and address) must be provided to the couple or the person receiving the donated gamete.

    A relative belonging to the same generation or age group, or an unrelated person known or unknown to the couple, may act as a surrogate mother. The infertility clinic must not be a party to any commercial element in donor programs or in gestational surrogacy. This would obviously not apply to semen banks which would also be expected to keep track of possible oocyte donors. The financial terms for surrogacy must be settled between the couple and the prospective surrogate mother.

    Gametes produced by a person under the age of 21 shall not be used. The accepted age for a sperm donor shall be between 21 and 45 years and for the oocyte donor between 21 and 35 years. A surrogate mother should not be over 45 years of age. Normally, no more than three eggs or embryos would be transferred into a woman; situations under which this number may be increased have been specified in the guidelines.

    Semen from two individuals would not be permitted to be mixed.

    A child born through surrogacy must be adopted by the genetic (biological) parents, unless they can establish through genetic (DNA) fingerprinting (of which the records will be maintained in the clinic) that the child is theirs.

Surrogacy by assisted conception would normally be considered only for patients for whom it would be physically or medically impossible or undesirable to carry a baby to term. A child born through any ART procedure shall be deemed to be a legitimate child of the couple having been born in wedlock and with the consent of both the spouses. Therefore, the child shall have legal right to parental support, inheritance, and all other privileges of a child born to a couple through sexual intercourse.

A surrogate mother would be required to register in a hospital or a nursing home for delivery, only in her own name but giving the name, addresses and other relevant information of the biological parents of the child she is carrying. The birth certificate shall be in the name of the biological parents.

The guidelines prescribe the test that any donor or surrogate mother must go through before he or she is accepted for the stated purpose.

Children born through donor gametes shall not have any right whatsoever to know the identity (such as name, address, parentage etc.) of their genetic parent(s). A child thus born will, however, be provided all other information about the donor as and when desired by the child, when the child becomes an adult

Normally, no ART procedure shall be used on a woman below 20 years. For a woman between 20 and 30 years, two years of cohabitation/marriage without the use of a contraceptive would be required before the use of an ART procedure on her, excepting in cases where the man is infertile or the woman cannot conceive physiologically. This period would be reduced to one year for a woman over 30 years.

All infertility clinics of Level-IB, Level-2 and Level-3 would be required to have their own ethics committee constituted according to the ICMR ethical guidelines.

Egg sharing that would allow the expenses of infertility treatment using an ART procedure on an indigent couple, to be met by an affluent couple who would, in exchange, receive an egg from the indigent couple, would be encouraged.

The provision or otherwise of an ART procedure to a HIV— positive woman would be governed by the implications of the decision of the Supreme Court in the case of X-vs-Hospital 2 (1998)8 Section 296, or any other relevant judgement of the Supreme Court or the law of the country, whichever is the latest.

There would be no bar to the use of ART techniques by a single or unmarried woman, or a lesbian or gay couple,who wish to have a child, and no ART Clinic may refuse to offer its services to the above, provided other criteria mentioned in the document are satisfied. The child thus born will have all the legal rights on the woman or the man as any child has on any of its parents.

The guidelines recommend reimbursement for expenses incurred by a couple for treatment of infertility. The guidelines also recommend that these expenses should be covered by medical insurance.

Keeping in mind the overwhelming preference in the country for a male child and the consequent dramatic fall in the female: male ratio, all procedures aiming to give the couple a child of a particular sex such as the use of X- or Y-enriched fractions, preimplantation genetic diagnosis, or prenatal sex determination, are banned in the guidelines.

12. **The mechanism for implementation of the guidelines**. The guidelines specifies this mechanism in detail. There would be a national accreditation authority of which the composition is given in the guidelines. This authority would set up a national accreditation committee and a review committee of which the powers and responsibilities are defined in the document. The States would be welcome to set up their own State accreditation committees and review committees, the procedure for which is also mentioned in the guidelines.

The appellate authority for a decision of the national accreditation committee would be the national accreditation authority, and for a decision of the accreditation authority, the Supreme Court. The appellate authority for the State-level accreditation committee, would be the national accreditation committee.

No new infertility clinic may start operating unless it has obtained temporary license to do so. (This would be applicable after the guidelines have been approved by the Government of India and either an Executive Order or an Act of the Parliament passed in this respect.) The license would be confirmed only if the clinic obtains accreditation (permanent license) from the Centre or the State's appropriate accreditation authority within two years after obtaining the temporary license. The license must be renewed every seven years.

The existing infertility clinics would need to obtain a temporary license within six months of the notification of the accreditation committee, and appropriate accreditation (a permanent license) within two years of the notification.

If the infertility clinic (existing or new) that has applied for a temporary license to the appropriate accreditation authority, does not receive the license (or a reply) within two months of the receipt of the application from the concerned office of the authority, the infertility clinic would be deemed to have received the license. The same would apply to the permanent license.

Appendix

Patient Demographic Record

Female Card Information	Male Card Information
Name :	Name :
DOB : 00/00/0000	DOB : 00/00/0000
Age : Years	Age : Years
Occupation :	Occupation :

Contact Address	Local Contact Address

☐ Primary Infertility   ☐ Endocrine

☐ Secondary Infertility   ☐ Genetics

☐ Obstetric   ☐ BOH

☐ Gynecological   ☐ Well Women Clinic

☐ Allergies   ☐ Cardiac

☐ Medication   ☐ Hypothyroid

☐ TB   ☐ Hyperthyroid

☐ DM   ☐ Abdominal/pelvic surgery

☐ Ectopic Pregnancy   ☐ Ovarian Cystectomy   ☐ Endometriotic Cyst

   ○ Right ○ Left ○ Both   ○ Right ○ Left ○ Both   ○ Right ○ Left ○ Both

☐ Oophorectomy   ☐ Sterilization   ☐ Sterilization Reversal

   ○ Right ○ Left ○ Both   ☐ Salpingectomy   ☐ Salpingostomy

☐ Myomectomy   ○ Right ○ Left ○ Both   ○ Right ○ Left ○ Both

☐ Endometriosis   ☐ Adhesiolysis   ☐ Appendecectomy

☐ Endoscopy   ☐ Laparoscopy   ☐ Hysteroscopy
                     ☐ Diagnostic   ☐ Diagnostic
                     ☐ Operative   ☐ Operative

☐ Diabetes Mellitus   ☐ Endocrine
☐ Hypertension   ☐ Koch's
☐ Carcinoma   ☐ Infertility
☐ Alcohol   ☐ Smoking
☐ Asthma
☐ HTN
☐ Others

Changes in weight: Kg   ◯ Increased   ◯ Decreased
          Duration: Years
Changes in density and distribution of hair: Duration:

Married: ◯ Yes   ◯ No
     First Marriage   Duration: Years   Months
                                  ◯ Consanguineous
                                  ◯ Non consanguineous
     Second Marriage   Duration: Years   Months
                                  ◯ Consanguineous
                                  ◯ Non-consanguineous

Sexual Intercourse: ◯ Daily   ◯ 1/Week   ◯ 1/Month
                        ◯ 2-3/Week   ◯ 2-3 Month   ◯ Nil

☐ Vaginismus   ☐ OCP   ☐ Vasectomy
☐ Inactive   ☐ IUCD   ☐ Condoms
☐ Dysfunction   ☐ Sterilization   ☐ Safe Period

DOC: Last Menstrual Period: 00/00/0000   Menarche: Years

☐ Current Menstrual Cycle   ◯ Regular ◯ Irregular   ☐ Normal Flow
                              ☐ Amenorrhea   ☐ Menorrhagia
☐ Premenstrual Tension   ☐ Dysmenorrhea   ☐ Polymenorrhea
☐ Midovulatory Pain   ☐ Midovulatory Bleeding   ☐ Oligomenorrhea

☐ Vaginal Discharge
☐ Postcoital Bleeding   ☐ Dyspareunia
☐ Intermenstrual Bleeding   ☐ Pelvic Infection

ULTRASOUND

Place: Date: 00/00/0000

Day of Cycle: Scan Type: ◯ Abdominal   ◯ Vaginal

Sonologist:

Uterus: ☐ Normal Size and Shape   ☐ Fibroids

                ☐ Bicornuate   ☐ Adenomyosis

                ☐ Bulky   ☐ Infantile

Endo:

Right Ovary: Left Ovary:

   Measures   Measures

   Follicles   Follicles

   Cysts   Cysts

   Endocyst   Endocyst

   Others   Others

POD   Comments:

☐ Clear

☐ Fluid   ◯ Clear   ◯ Blood

☐ Hydrosalpinx

Diagnostic Laparoscopy

Place: Date of Admission:

DOC: Discharge:

Anesthesia: ◯ IV   ◯ LA   Anesthetist :

            ◯ GA   ◯ Spinal   Surgeon :

Distending Media: Methods: ◯ D.P. Method   ◯ T.P. Method

                                          ◯ S.P. Method

Uterus:

Position: ◯ Anteverted   Shape: ◯ Normal   Mobility: ◯ Free

        ◯ Retroverted   ◯ Bulky   ◯ Restricted

        ◯ Others   ◯ Infantile   ◯ Fixed

                             ◯ Others   ◯ Others

☐ Fibroids Adenomyosis: Endometriosis:

Tubes: ○ Patency   ○ Left   ○ Right   ○ Both

         ○ Blocked   ○ Left   ○ Right   ○ Both

         ○ Abnormal

		Left	Right	Both
☐	Distended	○ Left	○ Right	○ Both
☐	Hydrosalpinx	○ Left	○ Right	○ Both
☐	Pyosalpinx	○ Left	○ Right	○ Both
☐	Tortuous	○ Left	○ Right	○ Both
☐	Bulbous	○ Left	○ Right	○ Both
☐	Adherent	○ Left	○ Right	○ Both
☐	Tuberculosis	○ Left	○ Right	○ Both

Ovaries:

Right: ☐ Normal   Left: ☐ Normal

       ☐ Follicles   ☐ Follicles

       ☐ PCO   ☐ PCO

       ☐ Cystic   ☐ Cystic

       ☐ Endometriosis   ☐ Endometriosis

       ☐ Adherent   ☐ Adherent

Pouch of Douglas: ☐ Free

                     ☐ Obliterated

                     ☐ Endometriosis

                     ☐ Koch's

                     ☐ Fluid

                     ☐ Others

I.F. No: Name:

Operative Laparoscopy

Place: Date of Admission:

DOC: Discharge:

Anesthesia: ○ IV   ○ LA   Anesthetist:

            ○ GA   ○ Spinal   Surgeon:

Distending Media: Methods: ○ D.P. Method   ○ T.P. Method

                                           ○ S.P. Method

Uterus:

Position: ○ Anteverted   Shape: ○ Normal   Mobility: ○ Free

          ○ Retroverted   ○ Bulky   ○ Restricted

          ○ Others   ○ Infantile   ○ Fixed

                                 ○ Others   ○ Others

☐ Fibroids Adenomyosis: Endometriosis:

Tubes: ◯ Patency ◯ Left ◯ Right ◯ Both
　　　 ◯ Blocked ◯ Left ◯ Right ◯ Both
　　　　　 ◯ Abnormal ☐ Distended ◯ Left ◯ Right ◯ Both
　　　　　　　　　　　 ☐ Hydrosalpinx ◯ Left ◯ Right ◯ Both
　　　　　　　　　　　 ☐ Pyosalpinx ◯ Left ◯ Right ◯ Both
　　　　　　　　　　　 ☐ Tortuous ◯ Left ◯ Right ◯ Both
　　　　　　　　　　　 ☐ Bulbous ◯ Left ◯ Right ◯ Both
　　　　　　　　　　　 ☐ Adherent ◯ Left ◯ Right ◯ Both
　　　　　　　　　　　 ☐ Tuberculosis ◯ Left ◯ Right ◯ Both

Ovaries:

Right: ☐ Normal　　　　　Left: ☐ Normal
　　　 ☐ Follicles　　　　　　　☐ Follicles
　　　 ☐ PCO　　　　　　　　　☐ PCO
　　　 ☐ Cystic　　　　　　　　☐ Cystic
　　　 ☐ Endometriosis　　　　　☐ Endometriosis
　　　 ☐ Adherent　　　　　　　☐ Adherent

Pouch of Douglas: ☐ Free　　　　Note:
　　　　　　　　　☐ Obliterated
　　　　　　　　　☐ Endometriosis
　　　　　　　　　☐ Koch's
　　　　　　　　　☐ Fluid
　　　　　　　　　☐ Others

Operative Procedure

☐ Myomectomy　　　　　　Myoma resected hemostasis maintained
☐ Cauterization of Ovary ◯ Left ◯ Right ◯ Both　cautery at multiple points
☐ Tubal ligation　　　　 ◯ Left ◯ Right ◯ Both　fallope rings
☐ Adhesiolysis　　　　Adhesions resected
☐ Fulguration of Endometriosis　done with unipolar cautery

Diagnostic Hysteroscopy

Place:

Day of Cycle:

Anesthesia :   ◯ IV   ◯ GA

             ◯ LA   ◯ Spinal

Anesthesia :

Surgeon:

Distending Media: ◯ Glycine

                   ◯ Carbon Dioxide

                   ◯ Dextran

                   ◯ Others

Uterocervical Length: inches

Input: mL

Output: mL

Ostia

Left   Right

◯ Normal   ◯ Normal

◯ Blocked   ◯ Blocked

◯ Narrow   ◯ Narrow

◯ Debris   ◯ Debris

◯ Polyp   ◯ Polyp

◯ Blood Clots   ◯ Blood Clots

◯ Others   ◯ Others

Advice:

Findings: DOA: 00/00/0000

                DOD: 00/00/000

Uterine Cavity Findings

◯ Regular   ◯   Irregular

Fibroids   ☐

Polyps   ☐

Septum   ☐

Synechea   ☐

Adhesions   ☐

Endometrium

Normal   ☐

Endometritis   ☐

Hyperplastic   ☐

Scanty   ☐

Bald   ☐

Patchy   ☐

☐ Endometrial Biopsy

Posthysteroscopy Scan

◯ POD Fluid

◯ Adnexa Fluid [Left]

◯ Adnexa Fluid [Right]

Operative Hysteroscopy

Place: DOA: 00/00/0000

Day of Cycle: Findings: DOD: 00/00/0000

Anesthesia :   ◯ IV   ◯ GA   Uterine Cavity Findings

                ◯ LA   ◯ Spinal   ◯ Regular ◯   Irregular

Anesthesia :   Fibroids   ☐

Surgeon: Polyps   ☐

Distending Media: ◯ Glycine   Septum   ☐

                     ◯ Carbon Dioxide   Synechie   ☐

                     ◯ Dextran   Adhesions   ☐

                     ◯ Others   Endometrium

Utero C Length: inches   Normal   ☐

Input: mL   Endometritis ☐

Output: mL   Hyperplastic ☐

Ostia   Scanty   ☐

Left   Right   Bald   ☐

◯ Normal   ◯ Normal   Patchy   ☐

◯ Blocked   ◯ Blocked   ☐ Endometrial Biopsy

◯ Narrow   ◯ Narrow   Posthysteroscopy Scan

◯ Debris   ◯ Debris   ◯   POD Fluid

◯ Polyp   ◯ Polyp   ◯   Adnexa Fluid [Left]

◯ Blood Clots   ◯ Blood Clots   ◯   Adnexa Fluid [Right]

◯ Others   ◯ Others

Operative Procedure:

☐ Debris Clearance   ◯ Right   ◯ Left   ◯ Both

☐ Polypectomy

☐ Myomectomy   ☐ Adhesiolysis

☐ Septum Resection   ☐ Endometrial Ablation

☐ Synechiae Resection   ☐ Foreign Body Removal

Male Record

☐ Primary Infertility   ☐ Secondary Infertility

Marital Status

☐ Married

☐ First Marriage   Duration: Years   Months

           ◯ Consanguineous

           ◯ Non consanguienous

☐ Second Marriage   Duration: Years   Months

           ◯ Consanguineous

           ◯ Non consanguineous

Sexual Intercourse

◯ Daily   ◯ 1/Week   ◯ 1/Month

◯ 2-3/Week   ◯ 2-3/Month   ◯ Nil

Erection   ◯ Normal   ◯ Poor   ◯ Nil

Penetration   ◯ Normal   ◯ Difficult   ◯ Nil

Ejaculation   ◯ Normal   ◯ Premature   ◯ Delayed   ◯ Nil

Family History

☐ Diabetes/Mellitus

☐ Hypertension

☐ Carcinoma

☐ Asthma

☐ Endocrine

☐ Koch's

☐ Infertility

Personal History

☐ Smoking

☐ Alcohol

☐ Tobacco Chewing

Note:

Past History

☐ Mumps

☐ Filariasis

☐ Smallpox

☐ Tuberculosis

☐ Pelvic Injury

☐ Herniorrhaphy

☐ Vasectomy

☐ Epididymitis

☐ Genital Injury

☐ Hydrocele

☐ Treated Infertility

☐ Varicocele

☐ Orchitis

☐ Diabetes

☐ Hypertension

☐ Carcinoma

☐ Asthma

☐ Endocrine

☐ Koch's

T. Biopsy: ◯ Done   ◯ Not Done   ◯ Right ◯ Left ◯ Both

Vasogram: ◯ Done   ◯ Not Done

Hormonal Profile: ◯ Done ◯ Not Done

Doppler: ◯ Done ◯ Not Done

Others:

Height:	Weight:
Pulse:	B.P.:
Obesity:	Distribution:
Cyanosis:	Gynecomastia:
Lymphadenitis:	Midline defects:
RS:	Scrotum:
CVS:	Varicocele:
Surg. Scars:	Discharge:
Ext/Penis Size:	Hydrocele:
Genitalia:	

SEMEN ANALYSIS

Time: 00:00 AM

Name:

METHOD OF COLLECTION   Age   :

                                                    ABSTINENCE :

PHYSICAL EXAMINATION:

                                                    Viscosity   :

Liquefaction Time: Volume   :

CHEMICAL EXAMINATION

Fructose: pH: ASA: HOS:

MICROSCOPIC EXAMINATION:

Sperm Count: Total Count:

Motility of Spermatozoa:

	Grade	After/1 hr
Good Linear Progressive	III and IV	
Sluggish Linear Progressive	II	
Total Forward Progressive	IV + III + II	
Nonprogressive	I	
Nonmotile	O	

SPERMIOGRAM:

ABNORMAL HEAD		ABNORMAL NECK		ABNORMAL TAIL	
Giant Heads :	%	Bent Neck :	%	Short Tail :	%
Pin Heads :	%	Thick Neck :	%	Double Tail :	%
Round Heads :	%			Curled Tail :	%
Double Heads :	%			Long Tail :	%
Ragged Heads :	%				

Total number of abnormal spermatozoa

CELLULAR ELEMENTS:

Epithelial Cells: Pus Cells: RBCs:

MISCELLANEOUS CHARACTERS:

Granular Debris   :   Agglutination of Sperms   :

    Crystals   :   Clumping   :

IMPRESSION   :

SUGGESTION   :

Semen Culture and Sensitivity

Place: Date:

Organism: ◯ Growth in Culture

Sensitivity   ◯ No Growth in Culture

Treatment

IUI PROTOCOL SHEET

NAME: Age:

Investigations: Routine

Endocrine Profile Date:

Tubal Patency

Uterine Sounding Date:

Scan before Starting Stimulation

Previous Treatment:

HbsAg	HIV
FSH	LH

Right Tube: ☐ Patent ☐ Blocked

UCL   AV/RV

Indication:

Vaginal Infection   Semen Analysis

TSH   PRL   Date   Count

Left Tube: ☐ Patent ☐ Blocked

Difficult/Easy   Motility   ASA

Day	1	2	3	4	5	6	7	8	9	10	11	
Date												
Clomiphen citrate												
GnRHa												
Recagon 50												
FSH 75												
HMG 75												
HCG 5000												
Lt. Ovary (mm)												
Rt. Ovary (mm)												
Endometrium (mm)												
E2												
LH												
PROG												

Insemination data:

Date and Time of Rupture:

IUI on
1:
2:

Easy/Difficult:

Luteal Support:

Pregnancy test on:

Outcome:

INSEMINATION PROCEDURE

Name:

Attempt:

Day of Cycle:

Mucus:

Prepared Sample Quality

Count:

☐ Husband

Motility:

☐ Donor

Cannulae ☐ Metal ☐ Plastic

☐ Mixed

◯ Frozen ◯ Free

Quantity Inseminated:

Count:

Mode of Procedure

Motility:

☐ Easy

Media of Preparation

☐ Moderately difficult

☐ HAM F10

☐ Difficult

☐ Earls Bicarbonate

Techniques

☐ Others

☐ Simple wash ☐ Swim-up

☐ Layering ☐ Percoll

☐ Others

POD:

Luteal Support

☐ Uterogestan 1 bid × 2 Weeks

☐ Duphaston 10 mg bid × 2 Weeks

☐ Inj. hCG 5000 IU day 3 and 7 post-ovulation day

☐ Inj. hCG 2000 IU day 3 and 7 post-ovulation day

☐ Inj. Progesterone 100 mg OD × 2 Weeks

☐ Others

Outcome

☐ Pregnancy

☐ Failed to Conceive

☐ Blighted Ovum

☐ Missed Abortion

☐ Miscarriage

☐ IUD (Intrauterine death)

☐ Stillbirth

☐ Live Birth

IVF PROTOCOL SHEET

NAME:
Investigations: Routine Age: HbsAg Previous Treatment: HIV Indication: Vaginal Infection
Endocrine Profile Date: FSH LH TSH PRL
Uterine Sounding Date: UCL AV/RV Difficult/Easy

Semen Analysis
Date Count
Motility ASA

Date								
Dose								
E2								
LH								
PROG								

Scan Before Starting Stimulation

Day	1	2	3	4	5	6	7	8	9	10	11
Date											
GnRHa											
Recagon 50											
FSH 75											
HMG 75											
HCG 5000											
Lt. Ovary (mm)											
Rt. Ovary (mm)											
Endometrium(mm)											
E2											
LH											
PROG											

Egg collection on
Inform: OT
Embryologist
Semen Frozen: Yes/No
ET on:
Luteal support
D28 on:
Outcome:
Embryology date:
No. of eggs:
Fertilized
Cleaved:
Frozen:

Oocyte Retrieval

Name:

DOC:

Team :

T.O.S. :   T.O.E:

Route :   TV: ◯ Yes ◯ No   TA: Yes ◯ No ◯

IVS   :   ◯ Yes   ◯ No

Spinal: ◯ Yes   ◯ No

GA   :   ◯ Yes   ◯ No Anesthetist:

Right Ovary   Left Ovary

No of Follicle Aspirated: No of Follicle Aspirated:

No of Eggs Retrieved: No of Eggs Retrieved:

Complication:

EMBRYOLOGY

Name: Age:

Semen Data

	Sample I	Sample II
Specimen Date		
Time Produced		
Volume		
Count (mil/mL)		
Motility %		
Progression (1-4)		
Abnormal %		
Agglutination		
Clumping		
Viscosity +/++/+++		
Cells (mil/mL)		
Prep. Method		
Prep. Time		
Stock Motile (mil/mL)		
Motility %		
Progression (1-4)		
Dilution		
Prepared by		

EMBRYOLOGY RECORD

Name: Age:

Time: 00:00 AM   Media Batch: E2:   LH: Prog:

Stimulation: Drugs: Approx No Follicles:

Egg No.												
Oocyte Mat (1-5)												
Cum Mat (1-5)												
Insem Time/ICSI												
Sperm Origin												
Day 1 PN												
Grade A/B/C												
Frozen												
Day 2 cell Score												
Grade A/B/C/D												
Replaced/Frozen												
Day 3 cell Score												
Grade A/B/C/D												
Replaced/Frozen												

Embryos Replaced: Date: Time: Team:

Catheter: Comments:

Total Eggs: Fert: 2PN: Cleaved:

Frozen: State: Pronucleate:

Rec Code: Cleaved:

Proced.	◯	IVF	◯	ICSI
Egg	◯	OEg	◯	DEg
Sperm	◯ HS	◯ DS	◯	FS
TESE	◯	Fresh	◯	Frozen

EMBRYO TRANSFER

No. of Eggs: No. of Eggs Fertilized:
Name:
No. of Embryos Transferred:

Grade:
Day: D1 D2 D3

Date: Time: Team:

Catheter: Gynetics Rocket Wallace

Frozen:

Date: 00/00/000

Stage: Pronucleate Embryo Transferred:

Cleaved

Mucus: Transfer: Moderately Difficult

Difficult

Note: Easy

Luteal Support

☐ Uterogestan 1 bid × 2 Weeks
☐ Duphaston 10 mg bid × 2 Weeks
☐ Inj. hCG 5000 IU day 5 and 10 post ovulation day
☐ Inj. hCG 2000 IU day 3, 7 and 10 post ovulation day
☐ Inj. Progesterone 100 mg OD × 2 Weeks
☐ Others

Outcome

☐ Pregnancy
☐ Failed to Conceived
☐ Blighted Ovum
☐ Missed Abortion
☐ Miscarriage
☐ IUD (Intrauterine Death)
☐ Stillbirth
☐ Live Birth
☐ Others

THERAPEUTIC INSEMINATION: DONOR MARRIED RECIPIENT CONSENT FORM

We,..............and ....being husband and wife authorize to perform one or more artificial inseminations/Assisted Reproductive Techniques (ART) on the wife with the sperm obtained from an anonymous donor(s) for the purpose of making her pregnant.

We agree to rely on the judgment and discretion of the physicians to select an appropriate donor(s), whose characteristics are compatible with ours, possible. We will never seek to identify the donor(s), nor shall the donor be advised of the identity of either husband or wife. We understand and agree that it cannot be guaranteed that the same donor will be utilized for each insemination/ART. We also agree that donor sperm that has been frozen (for storage purposes) may be used.

We understand that there is no guarantee that these inseminations/ART will result in a pregnancy.

We further understand that within the normal human population a certain (approximately 4%) of children we are born with physical or mental defects, and that the we understand that there is no guarantee that these inseminations/ART will result in a occurrence of such defects is beyond the control of the physicians. We, therefore understand and agree that the physicians do not assume responsibility for the physical and mental characteristics of any child or children born as a result of artificial insemination/ART. We also understand that within the normal population approximately 20% of pregnancies result in miscarriages and that this may occur after donor insemination as well. Similarly, obstetrical complications may occur in any pregnancy. We also understand and accept that the artificial insemination/ART procedure carries with it the risk of sexually transmitted diseases including but not limited to gonorrhea, syphilis, herpes, hepatitis, and acquired immune deficiency syndrome (AIDS). This agreement therefore is not a contract to cure, a warranty of treatment, nor a guarantee of conception. By these presence, we do hereby absolve, release indemnity, protect and hold harmless from any and all liability for the mental or physical nature of character of any child or children so conceived or born, and for affirmative acts or acts of omission which may arise during the performance of this agreement.

We understand that, if a woman is artificially inseminated or undergone ART with the consent of her husband, the husband is treated in law as if he were the natural father of a child thereby conceived.

Thus further agreed that from conception, I....................., as husband accept the act of insemination as my own and agree.
a. That such child or children conceived or born shall be my legitimate children and heirs of my body, and
b. That I hereby waive forever any right which I might have to disclaim or omit the child or children as my legitimate heir or heirs, and
c. That such child or children conceived or born shall be considered to be in all respects, including descent and distribution of my property, a child or children of my body.

Husband..............   Wife.................
Date...........   Time   Witness...............
I consent to the above doctor-patient relationship.....................................
                                    (Doctor)

VOLUNTARY CONSENT FORM FOR IN VITRO FERTILIZATION/ICE/ET EMBRYO TRANSFER/GAMETE/INTRA FALLOPIAN TRANSFER/ZIFT

We, the undersigned, have been medically advised that our case of infertility could be treated by *in vitro* fertilization and embryo transfer (IVF-ET). The entire therapeutic procedures and their outcome as indicated below have been explained to us.

Procedures involved in *IVF-ET/IVF-ICSI-ET/GIFT/ZIFT*

The following procedures involved in IVF-ET/IVF-ICSI-ET/GIFT/ZIFT have been explained to us which we have understood.
1. The therapy involves treatment of the wife with hormones or drugs for stimulation of the ovary and maturation of oocytes (eggs).
2. Laparoscopic aspiration of oocytes/transvaginal oocyte retrieval under ultrasound guidance.
3. Collection of husband's semen by masturbation for IVF-ET/IVF-ICSI-ET/GIFT/ZIFT.
4. After fertilization *in vitro*, the fertilized eggs will be transferred to the uterus followed by hormonal treatment.

Failures at different stages:
1. The ovaries may not respond to the stimulating protocol.
2. The ovaries may not be accessible for egg collection.
3. The egg collection may be a failure.
4. The eggs may fail to fertilize in the laboratory.
5. The fertilized eggs may fail to cleave.
6. The embryos may fail to implant in the uterus, and a menstrual period occurs.
    The last failure point is the most common of all, for reasons that still largely unknown.

Complications which may occur include:
1. Overstimulation of the ovaries to produce an excessive number of egg follicles/fluid in the peritoneal cavity.
2. Bleeding or pain in the ovaries or bladder at the time of egg collection.
3. Complications of general anesthesia or spinal anesthesia if that is used.
    Having fully understood these procedures and their outcome, we voluntarily consent to participate in the IVF-ET/IVF-ICSI/GIFT/ZIFT procedures for treatment of our infertility.

Signature: Husband............... Doctor's Signature............
Wife................. Serial No...................
Witness..............

CARE OF ENDOSCOPE: RIGID SCOPE

- To be stored in foam (sponge) box containing formalin tablets.
- Cap of lens to be removed.
- Irrigation channels to be kept open.
- Care to be taken that the lens of the scope does not hit any hard surfaces.

Before Using the Scope

- Check the scope for any damage.
- Soak the scope and its accessories for 30 minutes in Cydex.
- Use sterile water/distilled water/normal saline to the wash scopes after soaking in Cydex.
- Flush biopsy channel and irrigation channel thoroughly in distilled water/sterile water/normal saline.
- Care to be taken that the instrument should not be overlapped/should not be mixed up with other instruments.
- Clean the lens and eyepiece with sterile cotton balls.

After Using the Scope

- Wash the scopes and accessories in tap water thoroughly.
- Remove blood clots from biopsy channel and irrigation channel with cleaning brushes.
- Check for the damages if there is any.
- If any damages found immediately inform the qualified service engineer.
- Wash the scopes in distilled water/sterile water/normal saline.
- Dry the biopsy channels and irrigation channels using 5 cc syringe by flushing air repeatedly.
- There should not be a drop of water inside the channel.
- Check the lens and eyepiece for any scratches or blood clots sticking on to it.
- Gently wipe the scopes with a water absorbable cloth and lubricate the moving parts for smooth performance with lubricants supplied by the company.
- Store it in a box containing formalin tablets.

FLEXIBLE SCOPES: FIBER OPTIC

Before Using the Scope

- Check the scope for any damages.
- Soak the scope and its accessories for 30 minutes in Cydex.
- Use sterile water, distilled water or normal saline to wash the scopes after removing it from Cydex.
- Flush the biopsy channel and suction channels thoroughly.
- Wipe the scope with a sterile cloth or towel gently.
- Check the biopsy valve for any damage.
- To avoid air-bubbles in irrigation channel flush in irrigation fluid before introducing to the patient.
- Check light source and connect the scope switch on the light source, check for image through eyepiece or video camera.

After Using the Flexible Scope

- Wipe the external surface using wet guaze.
- Remove the biopsy valve and wash it in water.
- Flush distilled water/normal saline in to suction channel and biopsy channel.
- Clean the biopsy channel and suction channel with cleaning brush.
- Flush-distilled water/normal saline in to suction channel and biopsy channel, repeat at least three times.
- Flush air to dry the biopsy channel using 5 cc syringe, do not use more pressure.
- Lubricate the moving parts with lubricants supplied by the respective company.
- Not to be stored in carry case.
- Flexible scopes to be kept in hanging position in a fully covered foam (sponge) cupboard.
- Image guide has to be checked and two number of black dots to be recorded everyday.
- Leakage test has to be performed after each case.

Index